TO THE BOOK REVIEW EDITOR

Herewith is your review copy of the book described below

Listed + Carded 2-4-85

COMPARATIVE PHYSIOLOGY OF SENSORY SYSTEMS,
L. Bolis, R.D. Keynes and S.M.P. Maddrell
(editors)

D0072141

PUBLISHER Cambridge University Press

PLACE OF PUBLICATION New York (Cambridge and London UK)

PUBLICATION DATE August 31, 1984

ISBN 0 521 250021

PRICE $99.50

Please retain this slip for checking details

We will appreciate receiving three copies of your printed review: one for the author, one for our UK office, and one for our files.

Publicity Department

CAMBRIDGE ■ UNIVERSITY PRESS

32 East 57th Street, New York, N.Y. 10022

Comparative physiology of sensory systems

Papers from the Sixth International Conference on Comparative Physiology, 'Comparative Physiology of Sensory Systems', held at Crans-sur-Sierre, Switzerland, 14–18 June 1982.

The Conference was made possible through the generous support of Fidia Research Laboratories.

Also through the support of the International Unions of Biological Sciences, Physiological Sciences, and Pure and Applied Biophysics, Lirca Laboratories, Synthelabs, Banque Cantonale du Valais, Varian, Wild & Leitz, Aldepha, the community of Chermignon, Winterthur Assurances/Crans-sur-Sierre.

Comparative physiology of sensory systems

Edited by

LIANA BOLIS

Professor and Chairman of General Physiology
University of Messina

R. D. KEYNES

Professor of Physiology, University of Cambridge

S. H. P. MADDRELL

Agricultural Research Council Unit of Insect
Neurophysiology and Pharmacology, Cambridge

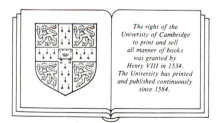

The right of the
University of Cambridge
to print and sell
all manner of books
was granted by
Henry VIII in 1534.
The University has printed
and published continuously
since 1584.

CAMBRIDGE UNIVERSITY PRESS

Cambridge

London New York New Rochelle

Melbourne Sydney

Published by the Press Syndicate of the University of Cambridge
The Pitt Building, Trumpington Street, Cambridge CB2 1RP
32 East 57th Street, New York, NY 10022, USA
296 Beaconsfield Parade, Middle Park, Melbourne 3206, Australia

First published 1984

Printed in Great Britain at The Pitman Press, Bath

Library of Congress catalogue card number: 83–14457

British Library Cataloguing in Publication Data

Comparative physiology of sensory systems.

1. Sense-organs – Congresses
I. Bolis, Liana II. Keynes, R.D.
III. Maddrell, S.H.P.
591.1′82   QP431

ISBN 0 521 25002 1

Contents

Contributors

Jorge M. Affanni: Instituto de Investigaciones, Facultad de Ciencios Exactos y Naturales, Ciudad Universitaria, Pabellon No. 2–4° Piso, 1428 Nunez, Argentina

Ferrante Aporti: Fidia Research Laboratories, Via Ponte della Fabbrica 3/A, 35031 Abano Terme, Italy

Jonathan Art: Physiological Laboratory, Downing Street, Cambridge CB3 3EG, UK

Curtis C. Bell: Neurological Sciences Institute of the Good Samaritan Hospital, 1015 N.W. 22nd Avenue, Portland, Oregon 97210, USA

P. R. Burgess: Department of Physiology, College of Medicine, The University of Utah, 410 Chipeta Way, Room 156, Research Park, Salt Lake City, Utah 84108, USA

Robert H. Cagan: Monell Chemical Senses Center, 3500 Market Street, Philadelphia, Pennsylvania 19104, USA

John Caprio: Zoology and Physiology Department, Louisiana State University & Mechanical College, Baton Rouge, Louisiana 70803, USA

L. W. Dodds: Neurology Service, Massachusetts General Hospital, Boston, Massachusetts, USA

Richard R. Fay: Parmly Hearing Institute, Loyola University, 6525 North Sheridan Road, Chicago, Illinois 60626, USA

J. S. Gage: Department of Physiology, Harvard Medical School, Cambridge 02138, Massachusetts, USA

Peter H. Hartline: Eye Research Institute, 20 Staniford Street, Boston, Massachusetts 02114, USA

Walter Heiligenberg: Scripps Institution of Oceanography, University of California, La Jolla, California 92093, USA

K. W. Horch: Department of Physiology, College of Medicine, The University of Utah, 410 Chipeta Way, Room 156, Research Park, Salt Lake City, Utah 84108, USA

D. E. Hornung: Biology Department, St Lawrence University, Canton, New York 13617, USA

R. Ientile: Università degli Studi di Messina, Piazza XX Settembre 4, 98100 Messina, Italy

A. J. Kalmijn: Scripps Institution of Oceanography, Ocean Research Division, A-020, University of California, San Diego, La Jolla, California 92093, USA

Nelson Y. S. Kiang: Eaton-Peabody Laboratory of Auditory Physiology, Massachusetts Eye & Ear Infirmary, 243 Charles Street, Boston, Massachusetts 02114, USA

Rainer Klinke: Zentrum der Physiologie, Klinikum der Johann Wolfgang Goethe-
    Universität, Theodor-Stern-Kai 7, D-6000, Frankfurt am Main 70, Germany
Masakazu Konishi: Division of Biology 216–76, California Institute of Technology,
    Pasadena, California 91125, USA
G. D. Lange: Marine Neurobiology Unit & Department of Neurosciences, University of
    California, San Diego, La Jolla, CA 92093, USA
Edwin R. Lewis: University of California, Department of Electrical Engineering and
    Computer Sciences, Berkeley, California 94720, USA
M. C. Liberman: Department of Electrical Engineering and Computer Science,
    Massachusetts Institute of Technology, Boston, Massachusetts, USA
P. J. Magistretti: Département de Pharmacologie, Ecole de Médecine, Université de
    Genève, 1211 Geneva 4, Switzerland
Claudine Masson: Laboratoire del Neurobiologie Sensorielle de l'Insecte, CNRS-INRA,
    91440 Bures-sur-Yvette, France
Axel Michelsen: Institute of Biology, Odense University, Campusvej 55, 5230 Odense M,
    Denmark
P. Moller: Département de Neurophysiologie Sensorielle, Laboratoire de Physiologie
    Nerveuse, CNRS-LPN3, 91190 Gif-sur-Yvette, France
Maxwell M. Mozell: Department of Physiology, College of Medicine, State University of
    New York, Upstate Medical Center, 766 Irving Avenue, Syracuse, New
    York 13210, USA
Gerhard Neuweiler: Zoologisches Institut der Universität München, Luisenstrasse 14,
    8 Munich 2, West Germany
Giuseppe Nistico: Università degli Studi di Messina, Piazza XX Settembre 4,
    98100 Messina, Italy
C. C. Northrop: Department of Otolaryngology, Harvard Medical School, Cambridge,
    Massachusetts 02138, USA
Shosaku Obara: Department of Physiology, Teikyo University School of Medicine,
    Kaga 2-11-1 Itabashi-Ku, Tokyo 173, Japan
M. E. Oliver: Eaton-Peabody Laboratory of Auditory Physiology, Massachusetts Eye &
    Ear Infirmary, 243 Charles Street, Boston, Massachusetts 02114, USA
Marco Piccolino: Istituto Neurofisiologia del CNR, Via San Zeno 51, 56100 Pisa, Italy
Christopher Platt: Department of Biological Sciences, University of Southern California,
    University Park, Los Angeles, California 90007, USA
Arthur N. Popper: Department of Anatomy, Georgetown University, 3900 Reservoir
    Road, NW, Washington D.C. 20007, USA
A. Pujia: Università degli Studi di Messina, Piazza XX Settembre 4, 98100 Messina, Italy
Werner Reichardt: Max-Planck-Institut für Biologische Kybernetik, 38 Spemannstrasse,
    D-7400 Tubingen 1, West Germany
François de Ribaupierre: Institut de Physiologie, Faculté de Médecine, Université de
    Lausanne, 7 Rue de Bugnon, 1011 Lausanne, Switzerland
Barry Roberts: Marine Biological Association of the United Kingdom, The Laboratory,
    Citadel Hill, Plymouth PL1 2PB, UK
R. Rubini: Fidia Research Laboratories, Via Ponte della Fabbrica 3/A, 35301 Abano
    Terme, Italy
L. G. Samartino: Instituto de Investigaciones, Facultad de Cientos Exactos y Naturales,
    Ciudad Universitaria, Pabellon No. 2–4° Piso, 1428 Nunez, Argentina
Olav Sand: The Centre for School Science, Department of Biology, University of Oslo,
    Post Box 1066, Blindern, Oslo 3, Norway
A. de Sarro: Università degli Studi di Messina, Piazza XX Settembre 4, 98100 Messina,
    Italy
Dietrich Schneider: Max-Planck-Institut für Verhaltensphysiologie, D-8131 Seewiesen,
    West Germany

Michel Schorderet: Département de Pharmacologie, Ecole de Médecine, Université de
      Genève, 1211 Geneva 4, Switzerland
J. Smolders: Zentrum der Physiologie, Klinikum der Johann Wolfgang Goethe-
      Universität, Theodor-Stern-Kai 7, D-6000 Frankfurt am Main 70, Germany
Heinrich Spoendlin: Universitätsklinik für Hals-Nassen- und Ohrenkrankheiten,
      Anichstrasse 35, 6020 Innsbruck, Austria
Y. Sugawara: Department of Physiology, Teikyo University School of Medicine, Kaga 2-
      11-1 Itabashi-Ku, Tokyo 173, Japan
Thomas Szabo: Département de Neurophysiologie Sensorielle, Laboratoire de Physiologie
      Nerveuse, CNRS-LPN3, 91190 Gif-sur-Yvette, France
G. Toffano: Fidia Research Laboratories, Via Ponte della Fabbrica 3/A, 35031 Abano
      Terme, Italy
R. P. Tuckett: Department of Physiology, College of Medicine, The University of Utah,
      410 Chipeta Way, Room 156, Research Park, Salt Lake City, Utah 84108,
      USA
G. Urna: Università degli Studi di Messina, Piazza XX Settembre 4, 98100 Messina, Italy
Rüdiger Wehner: Zoologisches Institut, Universität Zürich, Winterthurerstrasse 190,
      8057 Zürich, Switzerland
P. Witkovsky: Departments of Ophthalmology and of Physiology and Biophysics, New
      York University Medical Center, New York 10016, USA

Editorial Preface

The object of the International Conference on the Comparative Physiology of Sensory Systems held at Crans-sur-Sierre in June 1982, and sponsored by ICSV's Inter-Union Commission on Comparative Physiology representing the International Unions of Biological Sciences, Physiological Sciences, and Pure and Applied Biophysics, was to bring together experts on the functioning of the various parts of the sensory nervous system in different orders for the discussion of selected aspects of auditory systems, olfaction and taste, visual systems, the detection of magnetic and electric fields, and the maintenance of posture and the control of muscle movement. It became clear that there was much to be learnt from a comparison of the many ways in which information about the environment is acquired and processed in the animal kingdom, and the papers assembled in this volume not only illustrate the importance in studying a given sensory modality of choosing the right animal to work on, but also the value of adopting a comparative approach in this as in many other areas of biology.

Richard Keynes

1
Auditory systems

1.1

Lateral-line systems

OLAV SAND

The lateral-line organs are epidermal sense organs found in cyclostomes, fish, larval amphibians, aquatic adult urodeles and some adult aquatic anurans. The organs in the embryo develop from cells migrating from the pre and post auditory placodes, which are ectodermal thickenings on either side of the embryonic medulla oblongata (Stone, 1922, 1933; Landacre, 1927). The sensory cells of the lateral-line organs and the sense organs of the labyrinth, which arise from the central auditory placodes, show basic structural similarities. These sense organs are commonly referred to as the acousticolateralis system or the octavolateralis system.

In the first half of the previous century the accepted view was that the lateral line formed a system of glands for the production of mucus. This idea was not abandoned before Leydig (1850, 1851) concluded that the lateral line was a sense organ especially adapted for aquatic life. This work induced numerous studies on the sensory function of the lateral-line systems, and it was soon generally accepted that the lateral-line organs were mechanoreceptors (Parker, 1904). However, experimental results obtained mainly during the last three decades have led to division of the lateral-line systems into two groups, namely 'ordinary', or mechano-sensitive, lateral-line organs as opposed to 'specialized' lateral-line organs particularly sensitive to electrical stimuli (Dijkgraaf, 1963).

It has also been suggested that lateral-line organs may function as thermoreceptors (Hoagland, 1933, 1935; Sand, 1938; Murray, 1955a,b) and as chemoreceptors sensitive to different mono- and divalent cations (Katsuki, Hashimoto and Yanagisawa, 1970; Katsuki, Hashimoto and Kendall, 1971; Onada and Katsuki, 1972; Katsuki, 1973; Katsuki and

Onada, 1973; Nakagawa, Yoshioka and Katsuki, 1974; Yanagisawa, Taglietti and Katsuki, 1974; Yoshioka, Asanuma, Yanagisawa and Katsuki, 1978). However, most receptors are influenced by temperature and the ionic composition of their environment, and it is not clear if the reported thermo- and chemosensitivity of lateral-line systems are of any behavioral significance.

The present paper will be limited to the mechanosensitive lateral-line systems. This topic has been comprehensively reviewed in the past (Dijkgraf, 1963; Schwartz, 1974), and I will therefore concentrate on more recent experiments and not attempt to give a complete survey of the relevant literature. I will focus on the functional aspects of the lateral-line, with only a brief description of the structure of the organs, and the main emphasis will be on the peripheral part of the systems. However, the central processing of information from the octavolateral sense organs in fish, and the central nervous connexions involved, have been the topics of recent reviews (Northcutt, 1981; Roberts, 1981; Bullock, 1981).

Anatomy

The two main types of the mechanosensitive lateral-line organs, or neuromasts, are the freestanding superficial organs and the canal organs. The freestanding neuromasts are the only type found in cyclostomes, aquatic amphibians and some teleosts, whereas in most fishes the lateral-line system has partly been transformed into canal organs. The freestanding neuromasts commonly appear singly in fishes. However, in amphibians the neuromasts are usually distributed in small groups over the surface of the body and head, as indicated in Figure 1A for the mudpuppy (*Necturus maculosus*). These groups are commonly called stitches (Harris and Milne, 1966), and contain a variable number of neuromasts (Figure 1B).

The apical half of the neuromast contains the sensory cells, or hair cells, which are separated and surrounded by a large number of supporting cells. The peripheral layers of supporting cells are frequently called mantle cells (Flock, 1967). From the apical surface of the organ a transparent gelatinous cupula extends several hundred micrometers into the surrounding water. The cupula is secreted by the supporting cells, and the shape varies in different species. The mechanosensitive hair cells (Figure 1C) are pear-shaped and narrowing towards the apical end, from which a bundle of short stereocilia and a single kinocilium project into the cupula. The hair cells are thus mechanically coupled to the cupula, and the physiological stimuli for the lateral-line organs are

shearing displacements of the cupulae (Sand, 1937; Harris and van
Bergeijk, 1962; Harris and Milne, 1966; Flock, 1965). Each neuromast
contains two hair cell populations with opposite orientation (Flock and
Wersäll, 1962; Flock, 1967; Shelton, 1970; Jørgensen and Flock, 1973).
As a consequence of this, the neuromast as a whole shows strong
directional preference regarding the effect of cupular movements on the
afferent activity. The neuromasts receive both afferent and efferent
innervation, although efferent synapses of the lateral-line are more
abundant in fish than in amphibians (Flock, 1965).

A few species of temporary land-dwelling amphibians retain their
lateral-line system during the terrestrial phases (Noble, 1931; Dawson,
1936; Reno and Middleton, 1973). The lateral-line organs in these
species are partially dedifferentiated and overgrown by adjacent epidermal cells during the terrestrial phase, but this process is completely
reversible. The lateral-line system is the only special sensory system in
vertebrates which shows such cycles of regression and regeneration
during the life of the animal.

Figure 2A shows schematically the transformation of superficial

Figure 1. (A) Sketch of *Necturus maculosus* indicating the distribution
of stitches. (B) Schematical section through a stitch containing three
superficial neuromasts, each composed of hair cells, h, and supporting
cells, s, and surrounded by epithelial cells, e. The cupulae, c, extend
freely into the surrounding water. Two afferent fibres, a, innervate
each organ in amphibians. (C) Diagram of a single hair cell:
sc, stereocilia; kc, kinocilium; an, afferent nerve ending; en, efferent
nerve ending. (Redrawn from Sand et al., 1976 (A, B) and Flock,
1971 (C).)

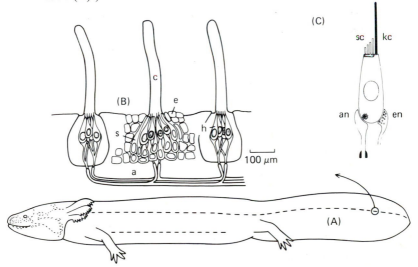

neuromasts into canal organs in fish. This transformation is never complete, and all fish with canal organs therefore also possess free neuromasts (Figure 2C). The pattern of lateral-line canals of the head region is rather complex and diversified in different species, whereas the trunk canals usually form a single line on each side of the body. The canal organs are situated at the bottom of the canals, where the dome-shaped cupulae are attached to oval discs of sensory epithelium. The system of canals usually communicates with the exterior through one pore near each organ, but in extreme cases, such as in the burbot (*Lota lota*), pores are present only in the head and tail ends of the canal system (Hyrtl, 1866).

Physiology

Receptor potentials and afferent synaptic transmission

The hair cells of the lateral-line are easily accessible compared to auditory and vestibular receptors, and the lateral-line organs have therefore been extensively used as a model for studying general hair cell

Figure 2. (A) Schematical cross-sections showing three successive stages in the transformation of superficial neuromasts into canal organs; 3a and 3b show sections through a canal organ and a pore, respectively. (B) Longitudinal canal section in the plane indicated in 3a. Black, epidermis and hair cells; dotted, cupulae. (C) Arrangement of canal pores (open circles) and free neuromasts (black dots) in *Phoxinus phoxinus*. The trunk canal is incomplete in this species. (Redrawn from Dijkgraaf, 1963.)

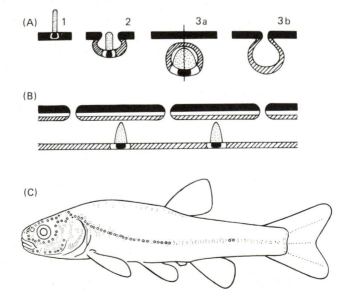

physiology. Receptor potentials in response to mechanical stimulation of hair cells were first recorded intracellularly from the neuromasts in *Necturus* (Harris, Frischkopf and Flock, 1969, 1970), and similar recordings have later been obtained from the lateral line of *Lota* (Flock, Jørgensen and Russell, 1973). Excitatory post-synaptic potentials have been recorded from afferent nerve fibers of the lateral-line organs in *Lota* (Flock et al., 1973; Flock and Russell, 1973a) and *Necturus* (Sand, Ozawa and Hagiwara, 1975). Sand et al. (1975) furthermore injected sinusoidal electrical current into the hair cells, causing potential fluctuations of the same amplitude as mechanically-induced receptor potentials. This treatment caused synchrony between the injected current and the afferent spikes, whereas ten times more intense current was insufficient to cause such synchrony when the afferent nerve terminals were injected directly. These experiments indicate both that a chemical synapse exists between the hair cells and the afferent terminals, and that the transmitter release is controlled by the receptor potentials. Bledsoe, Bobbin, Thalmann and Thalmann (1980) and Bobbin, Bledsoe, Chihal and Morgan (1981) have studied the release of amino acids from mechanically stimulated lateral-line organs in *Xenopus* and the actions of L-glutamate on these organs, and they have obtained circumstantial evidence in support of L-glutamate or a related compound being the afferent transmitter substance in the mechanosensitive lateral-line organs. However, the identity of the transmitter substance involved is still not unambiguously established.

Intracellular recordings of mechanically-induced receptor potentials in hair cells have recently been obtained from labyrinth organs in several species, including the basilar papilla of the inner ear of the lizard (*Gerrhonotus*) (Mulroy, Altmann, Weiss and Peake, 1974; Weiss, Mulroy and Altmann, 1974), the basilar papilla of the turtle (*Pseudemys*) (Fettiplace and Crawford, 1978, 1980; Crawford and Fettiplace, 1980, 1981), the frog sacculus (Hudspeth and Corey, 1977; Corey and Hudspeth, 1979; Hudspeth and Jacobs, 1979; Ashmore and Russell, 1982) and the guinea-pig cochlea (Russell and Sellick, 1977, 1978; Sellick and Russell, 1979, 1980). The lateral-line organs have thus lost their hegemony as a model system for investigation of hair cell physiology.

Efferent innervation

The mechanosensitive lateral-line organs receive efferent inhibitory innervation (Flock, 1965; Harris and Flock, 1967; Russell, 1968; Flock and Russell, 1973a,b). The efferent fibers are active just before and during active movement of the animal (Schmidt, 1965; Görner, 1967; Russell, 1971a, 1974; Roberts and Russell, 1972), thereby suppressing the activity in the afferent fibers from the lateral-line organs stimulated by these movements (Figure 3).

Electrical stimulation of the efferent fibers causes inhibitory post-synaptic potentials and conductance increase in the hair cells, which in turn leads to reduced synaptic potentials in the afferent terminals (Flock and Russell, 1976). It has also recently been suggested that efferent stimulation may alter the mechanical properties of lateral-line hair cells (Russell and Lowe, 1983). The lateral-line efferent synapses have properties characteristic of cholinergic synapses (Russell, 1971b), and it is now generally accepted that acetylcholine is the transmitter sub-stance.

The ionic milieu of the hair cells

A seemingly striking difference between the inner ear sense organs and the free neuromasts is the media to which the organs are exposed. The apical hair cell membranes in the mammalian labyrinth face an endolymph where K^+ (150 mM) is the predominant cation, and the endocochlear potential exceeds $+120$ mV (Johnstone and Sellick, 1972). The driving force for K^+ will thus be inward through the apex of the hair cell and outward through the cell body, and it is therefore reasonable to suggest that K^+ carries the receptor current. Russell and Sellick (1976) have measured the endocupular potential and the en-docupular K^+ and Cl^- activities in the superficial neuromasts of *Xenopus* using ion-selective microelectrodes. Their data showed that the cupulae preserved a microenvironment remarkably similar to that in the cochlea (Figure 4B, C). Cupular Cl^- and K^+ concentrations were in the range of 35–70 mM and 24–100 mM, respectively, whereas the endocupular potential varied between $+15$ and $+50$ mV. McGlone, Russell and Sand (1979) have recently measured endocupular Ca^{2+} concentrations between 2 and 30 μM in *Xenopus* (Figure 4D). These data

Figure 3. The response of efferent lateral-line fibres in *Xenopus laevis* to voluntary movements made by the animal. Upper trace, efferent impulses from a branch of the posterior lateral-line nerve; lower trace, voluntary movements monitored by a gramophone pick-up. (From Russell, 1971a.)

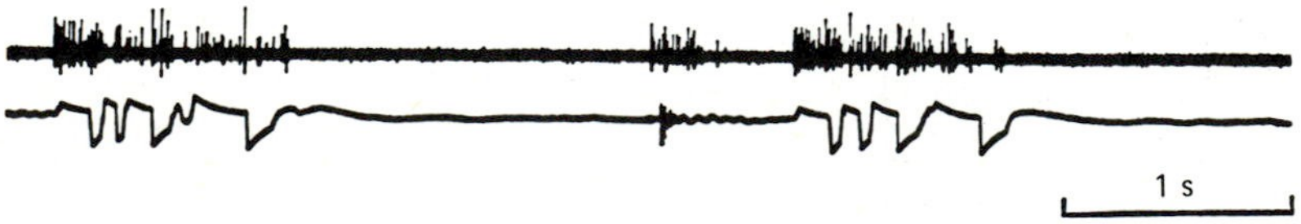

1 s

indicate the existence of an electrogenic K^+ pump actively maintaining the elevated K^+ concentration in the cupulae, whereas the Cl^- and Ca^{2+} ions are passively distributed. Even in the superficial neuromasts the bulk of the hair cell receptor current may thus be carried by K^+, although Ca^{2+} is essential for the mechanosensitivity of the hair cells both in these organs (Sand, 1975) and in the labyrinth (Valli, Zucca and Casella, 1979). The role of Ca^{2+} in the hair cell transduction process is obscure. It is possible that this ion controls the K^+ permeability of the apical hair cell membrane, or Ca^{2+} may even influence the mechanical properties of the hair cells (Sand, 1979).

Directional sensitivity of the canal organs

In amphibians with the neuromasts linearly arranged in stitches, the sensitivity is optimal for cupular movements either parallel to, as in *Necturus* (Harris et al., 1970), or at right angles to the stitch, as in *Xenopus* (Görner, 1963). The neuromasts of the canal organs have optimal sensitivity for cupular movements parallel to the canal (Flock, 1965). However, it is not clear which direction of external water movements will stir the canal fluid most efficiently. Katsuki, Yoshino and Chen (1951) and Dijkgraaf (1963) have suggested that the canal organs are particularly suited to detect local water movements perpendicular to the body surface, whereas Harris and van Bergeijk (1962) and Schwartz (1965) claimed that external water movements parallel to the canal are the effective stimulus. I have tested these possibilities using

Figure 4. Responses from double-barrel K^+, Cl^- and Ca^{2+} electrodes during insertion into lateral-line cupulae of *Xenopus laevis*.
(A) Diagram of the recording arrangement. c, cupula; v, potential electrode; i, ion-selective electrode. (B, C, D) Upper traces: responses from K^+ electrode (E_{K^+}), Cl^- electrode (E_{Cl^-}) and Ca^{2+} electrode ($E_{Ca^{2+}}$), respectively. Lower traces: potential records (endocupular potential). The bathing solution contained 1 mm KCl in (B) and (C) and 1 mm $CaCl_2$ in (D). (Modified from Russell and Sellick, 1976 (A, B, C) and McGlone et al., 1979 (D).)

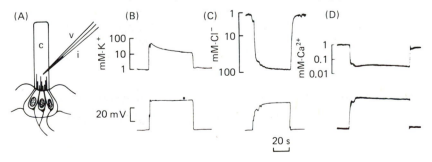

vibrating ball stimulation of the trunk lateral line in the roach (*Rutilus rutilus*) (Sand, 1981).

The water displacements caused by a vibrating sphere are easily predictable (Harris and van Bergeijk, 1962), as illustrated in Figure 5. The vectors beneath the ball indicate the displacements at different points along a straight line in a plane at a distance of $2r$ from the ball centre when the ball is vibrated parallel to the line or perpendicular to the plane. In the experiment presented in Figure 6, I was recording the afferent activity from a lateral-line nerve fiber responding to water motion in a restricted area surrounding a particular canal pore. The afferent response was measured as the difference between the highest and lowest probability for the occurrence of a spike during a stimulus cycle, or in other words, as the degree of synchrony between the vibrational stimulus and the spike activity. The fish was lying on its side, and the vibrating ball was moved along straight above the canal close to the sensitive spot. The vertical distance between the fish surface and the ball was 3.4 mm, or $2r$. The figure compares the response to horizontal ball vibrations parallel to the canal and vertical vibrations perpendicular to the skin. By comparing Figures 5 and 6 it is seen that the response to both these two modes of stimulation closely follows the horizontal vibration component at the fish surface just above a particular pore, with regard to both amplitude and phase. The data thus show that the

Figure 5. Displacement field caused by a vibrating sphere. Equations from Harris and van Bergeijk (1962). The vectors indicate the direction and relative amplitude of the displacements at different points along a straight line in a plane at a distance of $2r$ from the sphere center. (A) Ball vibrations parallel to the line. (B) Ball vibrations perpendicular to the plane. The distances between the points and the projection of the sphere center on to the plane are marked on the figure. (From Sand, 1981.)

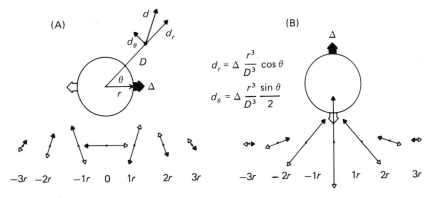

$$d_r = \Delta \frac{r^3}{D^3} \cos \theta$$

$$d_\theta = \Delta \frac{r^3}{D^3} \frac{\sin \theta}{2}$$

canal organ is optimally sensitive to water vibrations in a plane parallel to the skin surface.

The directional sensitivity to vibrations in this plane is displayed in Figure 7, where 0° represents vibrations parallel to the canal. It is clearly a cosine relationship between the response and the direction of vibration, with motions parallel to the canal being most effective. These results support the existence of a viscous coupling between vibrations in the external water and the canal fluid. This is in agreement with Denton and Gray (1983), who observed a similar directional relationship between the liquid displacements inside the lateral-line canals of the sprat (*Sprattus sprattus*) and the outside water movements relative to the fish. Furthermore, the ratio of the displacements inside the canal to the external water movements falls proportionately with frequency below 80 Hz. Compared with the superficial neuromasts, the canal lateral-line

Figure 6. (A) Synchronization between spike activity of a trunk lateral line fiber in *Rutilus rutilus* and mechanical stimulation by a vibrating sphere at different positions along the canal. The individual canal pores are indicated on the abscissa. Data for horizontal vibrations (○) parallel to the canal and vertical vibrations (●) perpendicular to the skin are compared. (B) Original recordings, giving the probability for spike occurrence as a function of stimulus phase, for both types of stimulation recorded at the ball positions indicated by roman numbers in (A). Distance between canal and ball center was 2r (3.4 mm). Compare the response nulls and maxima and the response phase shifts with the horizontal displacement components in Figure 5. Stimulation frequency was 50 Hz. (From Sand, 1981.)

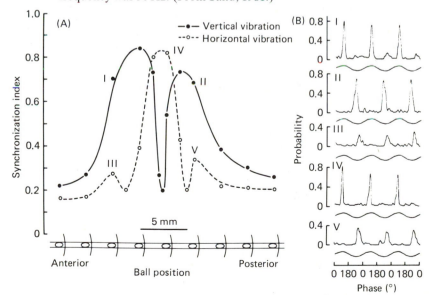

will thus perform high-pass filtering of the relative motion between the fish and the surrounding water.

Functional significance of the lateral-line mechanosensitivity

The functional significance of the mechanosensitivity of the ordinary lateral-line organs is still not settled. Experimental evidence unambiguously shows that these organs may detect local water movements and surface waves. Judging from the descriptions in most dictionaries and biology textbooks, it is also generally believed that the lateral line is a detector of propagated low-frequency sound waves. However, in light of the available experimental evidence, this latter notion ought to be abandoned.

Sensitivity to local water movements

The structure of the lateral-line organs strongly indicates sensitivity to water currents impinging locally on the fish, or to movements of the outside water relative to the fish skin. Hofer (1908) was the first to show this directly, and he concluded that the fish could 'feel at a distance' with the lateral-line. His results were later confirmed by several authors and extended to numerous species of both fish and amphibians (for review, see Dijkgraaf, 1963). Dijkgraaf in particular

Figure 7. Recordings from a trunk lateral-line fiber in *Rutilus rutilus* showing the synchronization (probability for spike occurrence as a function of stimulus phase) between afferent activity and ball vibration parallel to the skin surface. The recordings were obtained at different angles between the canal axis and the vibration direction. The ball center was positioned 2*r* above a sensitive pore. Vibrations parallel to the canal corresponds to 0°. Stimulation frequency was 50 Hz. (From Sand, 1981.)

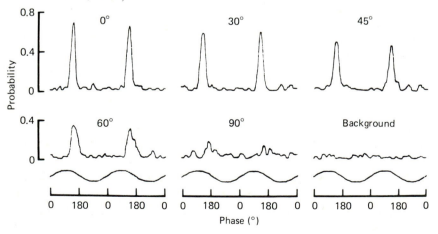

has been a strong advocate for the concept 'distance–touch' (Dijkgraaf, 1934, 1947, 1952a, 1960). He has shown convincingly that the displacement of water caused by a moving fish, or the 'damming' phenomenon, is the basis for close-range obstacle detection in blinded fish. Changes in the self-produced damming pattern around the moving fish, caused by the obstacle, then act as stimuli for the lateral-line. It should be stressed that the range of this 'distance–touch' seems to be limited to a few centimeters.

The different species of blind cavefish are especially dependent on this mechanism for detection of stationary objects in the surroundings. von Campenhausen, Riess and Weissert (1981) and Weissert and von Campenhausen (1981) have recently studied the behavior of the Mexican blind cave fish (*Anoptichthys*). When exploring a new object placed in the tank, the fish accelerates when approaching and then glides closely past the object without tail movements. This performance is repeated, and the fish may glide along different sides of the object. The fish frequently rotates sideways shortly before swimming above the object, thus facing its body side towards the object when passing. From conditioning experiments it was concluded that the fish detects bars with diameters down to two millimeters when passing at a distance of a few millimeters. In light of the function of the efferent innervation of lateral-line organs, it is interesting that the fish halts active muscle movements during passage of the object.

The water displacements generated by moving objects may of course also be detected at close range by stationary or moving fish. Any rigid object moved through the water will evoke a trailing turbulent current in addition to the general damming displacements. Such turbulence in connexion with swimming fish has been observed directly using different techniques (Rosen, 1959; Aleev and Ovcharov, 1969; McCutchen, 1976, 1977). Figure 8A presents an example from McCutchen (1977). The fish swims in thermally-stratified water, and discontinuities in temperature, and hence refractive index, are visualized in shadowgraphic projection. In addition to such a necklace of vortices caused by the movement of a fish through the water, it has been predicted that stronger vortices are produced by flapping of the fish tail (Gray, 1968; Lighthill, 1969; Weihs, 1972, 1973, 1975), leaving a double row of opposedly-spinning vortices behind the fish (Figure 8B). The existence of thrust vortices has been disputed, but Partridge and Pitcher (1979) have recently demonstrated such vortices behind swimming cod, in positions predicted by Weihs (1975).

Swimming fish thus seem to be rich sources for lateral-line stimulation of their neighbors. It is therefore surprising that most studies concerned with schooling in fish conclude that school organization and synchrony depend mainly on vision, whereas lateral-line sensation is unimportant (Parr, 1927; Bowen, 1931; Schlaifer, 1942; Breder, 1951, 1959; Atz, 1953; Hunter, 1969; Shaw, 1962, 1970). However, this conclusion has recently been challenged by Pitcher, Partridge and Wardle (1976), Partridge and Pitcher (1980) and Partridge (1981). In their studies the schooling performance of saithe (*Pollachius virens*) was investigated after blindfolding or sectioning of the lateralis nerves. The results showed that blinding had little effect on the position of the experimental fish within the school, whereas cutting the lateralis nerves altered the position relative to neighbors. Furthermore, the importance of the lateral-line in transmission of fright responses and sudden velocity changes within a school was also demonstrated. In normal schools fish responded with similar latencies to startling objects, whereas the latency increased with the distance from the disturbance in schools of lateralis-sectioned fish. It was concluded that school structure and dynamics depend upon both vision and lateral-line sensation, the latter being primarily important for monitoring the swimming direction and speed of neighbors. Several species with a pronounced schooling behavior lack the trunk lateral-line canals (i.e. the clupeids), but superficial neuromasts are still present along the body sides of these fish (Blaxter, Gray and Best, 1983).

It should finally be stressed that the rheotactic response most fish display in a gross water current is not dependent on the lateral-line, but on visual or tactile stimuli (Lyon, 1904; Parker, 1904; Dijkgraaf, 1934). However, the lateral-line may of course be stimulated by the turbulence

Figure 8. (A) Shadowgraph showing the turbulent wake left by a swimming 3.5-cm-long *Brachydanio rerio*. (From McCutchen, 1977.) (B) Sketch illustrating the double row of opposedly spinning vortices caused by the tail flapping of a swimming fish. (Redrawn from Weihs, 1973.)

(A)   (B)

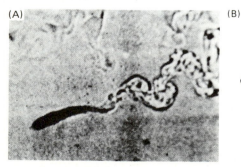

and steep gradients in current velocity which for instance occur in streams with stony bottoms.

Sensitivity to surface waves

The propagation of surface waves is very different from that of under-water sound. Surface waves are transverse waves and the propagation velocity depends on the frequency. The minimum propagation speed is $23 \, \text{cm s}^{-1}$ at 13.4 Hz, corresponding to a wavelength of 1.7 cm (Schwartz, 1967). The wavelength of under-water sound of the same frequency exceeds 100 m. Furthermore, particle motion below the surface induced by surface waves is not linear, but elliptical.

Schwartz (1965, 1967, 1970, 1971) and Schwartz & Hasler (1966) have shown beyond doubt that surface-feeding fish are able to detect and locate sources of surface waves, and that the lateral-line organs on the head are the sensors involved. Schwartz (1971) studied the threshold amplitudes for surface waves in several species, and he found optimal sensitivity in the frequency range 10–40 Hz, with the lowest threshold amplitudes around $2 \, \mu\text{m}$. However, recent behavioral (Bleckmann, 1980) and electrophysiological (Bleckmann and Topp, 1981) studies of the lateral-line sensitivity in *Aphocheilus* have revealed threshold amplitudes at least two orders of magnitude below these values. *Aphocheilus* furthermore showed optimal sensitivity around 100 Hz.

The clawed toad *Xenopus* also detects surface waves using the lateral-line (Kramer, 1933; Dijkgraaf, 1947; Görner, 1973). Görner (1976) determined the detection threshold for surface waves in *Xenopus* to be $0.2 \, \mu\text{m}$, and he also showed that both the lateral-line and the labyrinth are involved in wave detection by this animal.

The ability of surface-feeding fish to determine the direction to the wave source depends on the interaction of symmetrically-located head lateral-line organs, and differences in arrival time and amplitude of the wave between the two sides of the head provide the necessary information (Schwartz, 1965; Schwartz and Hasler, 1966). However, these fish are also able to determine the distance to a wave source when confronted with single wave pulses produced by insect prey or the dipping of a rod into the water (Schwartz, 1971; Bleckmann, 1980). This ability persists if all lateral-line organs except one are removed (Bleckmann and Schwartz, 1982), whereas the distance determination is abolished if monofrequent wave signals are presented (Bleckmann, 1980).

Figure 9 shows a wave train produced by a 5-ms click-like water disturbance recorded at different distances from the source (Bleckmann and Schwartz, 1982). Such a train consists of waves of different amplitudes and frequencies, and the wave pattern changes dramatically during propagation. Due to their higher velocity, the high-frequency waves (up to 190 Hz) are present only at the signal front after a distance of 2–3 cm has been covered. The damping of surface waves increases with frequency (Lang, 1980), and the high-frequency wave portions therefore gradually disappear with increasing distance from the wave source. At the same time new wave cycles within the signal are produced constantly, prolonging the train and lowering its frequency content during propagation. Only the first 8–10 wave cycles of a total wave signal are utilized for source localization in *Aplocheilus* (Bleckmann and Schwartz, 1981). This species has an acute ability to discriminate between surface waves of different frequencies (Bleckmann, Waldner and Schwartz, 1981), and Bleckmann and Schwartz (1982) have recently suggested that the fish utilizes the frequency modulation within a wave train as the source of information for distance determination.

Sensitivity to low-frequency sound
Behavior studies. An impressive number of behavior studies have indicated that the lateral-line organs are sensitive detectors of

Figure 9. Surface wave train produced by a 5-ms click-like water disturbance recorded at 5, 10 and 15 cm from the source. Note the differences in relative amplitude calibration. (From Bleckmann & Schwartz, 1982.)

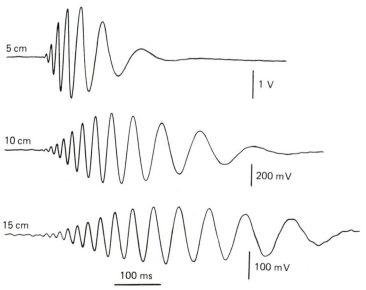

low-frequency vibrations or sound (Parker, 1904, 1909; Parker and van Heusen, 1917; Dye, 1921; Kramer, 1933; Kuiper, 1956; Kleerekoper and Roggenkamp, 1959; Maliukina, 1960; Backus, 1963; Tavolga and Wodinsky, 1963; Wisby, Richard, Nelson and Gruber, 1964; Wodinsky and Tavolga, 1964; Weiss, 1967, 1969; Cahn, Siler and Wodinsky, 1969; Cahn, Siler and Auwarter, 1971; Offutt, 1974). However, in none of these cases was involvement of the lateral-line shown beyond doubt. The stimuli employed in several of the studies are bound to have caused surface waves, for instance when the fish were stimulated by rocking movements of the tank. It is not easy to eliminate the lateral-line organs completely without damaging other receptors, and many of the experiments were hampered by dubious extirpation techniques. Auditory studies in fish, using conditioning techniques, have repeatedly revealed dual thresholds in the low-frequency range (Tavolga and Wodinsky, 1963; Wodinsky and Tavolga, 1964; Cahn et al., 1969, 1971; Offutt, 1974), and this phenomenon has been interpreted to indicate switching between inner ear and lateral-line sensation. This conclusion is speculative, however, since none of the experiments involved elimination of the lateral-line.

A few behavior studies have, on the other hand, led to the conclusion that lateral-line organs are insensitive to sound (Parker, 1902; Hofer, 1908; Regnart, 1928; von Frisch and Stetter, 1932; Reinhardt, 1935; Dijkgraaf, 1950, 1952b, 1967; Schuijf and Siemelink, 1974). All these studies involve extirpation experiments, and elimination of the lateral-line organs never reduced the sensitivity to sound or vibrations. Schuijf and Siemelink (1974) and Schuijf (1975) have furthermore demonstrated that directional hearing in fish is linked to the labyrinth receptors, and not to the lateral-line as suggested by van Bergeijk (1964). There is thus a complete lack of behavior experiments proving unambiguously that the lateral-line participates in sound reception at some distance from the source.

Electrophysiological studies. In contrast to the bewildering disagreement among the behavioral studies, the available electrophysiological data show nearly unanimously that the lateral-line is a sensitive vibration detector (Hoagland, 1933, 1934; Schriever, 1935; Sand, 1937; Suckling and Suckling, 1950, 1964; Katsuki et al., 1951; Jielof, Spoor and de Vries, 1952; Kuiper, 1956; Harris and van Bergeijk, 1962; Suckling, 1962; Flock, 1965; Horch and Salmon, 1973; Tavolga, 1977; Kroese, van der Zalm and van den Bercken, 1978; Bleckmann and Topp, 1981; Sand, 1981). These experiments involved recording of afferent activity or microphonic potentials from the lateral-line canal. The stimuli employed were sound, oscillatory water currents, vibrating objects close to the organ, vibration applied to the fish body or direct vibration of the cupulae. Figure 10 presents a lateral-line vibrogram for the roach (Sand, 1981), which displays the typical pattern emerging from these studies. The lateral-line organs of the different species show optimal sensitivity to vibrational stimuli within the frequency range 50–100 Hz, with threshold values usually between 0.1 and 0.5 μm. However, in all these cases the fish were exposed to stimuli very different from natural sound stimulation. Surface ripples probably occurred when sound stimuli were applied, and the fish were usually firmly clamped, which facilitates relative movements between the water and the fish surface. Such relative movements were of course predominant during stimulation with oscillatory objects or water currents applied locally.

There is a striking lack of firm data on sensitivity to sound stimulation

Figure 10. Thresholds for the afferent response of trunk lateral line fibers in *Rutilus rutilus* to local water vibrations. Data from five fish are included. (From Sand, 1981.)

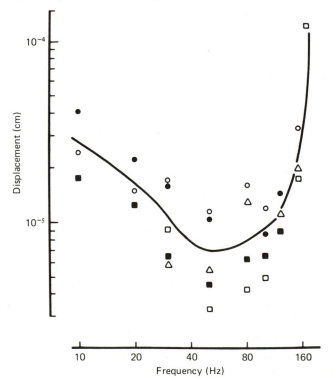

in a situation where the fish is free to move with the water mass. However, Cahn, Siler and Fujiya (1973) were unable to find lateral-line responses to sound stimuli in fish freely suspended in a standing wave tube.

Present views on the lateral line and sound reception

Several fairly recent studies claim a biologically significant role for the lateral-line in low-frequency sound detection (Suckling and Suckling, 1964; Weiss, 1967, 1969; Offutt, 1974; Horch and Salmon, 1973), although most investigators in the field today are more sceptical. The increasing number of fish audiograms recently obtained under free-field conditions show displacement thresholds far below the common thresholds for the lateral-line (Chapman and Sand, 1974), precluding any involvement of the lateral-line in the detection of low-intensity sounds. Most biologically significant sounds perceived by fish are, on the other hand, certainly well above the threshold intensities for the inner ear, and it is almost generally accepted that the lateral-line is bound to be stimulated in a sound field provided the sound energy suffices to create water displacements above the threshold values determined in the electrophysiological experiments (Harris and van Bergeijk, 1962; van Bergeijk, 1964; Tavolga, 1971, 1976; Popper and Fay, 1973; Schwartzkopff, 1976).

This conclusion is, however, wrong. A fish under water is nearly acoustically transparent and will vibrate with the same phase and amplitude as the surrounding water particles when exposed to sound. The otoliths have a specific density of about 2.9 (de Vries, 1950). These dense structures will therefore lag behind the oscillations of the sensory epithelia when exposed to sound, causing the appropriate shearing stimulation of the hair cells. The otolith organs are thus well adapted to detect far-field sound, and the presence of a swimbladder will only enhance this inherent ability (Sand and Enger, 1973). The cupulae of the lateral-line organs, on the other hand, have a specific density of about 1.0 (Jielof et al., 1952), which is close to that of the surroundings. No relative movements between the cupulae and the sensory cells will therefore occur during the gross vibration of fish and neighboring water in a sound field at some distance from the source. This will be the situation even well within the near field of a sound source. Dijkgraaf (1963) reached the same conclusion two decades ago, and in a series of later papers he has repeatedly argued against a possible use of the lateral-line in detection of propagated sound (Dijkgraaf, 1964, 1967, 1974).

The relationship between the movements of fish and water extremely close to the sound source has recently been studied by Denton and Gray (1982). Freshly killed fish of several species were suspended by fine threads in a seawater tank at various distances and angles with respect to the source. The resulting displacements of fish and water were measured optically. Figure 11 shows movement of water and of a sprat (*Sprattus sprattus*) with its long axis oriented radially to a pulsating source. At any particular distance from the source the longitudinal components of the fish displacements were constant along the fish, showing that the fish behaves as a rigid body longitudinally. The movements of the water particles, on the other hand, decrease in a predictable way (Harris, 1964). It is seen that at one position along the fish there is no relative movement between the fish and surrounding water, whereas relative movements of opposite phase occur on each side of this null position. This fact may give a hint as to why most fish and aquatic amphibians have their lateral-line organs distributed along the whole length of the

Figure 11. Movements of a *Sprattus sprattus* (●) and surrounding water (○) close to a pulsating source (12 Hz). The fish was oriented with its long axis in the axis of source vibration at three different distances from the source. Vertical lines indicate the corresponding positions of the snout. The longitudinal displacements of the fish skin and surrounding water were measured optically at different points along the fish. Horizontal lines show expected motions for a longitudinally rigid fish. (Redrawn from Denton & Gray, 1982.)

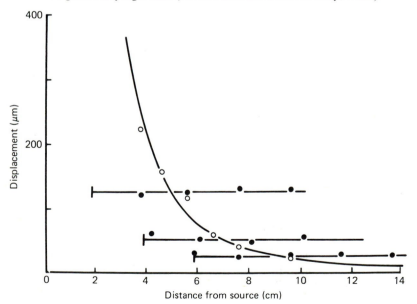

body. The relative movements between the fish and surroundings fall off dramatically with increasing distance from the source. Denton and Gray (1982) suggested that such movements are able to stimulate the lateral-line organs only within the distance limit of a few body lengths, which is merely a small fraction of the nearfield at the frequencies in question.

Figure 12. Comparison between the trunk lateral line response (maximum probability for spike occurrence during a stimulus cycle) in *Rutilus rutilus* to vibrating ball stimulation (upper and lower recordings) and to sound stimulation at different pressure/displacement ratios in an acoustic tube (middle recordings). Note the markedly reduced response to sound-induced water displacement compared with the response to local ball vibration. During sound stimulation the fish was positioned parallel to the long axis of the acoustic tube. Stimulation frequency was 50 Hz. (From Sand, 1981.)

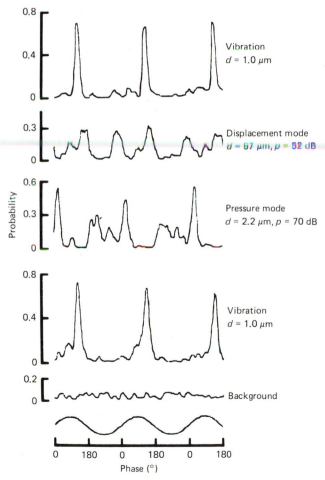

Several authors have reported maximum response distances of only a few centimeters for reactions proposed to depend on lateral-line stimulation (Wunder, 1927; von Frisch and Dijkgraaf, 1935; Reinhardt, 1935; Tavolga, 1976).

I have recently recorded the activity of the trunk lateral-line nerve in the roach with implanted electrodes, and compared the response to local water movements caused by a vibrating sphere close to the organ with the response to gross vibrations of fish and surrounding water (Sand, 1981). This latter stimulus condition simulates the situation a fish will encounter at some distance from a sound source, and the appropriate stimulus was obtained in an acoustic tube fitted with loudspeakers in both ends. Driving the loudspeakers 180° out of phase (displacement mode) causes large and uniform displacements throughout the tube, whereas driving the speakers in phase (pressure mode) causes large and uniform sound pressure combined with very low displacements (Hawkins and MacLennan, 1976). Figure 12 displays the afferent responses to these stimuli in the same animal. The upper record shows the response to a modest displacement of 1 μm parallel to the canal caused by local ball vibrations at 50 Hz. The fish was thereafter freely suspended parallel to and centrally in the tank. The whole water column, including the fish, was then vibrated at 57 μm. The otolith organs must have been excessively stimulated by these immense displacements. However, the lateral-line response decreased markedly compared to the previous 1-μm vibrations. Switching the acoustic tube to the pressure mode increased the pressure from 52 dB to 70 dB, while the displacements decreased to 2.2 μm. This caused the lateral-line response to increase, in spite of the reduced displacements. The last recording is a control repeating the vibrating ball stimulation after termination of the tank experiments.

These data indicate strongly that the lateral-line will be insensitive to particle motion at some distance from a sound source. However, the increased response when the acoustic tube was driven in pressure mode indicates that it is likely that the lateral-line may respond to sound pressure-induced swimbladder pulsations. The pressure threshold for the response was found to be about +40 dB, which is more than 70 dB above the lowest acoustic thresholds in teleosts (Hawkins, 1981). The sensitivity to sound-induced swimbladder pulsations therefore seems to be too low to justify any role of the lateral-line in the detection of sound pressure under natural conditions.

However, in the clupeids the central part of the elaborate head lateral-line canal system is separated from the inner ear perilymph by the flexible lateral recess membrane (Denton and Blaxter, 1976). The perilymph is in direct contact with the gas-filled bullae, which are extensions of the swimbladder. This arrangement (Figure 13) makes the auditory parts of the inner ear in clupeids extremely sensitive to sound pressure, and it seems likely that also the head lateral-line system may benefit from this anatomical specialization (Denton, Gray and Blaxter, 1979; Gray and Denton, 1979). Gray (1983) has recently recorded from the lateral-line nerves in sprat during independent pressure and displacement stimuli, and he observed clear afferent responses to moderate pressure stimulation. It is probable that similar anatomical arrangements also exist in other fish, but these possible exceptional cases should not obscure the general conclusion from this review.

The adequate stimulus for the mechanosensitive lateral-line systems is close-range water motion, causing relative movements between the

Figure 13. (A) The position of the two gas-filled bullae and the main lateral line canals (black) in the clupeids. (B) Diagram of the relationships between the swimbladder, ear, and the lateral line canals: b, bulla; bm, bulla membrane; e, endolymph; f, fenestra; ll, lateral line canal; lrm, lateral recess membrane; p, perilymph; pcd, pre-coelomic duct; sb, swimbladder; um, utricular macula. (From Blaxter et al., 1981 (A), and redrawn from Denton and Blaxter, 1976 (B).)

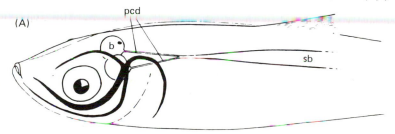

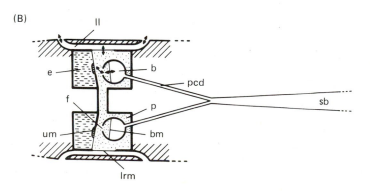

surface of the fish and the surroundings. Sound will not fulfill this requirement if the animal is positioned more than a few body lengths from the source. This insensitivity to propagated sound may even be beneficial to the lateral-line, since its responses to the appropriate stimuli will be undisturbed by most of the background noise in the sea (Denton and Gray, 1982).

References

Aleev, Y. G. and Ovcharov, O. P. (1969). The development of vortex formation processes and the characteristics of the boundary layer in the movement of fishes. (In Russian.) *Zool. Zh. 48*: 781–90.

Ashmore, J. F., and Russell, I. J. (1982). Effect of efferent nerve stimulation on hair cells of the frog sacculus. *J. Physiol., Lond. 329*: 25–6P.

Atz, J. W. (1953). Orientation in schooling fishes. In *Proceedings of a Conference on Orientation in Animals*, ed. T. C. Schneirla, pp. 115–30. Washington, D.C.: Office of Naval Research.

Backus, R. H. (1963). Hearing in elasmobranchs. In *Sharks and Survival*, ed. P. W. Gilbert, pp. 243–54. Boston: Heath.

van Bergeijk, W. A. (1964). Directional and nondirectional hearing in fish. In *Marine Bio-Acoustics*, ed. W. N. Tavolga, pp. 281–99. Oxford: Pergamon Press.

Blaxter, J. H. S., Denton, E. J., and Gray, J. A. B. (1981). Acousticolateralis system in clupeid fishes. In *Hearing and Sound Communication in Fishes*, ed. W. N. Tavolga, A. N. Popper and R. R. Fay, pp. 39–59. New York: Springer-Verlag.

Blaxter, J. H. S., Gray, J. A. B., and Best, A. C. G. (1983). Structure and development of the free neuromast and lateral-line system of the herring. *J. Mar. Biol. Ass. UK 63*: 247–60.

Bleckmann, H. (1980). Reaction time and stimulus frequency in prey localization in the surface-feeding fish *Aplocheilus lineatus*. *J. Comp. Physiol. 140A:* 163–72.

Bleckmann, H., and Schwartz, E. (1981). Reaction time of the topminnow *Aplocheilus lineatus* to surface waves determined by video- and electromyogram recordings. *Experientia 37:* 362–3.

Bleckmann, H., and Schwartz, E. (1982). The functional significance of frequency modulation within a wave train for prey localization in the surface-feeding fish *Aplocheilus lineatus* (Cyprinodontidae). *J. Comp. Physiol. 145A:* 331–9.

Bleckmann, H., and Topp, G. (1981). Surface wave sensitivity of the lateral-line system of the topminnow (*Aplocheilus lineatus*). *Naturwissenschaften 68:* 624–5.

Bleckmann, H., Waldner, I., and Schwartz, E. (1981). Frequency discrimination of the surface-feeding fish *Aplocheilus lineatus* – a prerequisite for prey localization? *J. Comp. Physiol. 143A:* 485–90.

Bledsoe, S. C. Jr., Bobbin, R. P., Thalmann, R., and Thalmann, I. (1980). Stimulus-induced release of endogenous amino acids from skins containing the lateral line organ in *Xenopus laevis*. *Expl Brain Res. 40:* 97–101.

Bobbin, R. P., Bledsoe, S. C. Jr., Chihal, D. M., and Morgan, D. N. (1981). Comparative actions of glutamate and related substances on the *Xenopus laevis* lateral line. *Comp. Biochem. Physiol. 69C:* 145–7.

Bowen, E. S. (1931). The role of sense organs in aggregations of *Ameiurus melas. Ecol. Monogr. 1:* 1–35.

Breder, C. M. (1951). Studies on the structure of the fish school. *Bull. Am. Mus. Nat. Hist. 98:* 7–28.

Breder, C. M. (1959). Studies on social groupings in fishes. *Bull. Am. Mus. Nat. Hist. 117:* 397–481.

Bullock, T. H. (1981). Comparisons of the electric and acoustic senses and their central processing. In *Hearing and Sound Communication in Fishes*, ed. W. N. Tavolga, A. N. Popper and R. R. Fay, pp. 525–71. New York: Springer-Verlag.

Cahn, P. H., Siler, W., and Auwarter, A. (1971). Acousticolateralis system of fishes: cross-modal coupling of signal and noise in the grunt, *Haemulon parrai. J. Acoust. Soc. Am. 49:* 591–4.

Cahn, P. H., Siler, W., and Fujiya, M. (1973). Sensory detection of environmental changes by fish. In *Responses of Fish to Environmental Changes*, ed. W. Chavin, pp. 363–88. Springfield: Charles C. Thomas.

Cahn, P. H., Siler, W., and Wodinsky, J. (1969). Acousticolateralis system of fishes: tests of pressure and particle velocity sensitivity in grunts, *Haemulon sciurus* and *Haemulon parrai. J. Acoust. Soc. Am. 46:* 1572–8.

von Campenhausen, C., Riess, I., and Weissert, R. (1981). Detection of stationary objects by the blind cave fish *Anoptichthys jordani* (Characidae). *J. Comp. Physiol. 143A:* 369–74.

Chapman, C. J., and Sand, O. (1974). Field studies of hearing in two species of flatfish *Pleuronectes platessa* (L.) and *Limanda limanda* (L.) (Family Pleuronectidae). *Comp. Biochem. Physiol. 47:* 371–86.

Corey, D. P., and Hudspeth, A. J. (1979). Ionic basis of the receptor potential in a vertebrate hair cell. *Nature 281:* 675–7.

Crawford, A. C., and Fettiplace, R. (1980). The frequency selectivity of auditory nerve fibres and hair cells in the cochlea of the turtle. *J. Physiol., Lond. 306:* 79–125.

Crawford, A. C., and Fettiplace, R. (1981). An electrical tuning mechanism in turtle cochlear hair cells. *J. Physiol., Lond. 312:* 377–412.

Dawson, A. B. (1936). Changes in the lateral line organs during the life of the newt, *Triturus viridescens*. A consideration of the endocrine factors involved in the maintenance of differentiation. *J. Exp. Zool. 74:* 221–37.

Denton, E. J., and Blaxter, J. H. S. (1976). The mechanical relationships between the clupeid swimbladder, inner ear and lateral line. *J. Mar. Biol. Ass. UK 56:* 787–807.

Denton, E. J., and Gray, J. A. B. (1982). The rigidity of fish and patterns of lateral line stimulation. *Nature 297:* 679–81.

Denton, E. J., and Gray, J. A. B. (1983). Mechanical factors in the excitation of clupeid lateral lines. *Proc. Roy. Soc., Lond. B218:* 1–26.

Denton, E. J., Gray, J. A. B., and Blaxter, J. H. S. (1983). The mechanics of the clupeid acoustico-lateralis system: frequency responses. *J. Mar. Biol. Ass. UK 59:* 27–47.

Dijkgraaf, S. (1934). Untersuchungen über die Funktion der Seitenorgane an Fischen. *Z. vergl. Physiol. 20:* 162–214.

Dijkgraaf, S. (1947). Über die Reizung des Ferntasinnes bei Fischen und Amphibien. *Experientia 3:* 206–8.

Dijkgraaf, S. (1950). Untersuchungen über die Funktionen des Ohrlabyrinths bei Meeresfischen. *Physiol. Comp. Oecol. 2:* 81–106.

Dijkgraaf, S. (1952a). Bau und Funktionen der Seitenorgane und des Ohrlabyrinths bei Fischen. *Experientia 8:* 205–16.

Dijkgraaf, S. (1952b). Über die Schallwahrnehmung bei Meeresfischen. *Z. vergl. Physiol.* *34:* 104–22.

Dijkgraaf, S. (1960). Hearing in bony fishes. *Proc. Roy. Soc. Lond. B152:* 51–4.

Dijkgraaf, S. (1963). The functioning and significance of the lateral-line organs. *Biol. Rev. 1963:* 51–105.

Dijkgraaf, S. (1964). The supposed use of the lateral-line as an organ of hearing in fish. *Experientia 20:* 586–7.

Dijkgraaf, S. (1967). Biological significance of the lateral-line organs. In *Lateral Line Detectors*, ed. P. H. Cahn, pp. 83–95. Bloomington: Indiana University Press.

Dijkgraaf, S. (1974). Problems in the field of lateral-line functioning. *Atti Acad. Sci. Ferrara 51:* 1–5.

Dye, W. J. P. (1921) The relation of the lateral line organs of *Necturus* to hearing. *J. Comp. Psychol. 1:* 469–71.

Fettiplace, R., and Crawford, A. C. (1978). The coding of sound pressure and frequency in cochlear hair cells of the terrapin. *Proc. Roy. Soc., Lond. B203:* 209–18.

Fettiplace, R., and Crawford, A. C. (1980). The origin of tuning in turtle cochlear hair cells. *Hearing Res. 2:* 447–54.

Flock, Å. (1965). Electromicroscopical and electrophysiological studies on the lateral line canal organ. *Acta Otolaryngol.* Suppl. *199:* 1–90.

Flock, Å. (1967). Ultrastructure and function in the lateral line organs. In *Lateral Line Detectors*, ed. P. H. Cahn, pp. 163–97. Bloomington: Indiana University Press.

Flock, Å. (1971). Sensory transduction in hair cells. In *Handbook of Sensory Physiology*, vol. *1*, ed. W. Lowenstein, pp. 396–441. Berlin: Springer-Verlag.

Flock, Å., Jørgensen, J. M., and Russell, I. J. (1973). The physiology of individual hair cells and their synapses. In *Basic Mechanisms in Hearing*, ed. A. Møller, pp. 273–306. New York: Academic Press.

Flock, Å., and Russell, I. J. (1973a). Efferent fibres: postsynaptic action on hair cells. *Nature, New Biol. 243:* 89–91.

Flock, Å., and Russell, I. J. (1973b). The postsynaptic action of efferent fibres in the lateral line organ of the burbot *Lota lota. J. Physiol., Lond. 235:* 591–605.

Flock, Å., and Russell, I. J. (1976). Inhibition by efferent nerve fibres: action on hair cells and afferent synaptic transmission in the lateral line canal organ of the burbot *Lota lota. J. Physiol., Lond. 257:* 45–62.

Flock, Å., and Wersäll, J. (1962). A study of the orientation of the sensory hairs of the receptor cells in the lateral line organs of fish, with special reference to the function of the receptors. *J. Cell Biol. 15:* 19–27.

von Frisch, K., and Dijkgraaf, S. (1935). Können Fische die Schallrichtung wahrnehmen? *Z. vergl. Physiol. 22:* 641–55.

von Frisch, K., and Stetter, H. (1932). Untersuchungen über den Sitz des Gehörsinnes bei der Elritze. *Z. vergl. Physiol. 17:* 686–801.

Görner, P. (1963). Untersuchungen zur Morphologie und Elektrophysiologie des Seitenlinienorganes des Krallenfrosches (*Xenopus laevis* Daudin). *Z. vergl. Physiol. 47:* 316–38.

Görner, P. (1967). Independence of afferent activity from efferent activity in the lateral line organ of *Xenopus laevis* Daudin. In *Lateral Line Detectors*, ed. P. H. Cahn, pp. 199–214. Bloomington: Indiana University Press.

Görner, P. (1973). The importance of the lateral line system for the perception of surface waves in the claw toad, *Xenopus laevis* Daudin. *Experientia 29:* 295–6.

Görner, P. (1976). Source localization with labyrinth and lateral line in the clawed toad (*Xenopus laevis*). In *Sound Reception in Fish*, ed. A, Schuijf and A. D. Hawkins, pp. 171–83. Amsterdam: Elsevier.

Gray, J. (1968). *Animal Locomotion*, 479 pp. London: Weidenfeld and Nicolson.

Gray, J. A. B. (1983). Interaction of sound pressure and particle acceleration in the excitation of the lateral-line neuromasts of sprats. (In preparation.)

Gray, J. A. B., and Denton, E. J. (1979). The mechanics of the clupeid acoustico-lateralis system: low frequency measurements. *J. Mar. Biol. Ass. UK 59:* 11–26.

Harris, G. G. (1964). Considerations on the physics of sound production by fishes. In *Marine Bio-Acoustics*, ed. W. N. Tavolga, pp. 233–47. Oxford: Pergamon Press.

Harris, G. G., and van Bergeijk, W. A. (1962). Evidence that the lateral line organ responds to water displacements. *J. Acoust. Soc. Am. 34:* 1831–41.

Harris, G. G., and Flock, Å. (1967). Spontaneous and evoked activity from the *Xenopus laevis* lateral line. In *Lateral Line Detectors*, ed. P. H. Cahn, pp. 135–61. Bloomington: Indiana University Press.

Harris, G. G., Frishkopf, L., and Flock, Å. (1969). Receptor potentials in the hair cells of mudpuppy lateral line. *J. Acoust. Soc. Am. 45:* 300–1.

Harris, G. G., Frishkopf, L., and Flock, Å. (1970). Receptor potentials from hair cells of the lateral line. *Science 167:* 76–9.

Harris, G. G., and Milne, D. C. (1966). Input–output characteristics of the lateral line sense organ. *J. Acoust. Soc. Am. 40:* 32–42.

Hawkins, A. D. (1981). The hearing abilities of fish. In *Hearing and Sound Communication in Fishes*, ed. W. N. Tavolga, A. N. Popper and R. R. Fay, pp. 109–37. New York: Springer-Verlag.

Hawkins, A. D., and MacLennan, D. N. (1976). An acoustic tank for hearing studies on fish. In *Sound Reception in Fish*, ed. A. Schuijf and A. D. Hawkins, pp. 149–69. Amsterdam: Elsevier.

Hoagland, H. (1933). Electrical responses from the lateral-line nerves of catfish. I. *J. Gen. Physiol. 16:* 695–714.

Hoagland, H. (1934). Electrical responses from the lateral-line nerves of catfish. III. *J. Gen. Physiol. 17:* 72–82.

Hoagland, H. (1935). Electrical responses from the lateral-line nerves of fishes. V. Responses in the central nervous system. *J. Gen. Physiol. 18:* 89–91.

Hofer, B. (1908). Studien über die Hautsinnesorgane der Fische. I. Die Funktion der Seitenorgane bei den Fischen. *Ber. K. Bayer. biol. Versuchsstation München 1:* 115–64.

Horch, K., and Salmon, M. (1973). Adaptations to the acoustic environment by the squirrelfishes *Myripristis violaceus* and *M. pralinius. Marine Behav. Physiol. 2:* 121–39.

Hudspeth, A. J., and Corey, D. P. (1977). Sensitivity, polarity, and conductance change in the response of vertebrate hair cells to controlled mechanical stimuli. *Proc. Natn. Acad. Sci., USA 74:* 2407–11.

Hudspeth, A. J., and Jacobs, R. (1979). Stereocilia mediate transduction in vertebrate hair cells. *Proc. Natn. Acad. Sci. USA 76:* 1506–9.

Hunter, J. R. (1969). Communication of velocity changes in jack mackerel *Trachurus symmetricus* schools. *Anim. Behav. 17:* 507–14.

Hyrtl, J. (1866). Der Seitenkanal von *Lota. Sber. Akad. Wiss., Wien 53:* 551–7.

Jielof, R., Spoor, A., and de Vries, H. (1952). The microphonic activity of the lateral line. *J. Physiol., Lond. 116:* 137–57.

Johnstone, B. M., and Sellick, P. M. (1972). The peripheral auditory apparatus. *Q. Rev. Biophys. 5:* 1–57.

Jørgensen, J. M., and Flock, Å. (1973). The ultrastructure of lateral line sense organs in the adult salamander *Ambystoma mexicanum. J. Neurocytol. 2:* 133–42.

Katsuki, Y. (1973). The ionic receptive mechanism in the acoustico-lateralis system. In *Basic Mechanisms in Hearing*, ed. A. R. Møller, pp. 307–34. New York: Academic Press.

Katsuki, Y., Hashimoto, T., and Yanagisawa, K. (1970). The lateral-line organ of shark as a chemoreceptor. *Adv. Biophys. 1:* 1–51.

Katsuki, Y., Hashimoto, T., and Kendall, J. I. (1971). The chemoreception in the lateral-line organs of teleosts. *Jap. J. Physiol. 21:* 99–118.

Katsuki, Y., and Onada, N. (1973). The lateral-line organ of fish as a chemoreceptor. In *Responses of Fish to Environmental Changes*, ed. W. Chavin, pp. 389–411. Springfield: Charles C. Thomas.

Katsuki, Y., Yoshino, S., and Chen, J. (1951). Action current of the single lateral-line nerve fibre of fish. II. On the discharge due to stimulation. *Jap. J. Physiol. 1:* 264–8.

Kleerekoper, H., and Roggenkamp, P. A. (1959). An experimental study on the effect of the swimbladder on hearing sensitivity in *Ameiurus nebulosus* (LeSueur). *Can. J. Zool. 37:* 1–8.

Kramer, G. (1933). Untersuchungen über die Sinnesleistungen und das Orientierungsverhalten von *Xenopus laevis* Daud. *Zool. Jb. Abt. Allgemeine Zool. Physiol. Tiere 52:* 629–76.

Kroese, A. B. A., van der Zalm, J. M., and van den Bercken, J. (1978). Frequency response of the lateral-line organ of *Xenopus laevis. Pflügers Archiv 375:* 167–75.

Kuiper, J. W. (1956). *The Microphonic Effect of the Lateral Line Organ*. Groningen: Publication of the Biophysical Group of the 'Natuurkundig Laboratorium'.

Landacre, F. L. (1927). The differentiation of the preauditory and postauditory primitive lines into preauditory and postauditory placodes, lateralis ganglia and migratory lateral-line placodes in *Ambystoma jeffersonianum. J. Comp. Neurol. 44:* 29–59.

Lang, H. H. (1980). Surface wave discrimination between prey and nonprey by the back swimmer *Notonecta glauca* L. (Hemiptera, Heteroptera). *Behav. Ecol. Sociobiol. 6:* 233–46.

Leydig, F. (1850). Über die Schleimkanäle der Knochenfische. *Arch. Anat. Physiol.* 170–81.

Leydig, F. (1851). Über die Nervenknöpfe in den Schleimkanälen von *Lepidoleprus, Umbrina* und *Corvina. Arch. Anat. Physiol.* 235–40.

Lighthill, M. J. (1969). Hydromechanics of aquatic animal propulsion. In *Annual Review of Fluid Mechanics*, vol. *1*, ed. W. R. Sears and M. van Dyke, pp. 413–46. Palo Alto: Annual Reviews.

Lyon, E. P. (1904). On rheotropism. I. Rheotropism in fishes. *Am. J. Physiol. 12:* 149–61.

Maliukina, G. A. (1960). Hearing in certain Black Sea fishes in connection with ecology and particulars in the structure of their hearing apparatus. (In Russian.) *Zh. obshch. Biol. 21:* 198–205.

McCutchen, C. W. (1976). Flow visualization with stereo shadowgraphs of stratified fluid. *J. Exp. Biol. 65:* 11–20.

McCutchen, C. W. (1977). Froude propulsive efficiency of a small fish, measured by wake visualisation. In *Scale Effects in Animal Locomotion*, ed. T. J. Pedley, pp. 339–63. London: Academic Press.

McGlone, F. P., Russell, I. J., and Sand, O. (1979). Measurement of calcium ion concentrations in the lateral line cupulae of *Xenopus laevis. J. Exp. Biol. 83:* 123–30.

Mulroy, M. J., Altmann, D. W., Weiss, T. F., and Peake, W. T. (1974). Intracellular electric responses to sound in a vertebrate cochlea. *Nature 249:* 482–5.

Murray, R. W. (1955a). Nerve endings as transducers of thermal stimuli in lower vertebrates. *Nature 176:* 698–9.

Murray, R. W. (1955b). The lateralis organs and their innervation in *Xenopus laevis. Q. Jl. Microsc. Sci. 96:* 351–61.

Nakagawa, K., Yoshioka, T., and Katsuki, Y. (1974). Effects of metallic ions on the lateral-line organs of bullfrog tadpoles. *Proc. Jap. Acad. 50:* 658–63.

Noble, G. K. (1931). *The Biology of the Amphibia.* New York: Dover Publishing Company.

Northcutt, R. G. (1981). Audition and the central nervous system of fishes. In *Hearing and Sound Communication in Fishes,* ed. W. N. Tavolga, A. N. Popper and R. R. Fay, pp. 331–55. New York: Springer-Verlag.

Offutt, G. C. (1974). Structures for the detection of acoustic stimuli in the Atlantic codfish, *Gadus morhua. J. Acoust. Soc. Am. 56:* 665–71.

Onada, N., and Katsuki, Y. (1972). Chemoreception on the lateral-line organ of an aquatic amphibian, *Xenopus laevis. Jap. J. Physiol. 22:* 87–102.

Parker, G. H. (1902). Hearing and allied senses in fishes. *Bull. US Fish Comm. 22:* 45–64.

Parker, G. H. (1904). The function of the lateral line organs in fishes. *Bull. US Bur. Fish. 24:* 185–207.

Parker, G. H. (1909). Influence of the eyes, ears, and other allied sense organs on the movements of the dogfish, *Mustelus canis* (Mitchill). *Bull. US Bur. Fish. 29:* 43–57.

Parker, G. H., and van Heusen, A. P. (1917). The reception of mechanical stimuli by the skin, lateral line organs and ears in fishes, especially in *Amiurus. Am. J. Physiol. 44:* 463–89.

Parr, E. A. (1927). A contribution to the theoretical analysis of the schooling behaviour of fishes. *Occ. Pap. Bingham Oceanogr. Colln 1:* 1–32.

Partridge, B. L. (1981). Lateral line function and the internal dynamics of fish schools. In *Hearing and Sound Communication in Fishes,* ed. W. N. Tavolga, A. N. Popper and R. R. Fay, pp. 515–22. New York: Springer-Verlag.

Partridge, B. L., and Pitcher, T. J. (1979). Evidence against a hydrodynamical function of fish schools. *Nature 279:* 418–19.

Partridge, B. L., and Pitcher, T. J. (1980). The sensory basis of fish schools: relative roles of lateral line and vision. *J. Comp. Physiol. 135A:* 315–25.

Pitcher, T. J., Partridge, B. L., and Wardle, L. S. (1976). A blind fish can school. *Science 194:* 963–5.

Popper, A. N., and Fay, R. R. (1973). Sound detection and processing by teleost fishes: a critical review. *J. Acoust. Soc. Am. 53:* 1515–28.

Regnart, H. C. (1928). Investigations on the lateral sense organs of *Gadus merlangus. Proc. Univ. Durham Phil. Soc. 8:* 55–60.

Reinhardt, F. (1935). Über Richtungswahrnehmung bei Fischen, besonders bei der Elritze (*Phoxinus laevis* L.) und beim Zwergwels (*Amiurus nebulosus* Raf.). *Z. vergl. Physiol. 22:* 570–603.

Reno, H. W., and Middleton, H. H. (1973). Lateral line system of *Siren intermedia* Le Conte (Amphibia: Sirenidae), during aquatic activity and aestivation. *Acta Zool. 54:* 21–9.

Roberts, B. L. (1981). Central processing of acousticolateralis signals in elasmobranchs. In *Hearing and Sound Communication in Fishes*, ed. W. N. Tavolga, A. N. Popper and R. R. Fay, pp. 357–73. New York: Springer-Verlag.

Roberts, B. L., and Russell, I. J. (1972). The activity of lateral line efferent neurons in stationary and swimming dogfish. *J. Exp. Biol. 57:* 435–48.

Rosen, M. W. (1959). Waterflow about a swimming fish. *Technical Publications of the United States Naval Test Station, China Lake, California*, NOTSTP 2298, 1–94.

Russell, I. J. (1968). Influence of efferent fibres on a receptor. *Nature 219:* 177–8.

Russell, I. J. (1971a). The role of the lateral line efferent system in *Xenopus laevis. J. Exp. Biol. 54:* 621–41

Russell, I. J. (1971b). The pharmacology of efferent synapses in the lateral line system of *Xenopus laevis. J. Exp. Biol. 54:* 643–58.

Russell, I. J. (1974). Central and peripheral inhibition of lateral line input during the startle response in goldfish. *Brain Res. 80:* 517–22.

Russell, I. J., and Lowe, D. A. (1983). The effect of efferent stimulation on the phase and amplitude of extracellular receptor potentials in the lateral line system of the perch (*Perca fluviatilis*). *J. Exp. Biol. 102:* 223–38.

Russell, I. J., and Sellick, P. M. (1976). Measurement of potassium and chloride ion concentrations in the cupulae of the lateral lines in *Xenopus laevis. J. Physiol., Lond. 257:* 245–55.

Russell, I. J., and Sellick, P. M. (1977). Tuning properties of cochlear hair cells. *Nature 267:* 858–60.

Russell, I. J., and Sellick, P. M. (1978). Intracellular studies of hair cells in the mammalian cochlea. *J. Physiol., Lond. 284:* 261–90.

Sand, A. (1937). The mechanism of the lateral sense organs of fishes. *Proc. Roy. Soc. Lond. B123:* 472–95.

Sand, A. (1938). The function of the ampullae of Lorenzini, with some observations on the effect of temperature on sensory rhythms. *Proc. Roy. Soc. Lond. B125:* 524–53.

Sand, O. (1975). Effect of different ionic environments on the mechano-sensitivity of lateral line organs in the mudpuppy. *J. Comp. Physiol. 102:* 27–42.

Sand, O. (1979). The role of Ca^{2+} in the hair cell transduction process. *Acta Physiol. Scand.* Suppl. *473:* 20.

Sand, O. (1981). The lateral line and sound reception. In *Hearing and Sound Communication in Fishes*, ed. W. N. Tavolga, A. N. Popper and R. R. Fay, pp. 459–80. New York: Springer-Verlag.

Sand, O., and Enger, P. S. (1973). Function of the swimbladder in fish hearing. In *Basic Mechanisms in Hearing*, ed. A. R. Møller, pp. 893–910. New York: Academic Press.

Sand, O., Ozawa, S., and Hagiwara, S. (1975). Electrical and mechanical stimulation of hair cells in the mudpuppy. *J. Comp. Physiol. 102:* 13–26.

Schlaifer, A. (1942). The schooling behaviour of mackerel – a preliminary experimental analysis. *Zoologica 27:* 75–80.

Schmidt, R. S. (1965). Amphibian acoustico-lateralis efferents. *J. Cell. Comp. Physiol. 65:* 155–62.

Schriever, H. (1935). Aktionspotentiale des *N. lateralis* bei Reizung der Seitenorgane von Fischen. *Pflügers Arch. ges. Physiol. 235:* 771–84.

Schuijf, A. (1975). Directional hearing of cod (*Gadus morhua*) under approximate free field conditions. *J. Comp. Physiol. 98:* 307–32.

Schuijf, A., and Siemelink, M. E. (1974). The ability of cod (*Gadus morhua*) to orient towards a sound source. *Experientia 30:* 773–5.

Schwartz, E. (1965). Bau und Funktion der Seitenlinie des Streifenhechtlings *Aplocheilus lineatus*. *Z. vergl. Physiol. 50:* 55–87.

Schwartz, E. (1967). Analysis of surface-wave perception in some teleosts. In *Lineral Line Detectors*, ed. P. H. Cahn, pp. 123–34. Bloomington: Indiana University Press.

Schwartz, E. (1970). Ferntasinnesorgane von Oberflächenfischen. *Z. Morphol. Tiere 67:* 40–57.

Schwartz, E. (1971). Die Ortung von Wasserwellen durch Oberflächenfische. *Z. vergl. Physiol. 74:* 64–80.

Schwartz, E. (1974). Lateral-line mechano-receptors in fishes and amphibians. In *Handbook of Sensory Physiology*, vol. III/3, ed. A. Fessard, pp. 257–78. Berlin: Springer-Verlag.

Schwartz, E., and Hasler, A. D. (1966). Perception of surface waves by the blackstripe topminnow *Fundulus notatus*. *J. Fish. Res. Bd Can. 23:* 1331–52.

Schwartzkopff, J. (1976). Comparative-physiological problems of hearing in fish. In *Sound Reception in Fish*, ed. A. Schuijf and A. D. Hawkins, pp. 3–17. Amsterdam: Elsevier.

Sellick, P. M., and Russell, I. J. (1979). Two-tone suppression in cochlear hair cells. *Hearing Res. 1:* 227–36.

Sellick, P. M., and Russell, I. J. (1980). The responses of inner hair cells to basilar membrane velocity during low frequency auditory stimulation in the guinea pig cochlea. *Hearing Res. 2:* 439–45.

Shaw, E. (1962). The schooling of fishes. *Scient. Am. 206:* 128–38.

Shaw, E. (1970). Schooling in fishes: critique and review. In *Development and Evolution of Behavior*, ed. L. R. Aronson, E. Tobach, D. S. Lehrman and J. S. Rosenblatt, pp. 452–80. San Francisco: Freeman.

Shelton, P. M. J. (1970). The lateral line system at metamorphosis in *Xenopus laevis* (Daudin). *J. Embryol. Exp. Morphol. 24:* 511–24.

Stone, L. S. (1922). Experiments on the development of the cranial ganglia and the lateral line sense organs in *Ambystoma punctatum*. *J. Exp. Zool. 35:* 421–96.

Stone, L. S. (1933). The development of lateral line sense organs in amphibians observed in living and vital stained preparations. *J. Comp. Neurol. 57:* 507–40.

Suckling, E. E. (1962). Lateral line in fish – possible mode of action. *J. Acoust. Soc. Am. 34:* 127.

Suckling, E. E., and Suckling, J. A. (1950). The electrical response of the lateral line system of fish to tone and other stimuli. *J. Gen. Physiol. 34:* 1–8.

Suckling, E. E., and Suckling, J. A. (1964). Lateral line as a vibration receptor. *J. Acoust. Soc. Am. 36:* 2214–16.

Tavolga, W. N. (1971). Sound production and detection. In *Fish Physiology*, ed. W. S. Hoar and D. J. Randall, pp. 135–205. New York: Academic Press.

Tavolga, W. N. (1976). Acoustic obstacle detection in the sea catfish (*Arius felis*). In *Sound Reception in Fish*, ed. A. Schuijf and A. D. Hawkins, pp. 185–204. Amsterdam: Elsevier.

Tavolga, W. N. (1977). Mechanisms for directional hearing in the sea catfish (*Arius felis*). *J. Exp. Biol. 67:* 97–115.

Tavolga, W. N., and Wodinsky, J. (1963). Auditory capacities in fishes. Pure tone thresholds in nine species of marine teleosts. *Bull. Am. Mus. Nat. Hist. 126:* 177–240.

Valli, P., Zucca, G., and Casella, C. (1979). Ionic composition of the endolymph and sensory transduction in labyrinthine organs. *Acta Otolaryngol. 87:* 466–71.

de Vries, H. (1950). The mechanics of the labyrinth otoliths. *Acta Otolaryngol. 38:* 262–73.

Weihs, D. (1972). Semi-infinite vortex trails, and their relation to oscillating airfoils. *J. Fluid Mech. 54:* 679–90.

Weihs, D. (1973). Hydrodynamics of fish schooling. *Nature 241:* 290–1.

Weihs, D. (1975). Some hydrodynamical aspects of fish schooling. In *Swimming and Flying in Nature*, ed. T. Y. Wu, C. J. Brokaw and C. Brenne. New York: Plenum Publishing Company.

Weiss, B. A. (1967). Sonic sensitivity in the goldfish (*Carassius auratus*). In *Lateral Line Detectors*, ed. P. H. Cahn, pp. 249–64. Bloomington: Indiana University Press.

Weiss, B. A. (1969). Lateral-line sensitivity in the goldfish (*Carassius auratus*). *J. Audit. Res. 9:* 71–5.

Weiss, T. F., Mulroy, M. J., and Altmann, D. W. (1974). Intracellular responses to acoustic clicks in the inner ear of the alligator lizard. *J. Acoust. Soc. Am. 55:* 606–19.

Weissert, R., and von Campenhausen, C. (1981). Discrimination between stationary objects by the blind cave fish *Anoptichthys jordani* (Characidae). *J. Comp. Physiol. 143A:* 375–81.

Wisby, W. J., Richard, J. D., Nelson, D. R., and Gruber, S. H. (1964). Sound perception in elasmobranchs. In *Marine Bio-Acoustics*, ed. W. N. Tavolga, pp. 255–68. Oxford: Pergamon Press.

Wodinsky, J., and Tavolga, W. N. (1964). Sound detection in teleost fish. In *Marine Bio-Acoustics*, ed. W. N. Tavolga, pp. 269–80. Oxford: Pergamon Press.

Wunder, W. (1927). Sinnesphysiologische Untersuchungen über die Nahrungsaufnahme bei verschiedenen Knochenfischarten. *Z. vergl. Physiol. 6:* 67–98.

Yanagisawa, K., Taglietti, V., and Katsuki, Y. (1974). Responses to chemical stimuli in the hair cells of the lateral-line organ of mudpuppy. *Proc. Jap. Acad. 50:* 526–31.

Yoshioka, T., Asanuma, A., Yanagisawa, K., and Katsuki, Y. (1978). The chemical receptive mechanism in the lateral-line organ. *Jap. J. Physiol. 28:* 557–67.

1.2

Hearing in insects

AXEL MICHELSEN

Textbooks of comparative physiology often contain a short description of hearing organs other than those of mammals. Insect ears – when mentioned – are generally dealt with in a few lines of text, in which it is stated that many insects can hear, but that the ears are primitive. The ears do not respond to the pressure components of sound, but to the movements of the oscillating air particles. The ears therefore have very little mass, and their suspension is very pliant so that the moving parts can follow the movements of the air exactly. A frequency analysis cannot be performed, and the ears are only suited for providing the animal with a rough idea of the direction to the sound source and of the coarse rhythmicity of the sounds.

Such summaries are very misleading, but one can find examples of ears where each of these statements is true. A sense of hearing has evolved independently at least a dozen times in different groups of insects, and the ears have further differentiated into a large number of functional types, making use of a wide variety of physical mechanisms. Some insect ears are built in a very simple way. For example, the ears of some moths just consist of one receptor cell attaching to a tympanal membrane. Other insect ears, however, contain more than a thousand receptor cells. Some hairs and antennae of insects respond to moving air particles. But the large majority of ears have tympanal membranes and respond to the pressure component of sound, and the mechanics of these ears are adapted to the detection of small changes in pressure. Although some insects cannot analyse the frequency of sound, several groups of insects are provided with frequency analysers of a surprising complexity. Furthermore, despite being in a difficult position with respect to analysis of the direction of sound, many insects have evolved

33

very complicated mechanisms for directional hearing, and some are also able to analyse time cues with great precision.

Sound communication and hearing in insects have been reviewed several times in recent years (e.g. Busnel, 1963; Elsner and Popov, 1978; Michelsen, 1974; Michelsen and Larsen, 1982; Michelsen and Nocke, 1974; Zhantiev, 1981). In the following, I shall not attempt to cover all aspects of the subject, but rather to mention a few areas which appear especially interesting to me. My special interest is in the biophysics of communication, and the selection of topics here reflects this preference.

Until recently, the differences and similarities within hearing organs were thought generally to reflect the evolutionary prehistory of the animals and thus to follow their systematic positions. However, we are now beginning to understand that some features of the hearing organs are simple consequences of the physical nature of sound. Furthermore, some insect ears are adapted for the reception of sounds from predators (e.g. the ultrasonic cries of hunting bats) and other ears for receiving conspecific songs. Ears used as bat-detectors can be fairly simple (Figure 1), because hearing organs can hardly avoid being very directional at high sound frequencies, and because the insects do not need to analyze the fine details of the ultrasonic bat-cries. It is not very interesting for the insect to know which kind of bat is approaching – the important thing to know is where the bat is (i.e. the direction and approximate distance to the bat). In contrast, insects often need a substantial capacity for analysis of the fine details of sound signals in order to be able to recognize a conspecific song in a chorus of many different songs. Bat-detecting insects do not need to be able to analyze the frequency content of the cries, and their ears therefore do not have this capacity (at least not in the ultrasonic range). Grasshoppers, crickets, bush crickets, mole crickets and various groups of bugs, on the other hand, all have frequency analysers with different receptor cells covering from two to no less than 24 frequency bands within the total frequency range covered by the ears (Figure 2). The cicadas appear to be the only exception from the general rule that communication between conspecific animals requires some capacity for frequency analysis.

The physical nature of sound is a major factor determining the kinds of signals available for communication and the ways in which they can be received and analysed. The behaviour of both sound-emitting systems and hearing organs depends very much upon the relationship between the wavelength of sound and the size of the sound emitter or receiver. For sound emission to be efficient, the diameter of the sound source should be of about the same order of magnitude as the wavelength (or larger). Large insects are not reasonably efficient sound emitters below a few kHz, and small insects must produce ultrasound if they are to make use of air-borne sound for long-distance communication. Very small insects have particular problems in communicating with each other, because the very high sound frequencies available to them are not suitable for penetrating an environment dominated by plants. They therefore often choose another strategy: they produce low-frequency songs by means of the same mechanisms as larger insects (e.g. stridulation or tymbals), but transmit the songs as vibrational signals through their host plants. The range of communication is limited, of course, to the size of the plant, but communication over distances of 1–2 m is possible with use of much less energy than that necessary for communication by air-borne sounds (Michelsen, Fink, Gogala and Traue, 1982). The vibration (displacement) amplitudes in the plants are

Figure 1. Some insect ears are built in a very simple way. The ear of the noctuid moth is used for detecting the cries of hunting bats and consists of a tympanal membrane (TM) backed by a tracheal air space (TAS). Two receptor cells (A) attach to the tympanum. They differ with respect to threshold, but have similar frequency sensitivities. (Reprinted by permission of the publishers from *NERVE CELLS AND INSECT BEHAVIOR*, by K. D. Roeder, Cambridge, Mass.: Harvard University Press, Copyright (©) 1963, 1967 by the President and Fellows of Harvard College.)

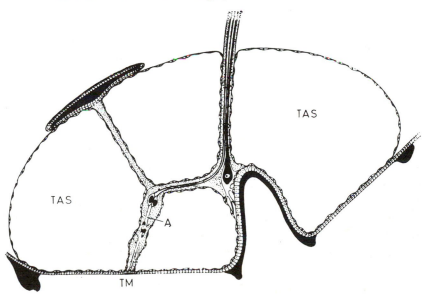

Figure 2. Bush crickets use their ears for detecting and analysing communication songs. (A) The ear (E) is in the front leg, just below the 'knee'. It receives sound both through a horn-shaped trachea (H), shown here in a section through the leg and thorax, and through slits in the leg cuticle. (B) A cross-section of the leg demonstrates the slits (S), the anterior and posterior tympana (AM and PM), the anterior and posterior tracheal branches (ATB and PTB) separated by a membrane (P), the receptor cells (SC) and spaces filled with blood (BC) and with muscle (MC). (C) Twenty-four receptor cells are arranged in a series along the wall of the anterior tracheal branch. The

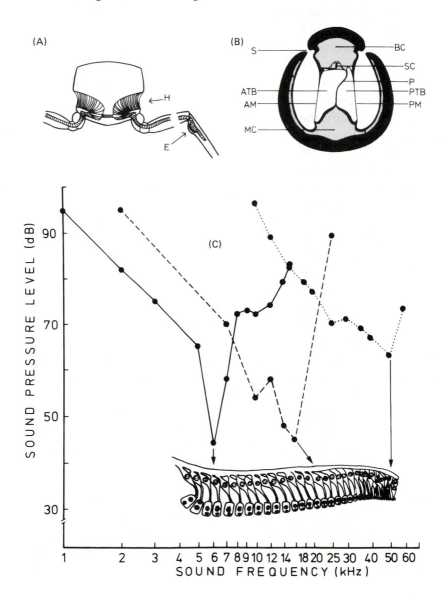

Caption for fig. 2 (*cont.*).
    cells have different frequency sensitivities and cover a frequency range
    of about one decade. The threshold curves of three cells are shown
    here. (From Michelsen and Larsen, 1978, and Zhantiev and
    Korsunovskaya, 1978.)

typically some hundred Ångströms, which is about two decades above
(100 times) the threshold of the vibration receptors (the subgenual
organs in the legs), but the plants cause considerable distortion of the
vibration signals (dispersion, reflections from the ends). Most of these
small insects appear to be deaf to air-borne sounds, but some respond to
both air- and substrate-borne signals. In recent years, it has been found
that larger insects (crickets, bush crickets) are much affected by
substrate-borne vibration also, which may considerably modify the
processing of auditory information in the CNS. Although biologists
normally try to treat the reception of air- and substrate-borne vibrations
as separate sensory modalities, the animals do not appear to do this.
Many biological sounds are so intense that they can cause the insects'
bodies or their substrate to vibrate with amplitudes well above the
thresholds of the vibration receptors. In such cases, it is not obvious,
which sense organs are the 'ears'.

    I mentioned that even large insects are forced to use sounds above
several kHz, if their sound emission is to be reasonably efficient. Muscle
contractions are too slow for driving the sound emitter directly, so the
animals have to use a frequency-multiplying device for transforming the
slow muscle contractions into high-frequency vibration (e.g. a stridulatory organ or a click generator). During stridulation, a so-called scraper
on one part of the body hits a series of cuticular teeth on another part of
the body. Each tooth impact gives rise to an impulse vibration. The
impulse vibrations may be used for driving a lightly-damped sound
emitter, which then radiates a pure tone signal. Alternatively, the sound
radiator may have so much mechanical damping that the impulses are
emitted without much distortion (Figure 3). The physics of these
processes is complicated and beyond the scope of this contribution, but
we may note that rather different kinds of ears are needed for analysing
the information carried by these very different kinds of sound. In the
first case, the animals emit fairly pure tones, which are normally also
rhythmical. Note that the resonating structures used by insects like
crickets for making these pure tones are solid structures which cannot be
much altered by action of the animal. In contrast to birds, for example,
the pure-tone singers among the insects cannot vary the frequency.
These insects therefore do not have any freedom in varying the

frequency parameter in their sound signals, but they have the advantage that a lightly damped resonator can generate vibration of very large amplitudes, so they can make very intense songs.

In the second case mentioned, the insects emit sound impulses corresponding to the impulse-like vibrations produced in frequency multipliers (Figure 3). Such impulses generally cover a broad frequency range, and for many years these songs were considered equivalent to amplitude-modulated noise. The behavioral information was thought to be carried by the pattern of amplitude modulation. It has been obvious for many years that the ears can easily signal the information about the slow rhythmicity in the songs to the CNS. Behavioral investigations in pure-tone singers like crickets have also shown that the coding of information is mainly in this rhythmicity. This is hardly surprising, but – of course – nice to know. In 1974, however, a very detailed analysis of the song patterns and stridulatory movements of gomphocerine short-horned grasshoppers demonstrated that the animals do not try to make the amplitude pattern as clear as possible (Elsner, 1974). In contrast, the fine patterns made by each of the animal's two 'instru-

Figure 3. The structure of the song of a gomphocerine short-horned grasshopper (*Chorthippus biguttulus*) and the terminology proposed by Elsner (1974). The time mark (↔): 15 s (sequence of 2nd order); 2.9 s (sequence of 1st order); 72.5 ms (chirp); 9.1 ms (syllable); 0.9 ms (impulse). (From Elsner, 1974.)

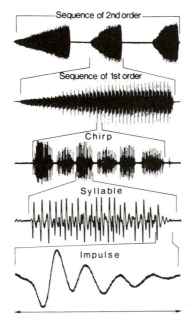

ments' (hindlegs and wings) are produced somewhat out of phase, so that the summated output is blurred. The resulting camouflage of the chirp and syllable pattern is not caused by sloppy coordination of the legs, since the phase shift between the legs is timed with precision of a millisecond. One may therefore speculate that the behavioral information could be carried also by another parameter: frequency. Detailed analysis of the song showed that the time interval between the impulses varies in a systematic way during a chirp (Figure 4). Furthermore, the maximum impulse rate is higher in normal animals (with two 'instruments') than in one-legged animals (compare b and c in Figure 4).

Although the spectrum of a single impulse of sound covers a broad frequency range, a series of such pulses may give rise to a line spectrum if the impulses are regularly spaced (Figure 5). In such a line spectrum, the fundamental frequency component is determined by the time interval between the impulses, and the other lines are harmonics of the fundamental one. During its stridulation, the insect changes the intervals between the impulses and thus changes the position of the maxima in the frequency spectrum. Such modulations of the impulse rate and of the positions of the fundamental and harmonic components of the spectrum have now been observed in the songs of several insects (Figure 6). The animals also vary the amplitude of the impulses in a

Figure 4. (a) Sequential histogram of impulse intervals in the courtship song of the short-horned grasshopper *Omocestus viridulus*. (b) and (c) The last part of the downstroke syllable in a normal animal (b) and in an animal with only one hindleg (c). (From Elsner, 1974.)

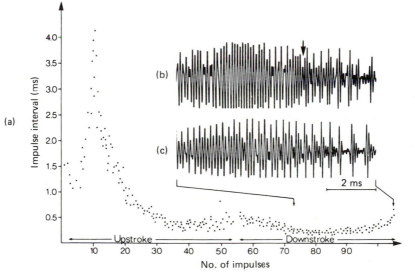

systematic way. But the problem is, whether they can detect the rapid variation in the amplitude of the impulses during the chirps. And are they also able to detect the even more rapid frequency modulations caused by changes in the time intervals between the individual impulses? We still do not know the answers, but we have made good progress in recent years in trying to find out.

In dealing with this complicated problem, we may divide it into some sub-problems. First, we may consider the analysing capacity of the ear. What we would like to know is not only that receptor cells can signal the intensity of a stimulus and slow changes in the intensity, but whether the cells are able to do this so fast that the fine details of the songs can be recorded by the receptor cells and signalled to the CNS. The same is true for the frequency-analysing capacity of the ear. Is it accurate enough and fast enough? In the CNS we would like to know whether the neuronal machinery is capable of handling the information, and whether the animals' brains are at all interested, i.e. whether the insects do in

Figure 5. The spectra of a single impulse (A, cf. Figure 3) and of a series of impulses. (B) Single-impulse sounds have their energy rather evenly distributed over a broad frequency range (components above 40 kHz have been removed by filtering). (C), (D) A series of regularly-spaced impulses has the energy concentrated in a few spectral lines. Note the difference between (C) (10 000 impulses s^{-1}) and (D) (2500 impulses s^{-1}). (Redrawn from Skovmand and Pedersen, 1978.)

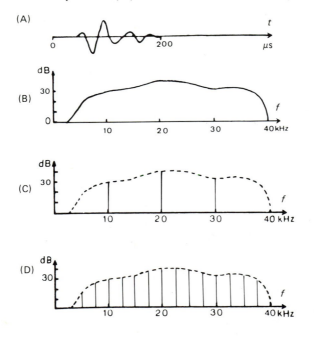

fact use these fine details in the songs for transmitting behavioral information.

One may attack such a complicated problem from various angles, but we have preferred to start with some behavioral work in order to learn whether these rapidly-changing sound parameters are used by the animals. This can be done nowadays with the help of digital computers, provided that one knows an expert in programming and signal analysis who can be persuaded to use his skills on such problems. We are so lucky to have such a colleague at the Technical University in Copenhagen. The procedure then is as follows. An impulse sound is recorded from a singing grasshopper and fed into the computer. It can now be repeated with the amplitudes and time intervals chosen by the programmer. In this way, one may produce a large number of artificial songs, which can then be tested on receptive animals in behavioral experiments. Short-horned grasshoppers are – like men – not very precise in their demands for sexual signals to be similar to the 'real thing'. They may respond to almost any kind of sound, if they have been isolated for some time and are in the right sexual mood. But if given the choice, they can be very selective, responding to much lower sound

Figure 6. Sonagraph of impulses and a long call from the leafhopper *Euscelis lineolatus*. This animal is about half a centimeter long and cannot emit air-borne sound with reasonable efficiency. Instead, it sends its signals as bending waves through the host plant. The signals shown here were recorded with a laser vibrometer about 23 cm from the singing animal, which was singing on a bean plant. Note the frequency modulation of the long call, in which the fundamental frequency component (about 300 Hz) is very weak. (From Michelsen et al., 1982.)

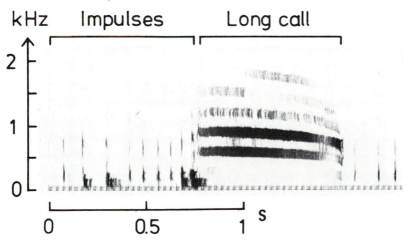

levels, when the artificial songs are getting closer to the natural song. From ethology it is even known that some artificial signals may be 'super-optimal', i.e. more efficient in releasing the behavior than the natural signal. So far, we have not seen this, but some of our artificial songs are now so good that the animals do not appear to distinguish them from the natural songs.

These experiments are done with the short-horned grasshopper *Omocestus viridulus*. The behavior of this species has been studied in considerable detail (Elsner, 1974). The song consists of a long series of identical chirps (cf. Figure 3). Each chirp is composed of two syllables, corresponding to one up and one down movement of the hind legs which are rubbing against the wings. Each wing carries a scraper and each leg a stridulatory file. The velocity of the leg movements varies markedly during each chirp, and – as already explained – this is equivalent to a frequency modulation of both the basic and harmonic frequency components. The basic frequency component, corresponding to the time interval between the tooth impacts, varies from about 250 Hz to 8 kHz.

The ears of locusts and short-horned grasshoppers contain four groups of receptor cells with different frequency sensitivities (Michelsen, 1971; Römer, 1976). As shown in Figure 7, three of the cell groups (named a–c) have their best frequencies between two and eight kiloHertz, whereas the fourth group (named d) is mainly sensitive to

Figure 7. The ear of short-horned grasshoppers and locusts contains four groups of receptor cells (called a, b, c, and d) with different frequency sensitivities. The figure shows the threshold curves of receptor cells in an isolated ear preparation (Michelsen, 1971). According to Römer (1976) the intact ear has rather similar frequency-analysing properties.

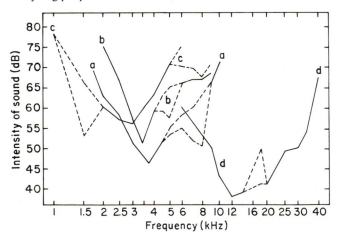

sounds above 10 kHz. The individual impulse (caused by a single tooth impact) has its main energy between 4 and 40 kHz (Figure 5), so it can be detected by all the receptor cells. A series of impulses with the range of time intervals found in *Omocestus* will always stimulate the high-frequency sensitive d-cells, but the impact on the other receptor cells will depend upon the position of the spectral maxima, i.e. upon the actual time intervals. During most of the chirp the time intervals are rather large, and the spectrum has a large number of maxima, so here a number of spectral maxima are always present within the frequency range covered by each of the groups of receptor cells. This is not so, however, at the end of the downwards movement of the leg, where the tooth impacts (and sound impulses) occur with very short intervals and with maximum amplitude. In this part of the song the basic frequency component varies from two to eight kiloHertz within a few milliseconds.

What does this mean in terms of stimulation of the receptor cells? Let us consider a group of cells tuned to four kiloHertz. These cells will be maximally stimulated when the tooth impact frequency is around two kiloHertz (by the first harmonic component of the spectrum) and again around four kiloHertz, but they will receive much less energy at other tooth impact frequencies. The three groups of receptor cells sensitive to sounds below 10 kHz will all be activated during the fast-frequency sweep, but not always simultaneously.

Do the animals in fact care about these, rather speculative details in the song? Yes, they do. Some years ago, when the first computer-generated songs were tested in behavioral experiments, it was shown that the animals seemed to prefer songs with a pattern of impulse-rate variation as close to the natural song as possible (Skovmand and Pedersen, 1978). Last summer, one of my students continued this work and found that attractive songs do not necessarily have to be very similar to the natural ones, but they have to cause a stimulation of the receptor cells which is very close to that caused by the natural song. The preliminary analysis of the data (Johansen, 1982) shows that the critical parameter is the timing of the stimulation of the individual groups of receptor cells in the ear during the fast-frequency sweep. Attractive songs appear to activate the different groups almost simultaneously (within a time interval of about one millisecond), whereas less-attractive songs tend to have a larger scatter in the time pattern.

There are several loose ends in this story, and the experiments are being continued this summer with a new series of artificial songs. There is no doubt that some songs are more attractive than others, but interpretation of the results in terms of the processing of sensory information in the ears and in the CNS is certainly not easy, because we are vastly ignorant about several basic features of the sensory processing. Space does not allow me to go into details, but I shall mention the most important problem briefly.

We have good reasons to assume that the receptor cells are responding to the amount of (vibrational) energy reaching them through the mechanical frequency filter, which is composed of the tympanum and its complicated system of cuticular bodies (to which the cells attach). We know that the mechanical parts of the ears are responding rather fast (Figure 8), and that the 'time constant' of this mechanical system is much smaller than that (those?) of the receptor cells (Schiolten, Larsen and Michelsen, 1981). We have not the slightest idea, however, what the time resolution is in the receptor cells or in the central neurons. We also do not know how the time resolution in the auditory pathway is improved by the redundancy in the signalling from a group of receptor cells. In other words: how much is the time resolution improved, when there are 10 receptor cells and not just one?

Figure 8. The time resolution in the tympanum of noctuid moths (cf. Figure 1) is investigated by observing the vibrational response (measured with laser vibrometry) to a pair of 16-μs acoustic impulses with impulse intervals (Δt) varying from 400 μs (in A) to 50 μs (in F). (From Schiolten et al., 1981.)

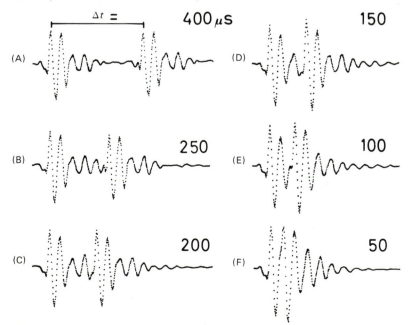

Simultaneously with the behavioral work mentioned, we have begun a biophysical and physiological study of the time resolution in some very simple ears in noctuid moths, where just one or two receptor cells attach to a tympanal membrane. These ears are so simple that one can reasonably hope to be able to control all the relevant parameters. The main problem in studies of time resolution is that time and frequency are intimately connected. A change in the time pattern of stimulation is also a change in the spectrum of the stimulus and thus a change in the amount of energy reaching the receptor cell through the mechanical frequency filter in front of the cell. We use patterns of very short (about 15 μs) acoustic impulses as stimuli and measure the vibrations in the ears with laser vibrometry. A Fast-Fourier-Transform analysis of the acoustic stimulus and of the vibrations activating the receptor cells is used for computing the changes of energy flow associated with the change in time pattern in the stimulus. I probably do not have to mention that numerous practical and theoretical problems have to be solved in order to perform the experiments in such a way that one can be quite sure of studying the time resolution and not changes in energy flow. But at least we now have a number of solved problems behind us, so we are beginning to feel optimistic about the prospects for improving our understanding of auditory processing sufficiently to answer some of the questions raised by the behavioral studies.

References

Busnel, R. G. (1963). *Acoustic Behaviour of Animals.* Amsterdam: Elsevier.

Elsner, N. (1974). Neuroethology of sound production in gomphocerine grasshoppers (Orthoptera: Acrididae). I. Song patterns and stridulatory movements. *J. Comp. Physiol. 88:* 67–102.

Elsner, N., and Popov, A. V. (1978). Neuroethology of acoustic communication. *Adv. Insect Physiol. 13:* 229–355.

Johansen, M. (1982). *Undersøgelse af signalbærende parametre ved den akustiske kommunikation hos markgræshoppen.* Ms-thesis. Odense University. 185 pp.

Michelsen, A. (1971). The physiology of the locust ear. *Z. vergl. Physiol. 71:* 49–128.

Michelsen, A. (1974). Hearing in invertebrates. In *Handbook of Sensory Physiology,* vol. V/1, pp. 389–422. Berlin: Springer.

Michelsen, A., and Larsen, O. N. (1978). Biophysics of the ensiferan ear. I. Tympanal vibrations in bushcrickets (Tettigoniidae) studied with laser vibrometry. *J. Comp. Physiol. 123:* 193–203.

Michelsen, A., and Larsen, O. N. (1982). Hearing and sound. In *Comprehensive Insect Physiology, Biochemistry and Pharmacology,* ed. G. A. Kerkut and L. I. Gilbert. Oxford: Pergamon (in press).

Michelsen, A., Fink, F., Gogala, M., and Traue, D. (1982). Plants as transmission channels for insect vibrational songs. *Behav. Ecol. Sociobiol. 11:* 269–81.

Michelsen, A., and Nocke, H. (1974). Biophysical aspects of sound communication in insects. *Adv. Insect Physiol. 10:* 247–96.

Roeder, K. D. (1967). *Nerve Cells and Insect Behavior.* Harvard University Press.

Römer, H. (1976). Die Informationsverarbeitung tympanaler Rezeptorelemente von *Locusta migratoria* (Acrididae, Orthoptera). *J. Comp. Physiol. 109:* 101–22.

Schiolten, P., Larsen, O. N., and Michelsen, A. (1981). Mechanical time resolution in some insect ears. I. Impulse responses and time constants. *J. Comp. Physiol. 143:* 289–95.

Skovmand, O., and Pedersen, S. B. (1978). Tooth impact rate in the song of a shorthorned grasshopper: a parameter carrying specific behavioral information. *J. Comp. Physiol. 124:* 27–36.

Zhantiev, R. D. (1981). *Bioacoustics of Insects.* Moscow University Press, 256 pp. (in Russian).

Zhantiev, R. D., and Korsunovskaya, O. S. (1978). Morphological organization of tympanal organs in *Tettigonia cantans* (Orthoptera, Tettigoniidae). *Zool. J. 57:* 1012–16 (in Russian).

1.3

Auditory function at the receptor level in reptiles

J. J. ART

In the auditory system of reptiles, the general features of afferent response are similar to those found in other terrestrial vertebrates. In the absence of any central control, each primary afferent is maximally sensitive to a narrow range of frequencies (Weiss, Mulroy, Turner and Pike, 1976; Manley, 1977; Klinke and Pause, 1980; Crawford and Fettiplace, 1980a), and any complex acoustic stimulus is transmitted to the CNS via a number of parallel channels. Recently, by recording intracellularly from hair cells in a number of species (Weiss, Mulroy and Altmann, 1974; Russell and Sellick, 1977; Hudspeth and Corey, 1977; Fettiplace and Crawford, 1978), it has been possible to begin to address at the receptor level the mechanisms by which mechanical vibrations of the tympanic membrane are transduced into electrical activity of the afferent fibres, and which features of the inner ear determine the frequency selectivity, or tuning, of afferent response.

In reptiles data are currently available from two species, an *in vivo* preparation of the alligator lizard, *Gerrhonotus multicarinatus* (Weiss et al., 1974), and an *in vitro* preparation of the turtle, *Pseudemys scripta elegans* (Fettiplace and Crawford, 1978). There are a number of advantages of these reptilian preparations over those of other vertebrates. Both preparations are extremely robust, and stable recordings can be made from a single hair cell for a number of hours. The basilar papilla, the homologue of the organ of Corti, is accessible over its entire length, making possible the examination of hair cells tuned to any frequency to which the animal is sensitive. Finally, given the limited high-frequency response in reptiles, the hair cell potentials can be faithfully reproduced using present recording techniques. These recordings are typically made with glass microelectrodes filled with either strong salt solutions or fluorescent dyes. The dyes permit the response patterns of various cell types within the papilla to be identified.

To date, the mechanisms involved in transduction and frequency selectivity have been examined by characterizing hair cell responses to acoustic stimulation, to the injection of extrinsic currents and to efferent stimulation. These data, in conjunction with measurements of the mechanical properties of the basilar membrane, have led to three conclusions. First, though the adequate stimulus of transduction is not yet known, the subsequent electrical events are consistent with the hypothesis that mechanical stimulation causes a conductance change in the hair cell membrane, and thereby modulates the hair cell voltage. Second, in both the turtle and the alligator lizard at least some of the mechanisms which confer frequency selectivity on auditory nerve fibres are local to the hair cells. Third, the hair cell tuning in turtles is not a static property, and can be modified under efferent control.

Papilla morphology

Within the class of reptiles, a remarkably diverse range of inner ear structures has evolved. Since recent reviews systematically address the variations in receptor morphology and afferent physiology of a number of reptilian families (Baird, 1970; Wever, 1978; Miller, 1980; Turner, 1980; Manley, 1981), we will concentrate on the two species for which intracellular data exists. Figure 1 shows transverse sections of the basilar papilla in the freshwater turtle and the alligator lizard. In the more primitive turtle (Figure 1A), the short papilla is supported on a thin and flexible basilar membrane which is approximately 700 μm long. The sensory epithelium consists of a single class of hair cells innervated by afferent and efferent fibres, and surmounted by a tectorial membrane (Mulroy, 1968; Miller, 1978). On the apical surface of each hair cell are 75–90 stereocilia, and a single eccentrically placed kinocilium, which defines the orientation of the cell. In the turtle the hair cells are all oriented with the kinocilium nearest the abneural side of the papilla. In the more derived alligator lizard (Figure 1B), the extremely short papilla (<400 μm) is supported on a somewhat thickened basilar bar (Mulroy, 1974). The epithelium can be divided grossly into two regions. In the apical, or tectorial, region there is an overlying tectorial membrane, and the abneurally oriented hair cells synapse with both afferent and efferent fibres. In the basal, or free-standing region, however, there are two oppositely oriented sets of hair cells, no tectorial membrane, and an absence of efferent innervation.

In addition to the gross differences between papillae as outlined above, there are systematic variations in morphological parameters along the length of reptilian papillae. These include variations in gross structures such as the width of the basilar papilla or tectorial membrane (Miller, 1980), as well as regional variations in receptor size and stereocilia length (Mulroy, 1974; Wever, 1978; Turner, Muraski and

Figure 1. Transverse sections through the basilar papilla of (A) the fresh-water turtle, *Pseudemys scripta elegans*, and (B) the free-standing and tectorial regions in the alligator lizard, *Gerrhonotus multicarinatus*. 20-μm scale bar applies to both parts of the figure. BM, basilar membrane; HC, hair cell; HP, habenula perforata; N, cochlear nerve; p, papillary bar thickness; SC, supporting cell; TM, tectorial membrane. (B modified from Mulroy, 1974.)

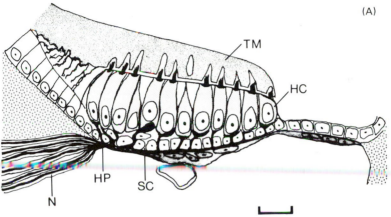

(A)

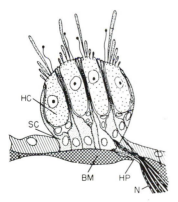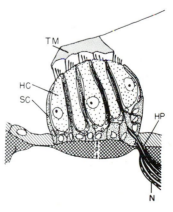

(B)

Nielsen, 1981). Such variation is of interest since in the mammalian cochlea a component of frequency selectivity and the tonotopic organization is thought to be imparted by gradients in the mechanical properties along the length of the cochlear partition (von Békésy, 1960). The unusual organization and afferent response properties of the granite spiny lizard (Turner et al., 1981) shown in Figure 2 serve to highlight the notion that the frequency selectivity and the tonotopic organization of the reptilian cochlea may result from more than systematic changes in the stiffness of the basilar membrane. In mammals the frequency map of afferent fibres is directly correlated with the distance along the cochlear partition. Afferents sensitive to the highest frequencies innervate the cochlea near the stapes in the basal portion, and those with low-frequency response innervate the apex. In this lizard, however, there are at least two tonotopic maps of frequency *v.* position oriented such that high-frequency fibres are found at either end of the papilla, with a low-frequency region in the centre (Figure 2C). In addition, instead of the usual monotonic progression in hair cell morphology along its length, the papilla has three distinct populations; the middle population has a tectorial membrane and the shortest stereocilia (Figure 2A). It is the inverse correlation between the cilia length and the characteristic frequency (CF) of afferent recordings in the two high-frequency regions, which supports the hypothesis that frequency selectivity may have more to do with cilia length and the presence or absence of tectorial structures, than with hair cell position on an anatomically graded basilar membrane.

Mechanoelectrical transduction

Transduction of the vibrations of the basilar membrane into potential changes developed across the hair cell membrane, the receptor potential, can be regarded as occurring in two stages: a stage where the vibrations of the cochlear partition are translated into movements of the stereocilia (the micromechanics), followed by a mechanoelectrical transduction of these movements into the receptor potential.

Micromechanics

The diversity of papilla morphologies in reptiles suggests that a variety of micromechanical sequences of transduction may exist. These processes appear to be least complicated in the tectorial free region of the lizard papilla, where ciliary movement would presumably be brought about by fluid coupling with the endolymph. The degree of coupling would necessarily be determined by ciliary bundle length, and,

Figure 2. Relation between cilium length and tonotopic map of afferent characteristic frequency in the granite spiny lizard. (A) Cilium length as a percentage of longest cilium (23 μm), versus position along papilla in a representative individual. (B) Schematic top view of papilla showing three hair cell populations. Arrows indicate orientation of hair cells in each region. (C) Tonotopic map of auditory nerve CF versus normalized position. Data pooled from eight animals. Inverse correlation between CF and cilium length can be seen for both free-standing regions, but no clear relation is evident in the tectorial region. (From Turner et al., 1981.)

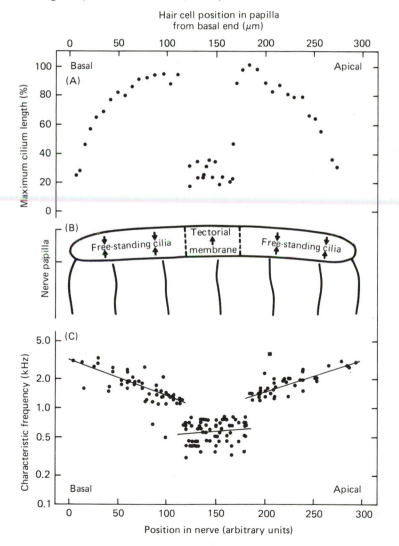

as we will consider later, it has been proposed that the micromechanics of the bundles could confer some degree of tuning on the hair cell responses (Weiss, Peake, Ling and Holton, 1978b).

In papillae which possess an overlying tectorial membrane the situation is even more complex. Traditionally (ter Kuile, 1900) it has been imagined that the tectorial membrane and the reticular lamina undergo a shear during vibration of the basilar membrane and that the ciliary movement is a consequence of this. In turtles the tectorial membrane appears to be attached to the apical surface of the supporting cells which surround each hair cell via a less-dense tectorial material (Baird, 1974), and consequently the ciliary bundles extend up into fluid-filled pockets. These bundles may also have a direct mechanical linkage to the tectorial membrane via the kinocilia (Miller, 1978), though the very tight direct coupling to each stereocilium typical of mammalian outer hair cells (Lim, 1972) has not been reported.

The only information we have on the micromechanical behaviour of a reptile papilla covered by a tectorial membrane is rather indirect, and comes from experiments in which the cochlear partition is displaced by a rigid probe (Crawford and Fettiplace, 1980b). For afferent fibres, sinusoidal vibrations of the basilar membrane as small as 1 Å at the CF can produce a vigorous discharge. At lower frequencies, however, the response decreases in a manner suggestive of apparent high-pass filtering between the basilar membrane motion and the afferent response. These observations might be accommodated either by proposing that transduction in turtle hair cells adapts as has been demonstrated in the frog saccule (Eatock, Corey and Hudspeth, 1979), or that in spite of the morphological evidence to the contrary, the coupling of the cilia to the tectorial membrane is primarily viscous.

Mechanoelectrical transduction

Reptilian hair cells have substantial negative resting potentials: −45 to −55 mV in turtle (Crawford and Fettiplace, 1980a) and −57 to −103 mV in the alligator lizard (Weiss, Altmann and Mulroy, 1978a). These measurements are made relative to the perilymph. The potential between endolymph and perilymph has been measured in a number of species (Schmidt and Fernández, 1962; Weiss et al., 1978a; Crawford and Fettiplace, 1980a), and the reported values between zero and 20 mV are considerably lower than those of mammals (Schmidt, 1963). In spite of these modest values the composition of the cochlear fluids seems very similar to those in mammals; the endolymph is rich in potassium and low in sodium ions, and the perilymph is rather similar to plasma with respect to alkali metal cations (Johnstone, Schmidt and Johnstone, 1963; Bosher and Warren, 1968; Peterson et al., 1978). It is not known whether the endolymph has the very low calcium concentration recently reported to exist in mammals (Bosher and Warren, 1978).

Our ideas about transduction in the cochlea have been largely guided by a model proposed by Davis (1958) in which he suggested that deflection of the ciliary bundles causes a conductance change in the apical membrane of the hair cell which gates the flow of the transducer current down the electrochemical gradients existing between the endo-lymph and the cell interior. Until the introduction of intracellular recording from hair cells it proved very difficult to gain any direct evidence for or against such a model.

Turtle hair cells respond to pure tones by producing a receptor potential that hyperpolarizes and depolarizes the cell on successive half cycles of the sound, and which may be up to 45 mV in peak-to-peak amplitude (Crawford and Fettiplace, 1980a). The results of one experiment which would be predicted from the Davis model are shown in Figure 3. The model suggests that the receptor potential should be suppressed completely if the hair cell is depolarized with extrinsic current to a potential that exactly balances the electromotive forces causing transducer current to flow. At more depolarized levels than this the current should flow again, but its direction will be reversed at any phase of the stimulus with respect to normal. This reversal phenomenon does indeed happen (Crawford and Fettiplace, 1979) when the interior of the cell is at zero or slightly positive with respect to the perilymph.

The identity of the ionic species that carry the transducer current in cochlear hair cells is unknown, although the reversal-potential measurements are consistent with potassium as the principal charge carrier, providing one makes the assumption that the intracellular potassium activity is close to that of endolymph. Similar conclusions have also been reached about the flow of current in the frog sacculus by Corey and Hudspeth (1979), though their results would suggest that the channels are not particularly selective for potassium over other monovalent cations.

Actual measurement of the transducer-conductance changes occurring during sound stimulation in hair cells is complicated by the presence in the cell membrane of other voltage and time-dependent conductances. The actions of these conductances can be circumvented by voltage-clamping of single hair cells and directly measuring the transducer current, as has been performed recently by Corey and Hudspeth (1979) in the frog saccule. No comparable measurements exist for any cochlear hair cell. However, it has been found that if turtle hair cells are treated on the perilymphatic surface with substances that are known to block voltage-sensitive potassium channels in nerve and muscle such as tetraethylammonium (TEA) (Armstrong and Binstock, 1965), or 4-aminopyridine (4-AP) (Meves and Pichon, 1977), the hair cell membrane shows little voltage-dependent behaviour and estimates of the

Figure 3. Reversal of average hair cell responses to tone bursts in turtle by steady current injection. Sound monitor is shown above the voltage records, and strength of injected current is given at the right of each trace. Frequency of stimulation was 77 Hz at 122 dB SPL re 20 μPa, and each trace is the average response of 32 presentations. The ordinate is the hair cell voltage, and the responses to current injection with and without sound stimulation are superimposed at each current intensity. Injection of 43 nA is sufficient to reverse the receptor potential at a mean membrane potential of +6 mV. The perilymph contained 14 mM TEA and 5 mM 4-aminopyridine. The CF of the cell was approximately 100 Hz. (From Crawford and Fettiplace, 1981b.)

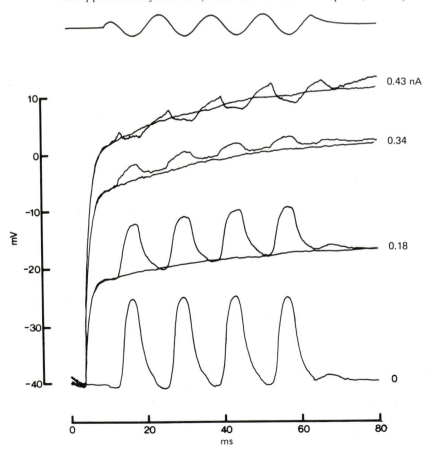

transducer current have been obtained (Crawford and Fettiplace, 1981b). This method carries the uncertainty that the pharmacological agents might also have interfered with the transducer channel. The maximum increase in conductance of the hair cell on its depolarizing phase of the receptor potential is about 5×10^{-9} mho and the maximum decrease on the hyperpolarizing phase is about one-fifth of this, giving a total conductance modulation of around 6×10^{-9} mho. These values are comparable to those obtained from the frog saccule (Corey and Hudspeth, 1979).

Saturation and rectification

At all frequencies examined the receptor potentials increase monotonically with the sound pressure of a tone, yet at intensities above 80 dB SPL (re $20 \, \mu$Pa) in the alligator lizard (Holton, 1981), and above 90 dB SPL in the turtle (Crawford and Fettiplace, 1980a) the receptor potential is effectively constant or saturated. This compressive non-linearity is seen in the mean value of the receptor potential (Holton, 1981), in the fundamental periodic component (Crawford and Fetti-place, 1980a; Holton, 1981) and in the higher harmonic components (Holton, 1981). Both hyperpolarizing and depolarizing phases of the receptor potential saturate at high sound-pressure levels (Crawford and Fettiplace, 1981b), but the magnitude of the saturated levels is asymmetric; the hyperpolarized level may be as little as one-tenth of that of the depolarized level.

The origins of this asymmetrical saturation appear complex. One factor which may contribute is the variation in driving force (the difference in potential between the reversal potential and the instantaneous membrane potential) at different phases of the receptor potential. In turtle hair cells where the responses close to the CF can be large, this factor substantially compresses the depolarizing phases of the receptor potential relative to the underlying conductance change (Crawford and Fettiplace, 1981b). Resistance changes in the non-transducer membrane may also contribute: hair cell current–voltage relationships show a decreasing resistance with depolarization and hence inward transducer currents develop proportionately smaller increments in the receptor potential with depolarization (Crawford and Fettiplace, 1981b). Moreover, the transducer conductance itself may be a non-linear function of ciliary displacements as is the case in the frog saccule (Hudspeth and Corey, 1977).

Though the micromechanical events which translate the basilar membrane vibration into ciliary motion could also contribute, it seems unlikely at least in the alligator lizard, that the receptor potential saturation is significantly affected by vibration of the basilar membrane. Mossbauer measurements of basilar membrane velocity (Peake and Ling, 1980) in the alligator lizard do not show saturated vibration amplitudes for sound intensities up to 80 dB SPL, and at higher sound pressures such non-linearities as exist are quite modest. These observations are, however, rather different from those made in mammals (Rhode, 1971; Rhode and Robles, 1974) where vibrational nonlinearities might be expected to influence the receptor potential of inner hair cells.

Tuning in the turtle cochlea

The response of a turtle hair cell to a low-intensity pure tone is shown in Figure 4A. The steady-state receptor potential is sinusoidal, and its amplitude is proportional to the sound pressure. At a given intensity, the largest response is obtained at a frequency that is characteristic for each cell. In turtles the papilla is tonotopically organized, and in juveniles of this species there is an e-fold change in CF along the papilla every 134 μm. The lowest CFs (about 50 Hz) are at the apical, or lagenar, end of the papilla, and the highest CFs (near 700 Hz) at the basal end.

The frequency selectivity of the receptor potential for this hair cell is shown in Figure 4C. Since turtle hair cells do not adapt in response to a sustained low-intensity tone, their frequency response can be characterized by continuous iso-intensity frequency sweeps. A maximum response of about 2 mV was obtained at 274 Hz, which defines the CF. A convenient index of the sharpness of tuning is the quality factor, or Q_{3dB}. This dimensionless variable is the ratio of the CF to the bandwidth of the curve at the points where the power of the response has fallen to

Figure 4. Response of a turtle hair cell to acoustic stimulation, or the injection of extrinsic currents. (A) Average receptor potential of the hair cell to tone bursts at 276 Hz, 55 dB SPL re 20 μPa (sound monitor is shown in the upper trace). (B) Average response to injection of depolarizing and hyperpolarizing current steps of 24 pA through the recording electrode. (C) Peak-to-peak amplitude of the sinusoidal response of the cell to a continuous tone during an iso-intensity frequency sweep at 51 dB SPL $\pm$ 1.5 dB re 20 μPa. Circles give the response of a tuned parallel resonator from eq. (20) (Crawford and Fettiplace, 1980a) using values of 274 Hz for the resonant frequency and 8.4 for the Q_{3dB}. Resting potential for the cell was -54 mV and the maximum peak response was 35 mV. (A and B from Fettiplace and Crawford, 1980; C from Crawford and Fettiplace, 1980a.)

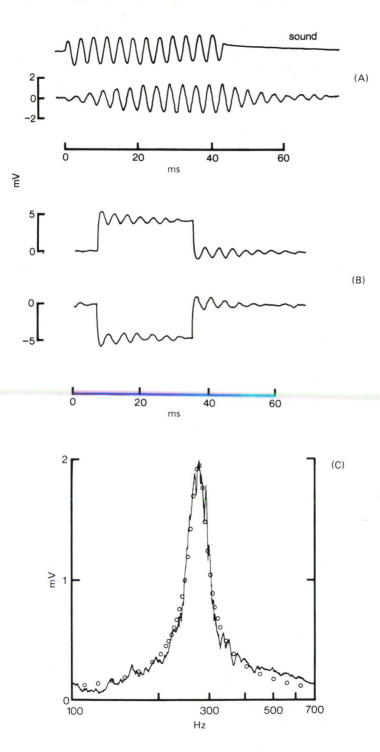

half the maximum value. Thus the higher the Q value, the sharper the tuning of the cell. The Q_{3dB} calculated in this way for the cell is 8.4.

The notion that the receptor potential is a linear function of the sound pressure for low-level stimulation is supported by the agreement of the tuning curve characteristics obtained by an iso-intensity frequency sweep, with the CF and Q_{3dB} values predicted from the transient response at the beginning and end of the abruptly gated tone burst shown in Figure 4A. The exponential growth and decay of the receptor potential at the onset and offset of the tone are similar to the behaviour one would expect from a simple tuned resonator stimulated at its frequency of free oscillation. When tone bursts at frequencies other than the CF are used, the transient at the beginning is more complex than that shown. However, regardless of the frequency of stimulation, the transient at the end is always at the CF of the cell. The time constant of decay of the oscillations after the burst can also be used to calculate the Q_{3dB} of an equivalent resonator. For the response shown in Figure 4A, the CF of the cell was 271 Hz and its Q_{3dB} was 9.6, values in close agreement with those derived from the iso-intensity sweep.

To explore further what mechanisms might impart frequency selectivity to the hair cell response, extrinsic currents can be injected through the recording electrode. The response of this same cell to small depolarizing and hyperpolarizing currents is shown in Figure 4B. Superimposed on the steady levels are a series of damped oscillations at both the onset and offset of the current step. These oscillations are quite unlike the behaviour one would expect from the passive properties of a cell membrane consisting only of resistance and capacitance. This behaviour is again reminiscent of a parallel resonant filter, and it implies that some property which is invoked by current injection has the behaviour of an inductor. From the frequency and rate of decay of the electrically induced oscillations, it is again possible to compute for this cell an electrical CF of 263 Hz and an electrical Q_{3dB} of 11.00.

Figure 5 shows the correlation between the frequency of oscillation during small extrinsic current steps, and the acoustic CF of the cells. The similarity between the electrical and acoustic response properties of these cells suggests an intriguing hypothesis about hair cell tuning. If the transducer current flowing during acoustic stimulation were subjected to the same filtering processes as are extrinsic currents, then the major features of frequency selectivity might be explained by the electrical properties of the hair cell. To explain the entire linear tuning curve it would be necessary to postulate that a rather broad filtering mechanism precedes the transducer current flow (Crawford and Fettiplace, 1981a).

The low-pass portion of the required filter would be consistent with what is known about the middle-ear mechanics in the turtle (Moffat and Capranica, 1978). The high-pass component, as suggested earlier, remains more problematical.

Tuning in the alligator lizard cochlea

Though suggestive, the hypothesis that major features of tuning can be addressed through the injection of extrinsic currents does not eliminate the possibility that basilar membrane motion might also reflect tuning. No direct evidence about the mechanical properties of the membrane is available from the turtle. Data from the alligator lizard support the view that in species with a short basilar membrane frequency, selectivity is unlikely to be imparted by differential motion of the membrane.

With recordings from primary afferents Weiss et al. (1976) demonstrated that, on the basis of CF, fibres could be divided into a low-frequency group with CFs from 200 Hz to 800 Hz innervating the tectorial region, and a high-frequency group with CFs between 900 Hz and 4 kHz innervating the free-standing region. Systematic mapping

Figure 5. A comparison in nine turtle hair cells of the frequency of voltage oscillation in response to extrinsic current injection plotted against the acoustic characteristic frequency. (From Fettiplace and Crawford, 1980.)

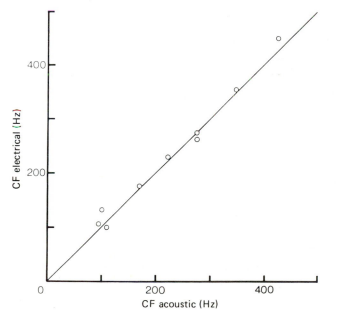

along the nerve parallel to the papilla showed that at least the free-standing region of the papilla was tonotopically organized with the lower-frequency fibres innervating it near the apical end, and the higher-frequency fibres innervating the basal end. In contrast, the measurements of basilar membrane vibration with Mössbauer techniques (Peake and Ling, 1980) shown in Figure 6 demonstrate that the iso-velocity response of the basilar membrane is broadly tuned with a best response centred at about 2 kHz. Comparison of three regions along the membrane reveals neither a tonotopic organization, nor even a simple dichotomy between the behaviours of the apical and basal extremes. This implies that there must be mechanisms subsequent to motion of the basilar membrane which impart the fibre tuning and tonotopic organization of the papilla. Again intracellular recordings

Figure 6. Iso-velocity tuning curves of basilar membrane motion from three alligator lizards. Position of each Mössbauer source on the basilar membrane is indicated in the sketch at the top. Each curve is the locus of points in sound pressure *v.* frequency which results in a specified velocity of the source. Velocity magnitudes for the curves are: 13, 0.5 mm s^{-1}; 14, 0.6 mm s^{-1}; 39, 0.8 mm s^{-1}. (From Peake and Ling, 1980.)

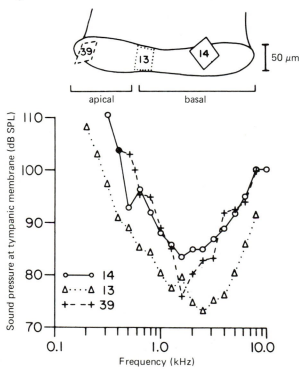

suggest that tuning is present in the receptor potential, and is a property local to each hair cell (Holton, 1981).

In the lizard the response is characterized not only by a periodic component at the stimulus frequency, but also by a steady depolarization of the cell. At a given frequency the amplitudes of both components increase as non-linear functions of the stimulus intensity. At a fixed intensity, the periodic component decreases relative to the maintained component at higher frequencies. Both components of the receptor potential demonstrate tuning, and the shape of the maintained component iso-response tuning curve most nearly resembles the afferent fibre tuning curves in this species (Holton, 1981). Except for a region immediately about the CF, a comparison of the maintained and periodic components in the lizard suggests that the periodic component is attenuated at 20 dB/decade relative to the maintained component for frequencies above 800 Hz (Holton, 1981). Though the electrical properties of the hair cell membrane were not examined directly, the responses to acoustic stimuli in the lizard are consistent with a model that the receptor potential is generated by a saturating non-linearity which is followed by a low-pass filter.

If the lizard hair cell membrane does behave as a low-pass filter, then this further implies that frequency selectivity is not only subsequent to the vibration of the basilar membrane, but also prior to the generation of the receptor potential. Thus tuning in the lizard would necessarily be different from the mechanism proposed for the turtle.

Discussion of tuning mechanisms

If a component of tuning in these two species is a local phenomenon specific to each hair cell, what mechanisms might be proposed to explain frequency selectivity? For convenience let us consider two possible mechanisms, one purely mechanical, and the other purely electrical. Though certainly not mutually exclusive, these two mechanisms are extremes of a possible spectrum in which varying amounts of mechanical and electrical interaction might be proposed.

Weiss et al. (1978b) have suggested that the tuning in the alligator lizard may be associated with the mechanical response of the stereocilia to the motion of the overlying fluid. In this scheme, frequency selectivity would be imparted by the micromechanics of ciliary motion. A given bundle of cilia would respond in a frequency-selective manner to apical fluid motion, and ciliary bundles of different lengths would be mechanically tuned to different characteristic frequencies. Such a proposition is morphologically plausible since in the tectorial free region of the papilla, hair cells at the low-frequency end have stereocilia as tall as 31 μm, while stereocilia at the high-frequency end are only 12 μm long (Mulroy, 1974).

On the other hand, Fettiplace and Crawford (1980) suggest that the filtering in turtle hair cells could take place subsequent to the transducer current as a consequence of the electrical properties of the cell membrane. A similar proposal has been made to explain the tuning mechanisms of electroreceptors in weakly electric fish (Hopkins, 1976). In electroreceptors the issue is somewhat clearer since no intermediate stage of mechanoelectric transduction takes place and presumably any frequency selectivity is due to the membrane properties of the receptor. Resonance phenomena similar to those seen in turtle hair cells have also been seen in other membrane systems. In the squid giant axon, for example, the subthreshold voltage oscillations are thought to be due to the kinetics of voltage-sensitive sodium and potassium channels (Hodgkin and Huxley, 1952; Mauro, Conti, Dodge and Schor, 1978). In turtle hair cells one possible explanation of the loss of frequency selectivity following application of TEA is that here, as in the nerve, the TEA blocked a voltage-sensitive potassium channel in the membrane that was associated with the resonant filter.

Efferent inhibition

Intracellular recordings, even with current injection, cannot by themselves distinguish whether the filtering is due solely to membrane properties of the cell, mechanical resonances, or in fact is a consequence of both. To explore further and isolate the components responsible, it will be necessary to change the mechanical and electrical properties of the cell and assess the effect on frequency selectivity.

One method of changing at least the electrical properties of the hair cell membrane would be via the direct efferent synaptic input to the basolateral cell surface. Figure 7 illustrates two components of a turtle hair cell response to efferent stimulation. In response to a train of eight electrical shocks to the efferent fibres, an inhibitory post-synaptic potential (IPSP) is produced in the cell (Figure 7A). The effect in this cell is prolonged, and the response to a single shock could last over 100 ms. Figure 7B shows the suppression of the receptor potential which accompanies the IPSP. When near-threshold tones at CF are used, a 15-fold reduction in the amplitude is seen on the peak of the IPSP. The reduction of the receptor potential when tones other than the CF are used is somewhat less.

This effect can be described as a desensitizing and a broadening of the frequency selective filter, and in turtle hair cells would be consistent with lowering of the quality of the resonant filter. Reversal experiments on the IPSP demonstrate that the synaptic event includes a conductance change to ions whose equilibrium potential is negative to the hair cell resting potential. If the tuning were determined at least in part by the membrane properties of the cell, then both the hyperpolarization and the increase in membrane conductance would be expected to decrease the frequency selectivity. The relative contributions of these two components remains to be determined.

Experiments such as these also suggest that not only is a component of the tuning of reptilian hair cells local, but in species with efferent innervation, it may be dynamically controlled as well. Clearly, in the presence of efferent activity, our usual notion that primary afferents are narrowly tuned would not necessarily be correct, and the precise degree of frequency selectivity would depend critically on the level of any

Figure 7. Effect of efferent stimulation on intracellularly recorded hair cell responses in the turtle. (A) Average of 172 responses to 8 efferent shocks, the timing of which are indicated by capacitive artifacts. (B) Average of 256 responses to tone bursts (465 Hz, 61 dB SPL re 20 μPa) plus 8 shocks with the same timing as for (A). Sound monitor is shown in the middle trace. The amplitude of the response was cut to one-fifteenth of its control size at the peak of the IPSP. For both traces the ordinate is the membrane potential relative to the resting potential (V_r) of -58 mV. (Art, Crawford, Fettiplace and Fuchs, unpublished observations.)

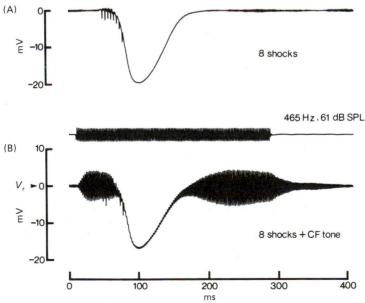

on-going efferent activity. A natural consequence of damping a highly-resonant hair cell filter would be to speed up the transient response of the cell as well. Thus efferents in the turtle cochlea appear to be able to modulate sensitivity, frequency selectivity, and the time resolution of the peripheral auditory apparatus. Isolating the functional role of such a system necessarily depends on determining under what behavioural circumstances the efferents are active.

Summary and conclusions

Some of the contributions to auditory physiology from the study of reptilian hair cells are as follows. The final event in the sequence of mechanoelectric transduction is a conductance change to ions with an equilibrium potential near zero millivolts. A major component frequency selectivity in the reptilian ear is local to the hair cell, and is not imparted by differential motion of the basilar membrane. Finally, in some cases it is possible to modify the local tuning and sensitivity under efferent control. This information should not be considered in isolation, however, and once the mechanisms involved in transduction and tuning have been examined in a number of species, it will be possible to determine which of these are fundamental to all auditory systems, and which might be accomplished by a variety of means.

I am indebted to my colleagues A. C. Crawford, R. Fettiplace and P. Fuchs and A. B. A. Kroese for their helpful comments on the manuscript. Preparation of the manuscript was supported by an NIH Post-doctoral fellowship, No. 5F32 NS6103-03.

References

Armstrong, C. M., and Binstock, L. (1965). Anomalous rectification in the squid giant axon injected with tetraethylammonium chloride. *J. Gen. Physiol.* *48:* 859–72.

Baird, I. L. (1970). The anatomy of the reptilian ear. In *Biology of the Reptilia,* ed. C. Gans and T. S. Parsons, pp. 193–276. London: Academic Press.

Baird, I. L. (1974). Anatomical features of the inner ear in submammalian vertebrates. In *Handbook of Sensory Physiology,* vol. V/1, ed. W. D. Keidel and W. D. Neff, pp. 159–212. New York: Springer-Verlag.

von Békésy, G. (1960). *Experiments in Hearing.* New York: McGraw-Hill.

Bosher, S. K., and Warren, R. L. (1968). Observations on the electrochemistry of the cochlear endolymph of the rat: a quantitative study of its electrical potential and ionic composition as determined by means of flame spectrophotometry. *Proc. R. Soc. Lond.* *B171:* 227–47.

Bosher, S. K., and Warren, R. L. (1978). Very low calcium content of cochlear endolymph, an extracellular fluid. *Nature 273:* 377–8.

Corey, D. P., and Hudspeth, A. J. (1979). Ionic basis of the receptor potential in a vertebrate hair cell. *Nature 281:* 675–7.

Crawford, A. C., and Fettiplace, R. (1979). Reversal of hair cell responses by current. *J. Physiol., Lond. 295:* 66P.

Crawford, A. C., and Fettiplace, R. (1980a). The frequency selectivity of auditory nerve fibres and hair cells in the cochlea of the turtle. *J. Physiol., Lond. 306:* 79–125.

Crawford, A. C., and Fettiplace, R. (1980b). Auditory nerve responses to mechanical deflections of the basilar membrane. *J. Physiol., Lond. 308:* 86P.

Crawford, A. C., and Fettiplace, R. (1981a). An electrical tuning mechanism in turtle cochlear hair cells. *J. Physiol., Lond. 312:* 377–412.

Crawford, A. C., and Fettiplace, R. (1981b). Non-linearities in the responses of turtle hair cells. *J. Physiol., Lond. 315:* 317–38.

Davis, H. (1958). A mechano-electric theory of cochlear action. *Ann. Otol. Rhinol. Laryngol. 67:* 789–801.

Eatock, R. A., Corey, D. P., and Hudspeth, A. J. (1979). Adaptation in a vertebrate hair cell: stimulus-induced shift of the operating range. *Soc. Neuro. Sci. Abstr.* (5), p. 19, No. 57.

Fettiplace, R., and Crawford, A. C. (1978). The coding of sound pressure and frequency in cochlear hair cells of the terrapin. *Proc. R. Soc. Lond. B203:* 209–18.

Fettiplace, R., and Crawford, A. C. (1980). The origin of tuning in turtle cochlear hair cells. *Hearing Res. 2:* 447–54.

Hodgkin, A. L., and Huxley, A. F. (1952). A quantitative description of membrane current and its application to conduction and excitation in nerve. *J. Physiol., Lond. 117:* 500–44.

Holton, T. (1981). Mechanoelectric transduction by cochlear receptor cells. Doctoral dissertation, Massachusetts Institute of Technology. 147 pp.

Hopkins, C. D. (1976). Stimulus filtering and electroreception: tuberous electroreceptors in three species of gymnotoid fish. *J. Comp. Physiol. 111:* 171–207.

Hudspeth, A. J., and Corey, D. P. (1977). Sensitivity, polarity, and conductance change in the response of vertebrate hair cells to controlled mechanical stimuli. *Proc. Natn. Acad. Sci. USA 74:* 2407–11.

Johnstone, C. G., Schmidt, R. S., and Johnstone, B. M. (1963). Sodium and potassium in vertebrate cochlear endolymph as determined by flame microspectrophotometry. *Comp. Biochem. Physiol. 9:* 335–41.

Klinke, R., and Pause, M. (1980). Discharge properties of primary auditory fibres in *Caiman crocodilus:* comparisons and contrasts to the mammalian auditory nerve. *Expl. Brain Res. 38:* 137–50.

Lim, D. J. (1972). Fine morphology of the tectorial membrane: its relationship to the organ of Corti. *Arch. Otolaryngol. 96:* 199–215.

Manley, G. A. (1977). Response patterns and peripheral origin of auditory nerve fibers in the monitor lizard, *Varanus bengalensis. J. Comp. Physiol. 118:* 249–60.

Manley, G. A. (1981). A review of the auditory physiology of the reptiles. In *Progress in Sensory Physiology 2,* ed. D. Ottoson, pp. 49–134. Berlin: Springer-Verlag.

Mauro, A., Conti, F., Dodge, F., and Schor, R. (1970). Subthreshold behavior and phenomenological impedance of the squid giant axon. *J. Gen. Physiol. 55:* 497–523.

Meves, H., and Pichon, Y. (1977). The effect of internal and external 4-aminopyridine on the potassium currents in intracellularly perfused squid giant axons. *J. Physiol., Lond. 268:* 511–32.

Miller, M. R. (1978). Scanning electron microscope studies of the papilla basilaris of some turtles and snakes. *Am. J. Anat. 151:* 409–36.

Miller, M. R. (1980). The reptilian cochlear duct. In *Comparative Studies of Hearing in Vertebrates*, ed. A. N. Popper and R. R. Fay, pp. 169–204. New York: Springer-Verlag.

Moffat, A. J. M., and Capranica, R. R. (1978). Middle ear sensitivity in anurans and reptiles measured by light scattering spectroscopy. *J. Comp. Physiol. 127:* 97–107.

Mulroy, M. J. (1968). Ultrastructure of the basilar papilla of reptiles. Doctoral dissertation, University of California.

Mulroy, M. J. (1974). Cochlear anatomy of the alligator lizard. *Brain Behav. Evol. 10:* 69–87.

Peake, W. T., and Ling, A. Jr. (1980). Basilar-membrane motion in the alligator lizard: its relation to tonotopic organization and frequency selectivity. *J. Acoust. Soc. Am. 67:* 1736–45.

Peterson, S. K., Frishkopf, L. S., Lechène, C., Oman, C. M., and Weiss, T. F. (1978). Element composition of inner ear lymphs in cats, lizards and skates determined by electron probe micro-analysis of liquid samples. *J. Comp. Physiol. 126:* 1–14.

Rhode, W. S. (1971). Observations of the vibration of the basilar membrane in squirrel monkey using the Mössbauer technique. *J. Acoust. Soc. Am. 49:* 1218–31.

Rhode, W. S., and Robles, L. (1974). Evidence from Mössbauer experiments for nonlinear vibrations in the cochlea. *J. Acoust. Soc. Am. 55:* 588–96.

Russell, I. J., and Sellick, P. M. (1977). Tuning properties of cochlear hair cells. *Nature 267:* 858–60.

Schmidt, R. S. (1963). Types of endolymphatic potentials. *Comp. Biochem. Physiol. 10:* 83–7.

Schmidt, R. S., and Fernández, C. (1962). Labyrinthine DC potentials in representative vertebrates. *J. Cell. Comp. Physiol. 59:* 311–22.

ter Kuile, E. (1900). Die Vebertragung der Energie von der Grundmembran auf die Haarzellen. *Pflügers Arch. ges. Physiol. 79:* 146–57.

Turner, R. G. (1980). Physiology and bioacoustics in reptiles. In *Comparative Studies of Hearing in Vertebrates*, ed. A. N. Popper and R. R. Fay, pp. 205–37. New York: Springer-Verlag.

Turner, R. G., Muraski, A. A., and Nielsen, D. W. (1981). Cilium length: influence on neural tonotopic organization. *Science 213:* 1519–21.

Weiss, T. F., Mulroy, M. J., and Altmann, D. W. (1974). Intracellular responses to acoustic clicks in the inner ear of the alligator lizard. *J. Acoust. Soc. Am. 55:* 606–19.

Weiss, T. F., Mulroy, M. J., Turner, R. G., and Pike, C. L. (1976). Tuning of single fibers in the cochlear nerve of the alligator lizard: relation to receptor morphology. *Brain Res. 115:* 71–90.

Weiss, T. F., Altmann, D. W., and Mulroy, M. J. (1978a). Endolymphatic and intracellular resting potential in the alligator lizard cochlea. *Pflügers Arch. 373:* 77–84.

Weiss, T. F., Peake, W. T., Ling, A. Jr., and Holton, T. (1978b). Which structures determine frequency selectivity and tonotopic organization of vertebrate nerve fibers? Evidence from the alligator lizard. In *Evoked Electrical Activity in the Auditory Nervous System*, ed. R. F. Naunton, and C. Fernández, pp. 91–112. New York: Academic.

Wever, E. G. (1978). *The Reptile Ear.* Princeton: Princeton University Press.

1.4

Sound detection and processing by teleost fish: a selective review

ARTHUR N. POPPER and RICHARD R. FAY

The literature on fish hearing has been reviewed extensively in recent years. The papers in the volume by Tavolga (1976a) provide an excellent guide to the older and more historical material. Papers by Moulton (1963), van Bergeijk (1967), Lowenstein (1971), Tavolga (1971), Hawkins (1973) and ourselves (Popper and Fay, 1973), along with the two volumes edited by Tavolga (1964, 1967) review the work on fish hearing leading up to the modern period. The more recent work has been discussed by Fay (1978a), Fay and Popper (1980), Popper (1983) and Popper and Coombs (1982). There are also extensive summaries of the work on fish audition, fish sound production and the lateral line in the volumes edited by Schuijf and Hawkins (1976) and by Tavolga, Popper and Fay (1981).

Our purpose here is not to review the literature again completely. Instead, we intend to provide a general outline of what is known about hearing in fishes, and to identify what we consider to be some of the most interesting and pressing questions that could occupy our research efforts for the next several years. In doing this we divide the topic of fish audition into four broad questions. First, what are the receptor organs of the ear and their structure? Second, what are the pathways of sound to the ear; what mechanical principles underly their operation, and what are the determinants of auditory sensitivity and the bandwidth of hearing? Third, what are the central acoustic pathways and how is acoustic information processed in the brain? Fourth, how do fish determine the location of a sound source and what are the behavioral and neural mechanisms involved?

Before going further, it is important to point out that there are over 25 000 extant fish species, and that the morphological physiological,

67

ecological, and behavioral variations among these species perhaps equal or exceed that of all other vertebrate groups combined. Thus, while it is tempting to form generalizations concerning fish audition, it is likely that there is no such thing as 'the' fish ear or hearing capabilities in 'the' fish. Furthermore, as recently argued (Platt and Popper, 1981a; Popper, Platt and Saidel, 1982), it is now not even clear that individual otolith organs have the single roles ascribed to them in the earlier literature.

Receptor organ morphology and function

The ears of most fish species are classically divided into the *pars superior* (utricle and semicircular canals) and the *pars inferior* (the saccule and lagena) (Figure 1) (e.g. von Frisch, 1938). The three otolith organs, the utricle, saccule and lagena are sac-like structures containing a single dense calcareous otolith lying close to a sensory epithelium that is part of the wall of the chamber. The sensory epithelia (or macula) has a large number (20 000 in a single saccular macula of a 3-cm-long kissing gourami – Saidel and Popper, 1983) of mechanoreceptors resembling the mammalian Type II vestibular hair cells (Wersäll, 1961). Each sensory hair cell has an apical ciliary bundle which consists of a large number (40 or more) of microvilli-like stereocilia and a single, eccentrically positioned, true cilium – the kinocilium (Figure 2). The stereocilia are generally graded in size, with the longest lying next to the kinocilium. The ciliary bundles project into holes in a thin, gelatinous, otolith membrane (Dale, 1976; Popper, 1977) which connects to both the sensory epithelium and the otolith, thereby effectively mechanically coupling the otolith to the sensory epithelium. Stimulation of the sensory hair cell arises from a relative motion between the otolith and the sensory epithelium. Since the ciliary bundles lie between these two structures, and are effectively attached to both, the motion results in a shearing of the ciliary bundle. Such shearing leads to a physiological response of the hair cell (Flock, 1965; Hudspeth and Corey, 1977) which depends in amplitude and sign on the direction of the stereociliary motion relative to the position of the kinocilium.

It has been suggested that the *pars superior* primarily responds to vestibular stimulation while the *pars inferior* has an auditory function (e.g. von Frisch, 1938; Lowenstein, 1971; many others). While it appears that the saccule and lagena are involved in sound detection in most species studied, the utricle in several groups of fishes may be an auditory structure. For example, a swimbladder extension to the utricle in the Clupeomorpha (herring-like fishes) results in its being a pressure-detecting organ (see Denton and Gray, 1980; Blaxter, Denton and

Figure 1. A medial view of the right ear of the herring, *Clupea harengus*, redrawn from Retzius (1881) (anterior to the left, dorsal to the top). This ear is typical of that found in teleosts other than the Ostariophysi. The *pars superior* consists of the three semicircular canals and the utricle (which is involved with audition in the herrings), while the *pars inferior* consists of the saccule and lagena. Each of the otolith chambers contains a single otolith and the various otic endorgans are innervated by branches of the eighth (octavus) nerve. Note that Retzius recognized that the saccular branch of the octavus nerve is divided into several parts. It has been shown (Saidel and Popper, 1983) that the anterior-most branch of the saccular nerve innervates horizontally-oriented cells, while the other branches innervate vertically oriented cells. aa, ap, ampullae of the anterior and posterior semi-circular canals; ca, cp, anterior and posterior semi-circular canals; ms, saccular macula; pl, lagenar macula.

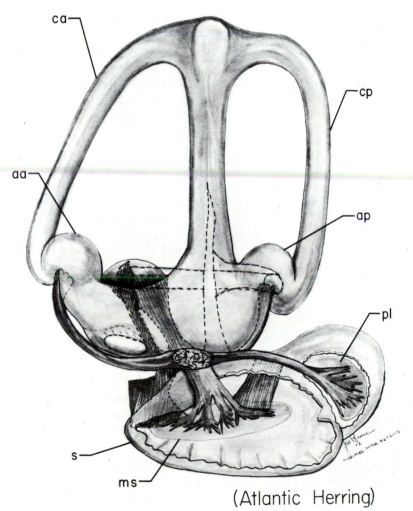

(Atlantic Herring)

Gray, 1981). While the evidence is less direct, it also appears that the excellent low-frequency hearing capabilities of a marine catfish, *Arius felis*, is related to the presence of a large utricle that may have the properties of an accelerometer tuned to low frequencies (e.g. 200 Hz) (Popper and Tavolga, 1981).

Observations on the shapes and ultrastructural features of the sensory epithelia have revealed levels of complexity and interspecific variation (e.g. Figure 3) for which functional correlates are not yet known. The epithelium of each organ is divided so that all cells in a particular region have their kinocilia on the same side of the ciliary bundles. Thus, all of the cells in one region are considered to be oriented in the same direction (Figure 2). In fishes of the superorder Ostariophysi (goldfish, carp, catfish and others with Weberian ossicles linking the swimbladder and ear; see below), hair cells of the saccule are oriented in two opposing directions (Platt, 1977; Jenkins, 1979, 1981; Popper and Tavolga, 1981), one dorsally and the other ventrally (Figure 3, top). The lagena and utricle also have oppositely-oriented groups, but since the border separating the two groups curves over the surface of the macula, the hair cells are generally oriented in various directions. Most other

Figure 2. Scanning electron micrographs of sensory epithelia showing the ciliary bundles on sensory hair cells in the kissing gourami. Left, Type F1 ciliary bundles (Popper, 1977). The F1 bundle has a kinocilium that is not too much longer than the longest stereocilia. Microvilli-covered supporting cells lie between the sensory cells. The F1 bundle is the most common of the various ciliary bundle types found in many species. Note that the ciliary bundles are organized into orientation groups, with all of the cells in a group having their kinocilia the same side of the ciliary bundle (arrows in figure). Right, Somewhat longer F3 ciliary bundles. These bundles are often found just inside of the periphery of a sensory region. They resemble, but are somewhat longer than, the F1 bundles. K, kinocilium; S, stereocilia.

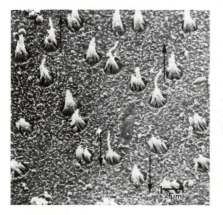
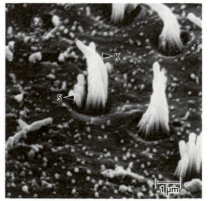

teleosts (often referred to by the non-taxonomic term, non-ostariophy-sans) have basically similar patterns of utricular and lagenar orientation to that encountered in the Ostariophysi. However, the non-ostariophy-san saccular pattern differs strikingly from that in the Ostariophysi (and in terrestrial vertebrates) in having hair cells oriented in four, rather than two, directions (lower four diagrams in Figure 3). In addition to vertically-oriented cells on the posterior end of the epithelium, as in the Ostariophysi, the non-ostariophysans (with a few notable exceptions – Popper, 1981) also have rostrally- and caudally-oriented cells at the rostral end of the saccular macula (Figure 3).

Ciliary bundles vary considerably in length at different epithelial regions. Furthermore, the distribution of the different-length ciliary bundles on the epithelial surface varies in different species (e.g. Popper, 1977; Platt and Popper, 1981a). Several different types of ciliary bundle can be identified, based on overall cilia length and on the relative lengths of stereocilia and kinocilia (Figure 2) (Popper, 1977; Platt and Popper, 1981a). In many non-ostariophysans, the very periphery of each sensory region contains type F2 ciliary bundles with long kinocilia and short stereocilia. These surround a narrow region containing F3 ciliary bundles (long kinocilia and long stereocilia). The bulk of the epithelium contains F1 ciliary bundles which resemble shortened F3 bundles. This distribution of different ciliary-bundle types, while fairly common among non-ostariophysans, is not found in all fishes. For example, the whole anterior end of the saccular macula in several ostariophysan species has F1 bundles, while the posterior end has F3 bundles (Platt, 1977; Popper and Tavolga, 1981). Most Myctophiformes (lantern fish) have F3 ciliary bundles over the whole saccular macula (Popper, 1977), and this pattern is also found in the taxonomically unrelated Clupeomorpha (Platt and Popper, 1981b).

There are few data on the functional significance of cilia length in fishes. In the goldfish (Furukawa and Ishii, 1967; Fay, 1978b) and the catfish, *Ictalurus punctatus* (Moeng, 1978; Moeng and Popper, in preparation), fibers innervating the anterior macular region, the area with F1 ciliary bundles, appear to have higher characteristic frequencies than neurons innervating the posterior end of the saccular macula where the longer F3 ciliary bundles are found. This potential correlation between ciliary bundle length and the tuning properties of innervating neurons is in accordance with data from reptiles (Turner, Muraski and Nielsen, 1981) and frogs (Lewis, Baird, Leverenz and Koyama, 1982). It has also been suggested that the F2 ciliary bundles at the margins of the maculae are in the early stage of development in sharks (Corwin, 1977,

Figure 3. Saccular hair cell orientation patterns found among teleost fishes (dorsal to the top, anterior to the right). SEM studies have shown that there are at least five different patterns among the extant species, with the bulk of the variability associated with the horizontally-oriented hair cells (Popper, 1981; Popper and Coombs, 1982). The vertical pattern is found in goldfish and all other Ostariophysi, while the four other patterns are only found in non-ostariophysans. The 'standard' pattern is found in such diverse species as salmon, cichlids, and some osteoglossids. The 'dual' pattern has horizontally-oriented cells at both the rostral and caudal ends of the macula. This pattern is commonly found among the Gadiformes (cods and relatives) and in several Perciformes. The 'alternating' pattern is found among the Elomorpha (eels and relatives) and in some osteoglossids. The 'opposing' pattern is frequently found in species that have specializations associated with the relationship between the swimbladder and inner ear that are thought to be involved with audition. Species include some squirrelfish (Fam. Holocentridae), some bubblenest builders (Fam. Anabantidae), and some osteoglossids. (From Popper, Platt and Saidel, 1982.)

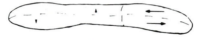

VERTICAL

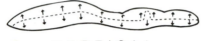

STANDARD

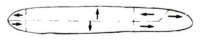

DUAL

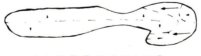

ALTERNATING

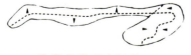

OPPOSING

1981) and amphibians (Lewis and Li, 1975), but this point has yet to be confirmed with fishes. Clearly, future experiments need to be directed at the functional differences between cells with different ciliary bundle sizes since the absolute sizes are likely to play a role in signal transduction in the ear.

Other structural features of the teleost ear, in addition to the different ciliary bundle lengths and hair cell orientation patterns, may have functional correlates with hearing (e.g. Platt and Popper, 1981a; Popper, 1983). These include the shape of the saccular otolith which, in most species, is highly complex and includes sculpturing along the edges (Figure 4). The saccular epithelium is often wide at the anterior end while it suddenly narrows out at the posterior region that contains vertically oriented sensory cells (Figure 3). Finally, regions of horizontally and vertically oriented hair cells in non-ostariophysans are separately innervated by two branches of the saccular nerve with little or no overlap (Saidel and Popper, 1983). This separation is maintained at least to the point where the saccular portion of the nerve enters the brainstem.

Structural variation

Although it is clear that the elegant relationships between taxonomy and the auditory portions of the ears found in reptiles (Wever, 1978; Miller, 1981) and amphibians (Lewis, 1981) are not found in fishes (Popper and Coombs, 1982) detailed examination of a group of species selected for taxonomic, behavioral and ecological diversity (Popper, 1976, 1977, 1978, 1980, 1981) has shown recurring patterns. The inter-specific diversity in the ear of fishes is primarily associated with the auditory portions of the ear (saccule and lagena in

Figure 4. The saccular (larger) and lagenar (smaller) otoliths from a parrotfish, *Scarus dubious*. The saccular otolith has a species-specific shape and is highly sculptured. The lagenar otolith is typical of many species. The medial side of the saccular otolith (left) has a deep groove, or sulcus, in which the saccular macula sits. (From Popper, 1981.)

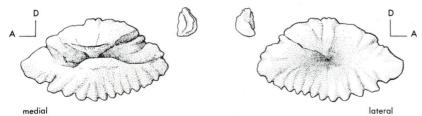

medial   lateral

most species). Substantial differences in the utricle depend on whether this organ primarily has an auditory or vestibular function (Popper and Platt, 1979; Platt and Popper, 1981a). This diversity includes inter-specific variation in the shape of the saccular otolith, the structural relationship between the otoliths and the sensory epithelia, the shapes, sizes and interconnections of the otolithic chambers, the distribution of the different length ciliary bundles, and the shape of the epithelia. Significantly, the ultrastructure of the cell bodies of the sensory cells themselves show little or no inter-specific variation (Popper, 1979; Popper and Hoxter, 1981).

The most striking case of inter-specific variation in the teleost ear appears to be associated with the orientation patterns of the sensory hair cells on the saccular macula. Examination of more than 75 species (reviewed in Platt and Popper, 1981a; Popper and Coombs, 1982) revealed no more than five distinct saccular hair cell orientation patterns. While it is likely that all patterns have not yet been identified (particularly considering that we have only sampled a small portion of all extant fishes), these five patterns seem to be widely distributed among most of the taxonomic groups studied (Popper and Coombs, 1982). The only variants from these patterns are found among non-teleosts such as the bowfin, *Amia calva* (Popper and Northcutt, 1983), the reedfish, *Polypterus bichir*, and the sturgeon, *Scaphirhynchus platorynchus* (Popper, 1978), as well as in a lungfish, *Protopterus* (Popper and Northcutt, in preparation). Variation is primarily associated with the way in which sensory cells are oriented along the horizontal axis of the animals.

The five recognized saccular patterns are shown in Figure 3. Each pattern may be found throughout a particular taxonomic group, or within several unrelated groups. For example, the 'vertical' pattern, found in all Ostariophysi (Platt, 1977; Jenkins, 1979; Popper and Tavolga, 1981), is also found in the unrelated Mormyriformes (elephant-nose fishes and relatives) (Popper, 1981). This convergence in auditory system structure between these two groups parallels converg-ence in electroreceptive structures between the mormyrids and one group of Ostariophysi, the gymnotids (Bullock, Northcutt and Bodz-nick, 1982). Similarly, the 'opposing' hair cell orientation pattern is found in several members of the squirrelfish family, the Holocentridae (Popper, 1977), in some bubble-nest builders, the Anabantidae (Popper and Hoxter, 1981; Saidel and Popper, 1983), and in some Osteoglosso-morpha (Coombs and Popper, 1982b) – a group of taxonomically unrelated species having swimbladder specializations for sound detection.

The taxonomic and functional significances of the different saccular patterns are not known, and remain an important area for study. Based upon the presence of similar patterns in fishes that are unrelated in a taxonomic sense to one another, it is likely that strong selective pressures have led to convergent evolution in the auditory portions of the ear. While similar ear patterns in different species may not reflect similarities in acoustic processing, we would argue that such is the case. How the different ear patterns vary functionally is still not clear and remains to be studied.

Sound pathways to the ear

Sound reaching the ear of a fish causes relative otolith movement via at least two pathways (von Frisch, 1938; Pumphrey, 1950; Dijkgraaf, 1960; van Bergeijk, 1967; Fay and Popper, 1974, 1975; Buwalda and Van der Steen, 1979; Fay, Hillery and Bolan, 1982). The 'direct' path involves acceleration of the ear by the particle motion component of the acoustic (or hydrodynamic) wave that passes relatively undisturbed through the fish's body. This motion is taken up by the various tissues at somewhat different amplitudes and phases, with the largest differences occurring between the dense otoliths and the underlying sensory tissue. In this accelerometer-like mode, stimulation is most likely proportional to the acceleration amplitude (see Lewis, this volume), and receptors respond to the particle motion waveform, including its directional characteristics. All otolith organs are stimulated via this direct route.

The 'indirect' path involves the response of the swimbladder (or any other nearby gas 'bubble') to the sound pressure waveform. As the swimbladder expands and contracts in rarefaction and compression phases, the movement of its walls may be transmitted to the ears via specialized routes (e.g. the Weberian ossicles, rostral swimbladder projections to the ear, etc.) in some species and not so specialized routes in others. Whether or not a given otolith organ is stimulated by the sound pressure waveform depends upon the efficiency of the sound-conducting pathway to that organ from the swimbladder. Van Bergeijk (1967) indicated that this mode of hearing could not be involved in sound source localization since the source of the sound, as far as the animal is concerned, is always the swimbladder, thereby stimulating the two ears directly and equally.

For any fish with a swimbladder (or with proximity to any gas–water interface including the water surface), sound could reach the ears by both the direct and indirect pathways. It is possible, therefore, that some auditory receptors receive information primarily about the sound pressure waveform, while others are subject to the particle acceleration waveform. In most cases, the possibility exists for an interaction (vector summation) of effects due to both pressure and particle motion. Since the amplitude and phase relations between these components of under-water sound vary as a function of sound source characteristics (e.g. distance and orientation relative to the fish, size, mode of motion, etc.), and as a function of local acoustic conditions (e.g. depth, proximity to the bottom or surface, etc. – Michelsen, 1978), it has been suggested that this dual sensitivity could provide the animal with high quality information about its acoustic environment. Whether this notion is a theorist's fantasy, or whether animals may process and use this informa-tion is not known. However, some data on sound localization and signal detection to be discussed in later sections encourage us to look more closely at these various possibilities.

Range and sensitivity of hearing

Enormous differences exist in the sensitivity and best frequency range of hearing among the 25 or so species which have been tested behaviorally. Figure 5 shows behavioral audiograms for seven species chosen to illustrate the best and worst sensitivities, and the narrowest and widest hearing bandwidths. Generally, greatest sensitivity (-30 to -50 dB re: 1 μbar) is associated with special adaptations for conducting the pressure-dependent movements of the swimbladder wall to the ear (usually the saccule). Poorest sound pressure sensitivity (generally above 0 dB re: 1 μbar) is associated with the lack of a swimbladder, or the lack of specialized conduction pathways to the ear.

The best known sound conduction specializations are the Weberian ossicles of the Ostariophysi. These bones link the anterior end of the swimbladder complex to the saccules of both ears. Other well-known adaptations generally include arrangements to bring anterior projec-tions of the bladder into close proximity with the ear, as in the mormyrids where a small bubble of air is associated with the ear itself (Stipetic, 1939), and in the clupeids where there is an extension of the swimbladder to the utricle (O'Connell, 1955; Blaxter et al., 1981). While it can be assumed that these structural modifications may increase sound pressure sensitivity over their absence, no biomechanical data yet explain the differences in sensitivity among those species having the various types of specializations for pressure detection.

Specializations for sensitivity and for increased bandwidth are not necessarily the same. For example, the marine catfish (*Arius felis*) has

Figure 5. Auditory sensitivity measures for seven teleost fishes demonstrating the variability in hearing range and sensitivity among different species. In each case, data were obtained in behavioral experiments and the mean thresholds are presented at each frequency in dB re: 1 dyne cm^{-2} (1×10^{-5} N cm^{-2}) and in dB re: 1 W cm^{-2} to facilitate comparison with tetrapod data. *Euthynnus affinis*, a tuna that has no swimbladder (Iversen, 1969), has a very narrow bandwidth and poor sensitivity. *Limanda limanda*, a flatfish, also does not have a swimbladder. (From Chapman and Sand, 1974.) All of the other species have a swimbladder. *Gadus morhua*, a cod, has good sensitivity but a relatively narrow bandwidth that may be associated with its not having any particular specializations for audition. (From Hawkins and Chapman, 1975.) *Adioryx xantherythrus* is a squirrelfish with no specializations and this is compared to *Myripristis kuntee*, another squirrelfish that has specializations in the connections between the swimbladder and the inner ear. *Myripristis* has far greater sensitivity and a wider bandwidth than *Adioryx*. (From Coombs and Popper, 1979.) Significantly, hearing in *Myripristis* is about as good as that found in two Ostariophysi, *Carassius auratus* (the goldfish) (from Fay, 1978a) and the Mexican blind cave fish, *Astyanax jordani*. (From Popper, 1970.)

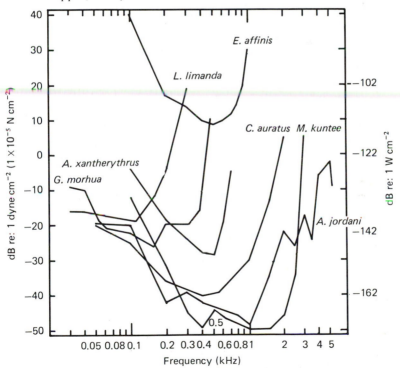

declining sensitivity above 200 Hz (Popper and Tavolga, 1981) in spite of a Weberian ossicle system which helps a related species, *Ictalurus nebulosus*, to have one of the widest bandwidths so far determined (Poggendorf, 1952). Electrophysiological studies on several species (Fay and Popper, 1974, 1975; Fay, 1981; Shen, Coombs, Fay, Popper and Saidel, 1982) have shown that the bandwidth of hearing measured behaviorally is similar to that of the otolith organs stimulated independently of their swimbladder. Thus, the otolith organs and more peripheral sound-conducting structures have apparently evolved together to determine the frequency range of hearing for a particular species.

Lateral line

Very early in the history of research on the lateral line (see Dijkgraaf, 1963, for a definitive review), it was considered likely that this system mediated this behavioral response to sound, particularly in the near-field (van Bergeijk, 1967), and particularly at low frequencies where near-field effects are relatively greater. While there is no doubt that hydrodynamic effects may stimulate the lateral line receptors (as in surface wave detection (Görner, 1976; Schwartz, 1967; Sand, 1981; Sand, this volume) it is unlikely that the lateral line is involved in the detection and processing of signals normally designated as 'sound' in laboratory and field studies. In a recent study Sand (1981) found best sensitivity to be about 3.3×10^{-6} cm at 50 Hz (with a very rapid decline in sensitivity toward 160 Hz) from the roach (*Rutilus rutilus*). (See Sand, this volume, for a detailed review of lateral line function and its relation to hearing.) Not only is this frequency range narrower than the 'hearing' range of even the less-sensitive species, sensitivity is at least 40 dB poorer than that of the otolith organs measured at 50 Hz by comparable methods (e.g. Fay, 1981). Sand concluded that the lateral line system would be relatively sensitive in an extreme near-field (where hydrodynamic motion, or flow, is at a high relative amplitude), but would be clearly out-performed by an otolith organ in detecting plane-wave displacements. In fact, in a rather intense sound field, the near-field produced by a swimbladder (in response to sound pressure fluctuations) would possibly be the most likely stimulus for a trunk lateral line receptor. Thus, while the lateral line could in this way indirectly respond to sound, the otolith organs are better adapted for this function, and the hypothetical usefulness of the lateral line in sound localization (van Bergeijk, 1967) would be minimal at best. Sand confined his conclusions to the trunk lateral line system, and to considerations of threshold sensitivity. The question remains open whether for supra-threshold stimuli the lateral line system may somehow contribute to signal processing capabilities in fishes. While there is continued interest in the lateral line receptor cell as a physiological preparation and as a cochlear hair cell model (Boston, 1981; Strelioff and Sokolich, 1981), we know almost nothing about how information is processed by the nervous system over time and space.

Other questions that need be considered include behavioral measures of sensitivity, the processing of directional information, and the specific contributions of the lateral line to orientation behavior and schooling (Burgess and Shaw, 1981; Partridge, 1981). Recent evidence shows that the head canal system of the lateral line is physically coupled to the fluid system of the inner ear in clupeids (Blaxter et al., 1981). This may indicate a functional relationship between the two systems. Finally, while it had been widely thought that the lateral line was innervated by the eighth, ninth or tenth cranial nerves (e.g. van Bergeijk, 1967), we now know that it has its own innervation (e.g. McCormick, 1981b; Northcutt, 1981; Bell, 1981b). Almost nothing is known about the CNS processing of lateral line input. While it is likely that information from the ear and lateral line converge somewhere in the CNS, the site, nature, and function of this convergence, if present, are not known.

Coding in the ear
Information processing – mechanical aspects
The early 'monolithic' view of the ear was that the otolith simply moved in linear pathways over the macula, and that all underlying hair cells were stimulated essentially similarly. There was no apparent basis for a Békésy travelling wave or any other phenomenon which could produce a frequency-dependent place of maximal stimulation; i.e. a place-principle of frequency representation. To the extent that a fish could distinguish one tonal frequency from another, some other principle of analysis had to be involved. The likely candidate was a temporal, or volley, principle.

This view has changed somewhat in recent years because of data from several different areas that indicate the ear is not as 'monolithic' as originally thought. First, as already mentioned, the saccule is organized in a complex fashion in many species showing intricate patterns of hair cell orientation and distributions of ciliary bundle lengths. Second, eighth nerve fibers of several species show variation in sensitivity, best frequency, and bandwidth – the basis for which is not yet clear. Third, data from intense tonal stimulation of the ear in two species show that different pure tones damage maximally, and thus are likely primarily to stimulate, different saccular and lagenar regions (Enger, 1981; Saidel and Popper, in preparation). Finally, evidence against the monolithic ear comes from studies on innervation of the saccule by showing that different parts of the macula are innervated by separate eighth nerve populations. This information from various ear regions may be processed separately within the CNS (Saidel and Popper, 1983).

Based on these observations, it would seem likely that the different patterns of hair cell orientation are adaptations that code the pathway of otolith movement over the macular surface. Particular orientations would be advantageous for coding otolith movement caused by swimbladder vibration (that is, coding the sound pressure waveform as described below), while others may best code the axis (or pathways) of a sound's particle motion as it impinges directly on the ear (see below). Such arrangements could effectively separate the sound pressure and particle motion waveforms (Buwalda, 1981), and thus play a role in sound localization, the enhancement of signal-to-noise ratio through directional filtering, and in the determination of sound wave impedance and source distance (Schuijf, 1981).

The interaction of sound pressure dependent and direct particle motion waveforms would result in complex relative motions between the otolith and the hair cells. This motion might ascribe something similar to a three-dimensional Lissajous pattern (an 'orbital') over the epithelial surface (Schuijf, 1981; Popper et al., 1982). Each orbital pattern is likely to change, depending upon the nature of the acoustic signal. Species-specific orbital patterns would also depend upon structures in the ear imposing limitations on its movement (e.g. the otolith membrane), by drag patterns imposed upon the complex sculptured surfaces of the otolith by inner-ear fluids, by species-specific shapes of the otoliths, and resonance characteristics of the otoliths. We then can hypothesize that signals varying in acoustic characteristics, such as direction, frequency, or impedance could produce different orbits with respect to the sensory surface, which would result in shearing patterns on the surface that vary temporally and spatially according to the signals. Biophysical measurements of the relative motions between the otolith and other structures of the ear are needed to add substance to these speculations (Sand and Michelsen, 1978).

Information processing in the eighth nerve

Recently, investigators have studied various aspects of responses from single units of the saccular and lagenar nerves (Enger,

1963; Furukawa and Ishii, 1967; Furukawa, Ishii and Matsuura, 1972; Fay, 1978b, 1980, 1981, 1982; Furukawa, 1978; Moeng, 1978; Fay and Olsho, 1979; Fay and Patricoski, 1980; Fay and Coombs, 1983; Fine, 1981; Hawkins and Horner, 1981; Horner, Hawkins and Fraser, 1981; Moeng and Popper, in preparation). In spite of the few species studied (in particular the goldfish, *Carassius auratus*, and cod, *Gadus morhua*), we make the following generalizations on eighth-nerve physiology.

First, substantial variation exists among neurons from a single species or individual in spontaneous activity rates and patterns, in adaptation rates, best frequency, bandwidth, sensitivity, directionality, phase locking, periodicity coding, and spike-rate v. intensity relations.

In goldfish, spontaneous rates range from 0 to over 300 impulses per second (ips), with some neurons showing irregular (Poisson) inter-spike interval distributions, and others showing regular (Gaussian) or burst (multi-model) distributions. The cellular mechanisms underlying the statistical variation of spontaneous rates are not known.

Adaptation rates may be slow or fast depending upon spontaneous rate, overall sound pressure level, and frequency content of the signal (Fay, 1981). The greatest adaptation is seen in non-spontaneous neurons stimulated at high frequencies. Intracellular studies of adaptation and the recovery from stimulation in saccular neurons have led Furukawa, Kuno and Matsuura (1982) to a model of neurotransmitter release at the hair cell where release sites with different thresholds are replenished at different rates. The considerable sensitivity of e.p.s.p. amplitude to small changes in stimulus level (Furukawa et al., 1982) most likely underlies the extreme sensitivity of goldfish saccular fibers (and behavioral detection) in response to amplitude modulated tones (Fay, 1980). Variation in adaptation rates probably accounts for the selective response of different saccular neurons to different stimulus envelope periodicities (Fay, 1980).

The frequency response areas of saccular fibers show great diversity, as illustrated in Figure 6. These tuning curves show variation in best frequency (100 to 800 Hz), and sensitivity (40 dB range) with bandwidths (Q_{10} dB) ranging from 0.5 to 1.5. While we have no data on the origin of this frequency selectivity, a mechanical resonance perhaps determined by a gradation of cilia length along the length of the saccule has been suggested as one basis, or by an electrical resonance of the hair cell as hypothesized for the terrapin by Fettiplace and Crawford (1978). In any case, the fact of peripheral frequency selectivity leaves open the possibility of a place-like analysis occurring in the fish ear.

All sound responsive saccular neurons studied show a robust tendency to phase lock to the stimulus waveform (Fay, 1978b,c; Moeng and Popper, in preparation). This observation is important since it means that neurons represent the precise details of the time course of sound pressure fluctuation as times between successive spikes. Phase locking accuracy in goldfish saccular neurons approaches that seen in mammalian auditory nerve for frequencies below 1000 Hz. Since fishes generally have hair cells that are oppositely oriented, both compression and rarefaction phases of the acoustic waveform are encoded in detail. The ability of goldfish to discriminate between transients, differing only in polarity, probably arises from this arrangement (Piddington, 1972; Furukawa, 1978). In goldfish, saccular fibers are most responsive to the

Figure 6. Tuning curves of representative single saccular nerve units of the goldfish. The sound pressure level necessary to produce a given small degree of phase-locking between the neural response and the stimulus waveform is plotted as a function of tone frequency for each unit. The dashed lines indicate units with generally low frequency sensitivity, and the solid lines indicate high-frequency sensitivity, with clear band-pass characteristics. The heavy solid line connecting symbols is behavioral sensitivity for the goldfish (Fay, 1969b.) The numbers labeling each curve identify the units. (From Fay, 1978b.)

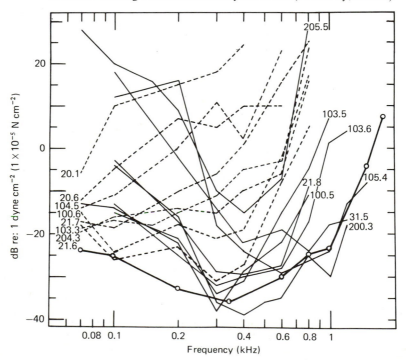

sound pressure waveform, while lagenar fibers respond best to whole body vibration (the accelerometer mode) (Fay, 1981). Phase locking in both organs thus preserves both of these independent waveforms in the time domain. Although the phase angle at which a neural response 'locks' onto a tonal stimulus (Fay and Olsho, 1979) varies, the origin and functional correlates of this are not clear.

The increase of neural firing with stimulus level in goldfish saccular fibers is quite variable (Figure 7). Non-spontaneous fibers generally show exceedingly steep rate-intensity functions, while spontaneous (or noise-driven) neurons show less-steep functions in which a doubling of sound power generally doubles spike rate. On the basis of data like those in Figure 7, Fay and Coombs (1983) have concluded that signal

Figure 7. Rate–intensity functions for two typical non-spontaneous saccular nerve units of the goldfish in response to an 800-Hz tone. The solid dots show the function in quiet, while the other curves in each panel show the function determined in the presence of continuous white noise at the individual sound pressure spectrum level (dB re: 1 dyne cm^{-2} Hz^{-1}, 1×10^{-5} N cm^{-2} Hz^{-1}). The number associated with each curve ($A =$) is the slope of the straight line (power function exponent) best fitting the data points near threshold. The horizontal line segments indicate the discharge rate to the noise alone. The intersection of this segment with the upwardly sloping segment defines the 'threshold' for response to the tone under each condition. The noise-masked functions are indistinguishable in form from those determined in quiet for spontaneously active neurons. (From Fay and Coombs, 1983.)

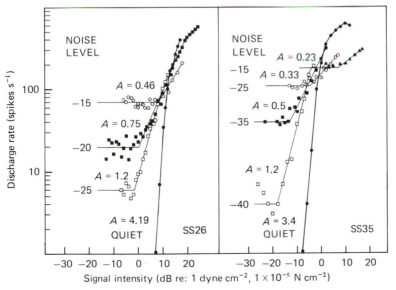

detection in quiet is mediated by non-spontaneous neurons, while detection of masked signals is caused by spike rate increments in on-going neural activity. The fact that signal to noise ratios (S/N) required for behavioral signal detection are equal to those required to increment an ongoing spike rate in saccular neurons demonstrates that masked signal detection is based on spike rate increments and not on phase locking which begins to occur at significantly lower S/N values, and that the frequency selective process which rejects noise and helps in signal detection are probably the tuning characteristics of peripheral neurons. Improving the signal to noise ratio for detecting signals in a noisy background is a great biological advantage gained from peripheral frequency selectivity.

Information processing – psychophysical analyses

The detectability of an auditory signal depends on several factors including stimulus frequency, intensity, duration, and the presence of other interfering or masking sounds (which may or may not be simultaneous with the signal). The relation between intensity and frequency for constant detectability (defined by behavioral audiograms) is shown in Figure 5.

Acoustic power is summed over time when signals are detected against a noise background in goldfish (Offutt, 1967) and cod (Hawkins, 1981) with a time constant greater than 500 ms in goldfish (Fay and Coombs, 1983). In this case, threshold drops three decibels for every doubling of duration, indicating equal energy at threshold. Under quiet conditions, however, very little (or unmeasurable) summation occurs indicating that brief signals are detected at a lower energy than longer signals (Popper, 1972). This behavior has its correlates in the shapes of the rate-intensity functions of single saccular units in goldfish (Fay and Coombs, 1983), and is consistent with a simple neural model of temporal summation developed for mammals (Zwislocki, 1969).

The effects of an interfering or masking sound on signal detection have been studied in a number of species for a variety of masker sounds. These experiments have been theoretically important because the results are used to make inferences about the characteristics of psychophysical 'auditory filters' used to detect signals (and reject noise). In general, the thresholds for tones masked by broad band noise indicate that noise power does not sum across the entire frequency range of hearing to interfere with the detection of a given tone (Chapman, 1973; Chapman and Hawkins, 1973; Fay, 1974a; Tavolga,

1974; Fay and Coombs, 1983), suggesting the existence of tuned filters. The power of masking also fails to summate completely over space to determine the detectability of a particle motion signal (stimulating the ear via the 'direct' accelerometer route which bypasses the swimbladder) (Chapman, 1973; Chapman and Johnstone, 1974; Hawkins and Sand, 1977; Buwalda, 1981). This means that masking will occur only to the extent that signal and masker share similar axes of particle motion (or originate from similar locations; the 'cocktail party effect'). Thus it appears that like mammals (Green and Yost, 1975), fishes use filtering in both the frequency and space domains to enhance signal detectability under noisy conditions.

Other masking studies have used tonal or narrowband noise maskers to more directly measure the shapes of the psychophysical 'auditory filter' (Buerkle, 1968, 1969; Tavolga, 1974; Hawkins and Chapman, 1975; Fay, Ahroon and Orawski, 1978; Hawkins and Johnstone, 1978; Coombs and Popper, 1982a). In general, all agree that masking is most effective when the masker is near the signal frequency, and that masking declines as the frequency separation between the masker and signal widens. Again, this is in qualitative agreement with data from birds and mammals and illustrates that some sort of frequency selectivity is operating in the auditory system. The dominant assumption is that such experiments demonstrate peripheral filtering processes, but this is not necessarily the case (Hawkins and Chapman, 1975; Fay et al., 1978), since the simultaneous presentation of masker and signal may produce effects such as amplitude modulation (beats) to which the auditory system is exquisitely sensitive (Fay, 1980; Furukawa et al., 1982).

One approach to this problem is to use 'non-simultaneous' masking paradigms in which the signal and masker do not overlap in time (Popper and Clarke, 1979; Coombs and Popper, 1982a). These results show, first, that a sound may have masking effects which extend forward in time (forward masking), and also backwards (in which case, signal detectability is degraded by a sound presented shortly after a brief signal sound has terminated) (Popper and Clarke, 1979). These effects attenuate rapidly with the temporal separation between signal and masker, in qualitative agreement with similar data from human observers (Houtgast, 1972). The study of Coombs and Popper (1982a) shows that filter functions determined using forward masking are more broadly tuned than those determined in simultaneous masking, suggesting that the detection of interaction products between signal and masker (e.g. beats) may have helped determine signal detectability in simultaneous masking.

Discrimination mechanisms

The greater portion of the experiments on auditory discrimination can be classified as intensity, frequency, or temporal discrimination. Most psychophysical data we have on the fundamental question of intensity discrimination are from the goldfish (Jacobs and Tavolga, 1967; Fay, 1980; Hall, Patricoski and Fay, 1981; Fay and Coombs, 1983). The differential intensive threshold (ΔI) for tones is smallest at 400 Hz (4 dB) and increases at higher and lower frequencies (Jacobs and Tavolga, 1967). Other measures show greater sensitivity (0.5 to 3.6 dB) depending upon overall sound pressure level, indicating a 'miss' to Weber's law (Hall et al., 1981). The ΔI for noise signals is duration dependent, ranging from 1.8 to 6 dB, but invariant with overall intensity (Fay and Coombs, 1983). These capabilities are quite consistent both quantitatively and qualitatively with similar measures for other vertebrates including man, and suggest similar underlying mechanisms. Neurophysiological studies on goldfish have shown that intensity discrimination behavior can be accounted for on the basis of processing spike rate increments in saccular fibers (Fay and Coombs, 1983).

More attention has been focused on the question of frequency (or time) discrimination since these data may be more directly related to hypotheses about time versus place coding in the ear. Overall, fishes are capable of detecting changes in pure tone frequency ranging from about 3% to about 20% (possibly more), depending on frequency and species. Several Ostariophysi, including the goldfish (Stetter, 1929; Jacobs and Tavolga, 1968; Fay, 1970), sea catfish (Tavolga, 1982), and the minnow *Phoxinus* (Stetter, 1929; Wohlfahrt, 1939; Dijkgraaf and Verheijen, 1950), show greatest sensitivity (3–7%). The several species tested which do not have specializations for sound pressure sensitivity appear to be slightly less sensitive with differential thresholds ranging from 8% to over 20% (Dijkgraaf, 1952; Pettersen, 1980, as cited by Enger, 1981). While the ostariophysans are an order of magnitude less sensitive to frequency changes than man, their performance falls within the non-human vertebrate range (Fay, 1974b).

The neural mechanisms underlying frequency discrimination capacities are not known. As discussed earlier, the finding that saccular neurons vary in best frequency, and the observation that intense sound stimulation causes frequency-dependent patterns of hair cell damage over the macular surface (Enger, 1981) suggest the possibility of a place-like principle of analysis in which frequency changes could be coded as a shift in the population of most-active fibers in the saccular nerve. No attempts have been made to evaluate this idea quantitatively.

The alternative hypothesis, that frequency is coded in the statistics of inter-spike-interval distributions within neural channels, has been evaluated in a series of psychophysical and neurophysiological experiments (Fay, 1978b, 1980, 1982; Fay and Passow, 1982). Neurophysiological data show that in the goldfish, the error made in discriminating one tone frequency from another (expressed as just noticeable difference in period), is highly correlated with the error with which saccular neurons represent pure tone period in times between spikes (Fay, 1978b). Further studies using amplitude-modulated and repeated-burst signals (in which animals are conditioned to detect changes in burst repetition rate) similarly show that temporal error in the representation of envelope periodicities in saccular fibers is highly correlated with (and in some conditions precisely equal to) the just discriminable change in repetition period (Fay, 1982; Fay and Passow, 1982). These data support the hypothesis that decisions about tone frequency or envelope modulation rate are made on information represented in the time domain (e.g. inter-spike intervals) (Mountcastle, Talbot, Sakata and Hyvarinen, 1969).

Other corroborating data come from psychophysical experiments (Fay, 1980; Fay and Passow, 1982) showing that performance in detecting periodicity or discriminating changes in sound burst rate when robust spectral cues are available is no different from that observed or expected when frequency domain cues are not available. This is evidence that the time domain cues in these discriminations are used by the organism, while the frequency domain cues are not. These results are consistent with observations that fishes normally use temporally-coded information in vocal communication in a social context (Myrberg and Spires, 1972; Spanier, 1979; Myrberg, Spanier and Ha, 1978).

Innervation of the ear and central projections

The innervation of the inner ear and the projections of afferent fibers of the ear and lateral line to the brain in fishes have only recently been studied experimentally. The lateral line along the trunk of the animal is innervated by the posterior lateral line nerve, while the canals on the head are innervated by fibers of the anterior lateral line nerve. Details concerning the innervation of the sensory cells of the lateral line are not available. Rather more data are available for the saccule of the inner ear. It has been demonstrated that sensory cells in the inner ear far outnumber the innervating fibers (Flock, 1964; Corwin, 1977; Popper and Northcutt, 1983). Dye injections of single saccular fibers have demonstrated different neuronal classes in the goldfish (Furukawa,

1978). One class innervates sensory cells of only one orientation group (ventral or dorsal), while another class innervates oppositely-polarized cells. These classes were predicted in neurophysiological studies (Furukawa and Ishii, 1967) from the appearance of units that responded to both the rarefaction and compression phases of an acoustic signal. Findings similar to those of Furukawa (1978) have been reported in several non-ostariophysans where individual fibers, for the most part, innervate hair cells in spatially restricted regions of the saccular epithelium (Saidel and Popper, 1983). Furthermore, the saccular branch of the eighth nerve divides in the non-ostariophysan teleost, with one branch going to horizontally-oriented cells and the other to vertically-oriented cells. This division is not found in Ostariophysi (Saidel and Popper, 1983).

Investigations of the central projections of the lateral line and eighth (octavus) nerve have recently been studied with modern neuroanatomical tracing techniques. Several investigators (Boord and Campbell, 1977; Boord and Roberts, 1980; Northcutt, 1980, 1981; Bell, 1981a,b; McCormick, 1981a,b, 1982; and others) have shown that the octavus

Figure 8. Lateral view of the brainstem of the bowfin, *Amia calva*, showing the position of the six nuclei associated with the otic (dark) and lateral line (hatch-marked) endorgans. Ant, anterior octavus nucleus; Caud, nucleus caudalis; CC, cerebellar crest; Desc, descending octavus nucleus; EG, eminentia granularis; Med, nucleus medialis; Mg, nucleus magnocellularis; NALL, anterior lateral line nerve; NVIIIa, anterior ramus of the eighth nerve; NVIIIp, posterior ramus of the eighth nerve; NIX, glossopharyngeal nerve; NX, vagus nerve; NPLL, posterior lateral line nerve; Post, posterior octavus nucleus; V–VII, trigeminal and facial nerves. Bar scale = 1 mm. (From McCormick, 1981a)

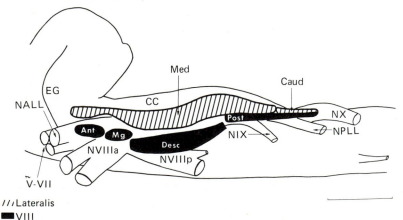

(eighth nerve) projections of the ear are largely separate from the projections of the lateral line at least within the medulla. It is also now clear that the lateral line nerves are not, as indicated in the early literature (e.g. van Bergeijk, 1967), part of any other cranial nerve.

At least five different nuclei are associated with the ear in bony fishes (Figure 8), although one of these nuclei is absent in non-teleost fishes (McCormick, 1981a, 1983a). Several additional nuclei, lying dorsal to those of the ear, are associated with the anterior and posterior lateral line nerves (Figure 8).

The specific projections of individual otic end organs to the various medullary nuclei are well known only in the mormyrid *Gnathonemus*, an electroreceptive fish (Bell, 1981a,b). In *Gnathonemus*, each of the otic endorgans projects to several different nuclei and any one nucleus may receive projections from more than one endorgan. Similar data have been found for other fishes that are not known to have sensory specializations (C. McCormick, 1983a,b; Meredith and Butler, 1983). These observations are in accord with the suggestions that otolith organ functions may overlap, and that a given otolith organ may have multiple functions (von Frisch, 1938; von Holst, 1950; Furukawa and Ishii, 1967; Budelli and Macadar, 1979; Fay and Olsho, 1979; Popper and Tavolga, 1981).

Higher-order projections of the otic and lateral line endorgans are only poorly known. However, investigations using neurophysiology (e.g. Grozzinger, 1967; Page, 1970; Knudsen, 1977; Echteler and Saidel, 1980; Fay, Hillery and Bolan, 1982; Finger and Bullock, 1982) demonstrate involvement of the torus semicircularis, diencephalon and telencephalon in responses to lateral line and inner ear stimulation. Neuroanatomical studies have revealed more specific information about the precise sites of projection of the various octavus nuclei of the medullary region. It now appears that one of these nuclei, the anterior octavolateralis nucleus, projects bilaterally to the midbrain auditory center, the torus semicircularis (possibly homologous to the mammalian inferior colliculus) (Northcutt, 1981), as does the main lateral line nucleus (Knudsen, 1977). However, at least in catfish, regions in the torus receiving input from the ear may be distinguished from regions receiving lateral line input (Knudsen, 1977). There is also evoked potential evidence in goldfish that the midbrain is not homogeneous with regard to relative sound pressure and particle motion sensitivity (Fay et al., 1982). Other octaval nuclei send descending projections to the spinal cord which descend as the vestibulospinal pathways (Northcutt, 1981). Neuroanatomical and physiological data indicate that the torus projects bilaterally to the diencephalon (Braford and McCormick, 1979; Finger, 1981), which in turn has projections to the telencephalon (Echteler and Saidel, 1981; Finger, 1981). The sites of termination of the otic and lateral line projections to the telencephalon are not known, although Northcutt and Braford (1980) suggest that only several of the numerous telencephalic nuclei are involved with these modalities. There is no evidence that the lateral line and octavus inputs converge extensively, at least to the level of the torus (Northcutt, 1981), although whether such convergence occurs at higher brain centers remains an open and important question.

Our knowledge of the function of the auditory CNS in fishes is still limited, particularly with regard to the physiology of the different regions of the brain. While there have been some earlier physiological studies (see above), these were done before investigators had a detailed understanding of the various brain regions associated with audition, and thus precise localization of recording sites within specific auditory centers was not possible. More extensive studies done in conjunction with modern neuroanatomical tracing techniques are now needed. Several major questions which are most interesting are: (1) how is the topography of the macular surface mapped onto the neural tissue, (2) how is periodicity of the acoustic stimulus mapped onto the neural tissue, (3) what are the projections of the ear and lateral line beyond the medulla, (4) to what extent do inputs from the various organs of the ear (and the two ears) converge, and (5) where, if at all, do the lateral line and inner ear projections converge?

Sound localization

It was originally doubted that fishes could localize a sound source in the usual sense without using near-field stimulation of the lateral line system (van Bergeijk, 1964, 1967). At that time, the behavioral evidence for localization ability was contradictory (see Tavolga, 1976b, for the history of this work), and the lateral line hypothesis seemed a reasonable way out of the controversy. In addition, it was evident that the ears were functionally too close together to make use of interaural time and intensity cues normally used by terrestrial vertebrates, particularly considering that the fish is closely impedance-matched to the water environment. In any case, it was recognized that to the extent sound stimulation was input to the ears via the pressure-sensitive swimbladder route, any interaural differences appeared to be impossible.

However, when Moulton and Dixon (1967) demonstrated directional behavioral responses which depended on the integrity of the auditory system (saccule) in goldfish, it became clear that the localization question had to be rethought. (See Schuijf, 1981, for the most recent ideas on this topic.) Subsequent behavioral studies on fishes (Fay, 1969a; Schuijf, Baretta and Wildschut, 1972; Popper, Salmon and Parvelescu, 1973; Chapman and Johnstone, 1974; Schuijf and Sieme-link, 1974; Schuijf, 1975; Schuijf and Buwalda, 1975; Hawkins and Sand, 1977; Schuijf, Visser, Willers and Buwalda, 1977) have helped to confirm that (1) fishes (primarily the cod) can be conditioned to discriminate between different sound sources with minimum audible angles ranging from 8 to over 20 degrees, depending on conditioning method and the signal-to-noise ratio, (2) the otolith organs of the ear are probably responsible for this behavior, (3) discrimination occurs in the median vertical as well as in the horizontal planes, and (4) fishes are not subject to 180° confusions.

One of the important observations made in behavioral studies is that the conditioned directional response of the cod could be inverted 180° by reversing the phase of the sound pressure field relative to a standing wave particle motion field impinging on the animal (Schuijf and Buwalda, 1975). These data and other theoretical considerations have led to the following view of localization mechanisms in fishes. The axis of particle motion is determined by a process termed 'vector detection' which depends on comparing activity across several channels innervating variously-oriented directionally-sensitive receptors. The process depends on the 'direct' detection of particle motion by the otolith organs responding in the accelerometer mode (Dijkgraaf, 1963). This information by itself is not complete since it is subject to a 180° ambiguity (Schuijf, 1975; Schuijf and Buwalda, 1975). In other words, knowing the axis of particle motion does not tell you which end of the axis points to the sound source. For example, a rarefaction pulse arriving from the left could not be discriminated from a compression pulse from the right. In order to determine the direction of wave propagation, Schuijf has suggested that the fish determines the phase (or timing) relations between the particle-motion waveform and the sound-pressure waveform, which depend on the direction of wave propagation with reference to the fish's body frame. This outline of a theory (see Schuijf and Buwalda, 1980; Schuijf, 1981) thus requires details of the particle motion and sound pressure wave form to be input simultaneously, and some mechanism for integrating the information. We do not know whether this integration occurs mechanically at the periphery, or centrally.

There are now neurophysiological data showing that single units of the goldfish (Fay and Olsho, 1979) and cod (Hawkins and Horner, 1981) eighth nerve are clearly directionally sensitive, and evidence for binaural interaction in the midbrain (Horner, Sand and Enger, 1980) in cod. In order for more progress to be made in understanding the physiological mechanisms of directional hearing, systematic neurophysiological studies on directional coding and representation must be carried out at several levels of the auditory system. This is a difficult prescription since the sound fields in these experiments must be both complex and very well controlled in terms of sound pressure level, particle motion amplitude and direction, and the phase relations between them.

Clearly, we are only beginning to understand sound localization and many questions remain to be asked about the specific behavioral capabilities of fishes and the function of the ear and CNS in localization. The most pressing questions are. Do species with different hair-cell orientation patterns localize sound with different acuity? How is directional information extracted by the CNS from the response of the ear? Is auditory space topography represented spatially in the brain?

Conclusions

In this paper we have touched upon some of the questions concerning fish hearing that need to be considered over the next several years. In preparing the 1980 Sarasota meeting (Tavolga et al., 1981) we did a thorough survey of the fish acoustic literature and we found that the growth in work in this area over the past 10 years has far exceeded all work to that time. More significantly, it becomes apparent from a survey of the literature that prior to the early 1970s the questions being asked about fish audition were relatively straightforward and included studies of what fish could hear and what they could discriminate. Interpretation of data was generally done in mammalian terms. Based upon these germinal studies and on data generated in the 1970s, new questions could be asked. We have become far more willing to 'throw out' constraints imposed by thinking in mammalian (or tetrapod) terms and we are now looking at the fish auditory system in a relatively new way. Thus, we are now in a position where the more complex types of questions we have proposed here can be realistically approached experimentally. Many of the questions we have posed here are inter-related to one another, and exploration of one topic will no doubt shed light on others.

We would like to acknowledge, with deep appreciation, the contributions of all of the participants at the 1980 Fish Hearing Conference in Sarasota Florida to the development of many of the ideas in this paper. We would also like to express particular thanks to our collaborators Drs Sheryl Coombs, Catherine A. McCormick, Christopher Platt, William M. Saidel, and William N. Tavolga for their influences on the development of the ideas presented here.

The work done in our laboratories has been supported by NIH grant NS-15090 from the National Institutes of Neurological Diseases and Stroke and by NSF grant BNS 80-09043 to ANP and by grants NS-15268 from NINCDS and BNS 81-11354 from NSF to RRF. Work has also been supported by Research Career Development Awards from NINCDS to ANP and RRF.

References

Bell, C. (1981a). Some central connections of medullary octavolateral centers in a mormyrid fish. In *Hearing and Sound Communication in Fishes*, ed. W. N. Tavolga, A. N. Popper and R. R. Fay, pp. 383–92. New York: Springer-Verlag.

Bell, C. (1981b). Central distribution of octavolateral afferents and efferents in a teleost (Mormyridae). *J. Comp. Neurol. 195:* 391–414.

Blaxter, J. H. S., Denton, E. J., and Gray, J. A. B. (1981). Acoustico-lateralis systems in clupeid fishes. In *Hearing and Sound Communication in Fishes*, ed. W. N. Tavolga, A. N. Popper and R. R. Fay, pp. 39–59. New York: Springer-Verlag.

Boord, R. L., and Campbell, C. B. G. (1977). Structural and functional organization of the lateral line system of sharks. *Am. Zool. 17:* 431–41.

Boord, R. L., and Roberts, B. L. (1980). Medullary and cerebellar projections of the statoacoustic nerve of the dogfish *Ecyliohinus canicila. J. Comp. Neurol. 193:* 57–68.

Boston, J. R. (1981). Modeling the effects of stimulus frequency and intensity on hair cell potentials. In *Hearing and Sound Communication in Fishes*, ed. W. N. Tavolga, A. N. Popper and R. R. Fay, pp. 507–13. New York: Springer-Verlag.

Braford, M., Jr, and McCormick, C. (1979). Some connections of the torus semicircularis in the bowfin, *Amia calva:* a horseradish peroxidase study. *Soc. Neurosci. Abstr. 5:* 139.

Budelli, R., and Macadar, O. (1979). Statoacoustic properties of utricular efferents. *J. Neurophysiol. 42:* 1749–63.

Buerkle, U. (1968). Relation of pure tone thresholds to background noise level in the Atlantic cod (*Gadus morhua*). *J. Fish. Res. Bd Can. 25:* 1155–60.

Buerkle, U. (1969). Auditory masking and the critical band in Atlantic cod (*Gadus morhua*). *J. Fish. Res. Bd Can. 26:* 1113–19.

Bullock, T. H., Northcutt, R. G., and Bodznick, D. A. (1982). Evolution of electroreception. *Trends Neurosci. 5:* 50–3.

Burgess, J. W., and Shaw, E. (1981). Effects of acoustico-lateralis denervation in a facilitative schooling fish: a nearest-neighbor matrix analysis. *Behav. Neur. Biol. 33:* 488–97.

Buwalda, R. J. A. (1981). Segregation of directional and non-directional acoustic information in the cod. In *Hearing and Sound Communication in Fishes*, ed. W. N. Tavolga, A. N. Popper and R. R. Fay, pp. 139–71. New York: Springer-Verlag.

Buwalda, R. J. A., and Van der Steen, J. (1979). The sensitivity of the cod sacculus to directional and non-directional sound stimuli. *Comp. Biochem. Physiol. 64A:* 467–71.

Chapman, C. J. (1973). Field studies of hearing in teleost fish. *Helgolander wiss. Meeresunters. 24:* 371–90.

Chapman, C. J., and Hawkins, A. D. (1973). A field study of hearing in the cod, *Gadus morhua* L. *J. Comp. Physiol. 85:* 147–67.

Chapman, C. J., and Johnstone, A. D. F. (1974). Some auditory discrimination experiments on marine fish. *J. Exp. Biol. 61:* 521–8.

Chapman, C. J., and Sand, O. (1974). Field studies of hearing in two species of flatfish, *Pleuronectes platessa* (L.) and *Limanda limanda* (L.) (Family Pleuronectidae). *Comp. Biochem. Physiol. 47A:* 371–85.

Coombs, S., and Popper, A. N. (1979). Hearing differences among Hawaiian Squirrelfish (family Holocentridae) related to differences in the peripheral auditory system. *J. Comp. Physiol. 132A:* 203–7.

Coombs, S., and Popper, A. N. (1982a). Comparative frequency selectivity in fishes: simultaneously and forward-masked psychophysical tuning curves. *J. Acoust. Soc. Am. 71:* 133–41.

Coombs, S., and Popper, A. N. (1982b). Structure and function of the auditory system in the clown knife fish, *Notopterus chitala. J. Exp. Biol. 97:* 225–39.

Corwin, J. T. (1977). Morphology of the macula neglecta in sharks of the genus *Carcharhinus. J. Morphol. 152:* 341–62.

Corwin, J. T. (1981). Postembryonic production and aging of inner ear hair cells in sharks. *J. Comp. Neurol. 201:* 541–53.

Dale, T. (1976). The labyrinthine mechanoreceptor organs of the cod *Gadus morhua* L. (Teleostei: Gadidae). *Norwegian J. Zool. 24:* 85–128.

Denton, E. J., and Gray, J. A. B. (1980). Receptor activity in the utriculus of the sprat. *J. Mar. Biol. Ass. UK 60:* 717–40.

Dijkgraaf, S. (1952). Über die Schallwahrnehmung bei Meeresfischen. *Z. vergl. Physiol. 34:* 104–22.

Dijkgraaf, S. (1960). Hearing in bony fishes. *Proc. Roy. Soc. Lond. B152:* 51–4.

Dijkgraaf, S. (1963). The functioning and significance of the lateral line organ. *Biol. Rev. 38:* 51–105.

Dijkgraaf, S., and Verheijen, F. (1950). Neue Versuche uber das Tonunterscheidungsvermogen der Elritze. *Z. vergl. Physiol. 32:* 248–56.

Echteler, S. M., and Saidel, W. M. (1981). Forebrain connections in the goldfish support telencephalic homologies with land vertebrates. *Science 212:* 683–5.

Enger, P. S. (1963). Unit activity in the fish auditory system. *Acta Physiol. Scand. 59* (Suppl. *210*): 1–48.

Enger, P. S. (1981). Frequency discrimination in teleosts – central or peripheral? In *Hearing and Sound Communication in Fishes*, ed. W. N. Tavolga, A. N. Popper and R. R. Fay, pp. 243–55. New York: Springer-Verlag.

Fay, R. R. (1969a). Acoustic sensitivity of the goldfish within the acoustic near field. Report No. 605, 1–11, US Navy Sub. Med Center, Groton, Conn.

Fay, R. R. (1969b). Behavioral audiogram for the goldfish. *J. Aud. Res. 9:* 112–21.

Fay, R. R. (1970). Auditory frequency discrimination in the goldfish (*Carassius auratus*). *J. Comp. Physiol. Psychol. 73:* 175–80.

Fay, R. R. (1974a). The masking of tones by noise for the goldfish. *J. Comp. Physiol. Psychol. 87:* 708–16.

Fay, R. R. (1974b). Auditory frequency discrimination in vertebrates. *J. Acoust. Soc. Am. 56:* 206–9.

Fay, R. R. (1978a). Sound detection and sensory coding by the auditory systems of fishes. *The Behavior of Fish and Other Aquatic Animals*, ed. D. Mostofsky, pp. 197–231. New York: Academic Press.

Fay, R. R. (1978b). Coding of information in single auditory nerve fibers of the goldfish. *J. Acoust. Soc. Am. 63:* 136–46.

Fay, R. R. (1978c). Phase-locking in goldfish saccular nerve fibres accounts for frequency discrimination capacities. *Nature 275:* 320–2.

Fay, R. R. (1980). Psychophysics and neurophysiology of temporal factors in hearing by the goldfish: amplitude modulation detection. *J. Neurophysiol. 44:* 312–32.

Fay, R. R. (1981). Coding in acoustic information in the eighth nerve. In *Hearing and Sound Communication in Fishes*, ed. W. N. Tavolga, A. N. Popper and R. R. Fay, pp. 189–221. New York: Springer-Verlag.

Fay, R. R. (1982). Neural mechanisms of an auditory temporal discrimination by the goldfish. *J. Comp. Physiol. 147:* 201–16.

Fay, R. R., Ahroon, W., and Orawski, A. (1978). Auditory masking patterns in the goldfish (*Carassius auratus*): psychophysical tuning curves. *J. Exp. Biol. 74:* 83–100.

Fay, R. R., and Coombs, S. (1983). Neural mechanisms in sound detection and temporal summation. *Hearing Res. 10:* 69–92.

Fay, R. R., Hillery, C. M., and Bolan, K. (1982). Representation of sound pressure and particle motion information in the midbrain of the goldfish. *Comp. Biochem. Physiol. 71A:* 181–91.

Fay, R. R., and Olsho, L. (1979). Discharge patterns of lagenar and saccular neurons of the goldfish eighth nerve: displacement sensitivity and directional characteristics. *Comp. Biochem. Physiol. 62A:* 377–86.

Fay, R. R., and Patricoski, M. L. (1980). Sensory mechanisms of low frequency vibration detection in fishes. In *Abnormal Animal Behavior Preceeding Earthquakes*, ed. R. Buskirk, Conference II. *U.S. Geological Survey Open File Report*, 80–453.

Fay, R. R., and Passow, B. (1982). Temporal discrimination in the goldfish. *J. Acoust. Soc. Am. 72:* 753–60.

Fay, R. R., and Popper, A. N. (1974). Acoustic stimulation of the ear of the goldfish (*Carassius auratus*). *J. Exp. Biol. 61:* 243–60.

Fay, R. R., and Popper, A. N. (1975). Modes of stimulation of the teleost ear. *J. Exp. Biol. 62:* 379–87.

Fay, R. R., and Popper, A. N. (1980). Structure and function in teleost auditory systems. In *Comparative Studies of Hearing in Vertebrates*, ed. A. N. Popper and R. R. Fay, pp. 1–42. New York: Springer-Verlag.

Fettiplace, R., and Crawford, A. C. (1978). Coding of sound pressure and frequency in cochlear hair cells of the terrapin. *Proc. Roy. Soc. Lond. 203:* 209–18.

Fine, M. (1981). Mismatch between sound production and hearing in the oyster toadfish. In *Hearing and Sound Communication in Fishes*, ed. W. N. Tavolga, A. N. Popper and R. R. Fay, pp. 257–63. New York: Springer-Verlag.

Finger, T. E. (1981). Nonolfactory sensory pathways to the telencephalon in teleost fish. *Science, 210:* 671–3.

Finger, T. E., and Bullock, T. H. (1982). Thalamic center for the lateral line system in the catfish, *Ictalurus nebulosus*: evoked potential evidence. *J. Neurobiol. 13:* 39–47.

Flock, Å. (1964). Structure of the macula utriculi with special reference to directional interplay of sensory responses as revealed by morphological polarization. *J. Cell Biol. 22:* 413–31.

Flock, Å. (1965). Electron microscopic and electrophysiological studies on the lateral line canal organ. *Acta Otolaryngol.*, Suppl. *199:* 1–90.

Furukawa, T. (1978). Sites of termination on the saccular macula of auditory nerve fibers in the goldfish as determined by intracellular injection of procion yellow. *J. Comp. Neurol. 180:* 807–14.

Furukawa, T., and Ishii, Y. (1967). Neurophysiological studies of hearing in goldfish. *J. Neurophysiol. 30:* 1377–403.

Furukawa, T., Ishii, Y., and Matsuura, S. (1972). Synaptic delay and time course of post synaptic potentials at the junction of hair cells and eighth nerve fibers of the goldfish. *Jap. J. Physiol. 22:* 617–35.

Furukawa, T., Kuno, M., and Matsuura, S. (1982). Quantal analysis of a decremental response at hair cell-efferent fibre synapses in the goldfish sacculus. *J. Physiol. 322:* 181–95.

Görner, P. (1976). Source localization with labyrinth and lateral line in the clawed toad (*Xenopus laevis*). In *Sound Reception in Fish*, ed. A. Schuijf and A. D. Hawkins, pp. 171–84. Amsterdam: Elsevier.

Green, D. M., and Yost, W. A. (1975). Binaural analysis. In *Handbook of Sensory Physiology*, Vol. V(2), ed. W. D. Keidel and W. D. Neff, pp. 461–80. Berlin: Springer-Verlag.

Grozinger, B. (1967). Elektro-physiologische Untersuchungen an der Horbahn der Schleie (*Tinca tinca* L.). *Z. vergl. Physiol. 57:* 44–76.

Hall, L., Patricoski, M., and Fay, R. R. (1981). Neurophysiological mechanisms of intensity discrimination in the goldfish. In *Hearing and Sound Communication in Fishes*, ed. W. N. Tavolga, A. N. Popper and R. R. Fay, pp. 179–86. New York: Springer-Verlag.

Hawkins, A. D. (1973). The sensitivity of fish to sounds. *Oceanography and Marine Biology Annual Review 11:* 291–340.

Hawkins, A. D. (1981). The hearing abilities of fish. In *Hearing and Sound Communication in Fishes*, ed. W. N. Tavolga, A. N. Popper and R. R. Fay, pp. 109–37. New York: Springer-Verlag.

Hawkins, A. D., and Chapman, C. J. (1975). Masked auditory thresholds in the cod *Gadus morhua* L. *J. Comp. Physiol. 103A:* 209–26.

Hawkins, A. D., and Horner, K. (1981). Directional characteristics of primary auditory neurons from the codfish ear. In *Hearing and Sound Communication in Fishes*, ed. W. N. Tavolga, A. N. Popper and R. R. Fay, pp. 311–28. New York: Springer-Verlag.

Hawkins, A. D., and Johnstone, A. D. F. (1978). The hearing of the Atlantic salmon, *Salmo salar. J. Fish. Biol. 13:* 655–73.

Hawkins, A. D., and Sand, O. (1977). Directional hearing in the median vertical plane by the cod. *J. Comp. Physiol. 122A:* 1–8.

Hillary, C., and Fay, R. R. (1982). Forward masking and suppression in the midbrain of the souther gray treefrog (*Hyla chrysoscelis*). *J. Comp. Physiol.* in press.

Horner, K., Hawkins, A. D., and Fraser, P. J. (1981). Frequency characteristics of primary auditory neurones from the ear of the codfish, *Gadus morhua* L. In *Hearing and Sound Communication in Fishes*, ed. W. N. Tavolga, A. N. Popper and R. R. Fay, pp. 223–41. New York: Springer-Verlag.

Horner, K., Sand, O., and Enger, P. (1980). Binaural interaction in the cod. *J. Exp. Biol.* 85: 323–31.

Houtgast, T. (1972). Psychophysical evidence for lateral inhibition in hearing. *J. Acoust. Soc. Am. 81:* 1885–94.

Hudspeth, A. J., and Corey, D. P. (1977). Sensitivity, polarity, and conductance change in the response of vertebrate hair cells to controlled mechanical stimuli. *Proc. Natn. Acad. Sci. USA 74:* 2407–11.

Iversen, R. T. B. (1969). Auditory thresholds of the scombrid fish (*Euthynnus affinis*), with comments on the use of sound in tuna fishing. *FAO Conference on Fish Behavior in Relation to Fishing Techniques and Tactics. FAO Fisheries Report,* No. 62, 849–59.

Jacobs, D. W., and Tavolga, W. N. (1967). Acoustic intensity limens in the goldfish. *Animal Behav. 15:* 324–35.

Jacobs, D. W., and Tavolga, W. N. (1968). Acoustic frequency discrimination in the goldfish. *Animal Behav. 16:* 67–71.

Jenkins, D. B. (1979). A transmission and scanning electron microscopic study of the saccule in five species of catfishes. *Am. J. Anat. 154:* 81–101.

Jenkins, D. B. (1981). The utricle in *Ictalurus punctatus*. In *Hearing and Sound Communication in Fishes*, ed. W. N. Tavolga, A. N. Popper and R. R. Fay, pp. 73–9. New York: Springer-Verlag.

Knudsen, E. I. (1977). Distinct auditory and lateral line nuclei in the midbrain of catfishes. *J. Comp. Neurol. 73:* 417–32.

Lewis, E. R. (1981). Evolution of inner-ear auditory apparatus in the frog. *Brain Res. 219:* 149–55.

Lewis, E. R., Baird, R. R., Leverenz, E. L., and Koyama, H. (1982). Inner ear: dye injections reveals peripheral origins of specific sensitivities. *Science 215:* 1641–3.

Lewis, E. R., and Li, C. W. (1975). Hair cell types and distributions in the otolithic and auditory organs of the bullfrog. *Brain Res. 83:* 35–50.

Lowenstein, O. (1971). The labyrinth. In *Physiology of Fishes*, vol. 5, ed. W. S. Hoar and D. J. Randall, pp. 207–40. New York: Academic Press.

McCormick, C. A. (1981a). Central projections of the lateral line and eighth nerves in the bowfin, *Amia calva. J. Comp. Neurol. 197:* 1–15.

McCormick, C. (1981b). Comparative neuroanatomy of the octavolateralis area of fishes. In *Hearing and Sound Communication in Fishes*, ed. W. N. Tavolga, A. N. Popper and R. R. Fay, pp. 375–82. New York: Springer-Verlag.

McCormick, C. A. (1983a). Organization and evolution of the octavolateralis area in fishes. In *Fish Neurobiology and Behavior*, ed. R. G. Northcutt and R. E. Davis, pp. 179–213. Ann Arbor: University of Michigan Press.

McCormick, C. A. (1983b). Central projections of inner ear endorgans in the bowfin, *Amia calva. Amer. Zool.*, in press.

Meredith, G. E., and Butler, A. B. (1983). Organization of eighth nerve afferent projections from individual endorgans of the inner ear in the teleost, *Astronotus ocellatus. J. Comp. Neurol.*, in press.

Michelsen, A. (1978). Sound reception in different environments. In *Sensory Ecology*, ed. M. A. Ali, pp. 345–73. New York: Plenum Press.

Miller, M. R. (1980). The reptilian cochlear duct. In *Comparative Studies of Hearing in Vertebrates*, ed. A. N. Popper and R. R. Fay, pp. 169–204. New York: Springer-Verlag.

Moeng, R. (1978). Characterization of saccular nerve responses in the catfish. *J. Acoust. Soc. Am. 64:* S85.

Moulton, J. M. (1963). Acoustic behaviour of fishes. In *Acoustic Behaviour of Animals*, ed. R. G. Busnel, pp. 655–93. Amsterdam: Elsevier.

Moulton, J. M., and Dixon, R. H. (1967). Directional hearing in fishes. In *Marine Bio-Acoustics, II*, ed. W. N. Tavolga, pp. 187–228. Oxford: Pergamon Press.

Mountcastle, V. B., Talbot, W., Sakata, H., and Hyvarinen, J. (1969). Cortical neuronal mechanisms in flutter vibration studied in unanesthetized monkeys. *J. Neurophysiol. 32:* 542–84.

Myrberg, A. A., Jr, Spanier, E., and Ha, S. J. (1978). Temporal patterning in acoustical communication. In *Contrasts in Behavior*, ed. E. Reese and F. Lighter, pp. 138–79. New York: J. Wiley and Sons.

Myrberg, A. A., Jr., and Spires, J. Y. (1972). Sound discrimination by the bicolor damselfish, *Eupomacentrus partitius. J. Exp. Biol. 57:* 727–35.

Northcutt, R. G. (1979). Primary projections of VIII nerve afferents in a teleost, *Gillichthys mirabilis. Anat. Rec. 193:* 638.

Northcutt, R. G. (1980). Central auditory pathways in anamniotic vertebrates. In *Comparative Studies of Hearing in Vertebrates*, ed. A. N. Popper and R. R. Fay, pp. 79–118. New York: Springer-Verlag.

Northcutt, R. G. (1981). Audition in the central nervous system of fishes. In *Hearing and Sound Communication in Fishes*, ed. W. N. Tavolga, A. N. Popper and R. R. Fay, pp. 331–55. New York: Springer-Verlag.

Northcutt, R. G., and Braford, M., Jr (1980). New observations on the organization and evolution of the telencephalon of the Actinopterygian fishes. In *Comparative Neurology of the Telencephalon*, ed. S. O. E. Ebbesson, pp. 41–98. New York: Plenum.

O'Connell, C. P. (1955). The gas bladder and its relation to the inner ear in *Sardinops caerulea* and *Engraulis mordax. Fish. Bull. 56:* 505–33.

Offutt, G. C. (1967). Integration of the energy in repeated tone pulses by man and the goldfish. *J. Acoust. Soc. Am. 41:* 13–19.

Page, C. H. (1970). Electrophysiological study of auditory responses in the goldfish brain. *J. Neurophysiol. 33:* 116–27.

Partridge, B. L. (1981). Lateral line function and the internal dynamics of fish schools. In *Hearing and Sound Communication in Fishes*, ed. W. N. Tavolga, A. N. Popper and R. R. Fay, pp. 515–22. New York: Springer-Verlag.

Piddington, R. W. (1972). Auditory discrimination between compressions and rarefactions by goldfish. *J. Exp. Biol. 56:* 403–19.

Platt, C. (1977). Hair cell distribution and orientation in goldfish otolith organs. *J. Comp. Neurol. 172:* 283–97.

Platt, C., and Popper, A. N. (1981a). Fine structure and function of the ear. In *Hearing and Sound Communication in Fishes*, ed. W. N. Tavolga, A. N. Popper and R. R. Fay, pp. 3–38. New York: Springer-Verlag.

Platt, C., and Popper, A. N. (1981b). Otolith organ receptor morphology in herring-like fishes. In *The Vestibular System: Function and Morphology*, ed. T. Gualtierotti, pp. 64–76. New York: Springer-Verlag.

Poggendorf, D. (1952). Die absoluten Horschwellen des Zwergwelses (*Amiurus nebulosus*) und Beitrage zur Physik des Weberschen Apparatus der Ostariophysen. *Z. vergl. Physiol. 34:* 222–57.

Popper, A. N. (1970). Auditory capacities of the Mexican blind cave fish (*Astyanax jordani*) and its eyed ancestor (*Astyanax mexicanus*). *Animal Behav. 32:* 552–62.

Popper, A. N. (1972). Auditory threshold in the goldfish (*Carassius auratus*) as a function of signal duration. *J. Acoust. Soc. Am. 52:* 596–602.

Popper, A. N. (1976). Ultrastructure of the auditory regions in the inner ear of the lake whitefish. *Science 192:* 1020–3.

Popper, A. N. (1977). A scanning electron microscopic study of the sacculus and lagena in the ears of fifteen species of teleost fishes. *J. Morphol. 153:* 397–418.

Popper, A. N. (1978). Scanning electron microscopic study of the otolithic organs in the bichir (*Polypterus bichir*) and shovel-nose sturgeon (*Scaphirhynchus platorynchus*). *J. Comp. Neurol. 181:* 117–28.

Popper, A. N. (1979). The ultrastructure of the sacculus and lagena in a moray eel (*Gymnothorax* sp.). *J. Morphol. 161:* 241–56.

Popper, A. N. (1980). Scanning electron microscopic study of the sacculus and lagena in several deep sea fishes. *Am. J. Anat. 157:* 115–36.

Popper, A. N. (1981). Comparative scanning electron microscopic investigations of the sensory epithelia in the teleost sacculus and lagena. *J. Comp. Neurol. 200:* 357–74.

Popper, A. N. (1983). Organization of the inner ear and auditory processing. In *Fish Neurobiology and Behavior*, ed. R. G. Northcutt and R. E. Davis, pp. 125–78. Ann Arbor: University of Michigan Press.

Popper, A. N., and Clarke, N. L. (1979). Non-simultaneous auditory masking in the goldfish *Carassius auratus*. *J. Exp. Biol. 83:* 145–58.

Popper, A. N., and Coombs, S. (1982). The morphology and evolution of the ear in Actinopterygian fishes. *Am. Zool. 22:* 311–28.

Popper, A. N., and Fay, R. R. (1973). Sound detection and processing by teleost fishes: a critical review. *J. Acoust. Soc. Am. 53:* 1515–29.

Popper, A. N., and Hoxter, B. (1981). The fine structure of the sacculus and lagena of a teleost fish. *Hearing Res. 5:* 245–63.

Popper, A. N., and Northcutt, R. G. (1983). Structure and innervation of the inner ear of the bowfin, *Amia calva*. *J. Comp. Neurol. 213:* 279–86.

Popper, A. N., and Platt, C. (1979). The herring ear has a unique receptor pattern. *Nature 280:* 832–3.

Popper, A. N., Platt, C., and Saidel, W. M. (1982). Acoustic functions in the fish ear. *Trends in Neurosci. 5:* 276–80.

Popper, A. N., Salmon, M., and Parvulescu, A. (1973). Sound localization by the Hawaiian squirrelfishes, *Myripristis berndti* and *M. argyromus*. *Animal Behav. 21:* 86–97.

Popper, A. N., and Tavolga, W. N. (1981). Sound detection and inner ear structure in the marine catfish, *Arius felis*. *J. Comp. Physiol. 144:* 27–34.

Pumphrey, R. J. (1950). Hearing. In *Physiological Mechanisms in Animal Behavior*, *Symp. Soc. Exp. Biol. 4:* 3–18.

Retzius, G. (1881). *Das Gehörorgan der Wirbelthiere*, vol. I. Stockholm: Samson and Wallin.

Saidel, W. M., and Popper, A. N. (1983). Spatial organization in the saccule and lagena of a teleost: hair cell pattern and innervation. *J. Morphol.*, in press.

Sand, O. (1981). The lateral-line and sound reception. In *Hearing and Sound Communication in Fishes*, ed. W. N. Tavolga, A. N. Popper and R. R. Fay, pp. 459–81. New York: Springer-Verlag.

Sand, O., and Michelsen, A. (1978). Vibration measurements of the perch saccular otolith. *J. Comp. Physiol. 123A:* 85–9.

Schuijf, A. (1975). Directional hearing of cod (*Gadus morhua*) under approximate free field conditions. *J. Comp. Physiol. 98:* 307–32.

Schuijf, A. (1981). Models of acoustic localization. In *Hearing and Sound Communication in Fishes*, ed. W. N. Tavolga, A. N. Popper and R. R. Fay, pp. 267–310. New York: Springer-Verlag.

Schuijf, A., Baretta, J. W., and Wildschut, J. T. (1972). A field investigation on the discrimination of sound direction in *Labrus berggylta* (Pisces: Perciformes). *Netherlands J. Zool. 22:* 81–104.

Schuijf, A., and Buwalda, R. J. A. (1975). On the mechanism of directional hearing in cod (*Gadus morhua* L.). *J. Comp. Physiol. 98:* 333–43.

Schuijf, A., and Buwalda, R. J. A. (1980). Underwater localization – a major problem in fish acoustics. In *Comparative Studies of Hearing in Vertebrates*, ed. A. N. Popper and R. R. Fay, pp. 43–77. New York: Springer-Verlag.

Schuijf, A., and Hawkins, A. D. (eds). (1976). *Sound Reception in Fish*. Amsterdam: Elsevier.

Schuijf, A., and Siemelink, M. E. (1974). The ability of cod (*Gadus morhua*) to orient towards a sound source. *Experientia 30:* 773–4.

Schuijf, A., Visser, C., Willers, A. F. M., and Buwalda, R. J. A. (1977). Acoustic localization in an ostariophysan fish. *Experientia 33:* 1062–3.

Schwartz, E. (1967). Analysis of surface-wave perception in some teleosts. In *Lateral Line Detectors*, ed. P. Cahn, pp. 123–34. Bloomington: Indiana University Press.

Shen, J., Coombs, S., Fay, R. R., Popper, A. N., and Saidel, W. M. (1982). Hearing in the jewel cichlid. *J. Acoust. Soc. Am. 71:* S49.

Spanier, E. (1979). Aspects of species recognition by sound in four species of damselfish, genus *Eupomacentrus* (Pisces: Pomacentridae). *Z. Tierpsychol. 51:* 301–16.

Stetter, H. (1929). Untersuchungen uber den Gehorsinn der Fische besonders von *Phoxinus laevis* L. und *Amiurus nebulosus* Raf. *Z. vergl. Physiol. 9:* 339–477.

Stipetic, E. (1939). Über das Gehororgan der Mormyriden. *Z. vergl. Physiol. 26:* 740–52.

Strelioff, D., and Sokolich, W. G. (1981). Stimulation of lateral-line sensory cells. In *Hearing and Sound Communication in Fishes*, ed. W. N. Tavolga, A. N. Popper and R. R. Fay, pp. 481–505. New York: Springer-Verlag.

Tavolga, W. N., ed. (1964). *Marine Bio-Acoustics*. Oxford: Pergamon Press.

Tavolga, W. N., ed. (1967). *Marine Bio-Acoustics, II*. Oxford: Pergamon Press.

Tavolga, W. N. (1967). Masked auditory thresholds in teleost fishes. In: *Marine Bio-Acoustics, II*, ed. W. N. Tavolga, pp. 233–45. Oxford: Pergamon Press.

Tavolga, W. N. (1971). Sound production and detection. In *Fish Physiology*, vol. V, ed. W. S. Hoar and D. J. Randall, pp. 135–205. New York: Academic Press.

Tavolga, W. N. (1974). Signal/noise ratio and the critical band in fishes. *J. Acoust. Soc. Am. 55:* 1323–33.

Tavolga, W. N., ed. (1976a). *Sound Reception in Fishes* – Benchmark Papers in Animal Behavior, vol. 7. Stroudsburg, Pa.: Dowden, Hutchinson & Ross.

Tavolga, W. N. (1976b). Acoustic obstacle detection in the sea catfish (*Arius felis*). In *Sound Reception in Fish*, ed. A. Schuijf and A. D. Hawkins, pp. 184–204. Amsterdam: Elsevier.

Tavolga, W. N. (1982). Auditory acuity in the sea catfish (*Arius felis*). *J. Exp. Biol. 96:* 367–76.

Tavolga, W. N., Popper, A. N., and Fay, R. R. eds (1981). *Hearing and Sound Communication in Fishes*. New York: Springer-Verlag.

Turner, R. G., Muraski, A. A., and Nielsen, D. W. (1981). Cilium length: influence on neural tonotopic organization. *Science 213:* 1519–21.

van Bergeijk, W. A. (1964). Directional and nondirectional hearing in fish. In *Marine Bio-Acoustics*, ed. W. N. Tavolga, pp. 281–99. Oxford: Pergamon Press.

van Bergeijk, W. A. (1967). The evolution of vertebrate hearing. In *Contributions to Sensory Physiology*, ed. W. D. Neff, pp. 1–49. New York: Academic Press.

von Frisch, K. (1938). Über die Bedeutung des Sacculus und der Lagena für den Gehörsinn der Fische. *Z. vergl. Physiol. 25:* 703–47.

von Holst, E. (1950). Die Arbeitsweise des Statolithenapparates bei Fischen. *Z. vergl. Physiol. 32:* 60–120.

Wersäll, J. (1961). Vestibular receptor cells in fish and mammals. *Acta Otolaryngologica* (Suppl.) *163:* 25–9.

Wever, E. G. (1978). *The Reptile Ear.* Princeton: Princeton University Press.

Wohlfahrt, T. A. (1939). Untersuchungen über das Tonunterscheidungsvermogen der Elritze (*Phoxinus laevis* Agass). *Z. vergl. Physiol. 26:* 590–604.

Zwislocki, J. (1969). Temporal summation of loudness: an analysis. *J. Acoust. Soc. Am. 46:* 431–41.

1.5

Spatial receptive fields in the auditory system

MASAKAZU KONISHI

The concept of a receptive field was first introduced by Hartline (1938) in his study of single optic fibers in the frog's retina. He wrote: 'No description of the optic response in single fibers would be complete without a description of the region of the retina which must be illuminated in order to obtain a response in any given fiber. This region will be termed the receptive field of the fiber. The location of the receptive field of a given fiber is fixed'. In the vertebrate visual, somatosensory and electroceptive systems the spatial distribution of receptors and its topographical projections onto central neural structures underlie the formation of single units' receptive fields and brain sensory maps. In these systems the peripheral receptors, by virtue of their spatial distribution, can encode the location of a stimulus. In contrast with these systems the spatial distribution of receptors in the auditory system is used to encode sound frequencies instead of locations. This fact would seem to preclude the formation of units' spatial fields in the vertebrate auditory system.

Although its theoretical significance was not recognized, the concept of a receptive field was applied to the auditory system particularly in connection with auditory–visual bimodal neurons, which responded both to visual and auditory stimuli located in the same restricted area in space (Wickelgren, 1971). Since this area, corresponding to a retinal area, is called a visual receptive field, it would seem justifiable to call it an auditory receptive field as well. However, the above consideration predicts that the neural mechanisms underlying an auditory receptive field should be completely different from those of a visual receptive field.

103

Receptive fields in the owl's auditory system

The anterolateral margin of the barn owl's midbrain nucleus, nucleus mesencephalicus lateralis dorsalis (MLD), the avian homolog of the inferior colliculus, contains neurons which respond only to an appropriate sound stimulus located in a small restricted area in space (Figure 1). These neurons share two other response properties: (i) the shape and size of this area are virtually independent of the nature and the intensity of the sound stimulus, and (ii) they respond selectively to the high-frequency end (5 to 8.7 kHz) of the barn owl's audible range. These units will be called here space-mapped neurons (Knudsen, Konishi and Pettigrew, 1977; Knudsen and Konishi, 1978a,b). The

Figure 1. The receptive field of an auditory neuron depicted from the observer's point of view. The owl is shown facing out from the center of the stimulus sphere (dashed globe) and the unit's receptive field (25° in azimuth by 62° in elevation) is projected onto the sphere (diagonally lined area). The unit was located in the owl's left hemisphere; its field dimensions were independent of stimulus intensity. Below and to the right are shown peristimulus-time histograms of the unit's responses to a sound stimulus presented at different locations within its receptive field. The stimulus was a 200-ms noise burst, 20 dB above threshold, delivered once per second. Each histogram is a 500-ms sample and represents 16 stimulus repetitions. Notice the increasing response vigor as the sound source approaches the center of the unit's receptive field. (From Knudsen, Konishi and Pettigrew, 1977.)

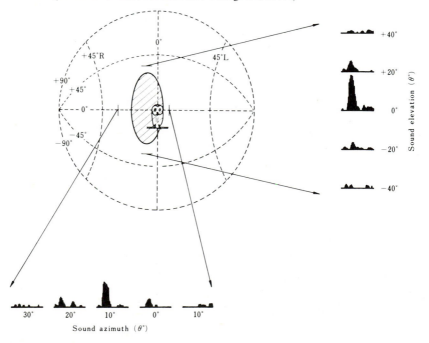

shape of an auditory receptive field is usually a vertically-elongated ellipse with a slight tilt to the owl's right. In rare cases, a unit's field is a narrow vertical band without any elevational boundary. The size of a receptive field ranges from 7 to 39° in azimuth and 23° to 'unrestricted' in elevation. Within a unit's field boundaries there is always an area, called the best area, where the unit shows the lowest threshold. The best area usually corresponds to the azimuthal center of the field, but it need not always correspond to the geometrical center of its elevational axis.

Figure 2. Effect of sound intensity and sound type on the receptive-field plots of space-mapped units. (A) Receptive fields of two units plotted with wide-band noise bursts at 10 dB (open circles) and 30 dB (closed circles) above threshold. The field of the unit on the left expands and the one on the right contracts at the higher sound intensity. Both units exhibited secondary areas behind the owl's head to 30-dB noise bursts. (B) Receptive fields of two units plotted with noise bursts. CF-tone bursts, and clicks, each presented at 30 dB above threshold. The unit on the left is typical of many units. The unit on the right represents the most extreme case of receptive-field variation owing to sound type. (From Knudsen and Konishi, 1978b.)

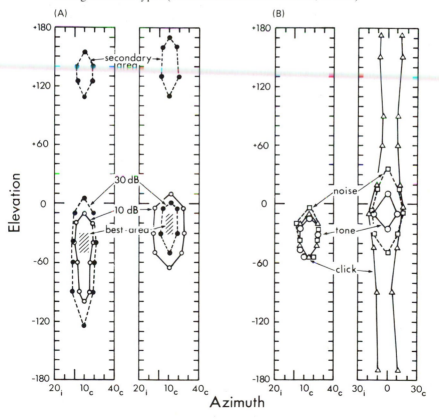

The size as well as the shape of a receptive field is little affected by changes in the intensity of the sound stimulus; an increase in sound intensity by as much as 20 dB may cause only a small expansion (2°) in the azimuthal borders of receptive fields. In some cases, an increase in sound intensity results in a slight decrease in the field size (Figure 2). Insensitivity to changes in sound intensity of this magnitude cannot be explained by the directionality of the owl's ears. Instead, some form of space-dependent neuronal processing must prevent sound stimuli located outside the unit's receptive field from exciting the unit. This process involves inhibition in which a sound outside the receptive field prevents the unit from responding to a sound inside it. Using two sound sources, inside and outside the field, it is possible to show that differences in sound intensity between them affect both the degree of

Figure 3. Center-surround receptive field organization of two space-mapped units in the MLD of the barn owl. Inhibitory areas are stippled; best areas are marked by a +. These fields were measured through use of 5-dB noise bursts from the driving speaker and 10-dB noise bursts from the roving speaker. A 5-dB increase in the noise level from the roving speaker caused the inhibitory areas to completely encircle the excitatory areas and to encompass large areas behind the owl's head. Above are the projections of the fields onto spherical coordinates of auditory space. Below are three-dimensional plots of the units' response to 10 noise bursts (*Y* dimension) as a function of the roving speaker's location (*X* and *Z* dimensions) plotted on linear coordinates. Both units were recorded in the anterior lateral portion of the right MLD. (From Knudsen and Konishi, 1978c.)

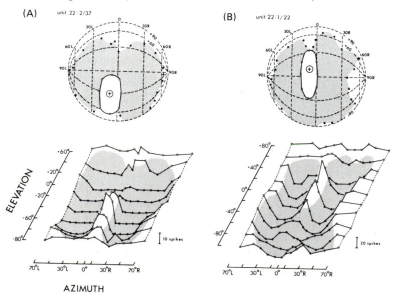

inhibition and the extent of the inhibitory surround. For any given unit, inhibition increases as the sound source moves in from the periphery and approaches the borders of its receptive field (Figure 3). As the source enters the unit's field, the effect of the sound changes from inhibitory to excitatory or neutral within a few degrees of movement. This transition is dramatic for azimuthal speaker movements, whereas transitions in elevation tend to be more gradual (Knudsen and Konishi, 1978c).

Receptive fields use binaural disparities

As discussed before, information from one ear is insufficient to define the location of sound. In fact, just as owls fail to localize sound with one ear, so do auditory receptive fields disappear when one ear is completely plugged. This indicates that the formation of receptive fields requires binaural cues. There are two kinds of binaural cues, intensity and time differences between the ears.

When one ear is in the 'shadow' of the head, it receives a less intense sound than the other ear, creating an interaural intensity difference or disparity. The same effects occur if the directionality of one ear differs from that of the other as in the barn owl. For high frequencies (6–8 kHz) the owl's ears show greater sensitivity differences in elevation than in azimuth: the right ear is more sensitive above the eye level, while the left ear is more sensitive below it. This vertical disparity is due to the vertically asymmetric positions of the ear-openings (Knudsen and Konishi, 1979).

The role of binaural intensity disparity in the formation of receptive fields can be easily demonstrated (Figure 4). Partial plugging of one ear which changes normal binaural disparities causes a shift in the location of a receptive field, meaning that the sound source must be moved to a new location in order to excite the unit: a left plug moves the field down and to the left of its original location, while a right plug moves it up and to the right of its original location. The magnitude of the field shifts increases with the density of the plugging material and the firmness of its placement in the ear canal. However, the shifts in elevation are about twice as large as the shifts in azimuth for all types of occlusion. Furthermore, when monaural occlusion alters the size of a receptive field, as is often the case, it is the vertical dimension of the field that is predominantly affected. These results indicate that both the elevational position and boundaries of a receptive field are determined by binaural intensity disparity (Knudsen and Konishi, 1980).

When a sound emanates from anywhere outside the mid-sagittal plane of the head, the sound paths to the two ears are different, creating an interaural difference in the time of arrival which will be called a transient time disparity. The arrival time refers to the time of arrival of the first wave of the signal. A binaural difference in arrival time obviously causes a binaural disparity in the rest of the signal waveform.

Figure 4. Shift in the location of space-mapped unit receptive field caused by monaural occlusion is demonstrated by two independent methods: conventional receptive-field plots (lower left) and spike counts to repetitive stimuli that were delivered at various locations in the unit's field (above and to the right). The stimulus was a wide-band noise burst presented at 20 dB above threshold for each condition. Occlusion was accomplished by means of a firmly placed clay plug. Spike totals for 10 stimulus presentations are plotted as a function of speaker location for three conditions: unplugged (filled circles), left ear plugged (open circles), and right ear plugged (open triangles). Totals were accumulated at regular 5° intervals in azimuth, and 5 or 10° intervals in elevation. Lines connecting points on the spike-count graphs are to enhance visual inspection of the data and are not intended to interpolate the unit's response to sounds located between the sampled points. Best area was quantified by fitting a parabolic curve to these data and determining the location of its maximum value. In the lower left, the receptive-field borders and best-area locations are plotted in azimuth and elevation for the three conditions. Unplugged best area is designated by an asterisk, right-plug best area by an R, and left-plug best area by an L. (From Knudsen and Konishi, 1980.)

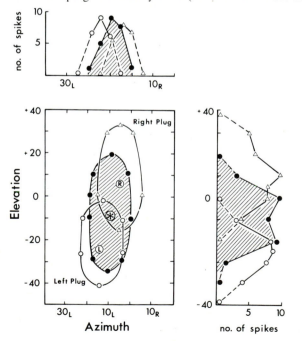

This will be called an ongoing time disparity and corresponds to a binaural phase difference in tonal signals. If the owl uses binaural time disparity, it must, due to its small head, be able to discriminate extremely small time differences. Measurement with small microphones installed near the owl's ear-drums shows that the time differences are in the microsecond range and that they vary as a function of sound azimuth.

By combining the free field and dichotic modes of stimulation, it is possible to examine the role of binaural time disparity in the formation of a receptive field. The free-field method with a movable speaker is used to determine the receptive field of a unit and then earphones are used to present dichotic stimuli so as to control binaural intensity and time disparities independently of each other.

The results of these experiments show that space-mapped neurons are tuned to a particular range of ongoing time disparity, while they are insensitive to variation in transient time disparity (Figure 5). They respond neither to monaural stimuli nor to binaural stimuli with ongoing time disparity set outside their tuned ranges. 'Wrong' ongoing time disparity often inhibits these neurons, as expected from the excitatory

Figure 5. Tuning of space-mapped neurons to binaural time disparity. Each space-mapped neuron is tuned to a specific range of ongoing time differences in the microsecond range. The tuning curves of the most and least sharply tuned neurons from MLD are shown. (From Moiseff and Konishi, 1981.)

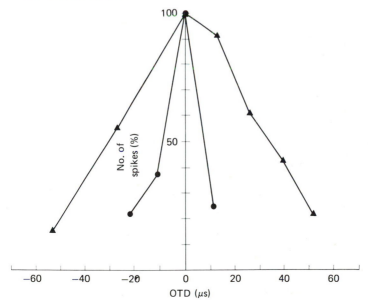

and inhibitory interaction mentioned above. The sharpness of tuning varies from unit to unit. Units with narrow azimuthal widths have narrow tuning curves. Since binaural temporal disparity varies as a function of sound azimuth, the azimuthal location of a unit's receptive field is related to the unit's most preferred ongoing time disparity (Figure 6). These results indicate that the azimuthal location as well as the width of a unit's receptive field is determined by the unit's tuning to a particular range of ongoing time disparity (Moiseff and Konishi, 1981).

Receptive field from neuronal AND gate

The space-mapped neuron is not excitable unless both binaural time and intensity disparities lie simultaneously within the range to which it is tuned. Thus, the neuron behaves like an AND gate and this is how a receptive field is formed (Figure 7).

A neural map of auditory space

The presence of spatial receptive fields in the owl's auditory system immediately poses the question of whether there is any systematic relationship between a unit's anatomical locus and the location of its receptive field; in other words, whether there is a neural map of auditory space. Systematic probing of the anterolateral margin of MLD reveals such a map (Figure 8). The azimuthal locations of receptive fields determined during a dorsoventral traverse across the nucleus tend

Figure 6. Ongoing time disparity determines receptive-field azimuth. The azimuthal center of a unit's receptive field is a linear function of the ongoing time disparity to which the unit responds best. Minus signs on the ordinate indicate the left side and those on the abscissa the left ear leading. (From Moiseff and Konishi, 1981.)

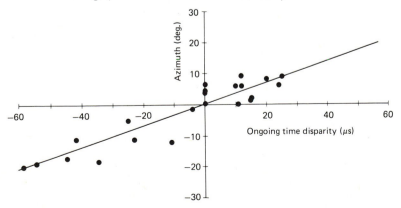

to be very similar; as the locus of penetration shifts posterolaterally along the anterolateral margin of the nucleus, receptive fields' azimuths gradually shift over a range of about 55° from ipsilateral 15° across the midline (0°) to contralateral 40°. Receptive fields' elevations change systematically with the depth of penetration, the dorsal, intermediate and ventral parts of the nucleus corresponding respectively to high, intermediate and low receptive fields' positions. Again few units have their receptive fields beyond about 40° above or below the horizontal plane (0° elevation). It is noteworthy that a disproportionate number of units have their receptive fields within 30° (15° on each side) of the midline of the face where the owl localizes sound most accurately (Knudsen and Konishi, 1978a,b).

It was pointed out earlier that auditory receptive fields differ from visual receptive fields in terms of the underlying neural connectivity involved. By the same token the neural map of auditory space is based on a principle which is entirely different from that underlying the map of visual space. The visual map owes its origin to the principle of topographical projection, whereas the auditory space map is derived from neural processing of binaural input (Konishi and Knudsen, 1982). Despite this basic difference, the auditory neurons are arranged so as to 'project' the positions of their receptive fields topographically to their anatomical loci. It is noteworthy that there is a visual–auditory bimodal map in the owl's optic tectum (Knudsen, 1982). This requires that the

Figure 7. Space-mapped neuron as an AND gate of intensity and time disparities. (A) Unit's receptive field, the vertical bar indicates the number of spikes obtained in 32-stimulus presentations. (B) Tuning of the same unit to ongoing time disparity. (C) Tuning of the same unit to binaural intensity disparity. In this case the unit responded only when both binaural time and intensity disparities lay simultaneously within the range shown in B and C. (From Moiseff and Konishi, 1981.)

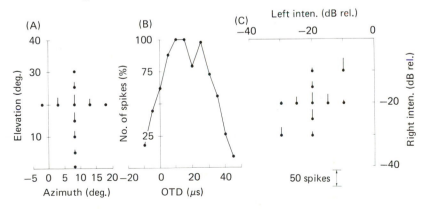

Figure 8. A neural map of auditory space. In the upper left, coordinates of auditory space are depicted as a globe surrounding the owl. Projected onto the globe are the receptive-field best areas (solid-lined rectangles) of 14 units that were recorded in four separate penetrations. The large numbers backed by the same symbols (dark diamonds, triangles, etc.) represent units from the same penetration; the numbers themselves denote the order in which the units were encountered. Penetrations were made with the electrode oriented parallel to the transverse plane of MLD at positions indicated in the horizontal section by solid arrows. Below and to the right of the globe are illustrated three histological sections through MLD in the horizontal, transverse, and sagittal planes. The stippled portion of MLD corresponds to the space-mapped region. Isoazimuth contours, based on field centers, are shown as solid lines in the horizontal and sagittal sections; isoelevation contours are represented by dashed lines in the transverse and sagittal sections. On each section, dashed arrows indicate planes of the other two sections. Solid, crossed arrows to the lower right of each section define the orientation of the section: a, anterior; d, dorsal; l, lateral; m, medial; p, posterior; v, ventral. OT denotes the optic tectum. (From Knudsen and Konishi, 1978a.)

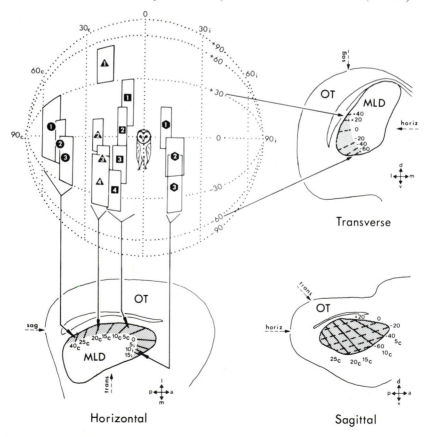

non-projectional auditory map be matched topographically with the projectional visual map. The significance of this matching is that these maps of different origin are functionally equivalent. This supports the idea that the map of auditory space is not an epiphenomenon but a method of encoding auditory space in the brain.

This research was supported by a National Institutes of Health grant.

References

Hartline, H. K. (1938). The response of single optic nerve fibers of the vertebrate eye to illumination of the retina. *Am. J. Physiol. 121:* 400–15.

Knudsen, E. I. (1982). Auditory and visual maps of space in the optic tectum of the owl. *J. Neurosci. 2:* 1177–94.

Knudsen, E. I., and Konishi, M. (1978a). A neural map of auditory space in the owl. *Science 200:* 795–7.

Knudsen, E. I., and Konishi, M. (1978b). Space and frequency are represented separately in auditory midbrain of the owl. *J. Neurophysiol. 41:* 870–84.

Knudsen, E. I., and Konishi, M. (1978c). Center-surround organization of auditory receptive fields in the owl. *Science 202:* 778–80.

Knudsen, E. I., and Konishi, M. (1979). Mechanisms of sound localization in the barn owl (*Tyto alba*). *J. Comp. Physiol. 133:* 13–21.

Knudsen, E. I., and Konishi, M. (1980). Monaural occlusion shifts receptive-field locations of auditory midbrain units in the owl. *J. Neurophysiol. 44:* 687–95.

Knudsen, E. I., Konishi, M., and Pettigrew, J. D. (1977). Receptive fields of auditory neurons in the owl. *Science 198:* 1278–80.

Konishi, M., and Knudsen, E. I. (1982). A theory of neural auditory space. In *Cortical Sensory Organization*, vol. 3, ed. C. N. Woolsey, Multiple Auditory Areas, chapter 7. Clifton, N.J.: Humana Press.

Moiseff, A., and Konishi, M. (1981). Neuronal and behavioral sensitivity to binaural time differences in the owl. *J. Neurosci. 1:* 40–8.

Wickelgren, B. G. (1971). Superior colliculus: some receptive field properties of bimodally responsive cells. *Science 177:* 69–71.

1.6

Auditory basis of echolocation in bats

GERHARD NEUWEILER

In this review mainly based on experiments from our own laboratories, the excellent performances in frequency and time analysis in the auditory system of echolocating bats are reported. Bats are mammals and possess a typical mammalian auditory system. The efficiency of echolocating bats is therefore discussed within the context of general mammalian auditory physiology.

Frequency analysis

In those bat species emitting broadband frequency-modulated (FM) or multiharmonic signals the audiograms recorded as thresholds of collicular evoked potentials are broadly tuned to a wide range of frequencies with shallow sensitivity maxima ranging from 20–30 kHz up to 150 kHz, depending on the frequency band emitted by the species. However, non-echolocating megachiropteran species also hear in the same frequency range as echolocating bats emitting broad band signals. Many echolocating and non-echolocating bats cannot be told apart by their hearing capacities (Figure 1). In fact most small mammals including cats would qualify as echolocators if good perception of high-frequency sounds above 20 kHz were a criterium.

The frequency fovea in horseshoe bats

The situation is different for a small group of bats which probe the nights with a unique echolocation sound (Figure 1). They emit a long (10–100 ms) pure tone of a species-specific frequency. This pure tone is frequently preceded by a short upward sweep and always terminated by a narrow downward frequency-modulated sweep. Bat species emitting this type of a combined constant frequency

115

(CF)-frequency-modulated (FM) signal are called CF-FM bats. All rhinolophid species so far investigated (*Rhinolophus ferrumequinum, Rh. rouxi, Rh. euryale, Rh. philippinensis, Rh. megaphyllus*), at least some of the hipposiderids, and the neotropical bat *Pteronotus parnellii* (Phyllostomatides) belong in this category.

CF-FM bats use the long pure tone as a carrier frequency for

Figure 1. Audiograms of non-echolocating and echolocating bats. Inferior colliculus (N_4)-evoked potential thresholds were recorded. Insets: Sonagrams of echolocation sounds. Black bars below audiograms indicate frequency range of the species' echolocation sound. Audiograms of bats emitting long pure tones (CF-FM bats) include narrow filters precisely tuned to the echo-frequency heard. Audiograms of bats emitting broad band signals (e.g. *Molossus ater*) and of non-echolocating bats are broadly tuned with minimal thresholds in the high frequency range. (After Grinnell and Hagiwara, 1972; Vater, Schlegel and Zöller, 1979; Neuweiler, 1970; Grinnell, 1970.)

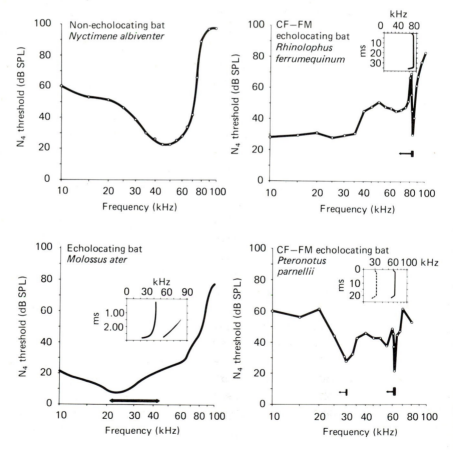

detecting fluttering targets, i.e. flying insects. When the echolocation pure tone bounces onto a wing-beating insect, Doppler shifts due to the speed and complex movements of their wings will impose small frequency and amplitude modulations onto the reflected pure tone echo. Thus fast and brisk movements of the prey and the periodicity of its wing beats are encoded onto the echo of the emitted carrier by distinct modulation patterns (Figure 8, p. 130).

The bats eliminate the effects of their own flight speeds from this movement-sensitive system. Depending on the bat's speed, echoes returning from any object will be Doppler shifted to higher frequencies (Schnitzler, 1967). The bat compensates for these Doppler shifts by lowering the emitted frequency by such an amount that the perceived echo frequency is always maintained at the same frequency, which we have called reference frequency (RF; Schuller, Beuter and Schnitzler, 1974; Figure 7, p. 128). This fixed reference frequency which can carry the modulations indicating prey is up to 200 Hz higher than that emitted in an echolocation sound of a non-flying specimen.

The broadly tuned audiograms of these CF-FM bats include a steep, narrow filter (Figure 1) precisely tuned to the specific CF-frequency band to which the echolocating species listens i.e. 82–84 kHz in *Rhinolophus ferrumequinum*, 84–86 kHz in *Rhinolophus rouxi* from Mysore in India, 103–104 kHz in *Rhinolophus euryale* and 61–63 kHz in *Pteronotus parnellii*. These species-specific auditory filters are extremely narrow with slopes to lower and higher frequencies amounting to 150 dB/kHz (Figure 1). The threshold difference between the center frequency of the filter and adjacent frequencies to which the bat is insensitive ranges between 30 and 40 dB. Filters of such a precise frequency specificity have not been reported in auditory systems of other echolocating bats or any other vertebrate.

As has been shown in *Pteronotus parnellii* (Pollak, Henson and Novick, 1972) and in horseshoe bats (*Rhinolophus*; Bruns, 1976b), these filters are of a cochlear nature and no additional central processing is mandatory for achieving the high-frequency selectivity in the CF-frequency band characteristic for each species. Therefore the question arises as to how this precise filtering is achieved.

In the mammalian cochlea the basilar membrane (BM) acts as a bank of mechanical low-pass filters. The place of maximum vibration for any frequency of sound is considered to be the site on the BM where that frequency is represented. High sound frequencies produce a maximal excursion of the BM in the basal parts and low ones in the apical region of the cochlea. Thus going from base to apex the frequencies represented gradually become lower, the octaves each covering roughly equal distances on the BM (Figure 2).

In the CF-FM bat *Rhinolophus ferrumequinum*, the horseshoe bat, frequency mapping by the swollen nuclei method (Bruns, 1976b) disclosed that the BM does not follow this uniform pattern of logarithmic frequency representation. The narrow frequency band of the filter adapted to the echolocation signal from 82 to 86 kHz is represented in the basal BM in a vastly expanded fashion covering a length of the basilar membrane otherwise reserved for a complete octave (e.g. 80 to 40 kHz). The narrow band of filter frequencies from 83 to 86 kHz or 3% of the total audible frequency range is spread over 3.2 mm or 20% of the total BM length amounting to 16.1 mm (Figure 2). On the generally accepted assumption that octaves cover equal distances on the basilar membrane this tiny frequency band should have covered only 0.16 mm instead of 3.2 mm.

Generally bats have long basilar membranes compared to other mammals of the same body weight, and lengthening of the cochlea has been associated with an expansion of the hearing range to higher

Figure 2. Frequency maps on the basilar membrane (BM) in different mammals. Lengths of BMs are drawn to scale. In horseshoe bats the BM is unusually long compared to a mammal of similar body weight and hearing range (mouse). In the horseshoe bat the frequency representation deviates from the expected logarithmic scaling by incorporation of an expanded representation of the echolocation frequencies 80–86 kHz (dashed lines, 'frequency fovea'). (After Keidel, 1967; Boudreau and Tsuchitani, 1973; Ehret, 1975; Bruns, 1976b.)

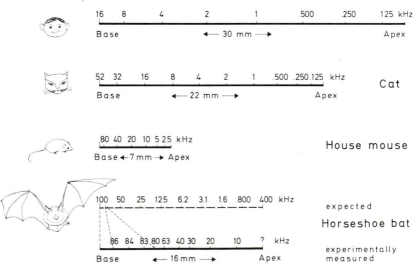

frequencies (Wever, 1974). House mouse and horseshoe bat have about the same body weight and both hear up to 100 kHz, yet the BM of the house mouse is only 7 mm long and that of the horseshoe bat 16 mm (Figure 2). However, the cochlea of *Hipposideros bicolor* is sensitive to frequencies up to 180 kHz with no loss on the low-frequency side, and spreads this vast frequency range over a total BM length of only 8.8 mm (Bruns, in press). Thus relative lengthening of the BM in mammals may not indicate an extension of the frequency range heard; instead it may reflect an expansion of the frequency scaling on the BM.

It is conceivable that for a given length of the traveling wave (two millimeters within the basal range in horseshoe bats as in cats and guinea pigs; Bruns, 1979) an expansion of the frequency representation on the BM would enhance frequency discrimination. By spreading out frequency ranges over a longer part of the BM a species might focus frequency analysis onto frequency bands of behavioral importance such as communication or echolocation signals. The case of the horseshoe bat would be an exceptionally conspicuous example of this general hypothesis in that this species focuses auditory analysis on the narrow band of the pure tone echoes between 82 and 86 kHz (Neuweiler, Bruns and Schuller, 1980).

This expansion of a narrow frequency band over a long part of the basilar membrane has profound consequences (Figure 3). Due to the frequency spreading, 25% of the cochlear receptor cells and 3400 of the 16 000 afferent fibres or 21% of the cochlear input to the ascending auditory pathway are assigned to 80–86 kHz or 6% of the total hearing range (Bruns and Schmieszek, 1980). This impressive over-representation of the narrow CF echo frequencies is maintained within the general cochleotopic arrangement in all auditory nuclei so far studied: nucleus cochlearis (Neuweiler and Vater, 1977), superior olivary complex (Schlegel, 1977), inferior colliculus (Pollak and Schuller, 1981), medial geniculate body (Engelstätter, 1981) and auditory cortex (Ostwald, 1978). In the other CF-FM bat, *Pteronotus parnellii*, studied in detail (Suga, Simmons and Jen, 1975; Suga and Jen, 1977; Pollak and Bodenhamer, 1981) the over-representation of the CF-echo frequency band of 61–63 kHz in the auditory nervous system is even more conspicuous. Thus a major portion of the auditory neuron population is analysing a narrowly restricted, but behaviorally most important frequency band. This appears as a striking analogy to the visual fovea where a small restricted spot of the visual field is also represented by a large portion of afferent fibres and spread over disproportionately large areas of the visual brain centers. In the same way as eye movements

track a visual stimulus of interest and fix it onto the fovea, CF-FM bats
actively compensate Doppler shifts of the entire echo by lowering the
emitted frequency, and thus fix the heard echo frequency within the
center frequency of their cochlear filter. Because of this analogy we
have called the expansion on the basilar membrane and the subsequent
over-representation in the nervous system of this narrow filter frequency
band an acoustical or frequency fovea (Schuller and Pollak, 1979).

Detailed and numerous studies in both mustache bat (*Pteronotus
parnellii*) and horseshoe bats have disclosed that neurons with best
frequencies (BF) within the specialized filter region feature exceptional-

Figure 3. The 'frequency fovea' in the auditory system of the horseshoe
bat, *Rhinolophus ferrumequinum*. (a) An electrode track through the
posterior part of the inferior colliculus. The position of each unit (left)
and its Best Frequency (right) are indicated. ND, no response to
acoustical stimulation. Neurons with BF between 83.4 and 85.3 kHz
are spread over three-fifths of the penetration. (b) Frequency
representation on the basilar membrane which is projected into the
transmodiolar plane. (c), (d) Frequency representation in spiral
ganglion and colliculus inferior. N, number of units recorded. (After
Pollak and Schuller, 1981; Neuweiler, Bruns and Schuller, 1980.)

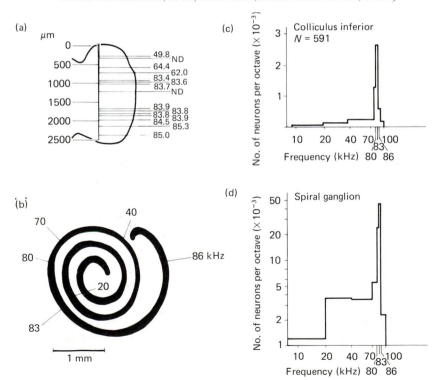

ly precise frequency selectivity as expressed by the so called Q-values (best frequency divided by the bandwidth of the tuning curve 10 dB above best frequency threshold: e.g. BF = 84 kHz, bandwidth 10 dB above threshold 0.2 kHz then $Q = 84/0.2 = 420$). The larger the Q-values the more precise the frequency selectivity. In all mammals so far studied, including echolocating bats emitting broad band signals, Q-values of auditory neurons rarely exceed 20. In CF-FM bats neurons with BFs within the specific filter band reach Q-values up to 500 (Figure 4). This steeply tuned filtering already exists at peripheral levels as shown by recordings of cochlear nucleus units, auditory nerve fibers and cochlear microphonics (Suga et al., 1975; Suga, Neuweiler and Möller, 1976; Neuweiler and Vater, 1976; Pollak et al., 1972). Since the length of the travelling wave is unaltered (two millimetres) an expanded representation of the frequencies on the BM necessarily results in narrower tuning curves of nerve fibers coming from that portion of the BM. This is demonstrated in Figure 4 where the tuning curves of peripheral units with BFs in the foveal region are drawn in the same expanded way as represented on the BM. When drawn on this 'real' scale the slopes of their tuning curves are normal as for units with lower BFs whereas their Q_{10dB} are 10–20 times higher than those of units with BFs represented on the normal part of the BM.

In the search for possible expanding mechanisms, striking morphological and physiological specializations have been found in the horseshoe bat, and these are mostly restricted to the basal part of the BM where the filter frequencies are represented:

Basilar membrane, mechanical systems (*Bruns, 1976a*)
(1) The basal part of the BM deviates from the general course of continuous widening and thinning from base to apex in that it narrows and remains extremely thick up to 4.3 mm from the base. At this site (where the lower-frequency slope of the filter is represented) the thickenings abruptly disappear, creating a sharp discontinuity in the thickness gradient of the BM (Figure 4). The enormous thickness of the basal BM is due mainly to a thickening of the pars pectinata supporting the outer hair cells (Figure 5).

(2) The basal part of the BM is mechanically weakly connected to the outer wall by a spiral ligament void of fibres and a very thin bony lamella (Figure 5a). This lamella expands into a bulky secondary spiral lamina adding a considerable mass to the outer anchoring system of the cochlea. In fact during high-frequency stimulation this mass also vibrates with only 5 dB lower amplitude than the BM itself (Figure 5a).

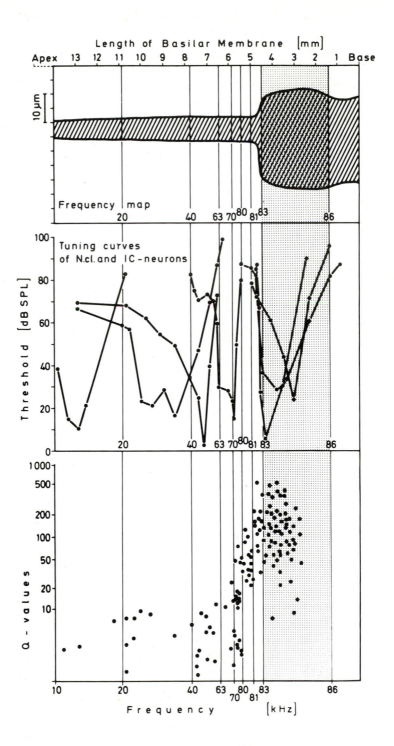

This suggests that the outer part of the basilar membrane and the loose anchoring system may act as a mechanical unit'.

(3) The rigid inner part of the basal BM carrying the inner hair cells is flexibly connected to the outer specialized one by only a thin sulcus. This may allow the inner and outer parts of the specialized basal BM to vibrate in a fairly independent manner (Bruns, 1980).

(4) In fact vibration measurements of the BM show that for frequencies within the filter region, which are represented on the specialized BM the inner and outer part may vibrate out of phase. For lower stimulus frequencies no such effect occurred (Wilson, 1977).

Receptor level (Bruns and Schmieszek, 1980; Bruns and Goldbach, 1980)

(1) There is no efferent innervation to the outer hair cells throughout the cochlea.

(2) In the basal region the first row of outer hair cells is shifted close to the inner hair cells (7 μm distance compared to 15 μm in other parts of the BM; Figure 6).

(3) In the basal part the surface of the inner hair cells is small and adjacent cells are widely separated by supporting cells. The inner hair cells do not form a continuous row as in other parts of the cochlea or as they do throughout the cochlea in other mammals (Figure 6B).

(4) In the basal part the stereocilia of the inner hair cells are extremely long (4.3 μm) whereas those of the outer hair cells are unusually short (0.8 μm).

(5) In the basal region the under surface of the tectorial membrane shows a conspicuous elevated zig-zag ridge with imprints exactly corresponding to the longest stereocilia of the first row of outer hair cells.

Figure 4. The filter or 'frequency fovea' tuned to the pure-tone part of the echoes in the horseshoe bat, *Rhinolophus ferrumequinum*. *Note:* the frequency on the abscissa is scaled as it is actually represented on the basilar membrane (BM). The stippled area marks the expanded representation of the pure-tone echo frequencies. Bottom graph shows the extremely high Q-values of cochlear nucleus and collicular neurons in the expanded region. Middle graph: in spite of the high Q-values the tuning curves of units with BF in the echo-frequency band show slopes similar to those of units with lower BFs when drawn in 'true scale' as the frequencies are represented on the BM. Upper graph shows coincidence of morphological specializations (thickness of BM is shown) with physiological data of the echo frequencies represented on that part of the BM (stippled area). (After Neuweiler et al., 1980; Suga, Neuweiler and Möller, 1976; Möller, Neuweiler and Zöller, 1978.)

All these mechanical and receptoral specializations occurring at the site of the cochlea where the foveal frequencies of 80–86 kHz are represented invite speculations on how these data can be made to fit into different models of frequency filtering in the cochlea. We shall refrain from this model-building here; however, the striking coincidence and convergence of these specializations onto the region of the BM where the echo frequencies are analysed suggest to us that they may be instrumental in the expansion of the filter frequencies on the basal part of the basilar membrane. This expanded representation is to a great extent responsible for the extremely narrow filtering qualities. The morphological specializations described may add yet unknown filtering mechanisms.

Pteronotus – *a case of converging evolution*

The movement-sensitive echolocation system of horseshoe bats, which consists of a narrowly tuned filter and of a feedback system

Figure 5. Structural specializations of the cochlea in the horseshoe bat, *Rhinolophus ferrumequinum*. (a) Cross-section through the specialized basal region (foveal region) of the cochlea. (b) For comparison, generalized cross-section through the basal turns of the cochlea of rat, mouse and bats emitting frequency-modulated echolocation sounds. BMA, arcuate zone of basilar membrane, carrying inner hair cells; BMP, pectinate zone of basilar membrane, carrying the outer hair cells; CC, Claudius cells; HC, Hensen's cells; LF, longitudinal fibers; PSL, primary spiral lamina; SSL, secondary spiral lamina; SL, spiral ligament; SV, stria vascularis; TM, tectorial membrane. As indicated below cross-section (a) the thick secondary spiral lamina SSL also vibrates considerably during high-frequency stimulation (above 80 kHz). (After Bruns, 1979.)

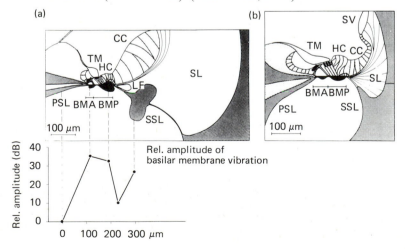

for compensating Doppler shifts induced by the bat's own flight speed, is a highly specialized mechanism. The other bat which uses the same echolocation technique is *Pteronotus parnellii*, the mustache bat, and one might expect to find the same specializations as in horseshoe bats.

Detailed morphological and physiological studies disclose only one similarity: in both species the filter becomes insensitive and shallow under heavy anesthesia. Otherwise there are marked differences. In *Pteronotus* none of the morphological peculiarities so obvious in horseshoe bat cochleae have been found (M. M. Henson, 1978). Frequency mapping by the same method as used in *Rhinolophus* failed since long lasting stimulation with the filter frequency results in widespread haircell damage throughout the basal turn. In fact the following comparisons of physiological cochlea data indicate that horseshoe bats and mustache bats apply different filter mechanisms:

(1) In *Pteronotus* the filter can easily be overdriven and eliminated for hours or days by overstimulation with the filter frequency (Pollak, Henson and Johnson, 1979). Horseshoe bats have no such susceptibility.

Figure 6. Arrangement of the inner and outer hair cells in the specialized basal part (b) and unspecialized middle part (a) of the cochlea in *Rhinolophus ferrumequinum*. Hair-cell arrangement in the middle region is typically mammalian with a continuous row of inner hair cells (left) separated by 15 μm from three rows of outer hair cells with V-shaped bundles of stereocilia. In the basal specialized part (b), however, the inner hair cells are widely spaced by supporting cells and the first row of outer hair cells is shifted towards the inner hair cells to lie within 7 μm of them. (Bruns and Goldbach, 1980.)

(B)

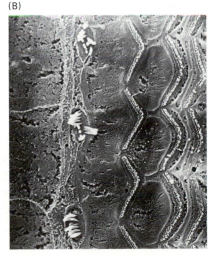

(A)

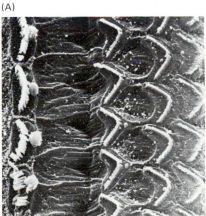

(2) In both species microphonics show fast phase changes. In *Pteronotus* they occur at the filter frequency whereas in horseshoe bats they are restricted to frequencies of the insensitivity peak separating the filter from the lower-frequency hearing range.

(3) At frequencies around the center frequency, microphonics show slow rising slopes and long-lasting slowly decaying oscillation after termination of the stimulus. In horseshoe bats such resonant effects are far less pronounced and in many recordings are missing.

(4) With stimuli of the same sound-pressure level the microphonics are largest at the center frequency in *Pteronotus*, whereas in horseshoe bats the amplitude is the same as for other frequencies. Yet for frequencies of the insensitivity peak the amplitudes reach a minimum (2–4: Henson, Schuller and Vater, 1981).

From these species-specific characteristics one might infer that the filter in *Pteronotus* shows typical features of a mechanical resonant filter. Whereas in *Rhinolophus* the data may indicate a sharply-tuned notch filter of insensitivity separating the narrow high-frequency filter from the low-frequency hearing region. In any case the cochlear filtering mechanisms are different in both echolocation systems although they produce the same specific effects.

These recent data have rather complicated the search for mechanisms responsible for the precise filtering. They clearly demonstrate that such a highly-specialized accomplishment as fluttering-target detection by echolocation has evolved independently twice, in the New (*Pteronotus parnellii*) and in the Old World (rhinolophids), by exploiting different capacities of the mammalian ear. These cochlear capacities, most probably inherent in any mammalian ear, have been refined and driven close to the theoretical limits of their capacities in the two species of bat considered. Studies of highly-specialized cases such as horseshoe and mustached bats demonstrate the large scope of specific efficiencies inherent in a basic design such as the mammalian frequency analyser, the cochlea. Depending on the species-specific behavioral requirements, certain aspects might become exaggerated and refined, whereas in an acoustically non-specialized mammal these potential capacities never show up. From these studies on mammals with specialized hearing we deduce the following hypothesis: The mammalian cochlea may be highly differentiated dependent on the species' acoustical behavior.

In the mammalian auditory system, frequency filtering is accomplished on the cochlear level only. No additional neuronal sharpening of the filter process is mandatory even when fine frequency discrimination is asked for. Over-representation of certain frequency bands within the cochleatopic frequency representation in auditory nervous systems results from a corresponding over-representation at the cochlear level as demonstrated by the frequency fovea in horseshoe bats. The first test for this hypothesis will be frequency mapping in the cochlea of the mustache bat.

Detection of frequency changes

As already mentioned CF-FM bats eliminate Doppler shifts of echoes caused by their own flight speed and maintain the heard echo frequency at the so-called reference frequency (RF) matching the center frequency of the cochlear fovea. The bat listens to the returning echo. When the echo frequency lies above the reference frequency the bat lowers the frequency of the subsequently emitted sounds by such an amount that the frequency of the next echo matches the reference frequency. Each bat has its individual reference frequency, which ranges between 82 and 85 kHz in *Rhinolophus ferrumequinum*.

When a horseshoe bat emitting echolocation sounds listens to electronically frequency-shifted playbacks it starts compensating for the experimentally induced frequency shifts by lowering the emitted frequency (Figure 7b). Only shifts above the reference frequency are compensated for (Schuller et al., 1974). This feedback mechanism provides a convenient way to test the detection of frequency shifts and hence frequency discrimination. It has been found that horseshoe bats detect and start to compensate for frequency shifts of only 50 Hz above the reference frequency. Thus frequency changes of only 0.06% are detected, demonstrating the precise narrow filter quality of the cochlear fovea. With the same precision the emitted frequency is controlled by the superior laryngeal nerve innervating the cricothyroid muscles, which precisely adjust the emitted frequency (Schuller and Rübsamen, 1981; Figure 8a).

As already mentioned CF-FM bats use the tonal signal for detecting fluttering prey by brisk frequency and amplitude changes imposed onto the echo carrier frequency. This requires high sensitivity of the auditory system for minor frequency and amplitude changes in the fovea frequency range.

Sensitivity to amplitude modulation appears to be a general feature of all neurons in cochlear nuclei and inferior colliculus. Irrespective of their Best Frequency modulation depths from 3 to 100% are encoded (Figure 8).

As one might expect cochlear nucleus neurons with BF within the

Figure 7. Control of the frequency emitted for compensating Doppler shifts of the entire echo induced by the horseshoe bat's own flight. (a) Superior laryngeal nerve fibers innervate the cricothyroid muscles controlling fine adjustment of the frequency emitted. Nerve activity is linearly correlated with frequency emitted. (b) Experimentally-induced positive frequency shifts (Δf, abscissa) are compensated for so that the heard echo frequency is kept constant at a so-called reference frequency (ca. 83 kHz in *Rhinolophus ferrumequinum*) with a precision of 50 Hz or 0.06%. Experimentally-induced frequency shifts of the echo below the reference frequency and positive shifts larger than 5–6 kHz are not compensated for. (From Schuller and Rübsamen, 1981; Schuller, Beuter and Schnitzler, 1974.)

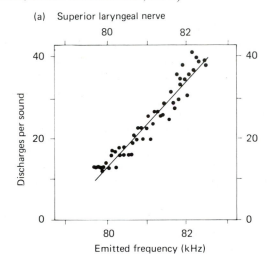

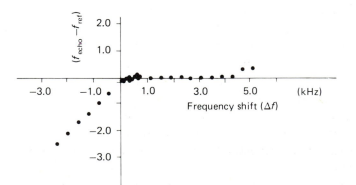

foveal frequency range of 82–86 kHz are particularly sensitive to narrow frequency modulations. These modulations may be as small as 20 Hz or 0.02% of the center frequency (Figure 8). The periodicity of modulations up to 1000 Hz is preserved in response patterns of cochlear nucleus neurons whereas in collicular neurons modulation frequencies larger than 500 Hz are no longer followed (Schuller, 1979; Vater, in press).

Cochlear nucleus neurons responding primary like-discharge patterns mirror very faithfully the time course of the modulated stimulus whereas phasic on-neurons respond to frequency changes within a certain band. When these changes occur periodically, as for instance in echoes from fluttering prey, these neurons are excellent encoders of the stimulus periodicity (Vater, 1982). Basically the sensitivity to modulations recurs at higher centers. However, mirror-like encoding of time courses is rarely seen; whereas responses to transients, such as amplitude and frequency slopes, are markedly enhanced (compare PST-histograms from cochlear nucleus and inferior colliculus neurons in Figure 8). Sensitivity to frequency modulation is best at low and medium sound intensities, that is, when the neuron is active within the steep slope of its dynamic range and away from the 100% saturation intensity (Pollak and Schuller, 1981). In the cochlear nucleus, neurons responding with a so-called build-up or complex discharge pattern do not react to frequency modulations. Since these types of neurons most probably are recorded from the dorsal cochlear nucleus we conclude that the capability for FM coding primarily comes from the ventral cochlear nuclei (Vater, 1982).

Enhancement of responses to transients from peripheral to central nuclei is a general feature of the auditory system and the response to modulations reflect common capacities of the auditory system in all mammals. The especially high sensitivity to frequency modulation depths of only 0.02% in neurons with BF within the foveal range of 82–86 kHz is readily explained by their narrow tuning. However, responses to modulations of many peripheral and higher-order neurons do not result simply from the shape of their tuning curves but also indicate complex neuronal interactions.

Time analysis

Binaural cues

The generally accepted 'duplicity-theory' postulates that interaural time differences can only be analysed by mammals with a large interaural distance whereas small mammals with closely-spaced ears have to rely on binaural intensity differences for evaluating

Figure 8. Encoding of frequency and amplitude modulations in neurons tuned to the echo frequencies in *Rhinolophus ferrumequinum*. Left column: responses to sinusoidal frequency modulations (SFM).

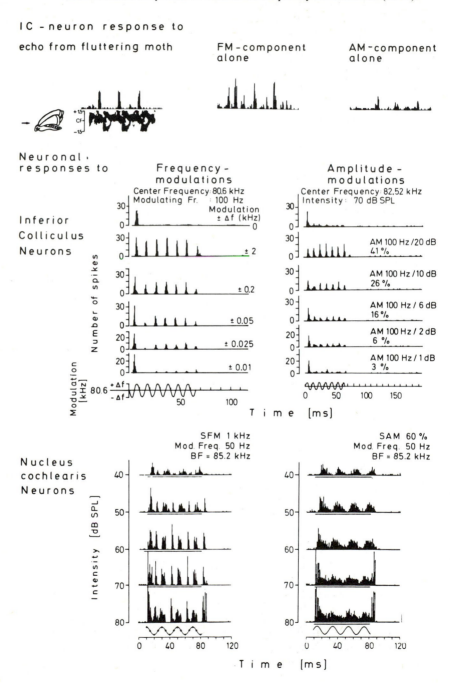

horizontal direction of a round source. This concept was associated with the findings of Irving and Harrison (1967) that small mammals do not have a medial olivary nucleus (MSO, e.g. bats) or only a vestigial one. The MSO is considered to be the site of interaural time difference analysis whereas the lateral olivary nucleus (LSO) is responsible for the analysis of interaural intensity differences and is consequently large in small mammals.

Contrary to these findings recent anatomical studies using HRP tracings in *Rhinolophus ferrumequinum* (Schweizer, 1981) and in *Pteronotus parnellii* (Zook and Casseday, 1980) clearly demonstrate an MSO which sends prominent projections to the ipsilateral inferior colliculus.

In the echolocating bat *Molossus ater*, Harnischfeger (1980) recorded single units from the superior olivary complex and histologically located 31 of them in the MSO and 10 in the LSO. As in the few other mammals so far investigated, all LSO neurons were excited by the ipsilateral ear and inhibited by the contralateral one (E/I-units), whereas MSO neurons were always excited contralaterally and excited (E/E-neurons) or inhibited by the ipsilateral ear (I/E-neurons). It is well established that the E/I-neurons which are so frequently recorded from the LSO are well suited for analysing interaural intensity differences.

Among the 11 I/E-units recorded in the MSO of *Molossus ater* there were four responding only phasically to binaural tone pulses. The spike-count functions of the excitatory contralateral input were non-monotonic with steep rising slopes (Figure 9). When the excitatory input was evoked with a stimulus intensity within the steep slope and the inhibitory ipsilateral input was added, full inhibition was reached within an ipsilateral input increase of only 5–10 dB above threshold. When these neurons were stimulated by a binaural intensity difference corresponding to inputs from the steep slopes of the dynamic range, minor delays of a few microseconds between the ipsilateral and contralateral

---

Caption for fig. 8 (*cont.*).

>   Both cochlear nucleus and collicular neurons encode SFM- periodicity over a wide range of stimulus intensities and for modulations as small as ±0.01 kHz or 0.12% of the center frequency. Right column: responses to sinusoidal amplitude modulations (SAM). Upper row: response of a collicular neuron to echoes returning from a fluttering moth. Arrow indicates direction of sound incidence (pure tone) onto the target. Below PST-histograms the spectrogram of the echo is shown reflecting the wing beats by modulations (±1.5 kHz around the emitted frequency (CF)). (From Vater, 1982; Schuller, 1979; Neuweiler et al., 1980).

Figure 9. In the bat *Molossus ater* medial olivary complex (MSO) neurons with high BFs encode binaural transient time differences in the microsecond range. Middle graph: Spike-count function of a MSO-neuron to binaural transient time differences (abscissa). Bar with arrowheads indicates time differences occurring at the bat's head due to the interaural distance. If the unit had responded to binaural phase

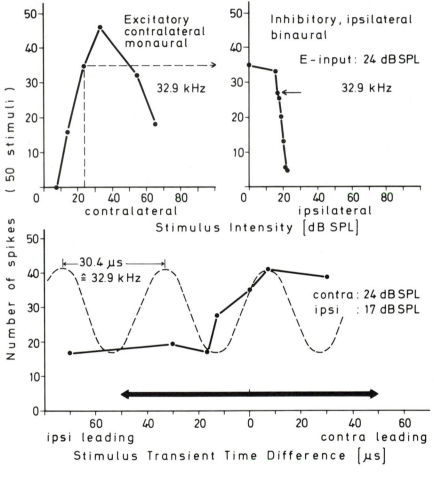

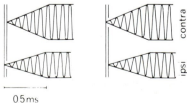

stimuli had dramatic effects. In these four MSO-neurons and in another eight of 78 inferior colliculus neurons, onset delays of the binaural tone pulses from -50 μs (ipsilateral leading) to $+50$ μs (contralateral leading) drove the neurons from minimal to maximal response. A $50\,\mu$s delay corresponds to the maximum possible delay in this bat species with an interaural distance of 1.7 cm (Figure 9).

Thus contrary to the dualistic concept, in this echolocating bat the analysis of minute interaural time differences within a biologically reasonable range of $\pm 50\,\mu$s, and hence sound localization by binaural timing cues, is at least neuronally feasible.

The encoding of binaural time differences in the microsecond range has already been described in other mammals (e.g. Brugge, Anderson and Aitkin, 1970, demonstrated neuronal effects of binaural time changes of only 2 μs in dorsal lateral lemniscus neurons of the cat); thus this specific sensitivity of auditory neurons is nothing new. New, however, is the fact, that in echolating bats neuronal responses to binaural time differences within the microsecond range may be elicited by pure tones with frequencies far above 5 kHz. In other mammals this neuronal sensitivity was assigned to binaural phase-difference stimulation with low frequencies. Phase, or as it is recently called, ongoing time difference, -sensitive neurons display a periodic discharge pattern when stimulated by continuously increasing binaural delays. The periodicity corresponds to the frequency of the binaural stimulus. In bats the binaural neurons were stimulated by tone pulses of 30 to 90 kHz (period length: 33 to 11 μs). None of the neurons sensitive to binaural time differences showed any periodic discharge pattern to continuously increasing delays (Figure 9). In fact when maximal discharge rates were reached by delaying the inhibitory input this activity level remained constant with longer delay. We therefore conclude that the MSO and

---

Caption for fig. 9 (*cont.*).

differences, the spike count function should show a periodic pattern with a period of 3.04 μs corresponding to the stimulus frequency of 32.9 kHz (dashed curve). Lowest graph shows schematically the envelopes of the binaural stimuli. Upper left: Non-monotonic spike count function for monaural excitatory stimulation at the MSO-unit's Best Frequency (32.9 kHz). Upper right: Spike-count function for simultaneous binaural stimulation (excitatory contralateral input: invariable at 24 dB SPL, ipsilateral inhibitory input variable) showing strong inhibition within a few dB of threshold of inhibition. Only units with excitatory/inhibitory binaural inputs responded to transient binaural time differences in the microsecond range. (After Harnischfeger, 1981.)

IC-neurons sensitive to binaural time differences in the microsecond ranges responded to the binaural differences in stimulus onset or transient time difference and not to phase or ongoing disparity. Thus at least in bats, due to this sensitivity to transient time differences, the well-documented neuronal sensitivity to binaural time disparities in mammals is extended to high-frequency stimuli up to 90 kHz.

Interestingly, all neurons displaying this sensitivity were I/E-neurons with narrow dynamic ranges for the monaural excitatory and inhibitory inputs, and which responded phasically with rarely more than one action potential. Apparently a delicate balance of inhibitory and excitatory events governs the discharge of these neurons. This balance may be easily offset by minor timing changes in the two differentially-acting inputs.

This timing effect is demonstrated in LSO neurons responding to binaural tone pulses with three to four evenly-spaced action potentials (chopper-neurons). Increasing contralateral stimulus intensities inhibit all action potentials except the first one. However, when the contralateral stimulus leads by about 0.4 ms the first discharge also disappears indicating that the latency of the inhibitory effect in the LSO ranges around 0.4 ms. This rather long latency may be due to additional delays which the contralateral inhibitory input for LSO undergoes in the medial nucleus of the trapezoid body. In contrast MSO receives both afferents directly from the ventral nuclei of the cochlear nucleus and hence differential interaction may occur within timing ranges which are small enough for coding naturally-occurring binaural differences.

We assume that sensitivity to timings in the microsecond range is not accomplished by just certain specialized species. Rather, it is our impression that it occurs when phasic neurons interact differentially. The degree of sensitivity may be enhanced by sequentially-repeating differential interactions. We suggest that timing sensitivity is a general capability of differentially-interacting neurons receiving precisely-timed afferent input. Precise time encoding would be the result of neuronal circuitry. It is hard to conceive that a single neuron provides the timing precision required. Even the so-called latency constant neurons frequently recorded in the auditory system of echolocating bats have minimal latency jitters of $\pm 100\,\mu s$ (Pollak, 1980).

In owls, Moiseff and Konishi (1981) recently demonstrated unequivocally that mesencephalic neurons react only to on-going time and not to transient time differences. They suggest that this sensitivity is achieved either by cross-correlation (but how then is cross-correlation neuronally realized?) or by averaging the on-going time difference over the sequence of stimulus waves. The latter mechanism is not applicable to bats since single-onset time differences are encoded. In this case we suggest that parallel averaging of the activity of a number of neurons excited simultaneously by a stimulus and converging onto one interacting unit may be a possible mechanism for improving precision in timing.

Time analysis for specific echolocational purposes

Bats locate a target by evaluating the azimuth, elevation and distance of the echo source. Azimuth is derived from binaural intensity and/or time disparities. It has recently been suggested that elevation angles are measured by phase differences of echo reflections occurring within the ear cones, especially by the tragus (Lawrence and Simmons, 1982). The tragus is a flap protruding into the opening of the conches in many bat species. However, such double and multiple echoreflections at the ear create complex interferences resulting in conspicuous and distinct changes of the echo-power spectrum. Thus the effect may also be analysed in the frequency domain.

The distance to an echo-reflecting target is measured by evaluating the time elapsed from the emission of the echolocation signal to the arrival of the echo. Ranging mechanisms are discussed extensively in a recent article by O'Neill and Suga (1982) on the role of the auditory cortex in echolocation.

Apart from these general requirements for time analysis of any echolocating system there exist additional timing effects adapted to specific purposes in echolocation.

As already described CF-FM bats control the frequency of the sound they emit by listening to the echo-frequency. If the latter is above the so-called reference frequency, which matches the cochlear filter, the bat lowers the frequency of the subsequently emitted sounds by a corresponding amount. This feedback system works only when the echo returns within about 20 ms after the onset of vocalization (Schuller, 1977). When the echo returns later, shifts of the echo frequency from the reference frequency are no longer compensated for. However, since the duration of the vocalization could not be manipulated, it is not clear whether the onset of vocalization opens a time window of 20 ms for frequency information to the vocalization system, or whether a minimal time of overlap between outgoing sound and returning echo is necessary. In any case, the compensation mechanism is restricted to an echo arrival time of up to 20 ms, corresponding to a distance of the reflecting target of up to about three meters.

In the inferior colliculus and in the medial geniculate body of

Figure 10. Long-lasting specific stimulation effects may enhance
responses to echoes in MGB and IC neurons of the horseshoe bat.
(a) Left column: a preceding pure-tone stimulus (straight line under
PST-histogram mimic of emitted echolocation sound) enhances
response to a frequency-modulated signal (SFM, mimic of echo from a
fluttering target) within a time window of 3 to 27 ms after pure tone
onset (Δt, ordinate). Enhancement is more prominent when frequency
of preceding pure tone is slightly below 'echo'-frequency (SFM)
corresponding to the auditory situation in a flying, echolocating

(a)   MGB—neuronal responses to vocalization-echo mimics

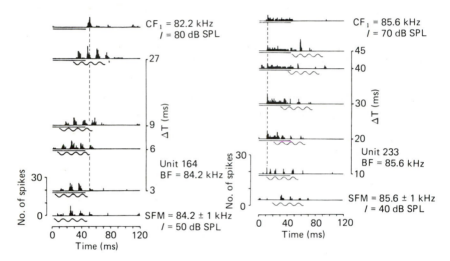

(b)   IC—neuronal responses to

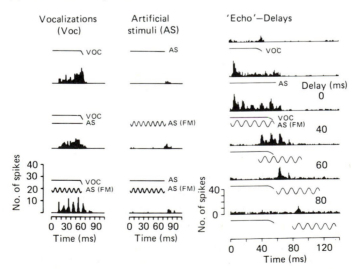

horseshoe bats we found a variety of neurons specifically adapted to hunting behaviour. A flying horseshoe bat pursuing a fluttering insect will hear both the emitted echolocation signal and overlapping returning echoes. Due to the Doppler effect compensation, the emitted frequency will always be up to 2.5 kHz lower than the carrier frequency of the echo, depending on the individual reference frequency of the bat. When the echo is returning from an insect with beating wings it will carry periodic frequency and amplitude modulations. In both nuclei we found neurons with short recovery times for the response to a second stimulus (echo) when the first stimulus contained frequencies up to 2.5 kHz lower than the echo. Within a certain time span from onset of the first tone the response to fainter second tones will even be enhanced when the louder first tone had a slightly lower frequency (Möller, 1978; Engelstätter, 1981). Other neurons display suppression of the response to a first pure tone (emitted sound) and enhancement of the response to periodic frequency modulations (echo from wing-beating insect) of a second tone when the second tone occurs not later than 20 ms after onset of the first stimulus (Figure 10a). For larger delays encoding of the frequency modulations are suppressed (Engelstätter, 1981).

Some collicular neurons only responded to frequency-modulated signals (echoes) when the bat had vocalized. The vocalization could not be replaced by an artificial stimulus of identical frequency, intensity and duration as the vocalized one. It seems that vocalization alters the responsiveness of certain neurons to frequency-modulated signals (Figure 10b). This effect could not be reproduced with mimics of the vocalized sound. The vocal influence was again restricted in time and

Caption for fig. 10 (*cont.*).

      horseshoe bat. (a) Right column: same enhancement effect in another neuron. Enhancement is restricted to a time span up to 20 ms after onset of pure tone stimulation. Responses to later signals are suppressed. In this neuron enhancement is best when both preceding and modulated 'echo'-signal have the same frequency. Note that intensity of the preceding pure tone is 30 dB higher than that of the modulated signal. (b) In some inferior colliculus neurons responses to sinusoidally-modulated signals are specifically enhanced by vocalizations. (b) left column: responses to vocalization alone (VOC) and to vocalization combined with simulated echoes (AS, pure tone of same frequency and intensity as pure tone part of VOC; AS(FM), same center frequency as AS, but sinusoidally-modulated by ±500 Hz). (b) middle column: responses to the same stimuli but without vocalization. (b) right column: responses to vocalizations and delayed simulated frequency-modulated echoes. As shown by the delays of the 'echo', the FM stimulus is only encoded during vocalization. (From Engelstätter, 1981; Schuller, 1979.)

occurred only within a distinct time span from the onset of vocalization (Schuller, 1979b, Figure 10b).

It has to be pointed out that all these specific effects were only detected in neurons with Best Frequencies within the narrow frequency range of the bat's own pure tone echolocation.

Conclusions

As in the auditory frequency analysis, we again suggest that the examples for time analysis from echolocating bats do not indicate auditory mechanisms which are specific only for bats. In our opinion they only disclose capacities principally inherent in the mammalian auditory system. Frequency analysis may be accentuated and refined in a restricted frequency band, but it is accomplished by cochlear mechanisms occurring in all mammals and most probably in all vertebrates. Binaural intensity and timing differences are analysed with the same interacting binaural inhibitory and excitatory activations as in other mammals. Specific timing effects, long-lasting inhibitions or enhancements which condition the responsiveness of auditory neurons to a selected set of behaviorally-relevant signals, are carried out by the same sequential interplay of excitatory and inhibitory activities on auditory neurons. Therefore the time course of excitatory and inhibitory activations of auditory neurons should be most relevant for understanding how the auditory system analyses complex auditory events such as sequences of echolocation signals or communication sounds. Unfortunately, investigations on the time course of neuronal activities have been vastly neglected so far. However, the striking examples from echolocating bats indicate an excellent capacity of the mammalian auditory system for time analysis.

Anatomical studies of the ascending auditory pathway in bats have shown that the projections from periphery to higher levels are principally the same as in other mammals studied (Schweizer, 1981). The structural pattern of sequentially-repeated inputs from cochlear nucleus to olivary complex, to lemniscal nuclei, and the convergence of projections from all these brain stem nuclei onto the inferior colliculus underline the potential capacities of timing analysis within the auditory system.

I should like to thank F. Althaus for drawing the figures and J. Manley for reading the manuscript and revising the English. The research reported here was supported by SFB45 Frankfurt and SFB 204, München.

References

Boudreau, J. C., and Tsuchitani, Ch. (1973). *Sensory Neurophysiology*. New York: van Nostrand Reinhold Comp.

Brugge, J. F., Anderson, D. J., and Aitkin, L. M. (1970). Responses of neurons in the dorsal nucleus of the lateral lemniscus of cat to binaural stimulation. *J. Neurophysiol. 33:* 441–58.

Bruns, V. (1967a). Peripheral auditory tuning for fine frequency analysis by the CF-FM bat, *Rhinolophus ferrumequinum*. I. Mechanical specializations of the cochlea. *J. Comp. Physiol. 106:* 77–86.

Bruns, V. (1967b). Peripheral auditory tuning for fine frequency analysis by the CF-FM bat, *Rhinolophus ferrumequinum*. II. Frequency mapping in the cochlea. *J. Comp. Physiol. 106:* 87–97.

Bruns, V. (1979). Functional anatomy as an approach to frequency analysis in the mammalian cochlea. *Verh. dt. zool. Ges. 1979:* 141–54.

Bruns, V. (1980). Basilar membrane and its anchoring system in the cochlea of the greater horseshoe bat. *Anat. Embryol. 161:* 29–50.

Bruns, V., and Goldbach, M. (1980). Hair cells and tectorial membrane in the cochlea of the greater horseshoe bat. *Anat. Embryol. 161:* 51–63.

Bruns, V., Henson, M. M.,Kraus, H. J., and Fiedler, J. (1981). Vergleichende und funktionelle Morphologie der Fledermauscochlea. *Myotis 18/19:* 90–105.

Bruns, V., and Schmieszek, E. (1980). Cochlear innervation in the greater horseshoe bat: demonstration of an acoustic fovea. *Hearing Res. 3:* 27–43.

Ehret, G. (1975). Masked auditory thresholds, critical ratios, and scales of the basilar membrane of the housemouse (*Mus musculus*). *J. Comp. Physiol. 103:* 329–41.

Engelstätter, R. (1981). Hörphysiologische Untersuchungen an Neuronen der aufsteigenden Hörbahn der echoortenden Fledermaus *Rhinolophus rouxi*. Dissertation of Fachbereich Biologie, University of Frankfurt/Main.

Grinnell, A. D. (1970). Comparative auditory neurophysiology of neotropical bats employing different echolocation signals. *Z. vergl. Physiol. 68:* 117–53.

Grinnell, A. D., and Hagiwara, S. (1972). Studies of auditory neurophysiology in non-echolocating bats, and adaptations for echolocation in one genus *Rousettus. Z. vergl. Physiol. 76:* 82–96.

Harnischfeger, G. (1980). Brainstem units of echolocating bats code binaural time differences in the microsecond range. *Naturwissenschaften 67:* 314–15.

Harnischfeger, G. (1981). Untersuchung binauraler Mechanismen des Richtungshörens im Intensitäts- und Zeitbereich an Stammhirnneuronen der echoortenden Fledermaus *Molossus ater*. Dissertation of Fachberich Biologie, University of Frankfurt/Main.

Henson, O. W., (1978). The basilar membrane of the bat, *Pteronotus p. parnelli. Am. J. Anat. 153:* 143–58.

Henson, O. W., Schuller, G., and Vater, M. (1981). Cochlear microphonic potentials in Doppler-shift compensating bats: a comparative study of mechanisms associated with frequency analysis and sharp tuning. *Fourth Midwinter Research Meeting of Association of Research in Otolaryngology*.

Irving, R., and Harrison, M. M. (1967). The superior olivary complex and audition: a comparative study. *J. Comp. Neurol. 130:* 77–86.

Keidel, W. D. (1967). *Kurzgefaβtes Lehrbuch der Physiologie*. Stuttgart: G. Thieme Verlag.

Lawrence, B. D., and Simmons, J. A. (1982). Echolocation in bats: the external ear and perception of the vertical position of targets. *Science 218:* 481–3.

Möller, J. (1978). Response characteristics of inferior colliculus neurons of the awake CF-FM bat *Rhinolophus ferrumequinum.* II. Two-tone stimulation. *J. Comp. Physiol. 125:* 227–36.

Möller, J., Neuweiler, G., and Zöller, H. (1978). Response characteristics of inferior colliculus neurons of the awake CF-FM bat, *Rhinolophus ferrumequinum.* I. Single-tone stimulation. *J. Comp. Physiol. 125:* 217–25.

Moiseff, A., and Konishi, M. (1981). Neuronal and behavioral sensitivity to binaural time difference in the owl. *J. Neurosci. 1:* 40–8.

Neuweiler, G. (1970). Neurophysiologische Untersuchungen zum Echoortungssystem der Großen Hufeisennase *Rhinolophus ferrumequinum. Z. vergl. Physiol. 67:* 273–306.

Neuweiler, G. (1980). Auditory processing of echoes: peripheral processing. In *Animal Sonar Systems,* ed. R. G. Busnel and J. F. Fish, pp. 519–48. New York: Plenum Press.

Neuweiler, G., Bruns, V., and Schuller, G. (1980). Ears adapted for the detection of motion, or how echolocating bats have exploited the capacities of the mammalian auditory system. *J. Acoust. Soc. Am. 68:* 741–53.

Neuweiler, G., and Vater, M. (1977). Response patterns to pure tones of cochlear nucleus units in the CF-FM bat, *Rhinolophus ferrumequinum. J. Comp. Physiol. 115:* 119–33.

O'Neill, W. E., and Suga, N. (1982). Encoding of target range and its representation in the auditory cortex of the mustached bat. *J. Neurosci. 2:* 17–33.

Ostwald, J. (1978). Tonotope Organisation des Hörcortex der CF-FM-Fledermaus *Rhinolophus ferrumequinum. Verh. dt. zool. Ges. 1978:* 198.

Pollak, G. D. (1980). Organizational and encoding features of single neurons in the inferior colliculus of bats. In *Animal Sonar Systems,* ed. R. G. Busnel and J. F. Fish, pp. 549–87. New York: Plenum Press.

Pollak, G. D., and Bodenhamer, R. D. (1981). Specialized characteristics of single units in inferior colliculus of mustache bat: frequency representation, tuning and discharge patterns. *J. Neurophysiol. 46:* 605–20.

Pollak, G. D., Henson, O. W., and Johnson, R. (1979). Multiple specializations in the peripheral auditory system of the CF-FM bat *Pteronotus parnellii. J. Comp. Physiol. 131:* 255–66.

Pollak, G. D., Henson, O. W., and Novick, A. (1972). Cochlear microphonic audiograms in the pure tone bat *Chilonycteris parnellii parnellii. Science 176:* 66–8.

Pollak, G. D., and Schuller, G. (1981). Tonotopic organization and encoding features of single units in the inferior colliculus of Horseshoe Bats: functional implications for prey identification. *J. Neurophysiol. 45:* 208–26.

Schlegel, P. (1977). Directional coding by binaural brainstem units of the CF-FM bat, *Rhinolophus ferrumequinum. J. Comp. Physiol. 118:* 327–52.

Schnitzler, H. U. (1967). Kompensation von Doppler-Effekten bei Hufeisen-Fledermäusen. *Naturwissenschaften 54:* 523.

Schuller, G. (1977). Echo delay and overlap with emitted orientation sounds and Doppler-shift compensation in the bat, *Rhinolophus ferrumequinum. J. Comp. Physiol. 114:* 103–14.

Schuller, G. (1979). Coding of small sinusoidal frequency and amplitude modulations in the inferior colliculus of 'CF-FM' bat, *Rhinolophus ferrumequinum. Exp. Brain Res. 34:* 117–32.

Schuller, G., Beuter, K., and Schnitzler, H. U. (1974). Response to frequency shifted artificial echoes in the bat *Rhinolophus ferrumequinum. J. Comp. Physiol. 89:* 275–286.

Schuller, G., and Pollak, G. D. (1979). Disproportionate frequency representation in the inferior colliculus of Doppler-compensating Greater Horseshoe bats: evidence for an acoustic fovea. *J. Comp. Physiol. 132:* 47–54.

Schuller, G., and Rübsamen, R. (1981). Laryngeal nerve activity during pulse emission in the CF-FM, *Rhinolophus ferrumequinum.* I. Superior laryngeal nerve. *J. Comp. Physiol. 143:* 317–21.

Schweizer, H. (1981). The connections of the inferior colliculus and the organization of the brainstem auditory system in the Greater Horseshoe Bat *Rhinolophus ferrumequinum. J. Comp. Neurol. 201:* 25–49.

Suga, N., and Jen, P., H.-S. (1977). Further studies on the peripheral auditory system of CF-FM bats specialized for fine frequency analysis of Doppler-shifted echoes. *J. Exp. Biol. 69:* 207–32.

Suga, N., Neuweiler, G., and Möller, J. (1976). Peripheral auditory tuning for fine frequency analysis by the CF-FM bat, *Rhinolophus ferrumequinum.* IV. Properties of peripheral auditory neurons. *J. Comp. Physiol. 106:* 111–25.

Suga, N., Simmons, J. A., and Jen, P. H.-S. (1975). Peripheral specialization for fine frequency analysis of Doppler-shifted echoes in the auditory system of the 'CF-FM' bat *Pteronotus parnellii. J. Exp. Biol. 63:* 161–92.

Vater, M. (1982). Single unit responses in cochlear nucleus of Horseshoe bats to sinusoidal frequency and amplitude modulated signals. *J. Comp. Physiol. 149:* 369–88.

Vater, M., Schlegel, P., and Zöller, H. (1979). Comparative auditory neurophysiology of the inferior colliculus of two Molossid bats, *Molossus ater* and *Molossus molossus.* I. Gross evoked potentials and single unit responses to pure tones. *J. Comp. Physiol. 131:* 137–46.

Wever, E. G. (1974). The evolution of vertebrate hearing. In *Handbook of Sensory Physiology*, Vol. V, 1, ed. W. D. Keidel and W. D. Neff, pp. 423–54. Berlin: Springer-Verlag.

Wilson, J. P. (1977). Towards a model for cochlear frequency analysis. In *Physiology of Hearing*, ed. E. F. Evans and J. P. Wilson, pp. 115–24. New York: Academic Press.

Zook, J. M., and Casseday, J. H. (1980). Ascending auditory pathways in the brainstem of the bat, *Pteronotus parnellii.* In *Animal Sonar Systems*, ed. R. G. Busnel and J. F. Fish, p. 1005. New York: Plenum Press.

1.7

Afferent innervation of the mammalian cochlea

N. Y. S. KIANG, M. C. LIBERMAN,
J. S. GAGE, C. C. NORTHROP, L. W. DODDS
and M. E. OLIVER

The mammalian endorgan for hearing, the cochlea, contains two types of sensory cells, inner hair cells (IHCs) and outer hair cells (OHCs). Both sets of hair cells receive primary afferent endings from neurons in the spiral ganglion which send axons into the central nervous system through the auditory nerve. There have been extensive studies describing electrophysiological recordings from auditory-nerve fibers in mammals (see e.g. Kiang, in press), but recently it has been demonstrated that all such recordings are from large axons of bipolar spiral ganglion neurons whose peripheral extensions exclusively innervate IHCs (Liberman, 1982). Nothing is known about the activity of the neurons that innervate the OHCs.

The cell bodies of these sensory neurons are located in the spiral ganglion within the cochlea. Following retrograde transport of horseradish peroxidase injected into the internal auditory meatus, ganglionic neurons can be traced directly to their target hair cells. From such material it is clear that there are distinct morphological differences between the cell bodies of OHC and IHC neurons with respect to cytoplasmic volume, process size and cell polarity (Kiang, Rho, Northrop, Liberman and Ryugo, 1982). The anatomical literature, at both the light- and electron-microscopic levels, abounds with descriptions of morphological differences among spiral ganglion neurons in a number of different species. The distinctions described have included large v. small, myelinated v. unmyelinated, filamentous v. non-filamentous, pseudomonopolar v. bipolar, and several others. However, comparison of such studies with our HRP material is made difficult by differences in the parameters studied, the histological techniques used and the sampling protocols employed.

The aim of the present study was to measure selected features of spiral ganglion cells in several mammalian species, in order to test the generality of the concept that there are two fundamentally different types of primary neurons in the peripheral auditory system of the mammal.

Methods

Cochleas from adult opossum (*Didelphis virginiana*), guinea pig (*Cavia cobaya*), squirrel monkey (*Saimiri sciureus*) and adult and neonatal human (*Homo sapiens*) and cat (*Felis catus*) were prepared for light microscopy. The cochleas from guinea pigs were control ears from animals with unilateral obliteration of the endolymphatic sac. The adult cat cochlea was the control side from an animal with the auditory nerve cut unilaterally. Following fixation with Heidenhain-Susa solution, decalcification and embedding in celloidin (Schuknecht, 1974), 20-μm-thick sections were cut and stained by Rasmussen's modification of the Bodian protargol method (Bodian, 1936): modifications include incubation in 0.25% protargol containing 6.6 g of copper per 100 ml. The reducer was 3% gelatin, 2% silver nitrate and 1% hydroquinone in an acetate buffer at pH 4.1.

In a separate series of experiments, spiral ganglion neurons in the adult cat were filled retrogradely with horseradish peroxidase (HRP) via iontophoretic injections into the internal auditory meatus. Following survival times of 24–36 h, cochleas were fixed with a buffered aldehyde solution, decalcified, embedded in gelatin, cut at 80 μm on a freezing microtome and reacted with diaminobenzidine. Details of the procedure are described elsewhere (Kiang et al., 1982).

Morphometry of spiral ganglion cells was accomplished by tracing the outlines of the cell body, its processes, nucleus and nucleolus using a drawing tube at an overall magnification of 2600 ×. Cells were included in the data-base only if the nucleus was visible. Tracings were then digitized with a Talos graphics tablet, and areas and diameters were determined by computerized planimetry.

Results

Spiral ganglion in the adult mammal

In recent years, morphological data have accumulated demonstrating that there are at least two different types of ganglion cells in the cat based on cell-body size, myelination, polarity, and cytoplasmic contents (Spoendlin, 1978). The hypothesis that these two neuronal types innervate different types of sensory cells (Spoendlin, 1971) has been verified by tracing the peripheral processes of single, HRP-labeled neurons in the spiral ganglion of the cat (Kiang et al., 1982). Important morphological features of the two neuronal types, as they appear in HRP material, are illustrated in Figures 1 and 2. The cell body of the type-I neuron (innervating IHCs) is typically large and usually bipolar in shape. The diameter of the central process is always larger than that of the peripheral process in the vicinity of the cell body. Ten to $100\,\mu m$ from the cell body, the myelinated peripheral and central processes become thick ($3-5\,\mu m$). The cell body of an OHC neuron (type II), on the other hand, tends to be smaller. Its processes are less likely to be strictly bipolar and are sometimes frankly pseudomonopolar (i.e. a single projection emerges from the cell body and divides into central and peripheral processes). The central and peripheral processes have nearly the same diameter in the vicinity of the cell body and gradually become even finer ($<0.5\,\mu m$) as they travel away from the cell. Both types of spiral ganglion neurons send their central processes deep into the internal auditory meatus towards the cochlear nucleus. The HRP data link type-II ganglion neurons to fine fibers that have the same diameter as does an unmyelinated fiber component seen in electron-microscopic analyses of the auditory nerve (Arnesen and Osen, 1978).

Figure 1. Camera lucida tracings of two HRP-filled afferent neurons from the middle turn of a cat cochlea. Each neuron was followed in serial sections from the HRP-injection site within the internal auditory meatus to the endings on hair cells. Only selected regions are illustrated in the figure; the portions omitted had no interesting special features such as branching. For the Type-I neuron, three segments of the cell are illustrated: a portion of the central axon close to the HRP-injection site, the region around the cell body in the spiral ganglion, and the terminal portion within the habenula perforata and the organ of Corti. For the Type-II cell, corresponding regions are shown except that an unbranched 580-μm segment that spiraled in the OHC region is not shown.

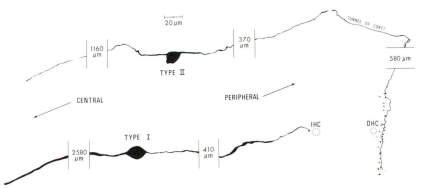

In a previous study of the morphology of HRP-filled spiral ganglion neurons, a measure of the relative sizes of the processes in the vicinity of the cell body was found to be a reliable indicator of the type of sensory cells innervated (Kiang et al., 1982). Process-size measurements are shown in Figure 3a for a sample of HRP-filled neurons traced to either IHCs or OHCs. Two of the neurons traced to OHCs were strictly

Figure 2. Photomicrographs of Type-I and Type-II ganglion cells from the middle turn of the cat cochlea as they appear following HRP injection and in protargol-stained material. Scale bar applies to all micrographs. The tracings beneath the photographs illustrate the conventions adopted for the cell morphometry shown in Figure 3 through 8. For cell-body size measurements, the cross-sectional area (stippling) was defined by extending the radius of curvature of the cell on either side of each process. Process size was defined as the minimum diameter seen within $10\ \mu m$ of the cell body. Nuclear and nucleolar sizes are defined as the maximum cross-sectional areas seen within the section.

HRP

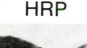

PROTARGOL

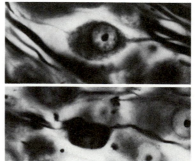

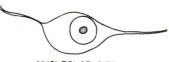

◄— PERIPHERAL   CENTRAL —►   ◄— PERIPHERAL   CENTRAL —►

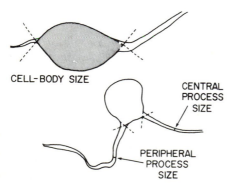

CELL-BODY SIZE

CENTRAL
PROCESS
SIZE

PERIPHERAL
PROCESS
SIZE

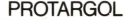

NUCLEOLAR SIZE

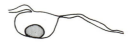

NUCLEAR SIZE

pseudomonopolar; most of the others traced to OHCs approached pseudomonopolarity in a way that is exemplified by the type-II HRP-filled neurons in Figure 2. In contrast, none of the neurons traced to IHCs were strictly pseudomonopolar and the great majority were strictly bipolar, as illustrated by the type-I neurons shown in Figure 2.

Although tracing of HRP-labeled neurons definitively identifies the sensory cells they innervate, the procedure is laborious and technically demanding, since unambiguous tracing requires cells to be intensely labeled and labeled processes to be sufficiently isolated so that no confusion exists in following the fibers. Thus, it is not easy to apply the technique to large numbers of neurons in many species, and impossible to use it in studying the human, because the HRP injections must be made in the living organism. In the present study a more routinely applicable histological technique was used to study spiral ganglion cell morphology. The protargol staining of serial celloidin sections was chosen, since in such preparations the neuronal processes and cell bodies are clearly stained, yet the cell body is not opaque, allowing study of certain organelles. Furthermore, in protargol material, one can study all ganglion cells rather than being limited to those that send central projections into the internal auditory meatus of cochlear nucleus where the HRP injections are made.

Measurements of central and peripheral process size for a sample of protargol-stained spiral ganglion neurons (Figure 3b) suggest that, in

Figure 3. Measurements of peripheral and central process sizes (as defined in the caption for Figure 2) for a population of HRP-filled neurons and a population of protargol-stained neurons from cat cochleas. The HRP-filled cells are gathered from eight cochleas from five cats, the protargol data from one cochlea. In this and all subsequent plots, cell samples are chosen from roughly the middle third of the cochlea. All scales are linear. The dashed line indicates equality of central and peripheral process diameters. No processes from spiral ganglion cells were traced to hair cells in protargol material.

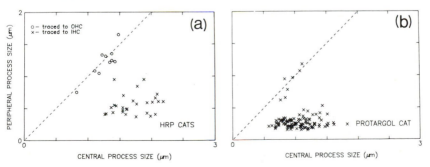

the cat, neurons innervating IHCs may be distinguished easily from those innervating OHCs without tracing peripheral connections. The data show a large group of neurons for which the central process is larger than the peripheral process and a small group of neurons with processes of roughly equal size. The consistently smaller size of the processes measured in the protargol material (compare Figures 3a and 3b) may arise because protargol stains neurofilaments within the process while the HRP reaction product fills the entire axoplasm (Ryugo and Fekete, 1982). The discrepancy might also be due in part to differences in fixation and embedding procedures (Merck, Reide, Löhle and Leupe, 1977).

The ratios of the cell process sizes are plotted in Figure 4 against cell size. In HRP material, the neurons traced to IHCs tended to have larger cytoplasmic areas (cell-body size) than those traced to OHCs (Figure 4a). However there was some overlap in sizes between the two neuronal types. Some of the overlap may have arisen because data from eight cochleas were pooled. Thus, data from a single animal might distinguish different groups of neurons more clearly than averaging data from many animals. Other sources of error can arise when non-spherical cells are viewed from different angles, as was the case here. Errors due to splitting of cells at section boundaries are unimportant for the HRP material since the sections were $80 \mu m$ thick and an entire cell had to be within the section to be included in the sample.

The splitting of cells at section boundaries is a more important consideration in the protargol material, since the sections were only $20 \mu m$ thick, and the criterion for inclusion in the sample was simply that the cell nucleus be present. Errors arising from different viewing angles, on the other hand, are less of an issue in the protargol material since only midmodiolar sections were used, thus roughly fixing the orientations of the cells.

Although there is a continuum in cell size among the HRP-labeled neurons, there is, nevertheless, a group of small neurons with quite different process-size ratios than those for the great majority of neurons which are larger. In the protargol data a similar group of small neurons constitutes less than 7% of the total number of cells (7 out of 105 cells) in Figure 4b. These small neurons in the protargol material also differed from larger neurons with respect to cell shape. Three of the small cells were definitely pseudomonopolar, and the other four approached pseudomonopolarity. One of the latter is pictured in Figure 2. Virtually all of the large neurons were bipolar. In interpreting statistics on cell polarity, one must bear in mind that a pseudomonopolar neuron can appear bipolar when viewed from the side of the cell away from the processes, whereas a bipolar neuron cannot be made to appear pseudo-monopolar by changing the viewing angle.

All of the small neurons in the protargol-stained material from the cat

Figure 4. Comparison of cell sizes and process-size ratios for samples of spiral ganglion cells from a number of species. Cell body size is measured as illustrated in Figure 2. For the human data (Figure 4f) only, circles represent data from pseudomonopolar cells. A cell is defined as pseudomonopolar only if there is no sign of cell convexity between the exiting peripheral and central process. Thus, neither of the Type-II cells illustrated in Figure 2 would be pseudomonopolar by this strict definition. Figures 4a and 4b represent the same cell samples as in Figures 3a and 3b, respectively. Figure 4c is based on a sample of both cochleas from one animal, Figure 4d on two cochleas from two animals, Figure 4e on two cochleas from one animal and Figure 4f on one cochlea from a 38-year-old male, without a history of hearing loss, who died from cancer of the bladder.

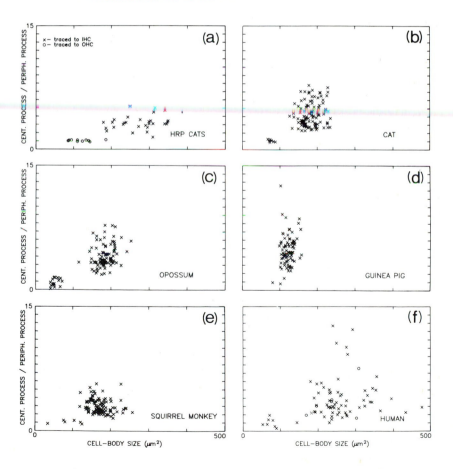

showed intensely dark cytoplasm (Figure 2), whereas the great majority of the larger neurons were pale-staining. A few large neurons stained as darkly as the small neurons. Since protargol stains neurofilaments, dark staining neurons in such material are presumably rich in this component.

Because all small neurons were intensely stained and often pseudo-monopolar, it was easy to estimate the total population of such cells in one cochlea. In a sample of every fifth section through one cochlea, 405 dark-staining small cells were counted. This result suggests that the total number of small neurons in the cat cochlea would be approximately 2000, or 4% of the total number of 50 000 auditory nerve fibers estimated for the cat (Gacek and Rasmussen, 1960). This percentage agrees well with Spoendlin's estimate that 5–10% of the afferent fibers (at the level of the organ of Corti) innervate the OHCs (Spoendlin, 1971).

Thus, even with all the sources of error inherent in measuring cell size in sectioned material discussed above, it appears that in protargol-stained material from the cat one can differentiate cells innervating IHCs from those innervating OHCs on the basis of cell size alone. The data in Figure 4 suggest that the same might be said of the opossum and, perhaps, the human. In both of these cases, as in the cat, most of the 'small' cells had intensely-stained cytoplasm. For the squirrel monkey, the incorporation of data on process-size ratio helps to isolate a discrete group of small cells, but in the guinea pig even the addition of that criterion appears insufficient for a convincing separation.

For the opossum and the squirrel monkey, only the small neurons were pseudomonopolar or approaching pseudomonopolarity. In the guinea pig the three neurons with the lowest ratio of central to peripheral process size were nearly pseudomonopolar (Figure 4d). These observations provide an added measure of confidence that the 'small-neuron' groups in other animals are not basically different from those in the cat. In the human material, on the other hand, the pattern of process polarity seems to be reversed. As illustrated in Figure 4f, many of the large cells were strictly pseudomonopolar. Furthermore, with one exception, all the small cells were strictly bipolar.

In histological preparations from which information on cell polarity or process dimensions is not readily available (e.g. Nissl stains or any thin- or ultrathin-sectioned material), it may be possible to substitute measures of nuclear morphology as aids in differentiating a clear small-neuron group (Figures 5, 6, 7). Since nuclear morphology is largely obscured in the HRP-filled cells, the HRP data in Figures 5 through 7 are of limited use in defining nuclear characteristics of cells definitively traced to either IHCs or OHCs. Nevertheless, plots of nuclear size v. cell size (Figure 5) from protargol material show a clear division into small- and large-neuron groups for all the species studied. In the protargol data, signs of a roughly linear relationship between cell size and nuclear size are present for the large neurons of cat, opossum, guinea pig and squirrel monkey. The lack of such a relationship in the human data may be partially due to unavoidable postmortem changes and the relatively poor fixation of the tissues which renders the cytoplasmic borders of many neurons indistinct.

Figure 5. Comparison of cell-body size and nuclear size for samples of spiral ganglion neurons from a number of species. The data in Figure 5a are taken from eight cochleas of six cats. The samples illustrated in the rest of this figure are as described for Figure 4, except that Figures 5d and 5e are based on only one cochlea.

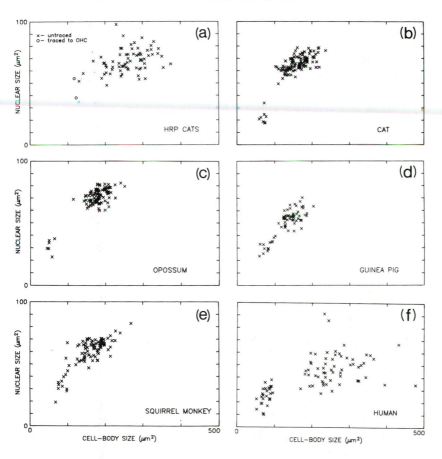

Measures of nuclear roundness (Figure 6) suggest that virtually all the nuclei of large neurons must be spherical, since cross-sections are almost always nearly circular. Nuclei of the small neurons, on the other hand, tend to be kidney-shaped, elliptical and even lobulated in cross-section. Were these lobulations, so clearly seen in the electron-microscopic literature, more easily resolved in the light microscope, the coefficients of nuclear roundness would be significantly lower for small neurons from several of these species, especially the cat. The coefficients of roundness also depend strongly on the cutting angle. For many types of non-spherical structures, circular cross-sections are possible in certain planes of section. Thus one would expect some heterogeneity in nuclear

Figure 6. Comparison of cell-body size and nuclear roundness (defined as the ratio of the measured nuclear area to the area of a circle with the same circumference). Cell samples are the same as those described for Figure 5.

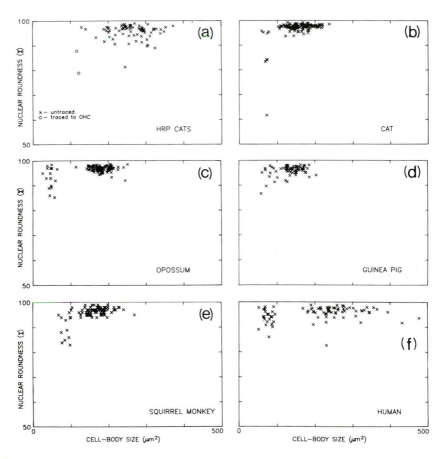

shape, as is seen among the small neurons of all species studied (Figure 6).

The size of the nucleolus (or nucleoli) can also be a useful indicator of neuronal type in certain species (Figure 7). Of all the area measurements, this is the one least susceptible to errors arising from the measured structure being split between two sections. Unfortunately, nucleoli could not be measured accurately in HRP-filled cells traced to OHCs (Figure 7a) due to the dark reaction product filling the cytoplasm. In the protargol material, comparison of nuclear size and nucleolar size easily separates the two groups of cells but with somewhat more difficulty for the animals having generally smaller cells.

Figure 7. Comparison of nuclear size and nucleolar size for samples of spiral ganglion cells in a number of species. Cell samples are the same as described for Figure 5, except that Figure 7c is also derived from only one cochlea.

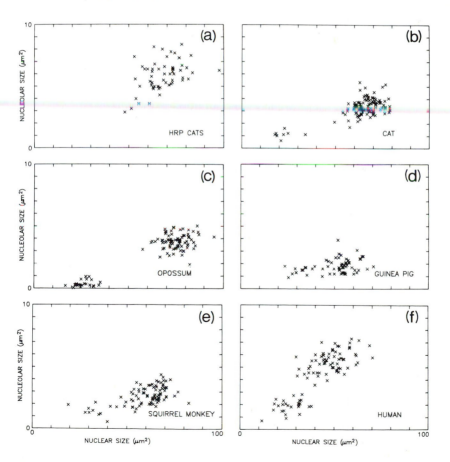

Data from neonatal animals

The foregoing data suggest that in adult mammals the cell bodies of neurons innervating OHCs are smaller than those innervating IHCs and are rarely strictly bipolar. This result is in conflict with much of the Golgi literature on the neuroanatomy of the peripheral auditory system which shows large, bipolar neurons innervating OHCs (Retzius, 1892; Lornte de Nó, 1937; Perkins and Morest, 1975). Since all the Golgi studies were on very young animals it becomes important to examine the morphological characteristics of protargol-stained spiral ganglion neurons in the neonate. This point is particularly crucial since Spoendlin (1981) reports that 'the type II cells with all their typical features are already present in the newborn kitten with the same percentages as in the adult cat'. Spoendlin's statement appears to be in conflict with a more systematic study on maturation of spiral ganglion cells (Romand, Romand, Mulle and Marty, 1980).

Figure 8. Comparison of cell-body size, process-size ratios, and nuclear size for samples of spiral ganglion cells from one cochlea of a two-hour neonatal kitten (Figures 8a and 8c) and from one cochlea of a one-day-old human male (Figures 8b and 8d), who died as a result of cardiac hypoplasia. As in Figure 4 the open circles represent data for pseudomonopolar cells. There are two points unplotted in Figure 8b. They have values of 107 v. 295 and 101 v. 238 for the *y* and *x* axes respectively.

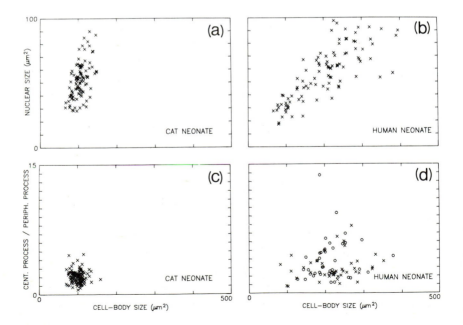

Morphometry of protargol-stained spiral ganglion neurons from a two-hour-old kitten and a one-day-old human are shown in Figure 8. Comparison of Figures 4 and 8 indicates that the conflict between the Golgi data and the present study does not arise because of the different techniques used. No combination of criteria, including the more subjective ones of cell darkness and degree of pseudomonopolarity, differentiated two discrete neuronal types in these neonatal specimens. It may be that Spoendlin's 'newborn kitten' was somewhat more mature than the usual neonate.

The data from the human neonate suggest that there are more pseudomonopolar large neurons present than in the adult. (Compare Figures 4f and 8d.) This finding is surprising in light of reports that in the *spinal* ganglia at early stages of development all the neurons, including those which will ultimately become pseudomonopolar, are bipolar with thick peripheral processes and thin central processes (Pannese, 1974). If pseudomonopolar *spiral* ganglion cells in the human also developed in a similar sequence, one would not expect the neonatal spiral ganglion to have more pseudomonopolar neurons than an adult cochlea, as is the case here.

Discussion

The idea that there are two kinds of neurons in the mammalian spiral ganglion, is not new (see Rasmussen, 1943). The earliest electron-microscopic description of mammalian spiral ganglion neurons described myelinated 'filamented' and 'granular' neurons in the rat and mentioned that the former type tends to be larger than the latter (Rosenbluth, 1962). Given that both of Rosenbluth's neuronal types were myelinated, the cells that he studied were probably all type-I cells in the modern formulation. It may be that his filamented cells correspond to those large cells that stain more darkly with protargol.

The first electron-microscopic descriptions of the small neurons were probably made on the guinea pig (Suzuki, Watanabe and Osada, 1963). In osmium-fixed and uranyl-acetate-stained material, most of the spiral ganglion neurons were seen as light bipolar cells of uniform size with a round or oval nucleus located to one side of the cell. The cell bodies were myelinated and one or several nucleoli were seen. A small number of comparatively dark neurons were also seen with nuclei that were often non-circular. In iron-hematoxylin stained material, bipolar neurons whose cell bodies and nuclei were smaller than the myelinated neurons were seen at the periphery of the ganglion. Most of these early observations on the guinea pig have withstood the test of later studies.

The finding that myelinated spiral ganglion neurons contain abundant ribosomes but few neurofilaments, whereas unmyelinated neurons contain few ribosomes and many neurofilaments, was added soon after the initial work (Nishimura, Kon, Awataguchi, Ishida and Yamamoto, 1965), and the fact that the central process was larger than the peripheral process in the bipolar myelinated neurons was noted (Thomsen, 1966). In all studies the number of unmyelinated neurons was small. Estimates ranged from 2–4% (Thomsen, 1966) to 10% (Kellerhals, Engstrom and Ades, 1967).

In later years, the general descriptions of two distinct neuronal types in the guinea pig were verified (Reinecke, 1967; Merck, Reide, Löhle and Cürten, 1977), although only a few studies attempted to explore possible exceptions (Trevisi, Testa and Riva, 1977). The theory that the two types of spiral ganglion neurons might differentially innervate inner and outer hair cells was not investigated in electron-microscopic studies in normal animals because of the difficulty of following small elements over long distances. Studying cats with transected auditory nerves, Spoendlin (1971) found that, while most of the ganglion cells degenerated, the remaining neurons (about 5% of the total population) were small and unmyelinated. Since the afferent endings on OHCs in these animals also appeared to survive, while most afferent endings on IHCs did not, he concluded that the small unmyelinated neurons (type II) supplied the afferent endings on OHCs while the large myelinated neurons (type I) gave rise to the afferent endings on IHCs. In a sequence of subsequent papers, Spoendlin elaborated on this idea, refining his descriptions of the two neuronal types in the cat (Spoendlin, 1973, 1974, 1975, 1978, 1979a,b). Meanwhile the original concept that there may be more than one type of *myelinated* neuron in the rat (Rosenbluth, 1962) was corroborated in the cat, in that some myelinated neurons appeared to show more neurofilaments, neurotubules and ribosomal clusters than others (Adamo and Diagneault, 1973).

Incorporating the present results with those of earlier studies, one may summarize the characteristics that distinguish the two types of spiral ganglion neurons in the normal adult cat (Table 1).

In attempting to determine from the literature how generally applicable these criteria might be to other species, one finds it difficult to separate true variations in morphology from differences that might be attributable to the use of different techniques, definitions or scientific standards. Many of the characteristics in Table 1 have not been carefully defined in terms that can be quantified. Descriptions of pseudomonopolarity, myelination, nuclear lobulation, staining properties, etc. have not received such definitive treatment even in one species.

Table 1. *Characteristics of Type-I and Type-II cells in the cat*

Cell characteristic	Type I	Type II
Peripheral innervation	Inner hair cell	Outer hair cell
Cell size	Large	Small
Nuclear size	Large	Small
Nucleolar size	Large	Small
Cell shape	Bipolar	Non-bipolar
Nuclear shape	Spherical	Kidney shaped, frequently lobulated
Presence of neurofilaments	Sparse	Abundant
Presence of ribosomes	Abundant	Usually sparse
Myelination of cell body	Yes	No
Cell processes within $10\,\mu m$ of cell body	Central > peripheral	Peripheral ≈ central
Central process away ($>100\,\mu m$) from cell body	Large myelinated	Small unmyelinated

The most serious challenge to the idea that the two neuronal types described for the cat are generalizable to all mammals comes from data on humans. Apparently most human spiral ganglion neurons, including the largest ones, are unmyelinated (Kimura, Ota, Schuknecht and Takahashi, 1976; Ylikoski, Collar and Palva, 1978; Ota and Kimura, 1980). This observation, coupled with the present finding of large, obviously pseudomonopolar cells in both the human adult and neonate, has raised the possibility that the human auditory nerve may differ in important ways from other mammals studied.

In interpreting these differences, one must consider that sectioned temporal bones from normal, healthy humans are difficult to obtain. There is evidence from animal experiments that in pathological conditions the characteristics of some type-I neurons change to resemble those of type-II neurons in that they lose their myelin sheaths, the nuclei become less round, and the cytoplasm becomes more filamentous (Ylikoski, Wersäll and Bjorkroth, 1974; Trevisi et al., 1977; Elverland and Mair, 1980). The present authors have observed that in at least two different chronic pathological conditions (one in a cat with a one-year survival from auditory-nerve section and one in a cat with a five-year survival from virtually total hair cell loss following ototoxic drug injection), the distinction between type-I and type-II neurons becomes much more difficult to make. Many dark-staining neurons are large and appear to be altered type-I cells. This finding fits with the doctrine that degenerating neurons show an increase in neurofilaments (Guillery, 1970) which would stain darkly with protargol.

Recently Spoendlin (1981) has recognized that his earlier work with the cut-nerve animals (Spoendlin, 1971) has to be reinterpreted because some of the 'type-II' neurons could have been degenerating type-I neurons. The use of pathological material to establish normal morphology must always be viewed cautiously and the final decision on how to interpret the extant human data must await analysis of material from more clearly normal specimens.

Some of the observations initially made on human material (such as synaptic endings on small cells) (Kimura et al., 1976) have later been confirmed and extended in animals (Kimura and Ota, 1981). In other instances, human data have been used to buttress arguments for certain theoretically important issues. A case in point is the issue of whether parasympathetic postganglionic cells exist in the spiral ganglion. Ross and Burkel (1973) reported finding multipolar cells in the rat cochlea which could be interpreted as such. Their published pictures, however, are far from convincing. The best evidence for multipolar cell in the spiral ganglion comes from Kimura, Ota and Takahashi (1979), who described finding a multipolar cell in a human cochlea. The cell was small and myelinated and was the only one of its type ever seen. The protargol method should be capable of demonstrating multipolar cells, even in the crowded conditions of normal spiral ganglia, but the present authors failed to find any multipolar cells in any of the normal animal cochleas. In our pathological material, on the other hand, a large number of neurons took on bizarre shapes, with swollen axonal process. In many cases, one or both of the processes emerging from the cell body bifurcated, producing multipolar cells with as many as five processes. In the neonatal human we found one cell which appeared to have three processes emerging from a single stalk. Our failure to find multipolar cells in normal adult material, and the ease with which we found them in pathological material, places the burden of proof on those who insist that multipolar cells are an essential component in the normal spiral ganglion.

For the moment, one can put the idiosyncrasies of the human data aside and ask whether there are 'unusual' findings in other species. For most, if not all, of the major characteristics in Table I there are no reliable data demonstrating strong exceptions. Certainly the bulk of the present results could be construed as supporting the general idea that the system of neurons innervating OHCs differs from that innervating IHCs in much the same way for all mammalian species, except perhaps for the human. The occasional cells that deviate from the general rules may be interpreted as examples of altered metabolic or functional state overlaid on a normal pattern that is fairly constant. Although there may be a consistent way to think about all of the existing anatomical data on mammalian spiral ganglion neurons, the subject of spiral ganglion cell morphology cannot be considered closed, and the difficult task of relating function to the morphology has hardly begun.

The authors wish to acknowledge the assistance of J. Rho, M. Curby, W. Sewell, B. Norris, E. Keithley, P. Dawley, and D. Dittman. This work was supported by US Public Health Service Grants 5 P01 NS 13126 and 1 R01 NS 18339.

Bibliography

Adamo, N. J., and Diagneault, E. A. (1973). Ultrastructural features of neurons and nerve fibres of the spiral ganglia of cats. *J. Neurocytol. 2:* 91–103.

Arnesen, A. R., and Osen, K. K. (1978). The cochlear nerve in the cat, topography, cochleotopy and fiber spectrum. *J. Comp. Neurol. 178:* 661–78.

Bodian, D. (1936). A new method for staining nerve fibers and nerve endings in mounted paraffin sections. *Anat. Rec. 65:* 89–95.

Elverland, H. H., and Mair, I. W. S. (1980). Hereditary deafness in the cat. *Acta Otolaryngol. 90:* 360–9.

Gacek, R. R., and Rasmussen, G. L. (1961). Fiber analysis of the statoacoustic nerve of guinea pig, cat and monkey. *Anat. Rec. 139:* 455–63.

Guillery, R. W. (1970). Light and electronmicroscopical studies of normal and degenerating axons. In *Contemporary Research Methods in Neuroanatomy*, ed. J. H. Nauta and S. O. E. Ebbesson, pp. 77–105. Berlin: Springer-Verlag.

Kellerhals, B., Engström, H., and Ades, H. W. (1967). Die Morphologie des Ganglion spirale cochleae. *Acta Orolaryngol.*, Suppl. *226.*

Kiang, N. Y. S. Peripheral neural processing of auditory information. In *Handbook of Physiology*, ed. I. Darian-Smith. Bethesda: The American Physiological Society. (In Press.)

Kiang, N. Y. S., Rho, J. M., Northrop, C. C., Liberman, M. C., and Ryugo, D. K. (1982). Hair-cell innervation by spiral ganglion cells in adult cats. *Science 217:* 175–7.

Kimura, R. S., and Ota, C. Y. (1981). Nerve fiber synapses on primate spiral ganglion. *Abstracts of the Fourth Association for Research in Otolaryngology Meeting.*

Kimura, R. S., Ota, C. Y., Schuknecht, H. F., and Takahashi, T. (1976). Electron microscopic cochlear observations in bilateral Meniere's disease. *Annls Otolaryngol. 85:* 791–801.

Kimura, R. S., Ota, C. Y., and Takahashi, T. (1979). Nerve fibers on spiral ganglion cells in the human cochlea. *Annls Otology-Rhinology-Laryngology 88:* Suppl. 62, 1–17.

Liberman, M. C. (1982). Single-neuron labeling in the cat auditory nerve. *Science 216:* 1239–41.

Lorente de Nó, R. (1937). The neural mechanism of hearing. I. Anatomy and physiology. (b) The sensory endings in the cochlea. *Laryngoscope 47:* 373–7.

Merck, W., Riede, U. N., Löhle, E., and Cürten, I. (1977). Eine ultrastrukturellmorphometrische Analyse des Ganglion spirale cochleae des Meerschweinchens. *Archs Oto-Rhino-Laryngol. 214:* 303–12.

Merck, W., Riede, U. N., Löhle, E., and Leupe, M. (1977). Einfluss verschiedener Pufferlösungen auf die Strukturerhaltung des Ganglion spirale cochleae. *Archs Oto-Rhino-Laryngol. 215:* 283–92.

Nishimura, T., Kon, I., Awataguchi, S., Ishida, M., and Yamamoto, N. (1965). Submicroscopic studies on the spiral ganglion in guinea pigs. *Hirosaki Med. J. 17:* 1–18.

Ota, C. Y., and Kimura, R. S. (1980). Ultrastructural study of the human spiral ganglion. *Acta Otolaryngol. 89:* 53–62.

Pannese, E. (1974). The histogenesis of the spinal ganglia. *Adv. Anat. Embryol. Cell Biol. 47:* 5–97.

Perkins, R. E., and Morest, D. K. (1975). Study of cochlear innervation patterns in cats and rats with the Golgi method and Normarski optics. *J. Comp. Neurol. 163:* 129–58.

Rasmussen, A. T. (1943). *Outlines of Neuroanatomy.* Dubuque, Iowa: Brown Publishing Co.

Reinecke, M. (1967). Elektronenmikroskopiche Untersuchungen am Ganglion spirale des Meerschweinchens. *Arch. klin. exp. Ohren-Nasen-und Kehlkopfheilk 189:* 158–67.

Retzius, G. (1892). Die Endingungsweise des Gehoernerven. In *Biol. Untersuch. 3:* 29–36.

Romand, R., Romand, M. R., Mulle, C., and Marty, R. (1980). Early stages of myelination in the spiral ganglion cells of the kitten during development. *Acta Otolaryngol. 90:* 391–7.

Rosenbluth, J. (1962). The fine structure of acoustic ganglia in the rat. *J. Cell Biol. 12:* 329–59.

Ross, M. D., and Burkel, W. (1973). Multipolar neurons in the spiral ganglion of the rat. *Acta Otolaryngol. 76:* 381–94.

Ryugo, D. K., and Fekete, D. M. (1982). Morphology of primary axosomatic endings in the anteroventral cochlear nucleus of the cat: a study of the end bulbs of Held. *J. Comp. Neurol.*

Schuknecht, H. F. (1974). *Pathology of the Ear.* Cambridge, USA: Harvard University Press.

Spoendlin, H. (1971). Degeneration behaviour of the cochlear nerve. *Arch. klin. exp. Ohren-Nasen-und-Kehlkopfheilkunde 200:* 275–91.

Spoendlin, H. (1973). The innervation of the cochlear receptor. In *Basic Mechanisms in Hearing,* ed. A. R. Møller and P. Boston, pp. 185–234. New York: Academic Press.

Spoendlin, H. (1974). Neuroanatomy of the cochlea. In *Facts and Models in Hearing,* ed. E. Zwicker and E. Terhardt, pp. 18–32. Berlin: Springer-Verlag.

Spoendlin, H. (1975). Retrograde degeneration of the cochlear nerve. *Acta Otolaryngol. 79:* 266–75.

Spoendlin, H. (1978). The afferent innervation of the cochlea. In *Evoked Electrical Activity in the Auditory Nervous System,* ed. R. F. Naunton and P. Fernandez, pp. 21–41. New York: Academic Press.

Spoendlin, H. (1979a). Sensory neural organization of the cochlea. *J. Laryngol. Otol. 93:* 853–77.

Spoendlin, H. (1979b). Neural connections of the outer haircell system. *Acta Otolaryngol. 87:* 381–7.

Spoendlin, H. (1981). Differentiation of cochlear neurons. *Acta Otolaryngol. 91:* 451–6.

Suzuki, Y., Watanabe, A., and Osada, M. (1963). Cytological and electron microscopic studies on the spiral ganglion cells of the adult guinea pigs and rabbits. *Archiv. Histol. Jap. 24:* 9–33.

Thomsen, E. (1966). Ultrastructure of the spiral ganglion of the guinea pig. *Acta Otolaryngol.,* Supplementum *224:* 442–8.

Trevisi, M., Testa, F., and Riva, A. (1977). Fine structure of neurons of cochlear ganglion of the guinea pig after prolonged sound stimulation of the inner ear. *J. Submicrosc. Cytol. 9:* 157–72.

Ylikoski, J., Collar, Y., and Palva, T. (1978). Ultrastructural features of spiral ganglion cells. *Arch. Otolaryngol. 104:* 84–8.

Ylikoski, J., Wersäll, J., and Bjorkroth, B. (1974). Degeneration of neural elements in the cochlea of the guinea pig after damage to the organ of Corti by ototoxic antibiotics. *Acta Otolaryngol.* Suppl. *326:* 23–41.

1.8

Efferent innervation of the cochlea

H. SPOENDLIN

An efferent innervation of the cochlea was first identified by Rasmussen in 1942. Using the Marchi method for staining nerve fibers he demonstrated the existence of an efferent olivo-cochlear bundle (OCB) in the cat, rat, and opossum (Rasmussen, 1942, 1946, 1953, 1960). This was essentially confirmed by Rossi and Cortesina with acetylcholinesterase (ACHE) histochemistry (1962, 1965) with a slightly different origin of the homolateral fibers. In addition to the olivo-cochlear fibers they described another efferent bundle originating in the reticular substance, the reticulo-cochlear bundle, which was confirmed in the rat (Brown et al., 1972) and might only be present in rodents. Ross (1969) presented an entirely different concept on the basis of ACHE histochemical studies in the mouse according to which the cochlear efferents are a part of the general visceral efferent system with post-ganglionic cells somewhere in the periphery, i.e. in the spiral ganglion and preganglionic neurons originating in various places in the medulla around the facial genu and the superior salivary nucleus. Although she maintains her view, claiming that degeneration studies and HRP studies on newborn kitten (Warr, 1975) are not conclusive (Ross et al., 1977), more recent studies with HRP injections leave no doubt that the efferents do originate in the superior olivary complex as originally described by Rasmussen.

According to Rasmussen the contralateral efferent olivo-cochlear fibers cross over at the floor of the IVth ventricle and join the homolateral olivo-cochlear fibers to enter the vestibular root. They reach the periphery together with the vestibular nerve. Only in the periphery, in the depth of the inner acoustic meatus, the efferent fibers pass over to the cochlear nerve through the anastomosis of Oort and

163

lead to the spiral ganglion in the upper basal turn as a compact bundle from where they continue as intraganglionic spiral bundles through all cochlear turns to the apex and the base of the cochlea giving off at regular intervals radial fibers to the Organ of Corti (Figure 1).

Engström (1958) was the first to suggest that the large vesicle-filled nerve endings at the outer hair cells (ohc) could be efferent; this was subsequently confirmed by degeneration studies (Iurato, 1962; Spoendlin and Gacek, 1963; Smith and Rasmussen, 1963) and histochemical demonstration of ACHE (Schuknecht, Churchill and Doran, 1959; Rossi and Cortesina, 1962). There are certainly some differences among different species but the system is basically the same in all species so far studied. This report relies mainly on the findings in the cat, which was mainly studied by the author and has a well-developed acoustic system for which most electrophysiological data are available. Differences in other species will be indicated when they are present and known.

Origin of olivo-cochlear efferent fibers

With the application of HRP techniques a clear and direct demonstration of the origin of the cochlear efferents was possible

Figure 1. Schematic representation of the general outlay of the homo- and contralateral olivo-cochlear neurons (interrupted lines) with their origin in the superior olivary complex. Arrows indicate the sites of possible selective lesions of the olivo-cochlear efferents: A, midline lesion of the contralateral neurons only; B, lesion in the vestibular root; C, lesion in the vestibular nerve of the homo- and contralateral olivo-cochlear bundle.

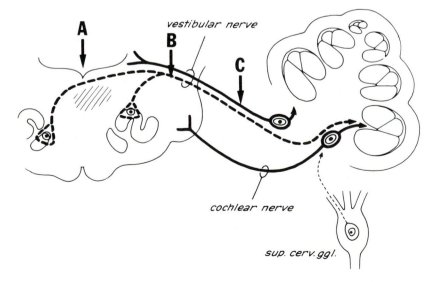

(Warr, 1975, 1978). After injection of HRP in the scala tympani the substance is taken up by the efferent endings and transported retrograde to the cells of origin, where it can be demonstrated by a histochemical method.

In the kitten Warr (1978) found one group of small cells in the lateral superior olivary nucleus (LSO) (85% contralateral and 15% homolateral), which he named the lateral group. Another group of larger cells was found in the medial nucleus of the trapezoid body (MNTB) (70% contralateral and 30% homolateral), the medial group. The number of labeled neurons was found to be around 1600, which is more than double the number indicated by Rasmussen. Occasionally also some facial neurons are labeled when HRP is spilled to the stapedius muscle, but they are easily distinguished from the olivo-cochlear fibers.

With a modified HRP technique of Mesulam we found similar figures in the adult cat as Warr had in the kitten with total numbers of about 1400 neurons (Spoendlin, 1981). This certainly represents a minimum number because it is uncertain whether all neurons are taking up the HRP, so the real number of neurons might be somewhat larger. In our material again the great majority (90%) of the neurons in the LSO is homolateral and the great majority of the neurons in the MNTB and periolivary nucleus (PON) (80%) is contralateral (Figures 2, 3, 4). In

Figure 2. Schematic representation of a longitudinal paramedial section of the brainstem of the cat. A and B indicate the plane of section to demonstrate the ganglion cells of the olivo-cochlear neurons shown in Figures 3 and 4.

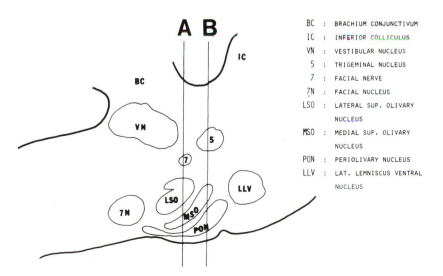

BC	:	BRACHIUM CONJUNCTIVUM
IC	:	INFERIOR COLLICULUS
VN	:	VESTIBULAR NUCLEUS
5	:	TRIGEMINAL NUCLEUS
7	:	FACIAL NERVE
7N	:	FACIAL NUCLEUS
LSO	:	LATERAL SUP. OLIVARY NUCLEUS
MSO	:	MEDIAL SUP. OLIVARY NUCLEUS
PON	:	PERIOLIVARY NUCLEUS
LLV	:	LAT. LEMNISCUS VENTRAL NUCLEUS

Figure 3. Schematic representation of a transverse section through the brainstem at the level of the LSO. The black dots indicate the cells of origin of the lateral group of the olivo-cochlear neurons, which are essentially associated with the ihc system. The size of the dots in Figure 3 and Figure 4 indicates the relative size of the ganglion cells. The numbers are actual counts of HRP-labeled cells in an adult cat.

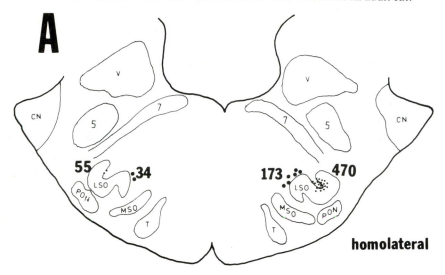

Figure 4. Schematic representation of a transverse section through the brainstem at the level of the MNTB and PON with the black dots, indicating the cells of origin of the olivo-cochlear neurons of the periolivary group, mainly associated with the ohc. The numbers represent actual counts of HRP-labeled cells in an adult cat.

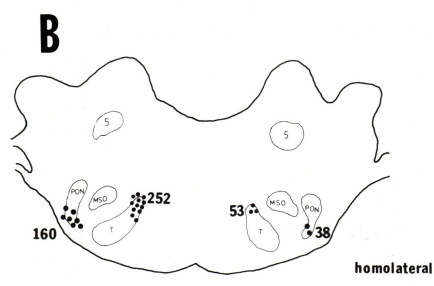

the adult cat the olivo-cochlear neurons do not present a uniform population of neurons. They constitute at least four groups of different types of ganglion cells. In the LSO the majority of ganglion cells is very small fusiform, mostly of bipolar appearance, with a diameter around 10 μm and located deep in the hilus of the S-shaped nucleus, whereas another smaller group of somewhat larger cells with usually more dendrites on one pole lies above and medial to the hilus (Figure 5). In the medial or periolivary group the majority of neurons sits within the MNTB and has medium-sized rounded ganglion cells with several short dendrites, whereas another somewhat smaller group of very large multipolar cells with long dendrites and diameters up to 20 μm is situated in the PON (Figure 6). Using this HRP-technique no cells could be found in the reticular substance or any other sites in the medulla in the cat. According to most recent findings of Warr (1982) in the rat, the small neurons of the LSO are exclusively homolateral and the larger neurons of the medial or periolivary group are exclusively contralateral in this animal.

Figure 5. LSO-associated olivo-cochlear neurons with one group of small fusiform cells deep within the hilus of the LSO and another group of somewhat larger cells superior and lateral to it. MSO, medial superior olivary nucleus.

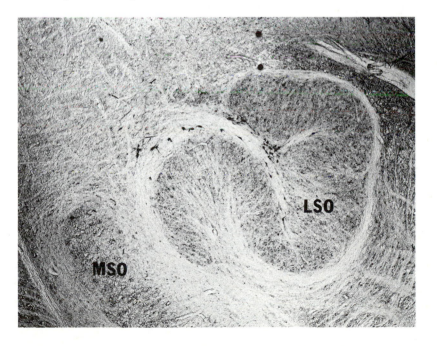

Figure 6. Periolivary olivo-cochlear neurons with one group of medium-sized, rounded, multipolar ganglion cells with short dendrites in the MNTB and another more lateral group in the PON of very large multipolar ganglion cells with longer dendrites.

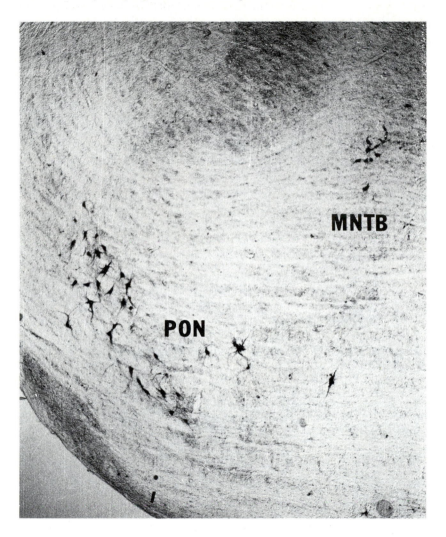

Pathways of the olivo-cochlear fibers

The original description of Rasmussen has generally been accepted and confirmed. All fibers of the contralateral superior olive cross the midline at the floor of the IVth ventricle as a compact bundle, where it can easily be demonstrated with HRP-techniques, and, at least in the cat, it does not seem that many fibers cross the midline in deeper areas of the medulla. At the level of the vestibular root the contra- and homolateral fibers join and run together through the vestibular nerve into the periphery.

The totality of efferent fibers can therefore best be reached and selectively transected in the vestibular nerve without damage to cochlear afferent neurons. Whether the few ACHE-positive fibers described in the cochlear nerve by Gacek, Nomura and Balogh (1965) belong to the olivo-cochlear bundle (OCB) is very uncertain. An ACHE-positive reaction is not enough evidence to establish the efferent nature of a fiber.

The fibers are best identified in the anastomosis of Oort and in the intraganglionic spiral bundle. There are myelinated and unmyelinated fibers in the anastomosis of Oort (Terayama et al., 1969). Osen (1981) found a majority of fibers to be unmyelinated and in an analysis of the intraganglionic spiral bundle we found similar relationships with two-thirds unmyelinated fibers, of which, however, some seem to belong to the adrenergic innervation originating in the superior cervical ganglion (Paradiesgarten et al., 1977). A fiber analysis of the intraganglionic spiral bundle in the upper basal turn of the adult cat clearly shows the group of the small unmyelinated fibers and the group of larger myelinated fibers (Figures 7, 8, 9, 10). In the newborn kitten only very few fibers are myelinated. Radiating fibers from the intraganglionic spiral bundle to the Organ of Corti can be demonstrated only by means of ACHE histochemistry or HRP-techniques. Already at this level in the osseous spiral lamina a certain degree of ramification of these fibers is taking place (Nomura and Schuknecht, 1965). In the osseous spiral lamina we find many unmyelinated fibers, which represent the unmyelinated efferents, the axons of the type II afferent neurons, and some adrenergic fibers (Spoendlin and Suter, 1976).

At the level of the habenula the efferent fibers are still very few as compared to the afferent cochlear neurons. In fiber counts at the level of the habenula we found no significant difference before and after elimination of the efferents (Spoendlin, 1970). Within the habenula the efferent fibers cannot be distinguished morphologically from the afferent fibers. Their identification is possible only when their course is followed further peripherally (Liberman, 1980a).

Distribution and endings in the Organ of Corti

After the suggestion of efferent terminals in the Organ of Corti on the basis of morphological criteria (Engström, 1958) the precise identification, the peripheral distribution pattern, and the numerical

Figure 7. Low-magnification EM picture of one intraganglionic spiral bundle in the upper basal turn of the adult cat with myelinated and unmyelinated (u) fibers of varying calibers and myelin sheath thickness. S, Schwann cell. The histogram of this particular bundle is shown in Figure 8.

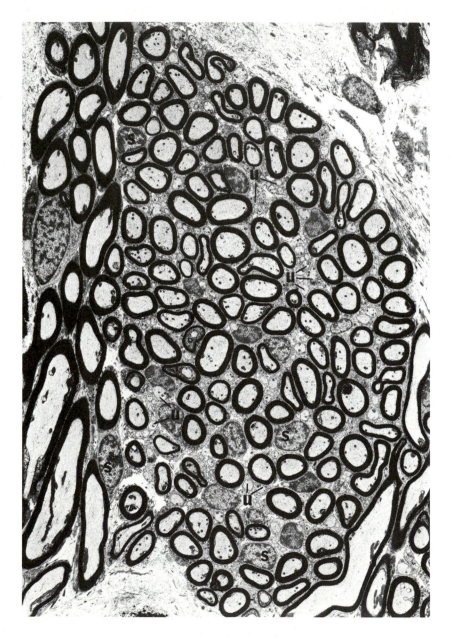

analysis of the cochlear efferents were done by means of degeneration studies in a number of different species: Iurato (1962, 1964) in the rat, Smith and Rasmussen (1963, 1965) in the guinea pig, Spoendlin and Gacek (1963) and Spoendlin (1966) in the cat, and Wright and Preston (1973) in the guinea pig.

Figure 8. Histogram of the nerve fibers in the intraganglionic spiral bundle of Figure 7. There are two main peaks, one for the small unmyelinated fibers (hatched columns) and the other for the larger myelinated fibers (gray columns).

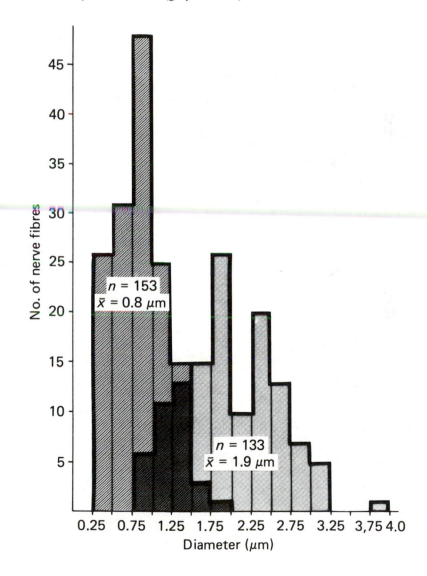

The cochlear efferents are subject to very fast Wallerian degeneration after section of their axons. This degeneration starts almost immediately after lesioning and is complete within a few days (Figure 11). The contralateral efferents can be selectively cut at the floor of the IVth ventricle (Kimura and Weisäll, 1962; Iurato, 1964; Spoendlin, 1970). The homo- and contralateral fibers can be completely eliminated within the vestibular root (Spoendlin and Gacek, 1963) or within the vestibular

Figure 9. Low-magnification EM-picture of two ohc (oH) of the basal turn of a guinea pig with a great number of large efferent nerve endings filled with synaptic vesicles and many mitochondria (e). In between these efferent endings are some smaller afferent nerve endings (a).

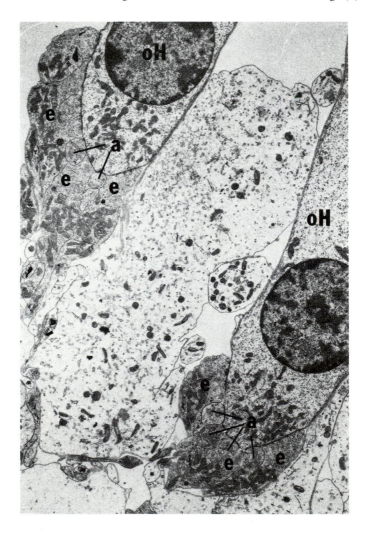

nerve (Spoendlin, 1966, 1969) (Figure 1). The best place to reach the totality of efferent fibers is the vestibular nerve because of easy identification of the vestibular nerve in the inner acoustic meatus and because all olivo-cochlear efferent fibers are associated with this nerve.

In such studies it was possible to show that all large vesiculated nerve endings, all upper tunnel radial fibers as well as the inner spiral and the tunnel spiral fibers belong to the olivo-cochlear efferent system since they degenerate and disappear completely after section in the vestibular nerve (Spoendlin, 1969) (Figure 12). Retrospectively, the semi-selective

Figure 10. Base of an ohc of the basal turn of an adult cat with large efferent nerve endings (e) having an enormous contact area with the outer hair cell (oH). The synaptic vesicles agglomerate and condense to form small spicules at the presynaptic membrane facing the hair cell which probably represent synapses (sy). In the cat the efferent nerve endings are always on the modiolar side of the hair cell base and the smaller afferent nerve endings (a) on the more distal side of the hair cell base. Adjacent to the contact with the efferent endings one always finds a subsynaptic cysterna (sc) in the hair cell.

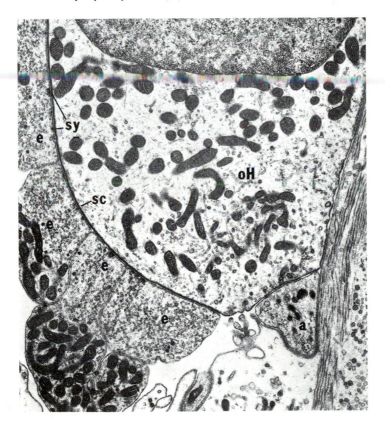

Maillet-stain using the Zink–Jodin–Osmium-technique can demonstrate very nicely the efferent nerve fibers and endings within the Organ of Corti (Engström et al., 1966; Spoendlin, 1968) (Figure 13).

The efferent innervation is not uniform throughout the cochlea. It is most abundant in the first row in the middle and upper basal turn, where anyway the highest innervation density of the cochlea exists (Spoendlin, 1972). The efferent innervation decreases towards the upper turns of the cochlea and is less in the second and third rows of outer hair cells. Whereas in the basal turn all ohc receive considerable efferent innervation, in the apical turn the ohc of the third row are frequently without any efferent nerve endings.

Figure 11. Base of an ohc (oH) of an adult cat four days after section of the olivo-cochlear fibers in the vestibular nerve. The efferent nerve endings (e) are in full degeneration whereas the afferent nerve ending (a) remains unchanged. The contact zone between ohc and efferent ending is collapsed and folded, but the subsynaptic cysterna (sc) is still there.

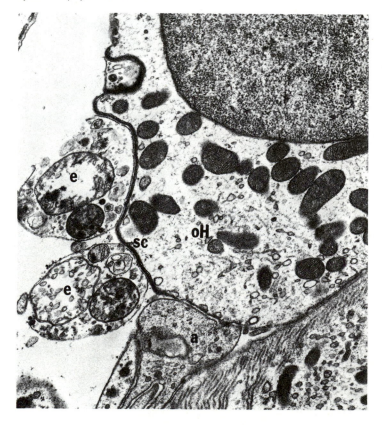

One of the most striking findings of electron-microscopic investigations of the ear was the enormous efferent innervation of the ohc. The efferent nerve endings are very large, filled with synaptic vesicles and rich in mitochondria (Figures 9, 10). The synaptic vesicles agglomerate and condense in certain places at the axon membrane facing the cell membrane of the ohc base. These vesicle condensations in the form of small spicules are considered as places of synaptic activity. Opposite the nerve ending there is always a subsynaptic cysterna parallel to the cell membrane within the ohc (Figure 10).

On the basis of serial sections we found six to ten large efferent nerve endings at the base of ohc in the basal turn of the cat and about an equal number of much smaller afferent nerve endings. These figures have recently been confirmed by means of serial sections using a high-voltage electron microscope, which enables one to observe very thick sections so that serial sectioning becomes much easier. The total number of efferent nerve terminals at the ohc has been estimated to be about 40 000 (Spoendlin, 1966).

Figure 12. Radial innervation schema of the Organ of Corti. The efferent fibers and endings, such as the inner spiral fibers (iS) and the tunnel spiral fibers (TS), the upper tunnel radial fibers (R) and the large endings at the base of the ohc (E) are represented by full black lines, whereas the afferent elements, such as the inner radial fibers (iR), the basilar fibers (b) and the outer spiral fibers (oS) are represented by hatched lines.

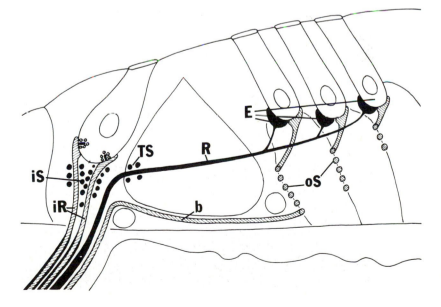

It is not only the relative number of the efferent nerve terminals which is surprising, but particularly the enormous contact area with the ohc, which in the first turn is about ten times as large as the contact area of the afferent nerve endings with the hair cell. In the cat there is morphological evidence for synaptic contacts exclusively with the hair cell but not with the afferent endings or dendrites associated with the hair cell (Figure 17, p. 180). The efferent and afferent nerve terminals are topographically well separated. The efferents lie almost always on the modiolar side and the afferents on the distal side of the hair cell base. This separation of efferent and afferent nerve endings and dendrites is not as clear in the rodents as it is in the cat (Figures 9, 10). In the guinea pig (Smith and Chester, 1961), for example, one finds also some efferent nerve endings, especially in the upper turns and outer rows, with synaptic contacts with afferent dendrites.

In many respects the cochlea of the cat presents strictly organized patterns with fewer exceptions than the cochleas of other species including man. The entire organ seems to be more developed with about twice as many cochlear neurons as in man.

The enormous contact area and the numerous synapses with the ohc certainly reflect the potential functional influence the efferents can have on the ohc.

Figure 13. Surface view of the Organ of Corti of the second cochlear turn of a normal adult cat stained after Maillet. With this semi-selective stain of efferent elements all efferent fibers and endings show black. Mainly, the efferent endings at the first row of ohc (1) are very large and abundant, whereas the efferent endings of the second and third rows are much less conspicuous. In addition, the tunnel-crossing upper tunnel radial fibers (R), the inner spiral fibers (iS) and the tunnel spiral fibers (TS) are clearly seen.

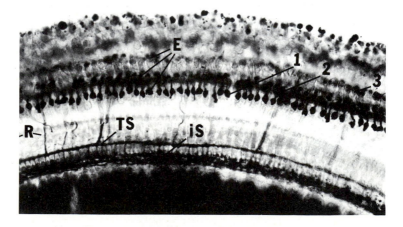

In the cat a clear separation of the tunnel crossing efferent and afferent fibers is found. The efferents cross at a middle level entirely free through the fluid, which fills the tunnel and must have extracellular character similar to the perilymph. They run as small fascicles of fibers with no sheathing whatsoever and with varying diameters (Figure 14). The afferent fibers on the other hand cross the tunnel as basilar fibers at the bottom, mostly hidden in invaginations of the supporting cell plasma membrane. All upper tunnel radial fibers belong to the efferents in the cat. They disappear completely after section of the OCB in the vestibular nerve as seen in tangential sections through the tunnel. They represent two-thirds of the tunnel-crossing fibers, which themselves represent about 15% of all fibers entering the Organ of Corti (Spoend-lin, 1972, 1978). In one cochlea they total about 5000, which is 10% of the entire cochlear nerve population. Here again the topographical separation of the afferent and efferent fibers is less strict in the rodents, where we find the tunnel-crossing fibers at many different levels and many afferent fibers running free through the tunnel at higher levels. The efferent fibers to the ohc take a direct radial course towards the ohc immediately after the habenula. After a minor degree of ramification they penetrate the inner pillars and cross the tunnel as upper tunnel radial fibers; thereafter they undergo considerable ramification before they terminate in the 40 000 large efferent nerve endings at the base of the ohc. Their distribution is essentially radial in the Organ of Corti. The caliber of these fibers ranges from 0.2 to 1.5 μm but most of them are relatively large with diameters of about 1 μm.

The efferents at the level of the ihc are quite different. They form the inner spiral fibers and the tunnel spiral fibers. They are small with diameters between 0.1 and 0.6 μm, the great majority about 0.2 μm (Figure 15). Their number increases from base to apex of the cochlea in contrast to the efferents of the ohc. Their number is mostly around 200 at any one place in the middle turn of the cat cochlea (Spoendlin, 1970). The spiral extensions and actual terminals are unknown. They form a plexus with the afferent dendrites, which penetrate through the spiral bundles on their way to the inner hair cells. Along their course these inner spiral fibers form varicous enlargements filled with synaptic vesicles partly surrounding the afferent dendrites (Figure 16). They have exclusively synaptic contacts with the afferent dendrites but not with the inner hair cells (Figure 17). In the rodents one finds some exceptions to this rule.

In reconstructions of this area Libermann (1980a,b) found that each afferent dendrite from the ihc has up to twenty synaptic contacts with

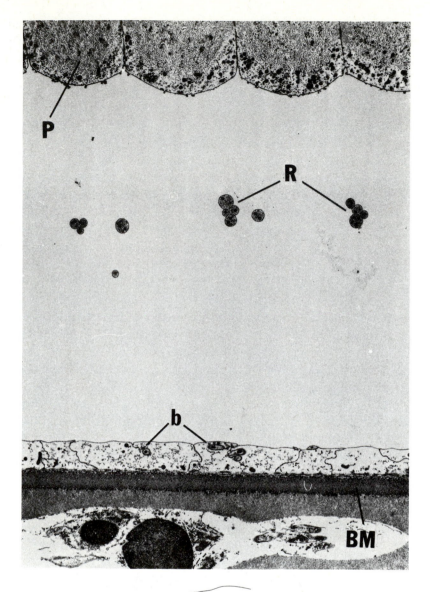

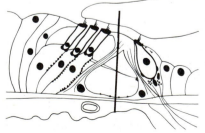

Figure 14. Longitudinal section through the tunnel of Corti of the basal turn of a normal adult cat with the efferent fascicles of the upper tunnel radial fibers (R) and the much smaller and fewer afferent nerve fibers (b) crossing the tunnel at the bottom hidden in invaginations of the supporting cells. P, pillar heads; BM, basilar membrane. All the upper tunnel radial fibers (R) disappear completely after total transection of the olivo-cochlear neurons within the vestibular nerve.

Figure 15. Radial section through the inner spiral fibers (iS), which usually are very small but from time to time have large varicosities filled with synaptic vesicles and show evidence of synaptic contacts with afferent dendrites (iR). iH, inner hair cell; a, afferent nerve endings; TS, tunnel spiral fibers; TR, tunnel radial fibers; of, afferent fibers for outer haircells.

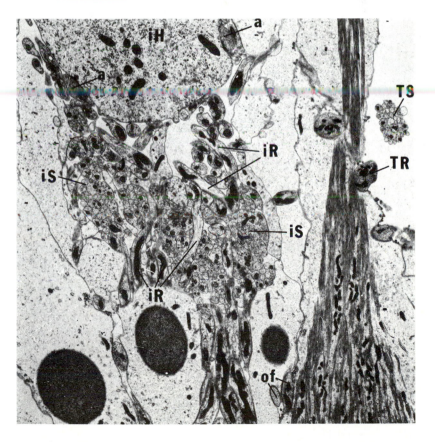

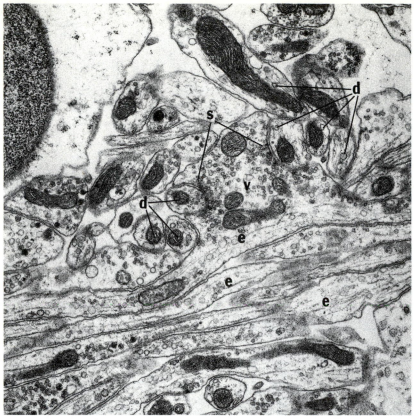

Figure 16

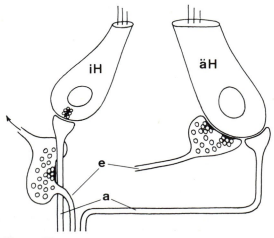

Figure 17

efferent inner spiral fibers. Even some afferents and efferents from the ohc occasionally have synaptic contacts with the inner spiral efferents and rarely some synaptic contacts between efferents and afferents are found just above the habenula.

Degeneration of the inner spiral fibers takes longer than for the efferents of the outer hair cells. They need about one week to degenerate and remnants of these fibers can be found in the form of myelin figures for many weeks. However, in due time the inner spiral fibers disappear completely after section of the vestibular nerve, leaving no doubt as to their efferent nature.

Efferent transmitter

All efferent fibers give a positive histochemical reaction for ACHE (Churchill, Schuknecht and Doran, 1956). This has been confirmed by many others in light (Schuknecht et al., 1959; Rossi et al., 1962; Ishii and Balogh, 1968; Ross, 1969) and electron-microscopic studies (Kaneko and Daly, 1968; Iurato, Luciano, Pannese and Reale, 1970) and certainly suggests a cholinergic system with acetylcholine as the transmitter.

On the other hand, Desmedt et al. (1960, 1961, 1963) found that they could block the effect of the efferents by the administration of strychnine and tetanus toxin. The fact that acetylcholine is increased in the perilymph after efferent stimulation (Fex, 1968; Guth et al., 1972) and that the efferents contain acetylcholinetransferase (Jasser and Guth, 1973) speaks in favor of acetylcholine being involved in the transmitting mechanism either as the transmitter or as an intermediate substance leading to the release of another transmitter.

Efferents for the inner hair cells and the outer hair cells as two different systems

There is some evidence that the efferents for the inner (ihc) and outer hair cells (ohc) belong to two different systems (Figures 18, 19).

Figure 16. Horizontal section through a portion of the inner spiral bundle (e) in a normal adult cat showing a varicous enlargement (v) of such a small inner spiral fiber (e) partly surrounding some afferent dendrites (d) and making synaptic contact (s) with them. These synapses are obviously 'en passant'.

Figure 17. Schematic representation of the synaptic contacts of the efferent fibers (e) within the Organ of Corti. At the level of the ohc they make contact almost exclusively with the sensory cells, whereas at the level of the ihc they make synaptic contacts exclusively en passant with the afferent dendrites (a) associated with the ihc.

Morphologically the efferents for the ohc are large and radial, and they synapse almost exclusively with the ohc. The efferents for the ihc area are small, they have a spiral distribution and they synapse exclusively with dendrites but not with the receptor cell. In addition they degenerate much more slowly than the efferents for the ohc system. There is also a difference in the developmental maturation. The

Figure 18. Horizontal innervation schema in the Organ of Corti of the cat. The afferents are indicated by full lines, the efferents by interrupted lines. The efferents for the ohc have essentially a radial distribution and an extensive ramification at the level of the ohc, whereas the efferents of the ihc system have essentially a spiral distribution, whose extent is not known yet. The afferent fibers, the majority of which are associated with the ihc, present a different distribution pattern with a radial distribution of fibers associated with the ihc and a spiral distribution of the few fibers associated with the ohc.

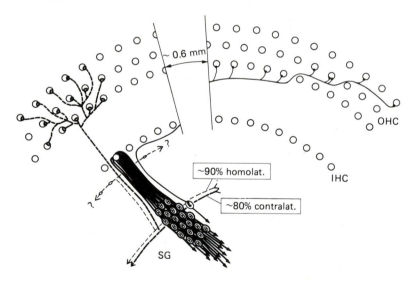

Figure 19. Schematic representation of the homo- and contralateral olivo-cochlear fibers to inner and outer hair cells.

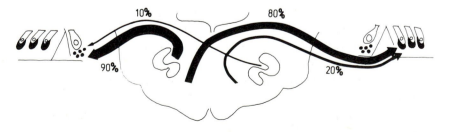

efferents of the ihc begin to form synapses with the afferent dendrites at birth whereas the efferents associated with the ohc do not form synaptic contacts with the hair cell until a week later (Pujol, Carlier and Devigne, 1978). The last important evidence was provided by a study of Warr and Guinan, 1979. Radioactive leucine or methionine was injected in the area of either the LSO or the MNTB using auditory-evoked potential recordings for orientation of the pipette. After 11–36 h the cochleas were evaluated by audioradiographic techniques and the silver grains in the area below the ihc and at the base of the ohc counted. After injection in the LSO silver grains were found almost exclusively in the ihc area, predominantly homolateral but also some contralateral. After injection in the MNTB most grains were found in the area of the ohc and only about 10% in the ihc region, which might be due to passage of the ohc efferents through this area.

These results are consistent with the degeneration studies according to which a midline lesion leads to degeneration of the majority of efferents of the ohc but has no effect (Iurato, 1964), or only a partial one (Spoendlin, 1970), on the efferents of the ihc area. Whether the myelinated efferent fibers belong to the contralateral and the unmyelinated to the homolateral system as has been suggested remains an open question. Considering that the olivo-cochlear efferent system consists of a number of different neuronal groups the situation might be more complex. However, after midline lesion the majority of the remaining nerve fibers in the intraganglionic spiral bundle are unmyelinated.

Functional significance

Stimulation of the crossed olivo-cochlear bundle was found to reduce the amplitude of the compound action potentials (CAP) (Galambos, 1956; Desmedt et al., 1961, 1962; Fex, 1962; Sohmer, 1965; Wiederhold et al., 1963, 1970) to a maximum of an equivalent of 30 dB sound pressure. The same effect can be found in single-fiber recordings (Wiederhold et al., 1970). Stimulation of the crossed olivo-cochlear fibers increases also the cochlear microphonics to an equivalent of 2–3 dB (Fex, 1959; Desmedt, 1962; Kittrell et al., 1969; Wiederhold et al., 1966). Only a few experiments with uncrossed olivo-cochlear bundle stimulations have been done and these show that the amplitude of the CAP is reduced correspondingly to reduction in sound pressure of 6 to 7 dB (Sohmer, 1966) but that the cochlear microphonics are not influenced.

The mode of action of the efferents might be by a change of the membrane resistance at the site of the synaptic contacts (Wiederhold, 1967); this would explain the decrease of action potentials and the increase of the receptor potential. Although the crossed olivo-cochlear fibers are predominantly associated with the ohc and the great majority of all afferent neurons are associated with the ihc, there is a clear effect of the stimulated crossed olivo-cochlear bundle on all afferent dendrites. This phenomenon can only be understood in connection with the general organization and functional significance of the ohc system (Spoendlin, 1980, 1981).

Although there are definite electrophysiologically recordable and measurable efferent effects on the cochlear potentials there is very scarce and conflicting evidence concerning the physiological significance of the efferents in the hearing process. The striking discrepancy between the extensive anatomical representation of the efferents in the Organ of Corti and the physiological effects has not yet been solved. A number of negative findings and the clinical observation that transection of the vestibular nerve in cases of Menière's disease did not induce any measurable changes of hearing led to the conclusion that the efferent system under normal conditions has no function (Pfalz, 1969). Such a situation, however, seems very unlikely since the efferent system is anatomically so well represented and highly developed that it is hardly conceivable that it would not have any functional significance. For a feedback system the latencies of more than 10 ms appear to be too long.

The evidence that the efferents are involved in a peripheral gating mechanism is uncertain (Irvine et al., 1972) and the observation that the peripheral adaptation of the cochlea is influenced by the efferents (Leibrandt, 1965) has not been confirmed. Interaural influences seem to occur at the level of second order neurons in the cochlear nucleus (Klinke et al., 1969). A number of behavioral experiments after transection of the crossed olivo-cochlear fibers have been reported. Dewson (1968) found an impaired ability of stimulus discrimination whereas Trahiotis and Elliott (1970) found similar effects in the cat. Igarashi, Alford, Gordon and Nakai (1979) on the other hand, found no effect on intensity and frequency discrimination in contrast to earlier findings of Capps and Ades (1968) in the squirrel monkey. Possible trophic functions are still hypothetical and the same is the case for eventual feed-forward systems, which have been demonstrated in the vestibular system.

References

Arnesen, A. R., and Osen, K. K. (1978). The cochlear nerve in the cat: topography, cochleotopy, and fiber spectrum. *J. Comp. Neurol. 178:* 661–78.

Brown, J. C., and Howlett, B. (1972). The olivo-cochlear tract in the rat and its bearing on the homologies of some constituent cell groups of the mammalian superior olivary complex: athiocholine study. *Acta Anat. 83:* 505–26.

Capps, M. J., and Ades, H. W. (1968). Auditory frequency discrimination after transection of the olivocochlear bundle in squirrel monkeys. *Expl Neurol. 21:* 147–58.

Churchill, J. A., Schuknecht, H. F., and Doran, R. (1956). Acetylcholinesterase activity in the cochlea. *Laryngoscope* (St Louis) 66: 1–15.

Desmedt, J. E., and LaGrutta, V. (1963). Function of the uncrossed efferent olivocochlear fibres in the cat. *Nature 200:* 472.

Desmedt, J. E., and Monaco, P. (1960). Suppression par la strychnine de l'effet inhibiteur centrifuge exercé par le faisceau olivo-cochléaire. *Arch. Intern. Pharmacodyn. 129:* 244–8.

Desmedt, J. E., and Monaco, P. (1961). Mode of action of the efferent olivocochlear bundle on the inner ear. *Nature 192:* 1263.

Desmedt, J. E., and Monaco, P. (1962). The pharmacology of a centrifugal inhibitory pathway in the cats acoustic system. *Proc. 1st Int. Pharmac. Meet. 8:* 183.

Dewson, J. H. (1968). Efferent olivocochlear bundle: some relationships to stimulus discrimination in noise. *J. Neurophysiol. 31:* 122–30.

Engström, H. (1958). On the double innervation of the sensory epithelia of the inner ear. *Acta Otolaryngol. 49:* 109–18.

Engström, H., Ades, H. W., and Anderson, A. (1966). *Structural Pattern of the Organ of Corti.* Stockholm: Almquist & Wiksell, 172 p.

Fex, J. (1959). Augmentation of cochlear microphonics by stimulation of efferent fibres to the cochlea. *Acta Otolaryngol. 50:* 540.

Fex, J. (1962). Auditory activity in centrifugal and centripetal cochlear fibres in cats. *Acta Physiol. Scand. 55:* 189.

Fex, J. (1968). Efferent inhibition in the cochlea by the olivo-cochlear bundle. In: Ciba Found. Symp. *Hearing Mechanisms in Vertebrates,* ed. A. V. S. de Reuck and J. Knight, pp. 169–86. London: Churchill.

Gacek, R. R., Nomura, Y., and Balogh, K. (1965). Acetylcholinesterase activity in the efferent fibers of the stato-acoustic nerve. *Acta Oto-laryngol. 59:* 541–53.

Galambos, R. G. (1956). Suppression of auditory nerve activity by stimulation of efferent fibers to cochlea. *J. Neurophysiol. 19:* 424–437.

Guth, P. S., Burton, M., and Norris, C. H. (1972). Release of acetylcholine by the olivocochlear bundles. *J. Acoust. Soc. Am. 52:* 143–4.

Igarashi, M., Alford, B. R., Gordon, W. P., and Nakai, Y. (1974). Behavioral auditory function after transsection of crossed olivo-cochlear bundle in the cat. II. Conditioned visual performance with intense white noise. *Acta Otolaryngol. 77:* 311.

Irvine, D. R. F., and Webster, W. R. (1972). Studies of peripheral gating in the auditory system of cats. *Electroencephalog. Clin. Neurophysiol. 32:* 545–56.

Ishii, D., and Balogh, K., Jr (1968). Distribution of efferent nerve endings in the Organ of Corti. Their graphic reconstruction in cochleae by localization of acetylcholinesterase activity. *Acta otolaryngol. 66:* 282–8.

Iurato, S. (1962). Efferent fibers to the sensory cells of Corti's Organ. *Expl Cell Res.* 27: 162–4.

Iurato, S. (1964). Fibre efferenti dirette e crociate alle cellule acustiche dell'Organo del Corti. *Monit. Zool. Ital.*, Suppl. 72: 62–3.

Iurato, S., Luciano, L., Pannese, E., and Reale, E. (1970). Histochemical localization of acetylcholinesterase (AChE) activity in the Organ of Corti after in toto incubation. In *Biochemical Mechanisms in Hearing and Deafness*, ed. M. M. Paparella. Springfield (Ill.): Ch. C. Thomas.

Jasser, A., and Guth, P. S. (1973). The synthesis of acetylcholine by the olivocochlear bundle. *J. Neurochem.* 20: 45–54.

Kaneko, Y., and Daly, J. F. (1968). Acetylcholinesterase on the nerve endings of outer hair cells and the tunnel radial fibers. *Laryngoscope* 78: 1566–81.

Kimura, R., and Wersäll, J. (1962). Termination of the olivocochlear bundle in relation to the outer hair cells of the Organ of Corti in guinea pig. *Acta Otolaryngol.* 55: 11–32.

Kittrell, B. J., and Dalland, J. I. (1969). Frequency dependence of cochlear microphonic augmentation produced by olivo-cochlear bundle stimulation. *Laryngoscope\78:* 228–38.

Klinke, R., Boerger, G., and Gruber, J. (1969). The alteration of afferent, tone-evoked activity of neurons of the cochlear nucleus, following acoustic stimulation of the contralateral ear. *J. Acoust. Soc. Am.* 45: 788–9.

Leibrandt, C. C. (1965). The significance of the olivocochlear bundle for the adaptation mechanism of the inner ear. *Acta Otolaryngol.* 59: 124.

Liberman, M. C. (1980a). Morphological differences among radial afferent fibers in the cat cochlea: an electron-microscopic study of serial sections. *Hearing Res.* 3: 45–63.

Liberman, M. C. (1980b). Efferent synapses in the inner hair cell area of the cat cochlea: an electron microscopic study of serial sections. *Hearing Res.* 3: 189–204.

Nomura, Y., and Schuknecht, H. F. (1965). The efferent fibers in the cochlea. *Ann. Otol.* 74: 289–302.

Paradiesgarten, A., and Spoendlin, H. (1976). The unmyelinated nerve fibres of the cochlea. *Acta Otolaryngol.* 82: 157–64.

Pfalz, R. K. J. (1969). Absence of a function for the crossed olivocochlear bundle under physiological conditions. *Arch. klin. Exp. Ohr.-, Nas.-Kehlk. Heilk.* 193: 89–100.

Pujol, R., Carlier, E., and Devigne, C. (1978). Different patterns of cochlear innervation during the development of the kitten. *J. Comp. Neurol.* 177: 529–35.

Rasmussen, G. L. (1942). An efferent cochlear bundle. *Anat. Rec.* 82: 441.

Rasmussen, G. L. (1946). The olivary peduncle and other fiber projections of the superior olivary complex. *J. Comp. Neurol.* 84: 141–219.

Rasmussen, G. L. (1953). Further observations of the efferent cochlear bundle. *J. Comp. Neurol.* 99: 61–74.

Rasmussen, G. L. (1960). Efferent fibers of the cochlear nerve and cochlear nucleus. In: Rasmussen, G. L., Windle, W. F. (Eds.): *Neural Mechanisms of the Auditory and Vestibular System*, ed. G. L. Rasmussen and W. F. Windle. Springfield (Ill.): Ch. C. Thomas.

Ross, M. D. (1969). The general visceral efferent component of the eighth cranial nerve. *J. Comp. Neurol.* 135: 453–78.

Ross, M. D., Nuttall, A. L., and Wright, C. G. (1977). Horseradish peroxidase acute ototoxicity and the uptake and movement of the peroxidase in the auditory system of the guinea pig. *Acta Otolaryngol.* 84: 187–201.

Rossi, G., and Cortesina, G. (1962). The efferent innervation of the inner ear. *Panminerva Med.* 4: 478.

Rossi, G., and Cortesina, G. (1962). Il 'Sistema efferente colinergico cocleovestibolare'. *Minerva Otorinolaringol. 12:* 1–63.

Rossi, G., and Cortesina, G. (1965). The 'Efferent cochlear and vestibular system' in *Lepus cuniculus* L. *Acta Anat. 60:* 362–81.

Schuknecht, H. F., Churchill, J. A., and Doran, R. (1959). The localization of acetylcholinesterase in the cochlea. *Arch. Otolaryngol. 69:* 549–59.

Smith, C. A., and Rasmussen, G. L. (1963). Recent observations on the olivocochlear bundle. *Ann. Otol. 78:* 489–506.

Smith, C. A., and Rasmussen, G. L. (1965). Degeneration in the efferent nerve endings in the cochlea after axonal section. *J. Cell Biol. 26:* 63–77.

Sohmer, H. (1965). The effect of contralateral olivocochlear bundle stimulation on the cochlear potentials evoked by acoustic stimuli of various frequencies and intensities. *Acta Otolaryngol. 60:* 59–70.

Sohmer, H. (1966). A comparison of the efferent effects of the homolateral and contralateral olivocochlear bundles. *Acta Otolaryngol. 62:* 74–87.

Spoendlin, H. (1966). *The Organization of the Cochlear Receptor.* Basel, New York: S. Karger.

Spoendlin, H. (1970). Structural basis of peripheral frequency analysis. In *Symposium on Frequency Analysis and Periodicity Detection in Hearing,* ed. R. Plomp and G. F. Smoorenburg. Leiden: Sijthoff.

Spoendlin, H., and Gacek, R. R. (1963). Electronmicroscopic study of the efferent and afferent innervation of the Organ of Corti in the cat. *Ann. Otol. 72:* 660–86.

Spoendlin, H. (1968). Ultrastructure and peripheral innervation pattern of the receptor in relation to the first coding of the acoustic message. In Ciba Found. Symp. *Hearing Mechanisms in Vertebrates,* ed. by A. V. S. de Rauck and J. Knight, pp. 89–119. London: J. & A. Churchill.

Spoendlin, H. (1969). Innervation patterns in the Organ of Corti of the cat. *Acta Otolaryngol. 67:* 239–54.

Spoendlin, H. (1972). Innervation densities of the cochlea. *Acta Otol. 73:* 235.

Spoendlin, H. (1978). Neuro-anatomy of the cochlea. *Audiologia e Foniatria 1:* 1–23.

Spoendlin, H. (1979). Neural connections of the outer haircell system. *Acta Otolaryngol. 87:* 381–7.

Spoendlin, H. (1981). HRP-studies on primary cochlear neurons. Poster Inner Ear Biology Workshop, Montpellier.

Spoendlin, H., and Suter, R. (1976). Regeneration in the VIIIth Nerve. *Acta Otolaryngol. 81:* 228–36.

Stopp, P. E., and Comis, S. D. (1979). Relationship of centrifugal fibres to 'Supporting' cells. *Arch. Otorhinolaryngol. 224:* 11–15.

Teryama, Y., Yamamoto, K., and Sakamoto, T. (1969). The efferent olivo-cochlear bundle in the guinea pig cochlea. *Ann. Otol. 78:* 1254–68.

Trahiotis, C., and Elliott, D. N. (1970). Behavioral investigation of some possible effects of sectioning the crossed olivocochlear bundle. *J. Acoust. Soc. Am. 47:* 592–6.

Warr, W. B. (1975). Olivocochlear and vestibular efferent neurons of the feline brain stem: their location, morphology, and number determined by retrograde axonal transport and acetylcholinesterase histochemistry. *J. Comp. Neurol. 161:* 159–82.

Warr, W. B. (1978). The olivocochlear bundle: its origins and terminations in the cat. In *Evoked Electrical Activity in the Auditory Nervous System,* ed. R. F. Naunton and C. Fernández, pp. 43–65. New York, San Francisco, London: Academic Press.

Warr, W. B. (1982). Personal communication.

Warr, W. B., and Guinan, J. J., Jr. (1979). Efferent innervation of the Organ of Corti: two separate systems. *Brain Res. 173:* 152–5.

Wiederhold, M. L. (1967). A study of efferent inhibition of auditory nerve activity (Ph.D. Thesis). Massachusetts Inst. Technol.

Wiederhold, M. L., and Chance, E. K. (1963). Effects of olivocochlear bundle stimulation on acoustically evoked potentials. *Mass. Inst. Technol. Res. Lab. Electron. Tech. Rept. 70:* 311–15.

Wiederhold, M. L., and Kiang, N. Y. S. (1970). Effects of electric stimulation of the crossed olivocochlear bundle on single auditory-nerve fibres in the cat. *J. Acoust. Soc. Am. 48:* 950–65.

Wiederhold, M. L., and Peake, W. T. (1966). Efferent inhibition of auditory-nerve responses. Dependence on acoustic-stimulus parameters. *J. Acoust. Soc. Am. 40:* 1427–30.

Wright, C. G., and Preston, R. E. (1973). Degeneration and distribution of efferent fibres in the guinea pig Organ of Corti. A light and scanning electron microscopic study. *Brain Res. 58:* 37–59.

1.9

Effect of ganglioside treatment on hearing loss in experimental diabetes in mice

F. APORTI, R. RUBINI and G. TOFFANO

One of the most significant complications of diabetes is the neuropathy affecting the motor, sensory and autonomic nervous systems. Lesions of the nervous system may result in anatomical alterations with clinical manifestations which develop slowly and take, in some cases, an irreversible course. With increasing duration of diabetes, there is increasing impairment of nerve conduction velocity (Kovar, 1973) essentially due to a neuroaxonal disorder although a role for segmental demyelination has also been suggested (Kirikae, 1944; Makishima and Tanaka, 1971). Gangliosides, an abundant component of neuronal membranes, seem to play an important role in the process of recovery of altered conduction velocity (for a review see Rapport and Gorio, 1981). Ganglioside treatment prevents the decrease of nerve conduction velocity in toxic polyneuritis (Aporti and Finesso, 1977), stimulates axonal sprouting during peripheral nerve regeneration (Ceccarelli, Aporti and Finesso, 1976; Gorio, Carmignoto, Facci and Finesso, 1980), and improves motor nerve conduction velocity in a model of experimental diabetic neuropathy (Gorio, Aporti and Norido, 1981).

Hearing loss is another complication of diabetes mellitus attributed to various factors acting on the stria vascularis, the endolabyrinthian fluids, the spiral ganglion, the axons and the central acoustical pathways. In the present study the effect of gangliosides has been investigated on the hypoacusia present in genetic or alloxan-induced diabetes.

Materials and methods
Alloxan-induced diabetes
Swiss mice, 18–20 g, were used and treated with a single dose of $90\,mg\,kg^{-1}$ of alloxan intravenously to kill β-cells and induce diabetes

(Saito, 1979). At 180 days after alloxan administration, mice were given intraperitoneally saline or different doses (from 2.5 to 25 mg kg^{-1}) of a ganglioside mixture extracted and purified from bovine brain (constituted by GM$_1$ 21%, GD$_{1a}$ 39%, GD$_{1b}$ 16%, GT$_{1b}$ 19%; nomenclature according to Svennerholm et al., 1980) for 30 days.

Acoustical–cortical evoked potentials (CER) were recorded by applying two Aesculap Michel 7.5 × 1.75 electrodes placed in the skin on the medial line of the cranium. The animals, blocked in a holder, were placed in a soundproof chamber, and unfiltered clicks, centered at 4 kHz, were presented at a rate of 3 s^{-1} via a Philips AD 0140/T4 loudspeaker placed 15 cm in front of the subjects. The acoustic potentials were amplified by a Tektronix 5A 22N preamplifier and mediated with a Nicolet model 1170 neuroaverager. The threshold was considered as the minimum sound intensity capable of producing an evoked potential.

Congenital diabetes

Diabetic mutant mice were from the inbred C57 BL/Ks strain (Jackson Labs, Bar Harbor, Maine, USA). The mutant diabetes is transmitted as an autosomal recessive gene with complete penetration in homozygote mice (db/db). Heterozygote mice (db/m) were used as controls. At the age of 150 days mice were injected intraperitoneally with 0.1 ml/10 g saline or with 10 mg kg^{-1} ganglioside mixture for 30 days.

Acoustical-evoked potentials for the brain-stem (BSER) were recorded as described above, with the only difference that the two electrodes were placed one on the medial line of the cranium and the other on the mastoid zone.

Results

In mice treated with alloxan, 210 days after drug injection there was extensive hearing loss, i.e. about 21% threshold increase during CER recording with respect to the control group. The threshold increase was significantly decreased by treatment with gangliosides. The effect of gangliosides was dose-dependent. At the highest dose of gangliosides, that is 25 mg kg^{-1}, there was complete recovery (Figure 1A). Similar results were obtained in P2 wave latencies. In alloxan-treated mice the latency increased by 24%, whereas in mice supplemented with gangliosides, 10 and 25 mg kg^{-1}, this latency increased by only 9% (Figure 1B).

By using a BSER technique it has been shown that in db/db mice the hearing loss is age-related. Sixty-day-old mice have a hearing loss of 12% (compared with db/m mice); loss is 22% at 100 days and 64% at 180 days (Figure 2A). After about 500 days the hearing loss is practically 100%. Mice at 180 days of age treated with gangliosides for 30 days showed a significant reduction of hearing loss (to 37%) (Figure 2B). The latency of BSER wave 2 was increased by 13.5% and 3% in saline- and ganglioside-treated db/db mice, respectively (Figure 3A). Analogous results were observed in the latency of wave 3, which was increased by 13% and 2% in saline- and ganglioside-treated db/db mice, respectively (Figure 3B). The increase in latency between waves 2 and 3 of BSER (i.e. nerve conduction velocity) reached 13.5% in saline-treated mice whereas there were no detectable variations in the ganglioside-treated group (Figure 3C).

Discussion

The present study has demonstrated that alloxan-induced or congenital (db/db mice) diabetes leads to hearing losses and that ganglioside treatment partly or completely repairs the functional damage.

Experimental diabetes apparently determines the same lesions as in the congenital form. Histological studies in alloxan-treated mice have shown that the decrease in conduction velocity of the sciatic nerve is

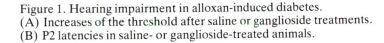

Figure 1. Hearing impairment in alloxan-induced diabetes.
(A) Increases of the threshold after saline or ganglioside treatments.
(B) P2 latencies in saline- or ganglioside-treated animals.

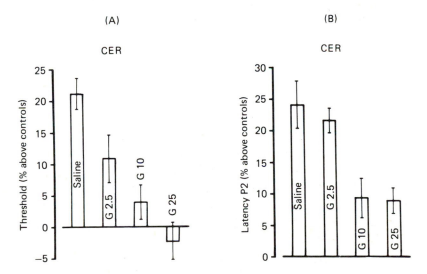

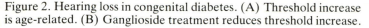

Figure 2. Hearing loss in congenital diabetes. (A) Threshold increase is age-related. (B) Ganglioside treatment reduces threshold increase.

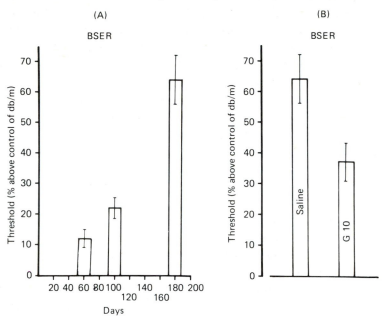

Figure 3. Hearing loss in congenital diabetes. (A) Latency increase of wave 2 in saline- or ganglioside-treated groups. (B) Latency increase of wave 3 in saline- or ganglioside-treated groups. (C) Increase in the latency between wave 2 and 3 in saline- or ganglioside-treated groups.

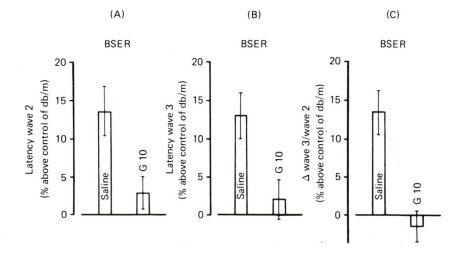

associated with an increase in the number of small-diameter myelinated fibers, a condition present also in db/db mice (Gorio et al., 1981). The increase in latency time for wave 2 indicates that in both cases the lesion occurs at the receptor site and/or at the acoustic nerve. Furthermore, the increased latency between waves 2 and 3 suggests the presence of alterations in the central acoustic pathways between the cochlea and the superior olivary nucleus. These suggestions are supported by histological observations (Makishima and Tanaka, 1971), which indicate the presence of both vascular and nervous lesions in the auditory apparatus and in the nervous system during diabetes.

The mechanism by which gangliosides exert their biological and pharmacological effect is still under investigation. Exogenous gangliosides bind to neuronal membranes with a defined kinetic (Toffano et al., 1980), and modify membrane properties, such as enhancement of the (Na^+, K^+)ATPase (Leon, Tettamanti and Toffano, 1981; Aporti et al., 1981) and of adenylate cyclase (Daly, 1981) activities. Parallel to this, gangliosides appear to counteract the depression of the cochlear electrical potential induced by ouabain (Aporti, Finesso, Molinari and Piccolo, 1977) and by ototoxic drugs such as streptomycin and ethacrine acid (Aporti, Finesso and Molinari, 1979). However, membrane excitability depends on the membrane resting potential and the latter in turn depends on the ion distribution across the membrane. A link cannot therefore be excluded between the molecular effects of gangliosides at the level of the enzyme activities regulating the ion distribution, such as the (Na^+, K^+)ATPase, and the cellular electrical responses underlying the pharmacological effects of the gangliosides.

In conclusion it appears that the hearing loss caused by diabetes is not irreversible, and that gangliosides may be used as a pharmacological tool for diabetic patients in addition to, or in replacement of, the conventional therapies.

References

Aporti, F., Facci, L., Pastorello, A., Siliprandi, R., Savastano, M., and Molinari, G. (1981). Brain cortex gangliosides and (Na^+, K^+)ATPase system of the stria vascularis in guinea pig. *Acta Otolaryngol. 92:* 433–7.

Aporti, F., and Finesso, M. (1977). Effetto dei gangliosidi nelle polinevriti tossiche sperimentali. *La Medicina del Lavoro 68:* 296–302.

Aporti, F., Finesso, M., and Molinari, G. (1979). Effect of exogenous gangliosides in experimental bradyacusia. In *2nd Midwinter Meeting of the Association for Research in Otolaryngology*, St Petersburg Beach, January 22–24.

Aporti, F., Finesso, M., Molinari, G. A., and Piccolo, L. (1977). Effect of gangliosides on the cochlear electrical activity. In *Colloque of Inner Ear Biology*, ed. M. Portmann and J. M. Aran, pp. 371–6. Paris: Inserm.

Ceccarelli, B., Aporti, F., and Finesso, M. (1976). Effects of brain gangliosides on functional recovery in experimental regeneration and reinnervation. In *Gangliosides Function: Biochemical and Pharmacological Implications*, ed. G. Porcellati, B. Ceccarelli and G. Tettamanti, pp. 275–93. New York: Plenum Press.

Daly, J. W. (1981). The effect of gangliosides on the activity of adenylate cyclase and phosphodiesterase from rat cerebral cortex. In *Gangliosides in Neurological and Neuromuscular Function, Development and Repair*, ed. M. M. Rapport and A. Gorio, pp. 55–66. New York: Raven Press.

Gorio, A., Aporti, F., and Norido, F. (1981). Ganglioside treatment in experimental diabetic neuropathy. In *Gangliosides in Neurological and Neuromuscular Function, Development and Repair*, ed. M. M. Rapport and A. Gorio, pp. 259–66. New York: Raven Press.

Gorio, A., Carmignoto, G., Facci, L., and Finesso, M. (1980). Motor nerve sprouting induced by ganglioside treatment. Possible implications for gangliosides on neuronal growth. *Brain Res. 197:* 236–41.

Kirikae, I. (1944). Hearing loss in diabetics. *Zeitforsch. Otol. 50:* 834–48.

Kovar, M. (1973). The inner ear in diabetes mellitus. *Department of Otorhinolaryngology, College of Physicians and Surgeons 35:* 42–52.

Leon, A., Tettamanti, G., and Toffano, G. (1981). Changes in functional properties of neuron membranes by insertion of exogenous ganglioside. In *Gangliosides in Neurological and Neuromuscular Function, Development and Repair*, ed. M. M. Rapport and A. Gorio, pp. 45–54. New York: Raven Press.

Makishima, K., and Tanaka, K. (1971). Pathological changes of the inner ear and central auditory pathway in diabetics. *Annals Oto-Rhino- and Laryngol. 80:* 218–28.

Rapport, M. M., and Gorio, A. (1981). *Gangliosides in Neurological and Neuromuscular Function, Development and Repair*. New York: Raven Press.

Saito, H. (1979). Hearing impairment in experimental alloxan diabetes mellitus. In *16th Workshop on Inner Ear Biology*, Bern, September 3–5.

Svennerholm, L., Fedman, P., Elwing, H., Holmgren, J., and Strannegard, O. (1980). Gangliosides as receptors for cholera toxin, tetanus toxin, and sendai virus. In *Cell Surface Glycolipids*, ed. C. C. Sweeley, pp. 373–90. Washington: American Chemical Society.

Toffano, G., Benvegnù, D., Bonetti, A. C., Facci, L., Leon, A., Orlando, P., Ghidoni, R., and Tettamanti, G. (1980). Interactions of GM_1 ganglioside with crude rat brain neuronal membranes. *J. Neurochem. 35:* 861–6.

1.10

Hearing mechanisms in caiman and pigeon

RAINER KLINKE and JEAN SMOLDERS

Primary afferent fibres of the auditory nerve of mammals are narrowly tuned to certain sound frequencies (see e.g. Evans, 1975, for review). It is not clear, however, how the frequency selectivity of the fibers is brought about. Receptor potentials of inner hair cells (IHCs) to which most of the afferent fibers contact, already possess this high selectivity (Russell and Sellick, 1978). Because of methodological difficulties there is, however, very little information available about the properties of the outer hair cells (OHCs) or the afferent fibers contacting them (Tanaka, Asanuma and Yanagisawa, 1980). As far as primary fiber or IHC tuning is concerned recent authors (Khanna and Leonard, 1982; Sellick, Patuzzi and Johnstone, 1982) describe that sharp tuning is already present in the basilar membrane kinetics. Apparently active processes influence basilar membrane (BM) mechanics, which are highly sensitive in a mammal. This vulnerability may be less in animals with lower metabolic activity. It is therefore of interest to see whether hearing organs of vertebrates lower than mammals allow more successful access. However, in most of the sub-mammalian vertebrates the inner ear is significantly different in morphology from the mammalian cochlea and it may also differ functionally. Fairly sharp frequency tuning curves have for example been determined in frogs and toads (e.g. Capranica and Moffat, 1975) where there is no BM. A tectorial membrane on the other hand is present (see e.g. Capranica, 1976). No traveling wave exists in the alligator lizard (Peake and Ling, 1980). In a portion of the papilla the hair cells are not covered with a tectorial membrane (see Mulroy, 1974; Wever, 1978) and the cilia are free-standing. Nevertheless afferent fibers from both parts of the papilla are frequency tuned, although the tuning properties differ. The examples show, however, that different tuning mechanisms may have evolved.

On the other hand the anatomy of the crocodilian and avian papilla basilaris resembles that of the mammalian cochlea in essential features (e.g. Baird, 1974; von Düring, Karduck and Richter, 1974; Leake, 1976, 1977; Takasaka and Smith, 1971; Tanaka and Smith, 1978; Hirokawa, 1978). Therefore the questions may be asked whether there are also functional similarities and whether insight into mammalian auditory physiology may be obtained by studying these more simple structures.

As far as morphology is concerned details from the caiman (*Caiman crocodilus*) inner ear are available. According to von Düring et al. (1974), von Düring (personal communication), Leake (1976, 1977) and Wever (1978) the papilla basilaris in the caiman is boomerang-shaped and about four millimetres in length. There are two populations of hair cells (IHCs and OHCs). There are some 20 to 30 hair cells per cross-section, with a majority of IHCs on the apical (lagenar) end of the papilla and a majority of OHCs on the basal end. The two hair cell populations are clearly distinguishable. Both carry stereocilia and one kinocilium which points towards the outer rim of the papilla. The length of cilia varies from 10 to 70 μm on the IHCs and from 5 to 30 μm on the OHCs. The smaller cilia are on the basal end of the papilla.

IHCs and OHCs are separately innervated and about 40% of the afferents contact the OHCs (von Düring, personal communication). The afferent fibers are unmyelinated within the papilla basilaris. In contrast to the mammal, both groups of fibers, those from the IHCs and those from the OHCs, are myelinated beyond the habenula. The diameters of the fibers in the auditory part of the eighth nerve are quite uniform and in the order of four micrometers. Therefore one should be able to record from fibers coming from both hair cell types.

There is also efferent innervation of the hair cells. Additionally, the hyaline cells, supporting cells lateral of the OHCs, receive rich efferent innervation.

The avian inner ear resembles closely the above-described caiman papilla basilaris (see Takasaka and Smith, 1971; Tanaka and Smith, 1978; Hirokawa, 1978). There are, however, intermediate hair cell types and less information about the innervation pattern is available.

Physiology of caiman afferent fibers

Basic properties of caiman primary auditory afferents have been described by Klinke and Pause (1980). In short, caiman afferents are sensitive down to 5 dB SPL, i.e. in the mammalian range. They possess characteristic frequencies (CFs) between 30 Hz and approximately 3 kHz. The tuning curves are non-symmetrical, the high-frequency (HF) slope being steeper than the lower-frequency (LF) slope. The sharpness of tuning as expressed by Q_{10dB} (Kiang, Watanabe, Thomas and Clark, 1965) varies between 1 and 6 (7 in a few cases) and is thus comparable to mammalian fibers of corresponding CF. HF-fibers are generally more sharply tuned than LF ones (for details see Klinke and Pause, 1980). It should be emphasized, however, that separation of fibers into two populations was not possible from these experiments except with regard to spontaneous activity (some 30% of the afferent fibers possess a spontaneous activity below 20 impulses s^{-1}). This means that from the caiman data also, no hypothesis about IHC/OHC function differences may be derived.

Temperature experiments in caiman

In the mammal the threshold of the primary afferents and the sharpness of tuning can be drastically impaired by a number of different noxious effects such as lack of energy (e.g. anoxia or cyanide poisoning), sound trauma, poisoning by ototoxic antibiotics and by diuretics (see e.g. Kiang, Moxon and Levine, 1970; Evans, 1974; Evans and Klinke, 1974; Robertson and Manley, 1974; Kiang, Libermann and Levine, 1976; Dallos et al., 1977; Dallos and Harris, 1978; Libermann and Kiang, 1978; Robertson and Johnstone, 1980; Cody and Johnstone, 1980; Klinke, Göttl and Roesch, 1981; Evans and Klinke, 1982a,b). In all the above experiments an elevation of fiber threshold and a loss of sharpness of tuning were reported. The applied noxious agents, however, had a rather crude effect. It was therefore decided to study this impairment by milder means, namely change of body temperature in caiman. It was expected that the temperature changes, by change of energy availability, would cause similar impairment of single fiber properties as for example cyanide poisoning (Evans and Klinke, 1974, 1982a) but with full reversibility in the case of this poikilothermic animal. Preliminary studies (Smolders and Klinke, 1977) and temperature studies in auditory fibers in other lower vertebrates reported by other investigators (Moffat and Capranica, 1976; Eatock and Manley, 1976, 1981) showed that temperature changes affect CF more than threshold. This result was not to be expected by analogy to the mammal data and therefore a more detailed study was undertaken.

The experimental technique was similar to that of Klinke and Pause (1980). Single fibers of the auditory nerve were located through a posterior approach. Neuronal responses to acoustic stimuli were computer evaluated. Additionally the head temperature of the caiman could be varied between 10° and 35°C. For this purpose a hollow copper plate was inserted deeply into the mouth of the animal and tubing was wrapped around head and neck. The copper plate and tubing could be perfused with hot (35°C) or cold (5°C) water. The inner ear temperature was monitored by a thermocouple placed on the bony wall of the otic capsule. Microelectrode recordings of single fibers were made between 12° and 35°C.

Figure 1. Spontaneous activity of 135 primary afferent fibers from one caiman ear as a function of temperature. The two fiber populations in respect to spontaneous activity can be clearly seen. All fibers are silent below 11°C.

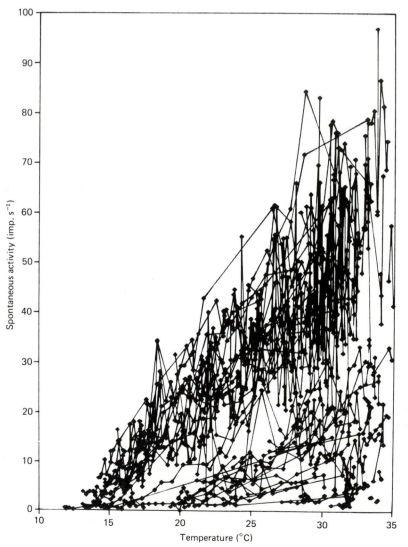

The spontaneous activity of 135 fibers from one animal in respect to inner ear temperature is shown in Figure 1. One can clearly see the two populations of fibers. The separation is maintained throughout the temperature range studied. The spontaneous activity rises *linearly* with temperature. The fibers become silent at about 11°C.

The CFs of the fibers shift downwards with lower head temperatures. An illustration is given in Figure 2. The tuning curves of the figure were automatically determined using the neuronal responses to randomized frequency-intensity pairs. Two-dimensional spatial filtering (Smolders, in preparation) was applied to the response area of the neurones and isorate functions were calculated. The tuning curve was defined as the isorate function with the rate 50% above the actual spontaneous activity at a given temperature.

Figure 2. Frequency-tuning curves of a caiman primary afferent determined at 29.8°, 25.1° and 19.9°C. The tuning curve is defined by an activity of the fiber 50% above the spontaneous activity at a given temperature.

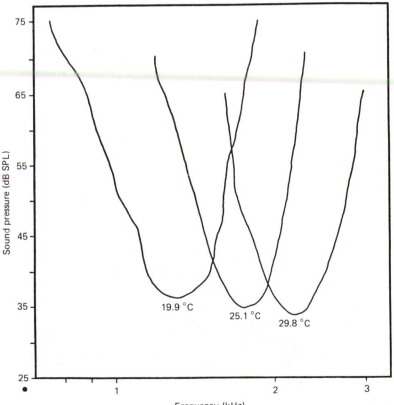

There is no hysteresis in the results, i.e. the CF of a fiber at a given temperature is independent from the sequence in which this particular temperature was reached. The shift of CF is about 1 oct/10°C in the medium temperature range. More precisely it amounts to about 0.14 oct/°C in the lower temperature range and to 0.02 oct/°C at higher temperature irrespective of the CF of the fiber. If the change of CF with temperature for a number of fibers is plotted on a linear frequency scale, however (Figure 3), one can see that there is a linear relationship between CF and temperature at least over the temperature range investigated. If one extrapolates these curves to lower temperatures all curves intersect at about 5°C where CF then would be zero. Sharpness

Figure 3. Shift of characteristic frequency of caiman primary afferents with temperature; linear frequency scale (see text).

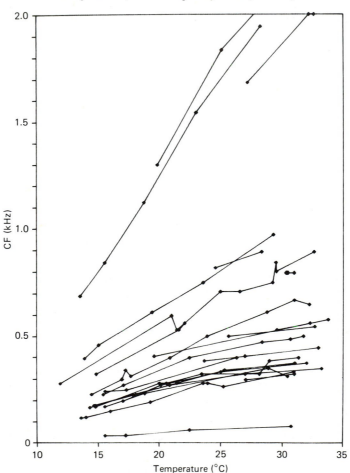

of tuning as expressed by Q_{10dB} does not change significantly with temperature.

In addition to the shift in CF there is a threshold elevation at lower temperatures and (not seen in Figure 2) also at higher temperatures. Minimal thresholds were found between 25° and 30°C. (The animals had been kept at a temperature of 27°C in the animal house. This raises the question whether the low thresholds found in this temperature range represent a temperature adaptation.)

In summary the effect of temperature changes in the caiman inner ear differs significantly from the influence of noxious agents on the mammalian cochlea. In the latter the CF shifts downwards with increasing impairment of hearing but the shift is only about half an octave for an elevation of threshold by 40–50 dB (see e.g. Cody and Johnstone, 1980). Threshold elevation is furthermore combined with loss of sharpness of tuning. In caiman the result of temperature changes is a uniform shift of the response area. No differential effects on the low-threshold CF part and the off-CF part of the tuning curve are seen.

One therefore has to conclude that temperature changes either influence mechanisms in the inner ear other than those affected by noxious agents or that there is a substantial difference between crocodilian and mammalian hearing mechanisms.

Temperature studies on pigeon primary afferents

The above conclusion leads to the question of the effect of cochlear temperature on tuning properties in birds and mammals. Therefore, single units were recorded from the cochlear ganglion in pigeons (Schermuly, 1982; Schermuly and Klinke, 1982; to be published). The ganglion was located through an approach via the recessus scalae tympani. This approach gives access to units with CFs between 125 and 2000 Hz. Cooling and warming of the head and monitoring of the cochlear temperature were done as for the caiman. Measurements were made between 27° and 39°C. Essentially the same results as in the caiman were obtained. An example is given in Figure 4, where the responses of a single unit at 30.2° and 37.4°C are plotted.

Shifts of CF with temperature range from 0.14 to 0.016 oct/°C in the lower- and high-temperature ranges, respectively. Thresholds increase with lower temperatures. Q_{10dB} is not significantly changed with temperature.

The similarity in results between the poikilothermic caiman and the homoiothermic pigeon raises the question as to how single mammalian afferents would react to temperature changes. Preliminary studies, using

Figure 4. Responses of a pigeon primary afferent fiber at 37.4 and 30.2°C. The mean spontaneous activity of the fiber is subtracted from the responses.

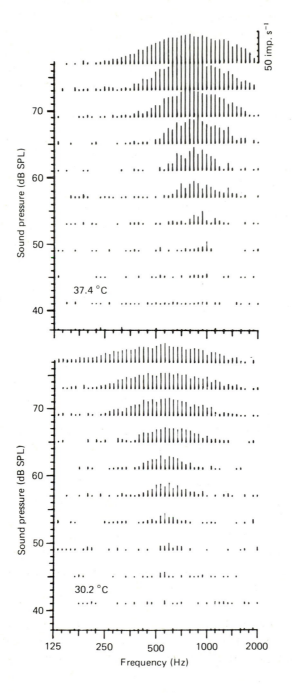

local warming of the hook portion of cats, the body temperature of which had been lowered, showed hardly any effect on fibers with CF above 20 kHz (Smolders and Klinke, 1977). The difference is not necessarily caused by species differences. It may also be a question of CF as the caiman and pigeon units recorded were all below 2 kHz. Therefore recordings from the ventral cochlear nucleus of the guinea pig have been performed (Gummer and Klinke, 1983) which allow stable recording over the necessary time of more than 30 min. Again, irrespective of CF (down to 0.8 kHz) the CF does not shift with temperature. Threshold elevation with lower temperature is significant however.

In another mammal – man – the perceived pitch in subjects with absolute pitch does not change with temperature (Emde and Klinke, 1977, to be published).

Is there a traveling wave in caiman papilla basilaris?

The significant influence of temperature on fiber tuning leads to the question of the functional basis of tuning. Is there a traveling wave in caiman (and bird) as is suggested by their inner ear morphology and the tonotopy of BM vibration in the chicken (von Békésy, 1960)? Are the inner ear mechanics significantly influenced by temperature? May tuning in these animals depend on cellular mechanisms instead of or in addition to a traveling wave mechanism and may it therefore be sensitive to temperature?

As a first approach, phase data of primary afferent fibers were studied according to the technique of Kim and Molnar (1979). The data show a continuous decrease in phase lag between the tonal stimulus and the neuronal spikes with CF, i.e. locus of origin, on the BM. The result is compatible with, but not conclusive evidence for, the existence of a traveling wave. Details will therefore not be described here and should be found elsewhere (Smolders and Klinke, 1981).

As a second step BM motion was measured in collaboration with Dr J. P. Wilson using his technique (Wilson, 1973; Wilson and Johnstone, 1975) of the capacitive probe (Smolders, Wilson and Klinke, 1982; to be published). With this approach the question of whether or not there is a traveling wave in the caiman can be reliably answered. A disadvantage is the need to drain the scala tympani. The influence of this draining on the results will be discussed later.

In the initial steps the animals were prepared for the experiment as described in Klinke and Pause (1980). To approach the inner ear, parts of the upper and lower jaw were removed as well as the mandibular muscles. Care was taken not to injure the tympanic membrane or the supporting structures. The bone of the skull was thinned with a dental drill and then removed with fine forceps to gain access to the middle ear cavities. In a second step the cochlear duct was opened by fine knives and forceps which exposed the basal two millimeters of the BM. More apical regions cannot be reached by this access as the BM is twisted.

Head temperature was controlled as in the above-described temperature studies. Inner ear temperature again was monitored with a thermocouple positioned at the lagenar part of the inner ear.

Acoustic stimulation was performed with a closed system using a B & K 1″ microphone, which was sealed to the external ear by a plastic tube and Vaseline. The upper lid normally covering the eardrum had been removed surgically.

Vibration of columellar footplate and BM were measured by the miniature capacitive probe (Wilson, 1973) and amplitude and phase evaluated by lock-in amplifiers. The capacitive probe was placed at different locations of the BM between 0 and 2 mm from a reference point close to the basal end where the limbic plate separates into the medial and lateral limbus. Stimulation frequencies between 20 Hz and 5 kHz were used.

The middle ear response of caiman is flat up to 500 Hz; between 500 Hz and 3 kHz there is a roll-off of 12 dB/oct, and above 3 kHz the amplitude decreases with about 25 dB/oct. The phase response shows increasing phase lag with frequency. The range exceeds the ± 0.25 cycles expected for a second-order system.

The BM of the caiman is suspended over a gap formed by a fibrocartilaginous U-shaped structure, the inner and outer limbus. This structure was found to vibrate much less (-20 dB) than the BM itself. Figure 5 illustrates the ratio of BM and columellar footplate motion as well as the phase relations for four different positions measured in the same ear. It is evident that there are systematic shifts of the amplitude peaks, HF slopes, and slopes of the phase response. HFs peak closer to the basal end and phase changes are more rapid with frequency for apical locations indicating longer delay times. The data therefore show that there is a tonotopic mapping and a traveling wave in caiman BM.

The values measured are influenced by the draining of the scala tympani. Refilling of the scala tympani with an electric insulator (liquid paraffin) shifts peaks and slopes to lower values by about 0.5 oct. It is likely that the values measured with liquid paraffin are closer to the natural condition than those measured in the partially drained scala.

The measurements were taken at different temperatures ranging from 9° to 38°C. In contrast to single-fiber tuning there was no significant influence of temperature on the mechanical properties of BM motion.

The conclusion from these series of experiments is, therefore, that a traveling wave does exist in caiman but that single-fiber tuning is not

Figure 5. (A) Ratio of basilar membrane (BM)/columellar footplate (CFP) displacement measured at four different locations on the BM of a caiman. (B) BM-CFP phase lag measured at the same locations as in (A).

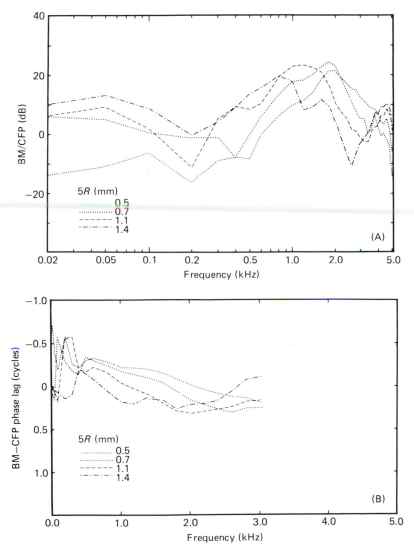

essentially based on the mechanics of the BM. Of course, recent measurements of BM motion in mammals (Khanna and Leonard, 1982; Sellick et al., 1982) have revealed a much sharper mechanical tuning than previous investigations. The assumption is that in earlier measurements cochlear function had been impaired by the surgical approach and that cochlear micromechanics consist of a passive and an active component more resistant and very susceptible to damage respectively. It may be that a similar system is present in the caiman inner ear and that the present investigations have measured the passive component which is largely independent of temperature. This, however, is improbable as response areas of primary afferents show a uniform shift with temperature and not a differential effect on the CF area and frequencies off CF. It may thus be that tuning in caiman is not based on a traveling wave but on a hair cell mechanism as discussed for the terrapin by Crawford and Fettiplace (1981). Other mechanisms, e.g. based on varying cilia length, are conceivable. This mechanism might depend on temperature. The traveling wave may be necessary to transport acoustic energy to the hair cells and may not play a role in the frequency tuning.

Is there an indication of an active process in the caiman inner ear?

Kemp (1978) has first described acoustic emissions from the human cochlea which are indicative for active processes occurring during the transduction process. These findings have been confirmed and extended (see e.g. contributions to the London Conference published in *Hearing Research 2*, 1980).

Attempts have been made to test whether similar emissions exist in the caiman inner ear (Strack, Klinke and Wilson, 1981; to be published). In an initial step the original Kemp technique was used. The ear was stimulated by clicks using a closed sound system. The sound pressure at the eardrum was recorded. By averaging techniques it was checked whether there is an oscillation in the sound pressure a few milliseconds after the click and whether this phenomenon has a non-linear intensity function. By this technique, however, no cochlear emissions in caiman could be demonstrated. Up to 10000 responses have been averaged. This negative result is not conclusive, however, as the cochlear emissions may be hidden in the oscillations of sound pressure caused by the click. Evidence for acoustic emissions can, however, also be gained by steady-tone stimulation (Kemp, 1979; Wilson, 1979). The emissions cause ripples in the intensity–frequency plot of the sound pressure at low stimulus intensities. Therefore a series of experiments with continuous-tone stimuli was carried out. The sound pressure at the eardrum was evaluated with a pair of quadrature lock-in amplifiers using the stimulation frequency as a reference. The above ripples in the sound pressure were found in the caiman ear as shown in Figure 6A, recorded with a stimulus intensity of 10 dB SPL. With higher stimulus intensities (see Figure 6B) these irregularities disappear and they are also absent in the dead animal at low and high intensities.

Also in caiman the peaks and dips in the sound pressure can be suppressed by a second tone as for example described by Kemp and Chum (1980). The sound intensity of the suppressor tone depends on

Figure 6. Sound pressure and phase at a caiman eardrum measured in a closed system. Stimulus intensity 10 dB SPL (A) and 50 dB SPL (B) at 1 kHz.

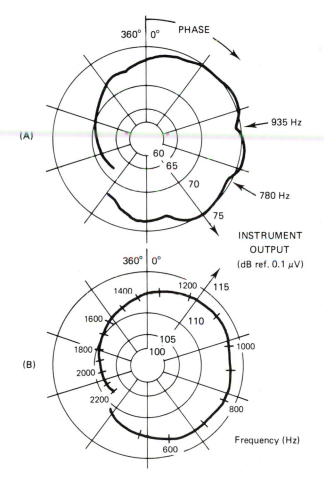

the frequency difference between suppressor and probe tone. The closer the frequencies the less intensity of the suppressor is needed for a certain amount of suppression.

Conclusion

The tuning of single auditory fibers of caiman and pigeon is as good or better than tuning in mammals of corresponding CF. In caiman and pigeon the CFs of the fibers shift, however, to considerably lower values with lower temperature. This is not the case for mammalian units. So there is a discrepancy between mammalian and sub-mammalian vertebrates which seems to indicate a substantial difference in cochlear function, regardless of whether the sub-mammalian creature is warm- or cold-blooded. A further argument is the absence of noxious effects of the ototoxic agent Furosemide on the pigeon inner ear (Schermuly, Göttl and Klinke, 1983) quite in contrast to the high sensitivity of the mammalian cochlea to this agent (see Evans and Klinke, 1982b). No doubt the above suggestion has to be verified more directly. Therefore, further experiments are in progress in this laboratory.

The above investigations were supported by the Deutsche Forschungsgemeinschaft (SFB 45). Ms R. Plotz is thanked for typing the manuscript.

References

Baird, I. L. (1974). Anatomical features of the inner ear in sub-mammalian vertebrates. In *Handbook of Sensory Physiology*, Vol. V/1, ed. W. D. Keidel and W. D. Neff, pp. 159–212. Berlin, Heidelberg, New York: Springer.

von Békésy, G. (1960). *Experiments in Hearing*. New York: McGraw-Hill.

Capranica, R. R. (1976). Auditory system – morphology and physiology of the auditory system. In *Frog Neurobiology*, ed. R. Llinás and W. Precht, pp. 552–75. Berlin, Heidelberg, New York: Springer.

Capranica, R. R., and Moffat, A. J. M. (1975). Selectivity of the peripheral auditory system of spadefoot toads (*Scaphiopus couchi*) for sounds of biological significance. *J. Comp. Physiol. 100:* 231–49.

Cody, A. R., and Johnstone, B. M. (1980). Single auditory neuron response during acute acoustic trauma. *Hearing Res. 3:* 3–16.

Crawford, A. C., and Fettiplace, R. (1981). An electrical tuning mechanism in turtle cochlear hair cells. *J. Physiol., Lond. 312:* 377–412.

Dallos, P., and Harris, D. (1978). Properties of auditory nerve responses in absence of outer hair cells. *J. Neurophysiol. 41:* 365–83.

Dallos, P., Ryan, A., Harris, D., McGee, T., and Özdamar, Ö. (1977). Cochlear frequency selectivity in the presence of hair cell damage. In *Psychophysics and Physiology of Hearing*, ed. E. F. Evans and J. P. Wilson, pp. 249–58. London, New York, San Francisco: Academic Press.

von Düring, M., Karduck, A., Richter, H.-G. (1974). The fine structure of the inner ear in *Caiman crocodilus*. *Z. Anat. Entw. Gesch. 145:* 41–65.

Eatock, R. A., and Manley, G. A. (1976). Temperature effects on single auditory nerve fiber responses. *J. Acoust. Soc. Am. 60:* S80.

Eatock, R. A., and Manley, G. A. (1981). Auditory nerve fibre activity in the Tokay Gecko. II. Temperature effect on tuning. *J. Comp. Physiol. A142:* 219–26.

Emde, C., and Klinke, R. (1977). Does absolute pitch depend on an internal clock? In *Inner Ear Biology 68,* ed. M. Portmann and J. M. Aran, pp. 145–6. Paris: INSERM.

Evans, E. F. (1974). The effects of hypoxia on the tuning of single cochlear nerve fibres. *J. Physiol., Lond. 238:* 65–7 P.

Evans, E. F. (1975). Cochlear nerve and cochlear nucleus. In *Handbook of Sensory Physiology*, Vol. V/2, ed. W. D. Keidel and W. D. Neff, pp. 1–108. Berlin, Heidelberg, New York: Springer.

Evans, E. F., and Klinke, R. (1974). Reversible effects of cyanide and furosemide on the tuning of single cochlear nerve fibres. *J. Physiol., Lond. 242:* 129–30 P.

Evans, E. F., and Klinke, R. (1982a). The effects of intracochlear cyanide and tetrodotoxin on the properties of single cochlear nerve fibres in the cat. *J. Physiol., Lond. 331:* 385–408.

Evans, E. F., and Klinke, R. (1982b). The effects of intracochlear and systemic Furosemide on the properties of single cochlear nerve fibres in the cat. *J. Physiol., Lond. 331:* 409–27.

Gummer, W. A., and Klinke, R. (1983). Influence of temperature on tuning of primary-like units in the guinea-pig cochlear nucleus. *Hearing Res.* (in press).

Hirokawa, N. (1978). The ultrastructure of the basilar papilla of the chick. *J. Comp. Neurol. 181:* 361–74.

Kemp, D. T. (1978). Stimulated acoustic emissions from within the human auditory system. *J. Acoust. Soc. Am. 64:* 1386–91.

Kemp, D. T. (1979). The evoked cochlear mechanical response and the auditory microstructure – evidence for a new element in cochlear mechanics. *Scand. Audiol.,* Suppl. *9:* 35–47.

Kemp, D. T., and Chum, R. A. (1980). Observations on the generation mechanism of stimulus frequency acoustic emissions – two tone suppression. In *Psychophysical, Physiological and Behavioural Studies in Hearing*, ed. G. van den Brink and F. A. Bilsen, pp. 34–42. Delft: University Press.

Khanna, S. M., and Leonard, D. B. G. (1982). Basilar membrane tuning in the cat cochlea. *Science 215:* 305–6.

Kiang, N. Y. S., Liberman, M., and Levine, R. A. (1976). Auditory nerve activity in cats exposed to ototoxic drugs and high-intensity sounds. *Ann. Otol. Rhinol. Laryngol. 85:* 752–69.

Kiang, N. Y. S., Moxon, E. C., and Levine, R. A. (1970). Auditory-nerve activity in cats with normal and abnormal cochleas. In *Sensorial Hearing Loss*, ed. G. E. W. Wolstenholme and Julie Knight, pp. 241–73. London: Churchill.

Kiang, N. Y. S., Watanabe, T., Thomas, E. C., and Clark, L. F. (1965). Discharge patterns of single fibers in the cat's auditory nerve. Res. Monograph No. 35, pp. 1–154. Cambridge, Mass.: MIT Press.

Kim, D. O., and Molnar, C. E. (1979). A population study of cochlear nerve fibers: comparison of spatial distributions of average-rate and phase-locking measures of responses to single tones. *J. Neurophysiol. 42:* 16–30.

Klinke, R., Göttl, K.-H., and Roesch, A. (1981). Testing strategy for ototoxic side effects. *Scand. Audiol.*, Suppl. *14:* 95–109.

Klinke, R., and Pause, M. (1980). Discharge properties of primary auditory fibres in *Caiman crocodilus*: comparisons and contrasts to the mammalian auditory nerve. *Expl Brain Res. 38:* 137–50.

Leake, P. A. (1976). Scanning electron microscopy of labyrinthine sensory organs in *Caiman crocodilus*. *Scanning Electron Microscopy* (Part V), pp. 277–83.

Leake, P. A. (1977). SEM observations of the cochlear duct in *Caiman crocodilus*. *Scanning Electron Microscopy*, Vol. II, pp. 437–44.

Liberman, M. Ch., and Kiang, N. Y. S. (1978). Acoustic trauma in cats. *Acta Oto-Laryngol.*, Suppl. *358:* 5–62.

Moffat, A. J. M., and Capranica, R. R. (1976). Effects of temperature on the response properties of auditory nerve fibers in the American toad (*Bufo americanus*). *J. Acoust. Soc. Am. 60:* S80.

Mulroy, M. J. (1974). Cochlear anatomy of the alligator lizard. *Brain Behav. Evol. 10:* 69–87.

Peake, W. T., and Ling, A., Jr (1980). Basilar membrane motion in the alligator lizard: its relation to tonotopic organization and frequency selectivity. *J. Acoust. Soc. Am. 67:* 1736–45.

Robertson, D., and Johnstone, B. M. (1980). Acoustic trauma in the guinea pig cochlea: early changes in ultrastructure and neural threshold. *Hearing Res. 3:* 167–79.

Robertson, D., and Manley, G. A. (1974). Manipulation of frequency analysis in the cochlear ganglion of the guinea pig. *J. Comp. Physiol. 91:* 363–75.

Russell, I. J., and Sellick, P. M. (1978). Intracellular studies of hair cells in the mammalian cochlea. *J. Physiol., Lond. 284:* 261–90.

Schermuly, L. (1982). Untersuchungen zur Temperaturabhängigkeit der Tuning-Eigenschaften primärer afferenter Fasern des Hörnerven bei Vögeln. Diplomarbeit Fachbereich Biologie, J. W. Goethe-Universität, Frankfurt.

Schermuly, L., and Klinke, R. (1982). Tuning properties of pigeon primary auditory afferents depend on temperature. *Pflügers Arch.*, Suppl. *394:* R63.

Schermuly, R., Gottl, K. H., and Klinke, R. (1983). Little ototoxic effect of Furosemide on the pigeon inner ear. *Hearing Res., 10:* 279–82.

Sellick, P. M., Patuzzi, R., and Johnstone, B. M. (1982). Measurement of basilar membrane motion in the guinea pig using the Mössbauer Technique. *J. Acoust. Soc. Am. 72:* 131–41.

Smolders, J., and Klinke, R. (1977). Effect of temperature changes on tuning properties of primary auditory fibers in caiman and cat. In *Inner Ear Biology*, ed. M. Portmann and J. M. Aran, *68:* 125–6. Paris: INSERM.

Smolders, J., and Klinke, R. (1981). Phase versus frequency in Caiman primary auditory fibres. Is there a travelling wave? In *Neuronal Mechanisms of Hearing*, ed. J. Syka and L. Aitkin, pp. 43–8. New York: Plenum Press.

Smolders, J., Wilson, J. P., and Klinke, R. (1982). Mechanical frequency analysis in the cochlear duct of *Caiman crocodilus*. *Pflügers Arch.*, Suppl. *392:* R51.

Strack, G., Klinke, R., and Wilson, J. P. (1981). Evoked cochlear responses in *Caiman crocodilus*. *Pflügers Arch.*, Suppl. *391:* R43.

Takasaka, T., and Smith, C. A. (1971). The structure and innervation of the pigeon's basilar papilla. *J. Ultrastruct. Res. 35:* 20–65.

Tanaka, K., and Smith, C. A. (1978). Structure of the chicken's inner ear: SEM and TEM study. *Am. J. Anat. 153:* 251–72.

Tanaka, Y., Asanuma, A., and Yanagisawa, K. (1980). Potentials of outer hair cells and the membrane properties in cationic environments. *Hearing Res. 2:* 431–8.

Wever, E. G. (1978). *The Reptile Ear*. Princeton: Princeton University Press.

Wilson, J. P. (1973). A sub-miniature capacitive probe for vibration measurements of the basilar membrane. *J. Sound Vibration 30:* 483–93.

Wilson, J. P. (1979). Subthreshold mechanical activity within the cochlea. *J. Physiol., Lond. 298:* 32–3P.

Wilson, J. P., and Johnstone, J. R. (1975). Basilar membrane and middle ear vibration in guinea pig measured by capacitive probe. *J. Acoust. Soc. Am. 57:* 705–23.

1.11

Functional organization of the medial geniculate body in cats

F. DE RIBAUPIERRE

In mammals the Medial Geniculate Body (MGB) is the last relay station of the auditory pathway leading to the neocortex. It receives its main input from the ipsilateral inferior colliculus (IC) upon which acoustical information has converged from two main parallel pathways. One ventral, which integrates the information coming from the two ears and is mainly involved in the localization of sound sources. The other, dorsal, probably deals with the identification of acoustical features. Thus the information converging on the MGB has already been processed in parallel through different circuits involving from two to five synapses. The afferent pathways are organized in a way that conserves the topological order of the sensory epithelium and the cochlea is represented one or more times at each relay. Acoustical frequencies are mapped onto the neuronal space, and most of the afferent centers are organized in parallel isofrequency sheets of neurons.

The MGB itself is a complex nucleus composed of different sub-nuclei identifiable by their neuronal morphology and afferent/efferent projections (Morest, 1964; Sousa-Pinto, 1973). We will restrict our presentation to the pars lateralis (PL) which is histologically organized in parallel sheets of neurons (Morest, 1965). The laminae are roughly parallel to the external border of the MGB and extend through its rostro-caudal axis. PL is the main afferent source of the primary auditory cortex (AI). Recent microelectrode mapping work (Merzenich, Knight and Roth, 1975; Reale and Imig, 1980) done on anesthetized cats has shown that layer IV of AI was tonotopically organized with isofrequency strips of cortex oriented perpendicular to the axis of frequency representation. AI is surrounded by three more complete cochlear representations: one anterior (AAF), one posterior (PAF), and one ventro-posterior

213

(VPAF). Each of these fields is tonotopically organized as the mirror image of its neighbors (see Figure 1).

Microinjections of retrogradely transported material into such isofrequency strips in AI will label columns of neurons within a whole lamina of PL (Diamond, 1978; Andersen, Knight and Merzenich, 1980) as represented schematically in Figure 1. Double-labeling technique using ortho- and retrogradely transported material has shown that thalamocortical and cortico-thalamic projections are always reciprocal and overlapping, and that strips of corresponding frequencies in AAF and in AI project roughly to the same laminae in PL, AI having a denser interconnection with PL than AAF (Andersen et al., 1980). There is as yet no published evidence that homofrequency regions in PAF and PVAF are connected similarly to PL. We will show later in this paper that it is probably the case.

It is clear that complex convergent–divergent projection patterns exist between a given lamina in PL and the four cortical isofrequency strips. If these four cortical fields are processing, in parallel, different aspects of the acoustical information, they should influence quite diversely the neurons belonging to a given lamina in PL. One might then expect that these neurons would display a great diversity in their response prop-

Figure 1. Schematic representation of connections between the pars lateralis (PL) of the MGB and the auditory cortex. Summary diagram established from published data using intracortical injections (Diamond, 1978; Andersen et al., 1980). AAF, anterior auditory field; AI, primary auditory cortex; PAF, posterior auditory field; VPAF, ventro-posterior auditory field. Filled square (■), low-frequency region of the cochlea representation; empty triangle (△), high-frequency region.

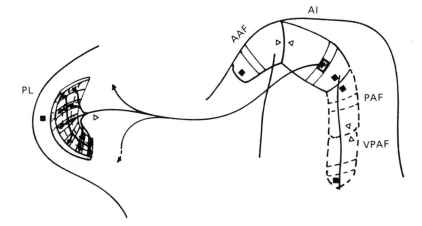

erties if descending cortical influences are not completely inhibited by a deep anesthetic state.

Cortico-thalamic projection and tonotopic organization of the pars lateralis of the MGB

Methodological approach

The MGB was reached through a stereotaxically oriented closed chamber system, the dura and the cortex being left intact. Single-unit recordings were obtained with glass-insulated tungsten microelectrodes on paralysed, nitrous-oxide anesthetized cats (Rouiller, de Ribaupierre and de Ribaupierre, 1979). Two different spike trains were simultaneously discriminated from the same microelectrode using an analog device. This method allows one to characterize functional properties of adjacent neuron pairs under exactly the same physiological conditions (Figure 2). After the neuronal properties had been established along an electrode penetration, the microelectrode was withdrawn, its guide being left in place. A microsyringe needle was inserted in the same guide down to a given depth in the track, where a controled microinjection of horseradish peroxidase (HRP) was performed.

In this way, all neurons projecting to the site of injection could later be traced back in serial histological sections.

The original data presented here are the results of a work in collaboration with P. Heierli, K. Horner, C. Ivarsson, Y. de Ribaupierre, E. Rouiller and A. Toros-Morel.

Tonotopic organization of PL

Single-unit studies of PL have shown that the characteristic frequencies (CF) of neurons are arranged in a way that is compatible with its laminar organization, with low frequencies laterally and high frequencies medially (Aitkin and Webster, 1971; de Ribaupierre, F., and Toros, 1976). In our experimental conditions, this tonotopic organization is far from being as regular as in the lower auditory centers (Morel, 1980; de Ribaupierre et al., 1980). On data pooled from many cats only about 40% of the neurons have their CF within the same octave as the one predicted by their anatomical position. One way to avoid the problem of comparing data from different animals is to compare the CF between each member of simultaneously recorded single-unit pairs. The average radius separating two units of the same pair has been shown to be in the order of $20\,\mu$m (Abeles, 1982). If the structure is strictly tonotopically organized, one would expect to find very similar CFs for units of the same pair. In Figure 3, the CF of one unit is plotted against the CF of the other unit for 432 pairs recorded in PL. It is clear that the scatter on both sides of the identity line is quite important, and the correlation coefficient of the linear regression is 0.76. One can compute what would be the distribution of the intra-pair CF

Figure 2. Single-unit pair recording techniques. Left side: different spike trains are recorded from the same microelectrode and are discriminated on line; according to their shapes, they make different clusters on a two-dimensional space. Responses are visualized as dot display (top right) with time on the abscissa and stimulus parameter on the ordinate (in this case a linear frequency increase from 0.2 to 2.2 kHz). The horizontal bar indicates occurrence of the 200-ms stimulus. Only cell A responded from 0.25 to 0.70 kHz. Low right: reconstruction of a vertical penetration going through PL. Positions of single-unit pairs are marked by small horizontal bar on the right of the track; on the left a small arrow indicates the place of HRP injection.

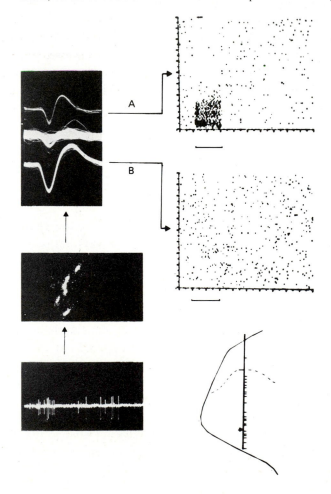

separations for a perfect tonotopic organization taking into account the radius (r) of a sphere into which two units can be recorded at a given place by the electrode tip and the width (d) of the neuronal space devoted to the representation of one octave. If $d = 2r$, the probability of finding an intra-pair CF difference of a given value is given by the curve in Figure 4A. With these assumptions, which are largely on the safe side, a CF separation greater than one octave cannot be found. This distribution is clearly much more narrow than the one obtained from our data represented by the histogram of Figure 4. This confirms that PL is not strictly tonotopically organized. One way to interpret these results is to admit the presence of a tonotopic main frame imposed by the afferents from the inferior colliculus upon which a random scatter of CF is imposed by local or cortical descending connections. Another more compelling interpretation would be to consider many superimposed tonotopically organized inputs, each being partially shifted in space compared to the principal cochlear representation. Our data can be well fitted by a model involving six overlaid cochlear representations, each shifted by one-third of an octave and having a progressively decreasing importance (continuous curve of Figure 4B). This model would provide a means for the nervous system to bring together, in an orderly manner,

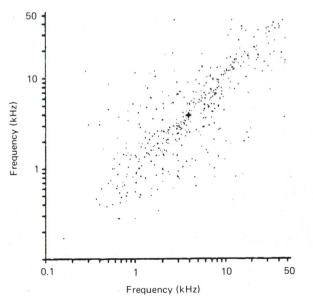

Figure 3. Characteristic frequency correlation scatter diagram for 432 single-unit pairs located in PL.

Frequency (kHz)

Frequency (kHz)

distant points of the cochlea, probably a necessary condition for the handling of complex acoustical stimuli.

Cortico-thalamic projections on PL

Projections to functionally defined points in PL have been studied quantitatively in a few experiments. Retrograde transport of HRP labels mainly pyramidal cells in layer VI and the superficial half of layer V, in the four tonotopically organized auditory cortical fields. Projection of labeled cells on the cortical surface was made from drawings of serial coronal sections for two experiments shown in Figure 5. In experiment A, the electrode track was in the lateral region of PL, and cells with low CF (300 Hz) were recorded in the region where the HRP injection was done. Comparing the mapping obtained with the idealized schematic Figure 1, one can interpret the results in the following way. The heaviest projection comes from the low-frequency region of AI; anterior to it there is a small spot of labeled cells which would correspond to the low-frequency region of AAF. The two regions are separated by a relatively large free area, which would correspond to the high-frequency representation in AI and its mirror image in AAF.

Figure 4. Probability distribution of intra-pair CF separation. (A) Expected distribution for a perfect tonotopically organized structure where the neuronal space devoted to one octave (dashed line of the insert drawing) is equal to the diameter of the sphere from which two units can be simultaneously recorded. Abscissa: frequency separation between the CFs of two units of the same pair, expressed in octave. (B) The bar histogram represents the intra-pair CF separation observed for a sample of 433 single-unit pairs recorded in PL. The smooth curve is the computed probability for a model consisting of six shifted overlaid cochlear representations (see text).

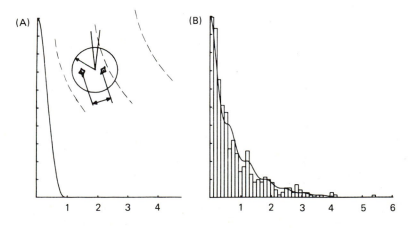

Figure 5. Reconstructions of cortical projections to PL. (A) HRP, 0.23 µl, was injected in the lateral border of PL where low-frequency units were recorded (arrow). Each cortical cell retrogradely filled with HRP is marked by a dot on the cortical reconstruction. Small horizontal bar = 1 mm on the cortex. (B) HRP, 0.08 µl, was injected more medially in PL at the place marked by the arrow where relatively high CFs were recorded.

(A)

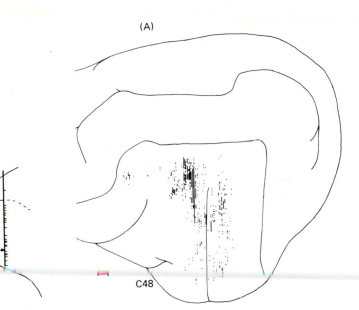

C48

(B)

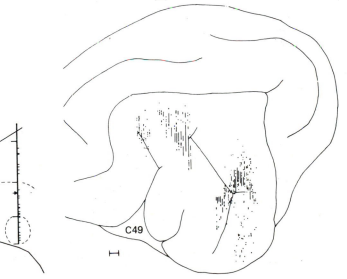

C49

Posteriorly to AI two other labeled regions are found, corresponding to PAF and VPAF. In experiment B (right side of Figure 5) the electrode track was placed more medially and cells with higher CF (6–10 kHz) were encountered where the HRP was injected. The cortical mapping obtained is somewhat complementary to the one obtained for low frequencies (Figure 5A): a smaller gap between AI and AAF and a larger gap between AI and PAF are explained by the mirror image representation of these auditory fields and their respective symmetry axis, which is at the high-frequencies representation for the AI–AAF limit and at the low frequencies for the AI–PAF border.

By counting the number of cells labeled, one can estimate the relative density of IC-afferents and cortical projections onto a small region of PL. The projections were found to be of the same order of magnitude (IC/total cortex = 1.5 in A and 0.5 in B). The densities of cortical projections originating from AAF, AI, and PAF + VPAF were found to be different and represented respectively 3, 73 and 24% of the total

Figure 6. Two possible interconnection diagrams between the four auditory fields and PL. (A) a point-to-point interconnection; (B) a convergent–divergent interconnection.

(A)

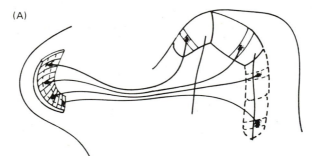

(B)

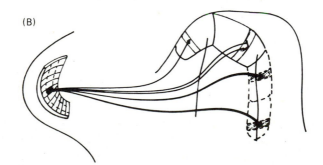

cortical projections for experiment A and 4, 37 and 59% for experiment B.

Two ways of interconnecting a two-dimensional sheet of neurons with four cortical areas are illustrated in Figure 6. The first (Figure 6A) would be a point-to-point connection without overlapping, each homolog cortical region being mapped on a different place in the corresponding lamina in PL. Our data can rule out this first model. On the contrary, cells from within strips of all the four auditory fields project to a limited portion of a PL lamina (Figure 6B). From their topographical distributions these strips belong to similar frequency representations. But if they are not in perfect register, they may represent a partial substrate for the model developed above of multiple, shifted overlaid cochlear representations. The fact that the relative densities of projections from these four cortical areas are not the same would be in agreement with the model, as well as the observation that the response latencies of cells having their CF outside the main tonotopic representation in PL tend to be longer on the average by a few milliseconds.

Evolution of functional properties along the rostro-caudal axis of PL

Response properties to click, tone, and noise bursts were studied for over 2000 single units located in PL, and analysed as a function of their rostro-caudal position (Toros et al., 1979). There appears to be a statistical inhomogeneity along this axis for different properties, some being more frequent anteriorly, others posteriorly, as illustrated schematically in Figure 7. The mean response latency to tone bursts shifts progressively from 29 ms to 15 ms going from posterior to anterior; the same evolution is true for latencies to noise bursts and clicks. Response patterns to these stimuli are also distributed differently: 'ON' and 'THROUGH' responses are most frequent anteriorly, 'OFF' and 'LATE' responses predominate posteriorly. The responsiveness to tone and broad-band stimuli is higher in the anterior half of PL, where more units are sensitive to all three types of stimuli tested. Whereas units sensitive only to tone and not to click and noise are more frequently encountered in the posterior half of PL, more broadly frequency-tuned units are found posteriorly. Most of the units have their dominant inputs from the contralateral ear, but the minority which have an ipsilateral dominance are found in the anterior half. Phase-locked responses to low-frequency tones are found essentially anteriorly as well as synchronization to click trains. Units giving transient responses or no responses to click trains are mostly located posteriorly.

Conclusion

The pars lateralis of the MGB appears to be made up of superimposed functionally heterogeneous populations of cells, the relative densities of which can vary locally. According to their frequency selectivity they are organized in parallel sheets within which a given frequency dominates but which is far from being the only one represented. Within such an 'isofrequency' sheet, other coding properties vary along the rostro-caudal axis in a way compatible with the presence of a more complex coding of the acoustical information in its posterior part. Cortical descending projections are quantitatively as important as collicular afferents. Part of the complexity and the heterogeneity of the responses observed must be due to the way the auditory thalamus and cortex are functionally linked together.

Figure 7. Schematic representations of the evolution of some functional properties along the rostro-caudal axis of PL.

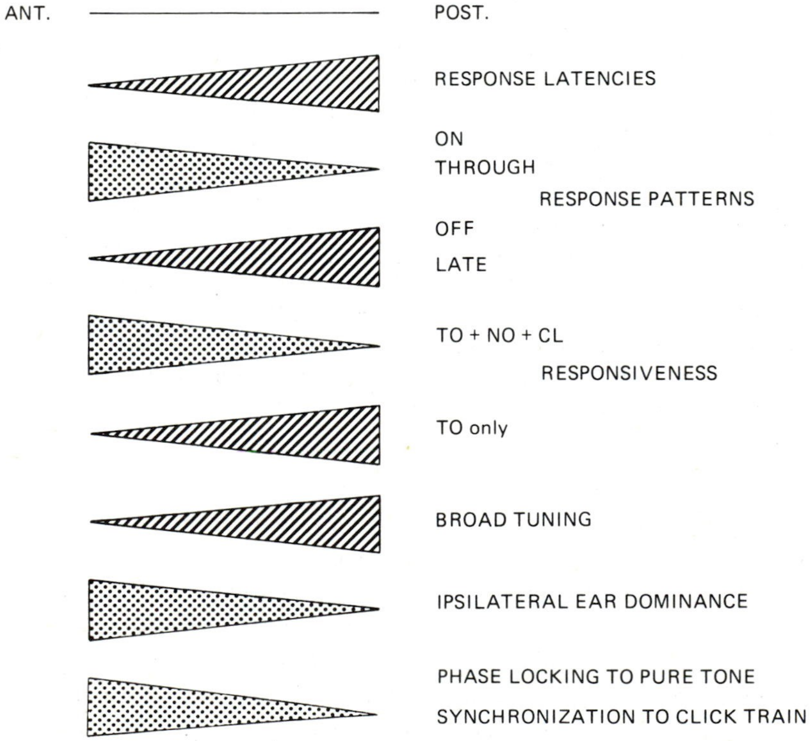

ANT. ———————————————— POST.

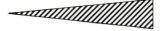
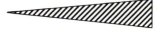

RESPONSE LATENCIES

ON
THROUGH
          RESPONSE PATTERNS
OFF
LATE

TO + NO + CL
          RESPONSIVENESS

TO only

BROAD TUNING

IPSILATERAL EAR DOMINANCE

PHASE LOCKING TO PURE TONE

SYNCHRONIZATION TO CLICK TRAIN

References

Abeles, M. (1982). *Local Cortical Circuits, an Electrophysiological Study*. Berlin: Springer.

Aitkin, L. M., and Webster, W. R. (1971). Tonotopic organisation in the medial geniculate body of the cat. *Brain Res. 26:* 402–5.

Andersen, R. A., Knight, P. L., and Merzenich, M. M. (1980). The thalamocortical and corticothalamic connections of AI, AII and the anterior auditory field (AAF) in the cat: evidence for two largely segregated systems of connections. *J. Comp. Neurol. 194:* 663–701.

Diamond, I. T. (1978). The auditory cortex. In *Evoked Electrical Activity in the Auditory Nervous System*, ed. R. F. Nauton and C. Fernandez, pp. 463–85. New York: Academic Press.

Merzenich, M. M., Knight, P. L., and Roth, G. L. (1975). Representation of cochlea within primary auditory cortex in the cat. *J. Neurophysiol. 38:* 231–49.

Morel, A. (1980). *Codage des Sons dans le Corps Genouillé Médian du Chat: Evaluation de l'Organisation Tonotopique de ses Différents Noyaux*. Thésis Université de Lausanne.

Morest, D. K. (1964). The neuronal architecture of the medial geniculate body of the cat. *J. Anat. 98:* 611–30.

Morest, D. K. (1965). The laminar structure of the medial geniculate body of the cat. *J. Anat. 99:* 611–34.

Reale, R. A., and Imig, Th. J. (1980). Tonotopic organization in auditory cortex of the cat. *J. Comp. Neurol. 192:* 265–91.

de Ribaupierre, F., and Toros, A. (1976). Single unit properties related to the laminar structure of the MGN. In *Afferent and Intrinsic Organization of Laminated Structures in the Brain. Expl Brain Res.*, Suppl. 1, ed. O. Creutzfeldt, pp. 503–5. Berlin: Springer.

de Ribaupierre, Y., Rouiller, E., Toros, A., Ivarsson, C., and de Ribaupierre, F. (1980). How strict is the tonotopic organization in the pars lateralis of the cat's medial geniculate body (MGB)? *Neurosci. Lett.*, Suppl. 5: 148.

Rouiller, E., de Ribaupierre, Y., and de Ribaupierre, F. (1979). Phase-locked responses to low frequency tones in the medial geniculate body. *Hearing Res. 3:* 65–77.

Sousa-Pinto, A. (1973). Cortical projections of the medial geniculate body in the cat. *Adv. Anat., Embryol. Cell Biol. 48*, Suppl. 2, 1–42.

Toros, A., Rouiller, E., de Ribaupierre, Y, Ivarsson, C., Holden, M., and de Ribaupierre, F. (1979). Changes of functional properties of medial geniculate body neurons along the rostro-caudal axis. *Neurosci. Lett.*, Suppl. 3: 5.

2
Olfaction and taste

2.1

Initial events influencing olfactory analysis

MAXWELL M. MOZELL and
DAVID E. HORNUNG

Prior to reaching the headspace above the olfactory epithelium in terrestrial animals, odorant molecules must be drawn over the sorptive surfaces of the non-olfactory nasal mucosa. In order to reach the olfactory receptors the odorant molecules must then partition across the air/mucosa interface and diffuse to the olfactory receptors. These physicochemical processes will likely influence the receptor access of different odorants differentially. It has been suggested, as discussed below, that this differential access might be one of the peripheral mechanisms of olfactory discrimination. However, even if not a basic mechanism for discrimination, it will still affect the number and time course of the odorant molecules reaching the receptors, thus impacting upon any other coding mechanism. Once an odorant molecule reaches the receptor, transduction can occur. If the olfactory system were like many other sensory systems, a given receptor cell would not be equally sensitive to all odorants. Receptor cells would instead be maximally excited by some odorants and less, or not at all, by others. Thus, a full description of the peripheral olfactory events must ultimately involve a description of the physicochemical processing affecting the access of the molecules to the receptors as well as the sensitivity of the receptor cells themselves.

Single-unit studies

The selective sensitivity of the receptors has received considerable attention. The expectation was that all chemicals exciting the same unit would have some discernible common property which, if identified, would aid in the classification of basic receptor cell types. This line of investigation began with Adrian's (1953, 1954) recordings from single

227

units in the olfactory bulb which he assumed would reflect the sensitivities of the receptors themselves. This work was followed by a number of investigations not only recording from single bulbar units but, more pertinently, recording extracellularly from single units of the epithelium (Gesteland, Lettvin, Pitts and Rojas, 1963; Shibuya and Shibuya, 1963; Matthews and Tucker, 1966; Matthews, 1972; Shibuya and Tucker, 1967; Takagi and Omura, 1963; Doving, 1966a,b; Getchell, 1974a; O'Connell and Mozell, 1969). By and large, these studies reached the same general conclusion, viz., although selective sensitivity was demonstrated in that each unit appeared to respond to a particular group of odorants, very few, if any, units responded to the same total group of odorants. This led Gesteland, Lettvin and Pitts (1965) to propose the concept of 'utter chaos', a concept suggesting that each receptor cell sees the world of odorants in its own particular way and that the total discharge pattern across all the receptor cells, which would differ for each odorant, encodes this world of odors.

To continue seeking a commonality in the sensitivities of the receptor cells several investigators treated their data with sophisticated statistical procedures. Doving (1966a,b, 1970) recorded the responses of single units in the olfactory bulb to a variety of chemicals and then, using a statistical approach, estimated the degree to which members of each possible pair of odorants produced similar responses across all units. This treatment allowed Doving to plot out the position of each odorant in an 'odor space' relative to every other odorant. Using Leveteau and MacLeod's (1969) recordings from glomeruli, Doving (1973, 1974) later analysed nineteen physical properties of odorant stimuli in relation to the neurophysiological response and determined that the five most important were: absorption energy, molecular length, air/oil partition coefficient, oil/water partition coefficient, and density. More recently, Chastrette (1981) mathematically found a combination of physicochemical variables that was able to reproduce all the significant features of an odorant classification based upon the discharges of frog olfactory receptor cells recorded by Duchamp, Revial, Holley and MacLeod (1974). Chasterette found the polarizability of the molecules, acid-base properties, and oil/water partition coefficient to be most important in reproducing this odorant classification. These statistical procedures have helped identify some physicochemical dimensions likely to be basic to olfactory receptor sensitivity. On the other hand, the expectation that receptor cells can be classified into basic types has not been met nor has the concept of 'utter chaos' been dispelled. Indeed, some investigators (Holley, Duchamp, Revial, Juge and MacLeod, 1974) have concluded that a basic classification of receptor cells does not exist.

Chromatographic-like effects

In recent years the attempt to understand how odorants are differentiated at the mucosal level has been undergoing a shift in emphasis. Instead of focusing on the responses of individual receptor cells, some investigators have become increasingly interested in the spatial and temporal activity patterns generated by the sheet of receptors across the entire olfactory mucosa. The concept that one of the mechanisms underlying olfactory discrimination might be the different spatiotemporal activity patterns produced across the mucosal receptor sheet by different odorants is not new. Adrian first suggested it in the early 1950s (Adrian, 1953, 1954) and it was later supported by Mozell (1970) and Moulton (1967). However, this concept did not seem to attract widespread support until rather recently. Pinching and Doving (1974) and Stewart, Kauer and Shepherd (1979) observed several spatially differentiated odorant-induced events in the olfactory bulb which seemed likely to result from precursory activity patterns generated along the olfactory mucosa. For instance, Pinching and Doving (1974) reported that when rats are exposed to odorants for relatively long periods of time, their olfactory bulbs show evidence of regional 'degeneration'. Those regions of 'degeneration' depend upon either the particular odorant included in the exposure (Doving and Pinching, 1973; Pinching and Doving, 1974) or, as some others believe (Laing and Panhuber, 1978), they depend upon the odorants missing in that exposure. In addition, Stewart et al. (1979) have shown topographical differences in the bulbar uptake of injected [^{14}C]2-deoxy-D-glucose (2DG) depending upon the odorant to which the animal was exposed.

These studies alone do not necessarily support the existence of different odorant-induced spatial activity patterns at the mucosal level. The various activity patterns observed at the level of the olfactory bulb could just as well be established by different groups of selectively sensitive receptor cells. These activity patterns could occur if each group of receptor cells, while being homogeneously distributed across the olfactory mucosa, projected to a particular region of the bulb. When, however, these 'degeneration' and 2DG studies were brought together with a number of anatomical and electrophysiological studies showing at least some degree of topographical projection of the mucosa onto the bulb (Land, 1973; Land and Shepherd, 1974; Costanzo and Mozell, 1976; Kauer, 1980), demonstrations that different odorants establish different spatiotemporal activity patterns across the mucosa began to attract more widespread attention.

The first indication in our laboratory of such odorant-specific spatiotemporal activity patterns across the mucosa came as a result of simultaneously recording summated multiunit discharges (Beidler, 1953) from different branches of the bullfrog's olfactory nerve. These recordings sampled the activity coming from two different mucosal regions on the roof of the olfactory sac. One branch, the most medial branch, served a region near the external naris and, therefore, reflected the activity of a mucosal region which is among the first in the olfactory sac contacted by the incoming odorized air. The other nerve branch, the most lateral, served a region overhanging the internal naris and thus reflected the activity of a mucosal region further along the flow path where the odorized air leaves the olfactory sac. The ratio of the summated discharge magnitude recorded from the lateral nerve branch (LB) to that from the medial nerve branch (MB) was used to compare the relative activity of the two regions in response to different odorants. The smaller this LB/MB ratio, the steeper was the gradient in the fall-off of mucosal activity from the external naris towards the internal naris. Each of the sixteen odorants tested (Mozell, 1970) produced a characteristic relative gradient of activity (LB/MB ratio) across the mucosa (see Figure 1 for examples). This effect remained consistent in any one frog, across frogs, and in the face of a rather wide range of odorant concentrations and presentation flow rates. In addition, for each odorant there was a different time interval between the onset of the summated discharges on the two nerve branches (Figure 1), and the longer the time interval for a given odorant the smaller was its LB/MB ratio. This parallel suggested that the time intervals and the LB/MB ratios which represent a possible spatiotemporal differentiation of

---

Figure 1. Traces of summated multiunit discharges showing the responses of one frog to a single presentation of each of four odorants at each of several concentrations expressed in partial pressure (Mozell, 1966.) (Multiply by 10^{-2} for mm Hg or 133 for $N\,m^{-2}$.) The upper response of each simultaneously recorded pair was from the lateral nerve branch and the lower was from the medial nerve branch. Although in this single array the octane response appears to be larger on the lateral nerve branch than on the medial nerve branch, in a later more comprehensive study (Mozell, 1970) the median octane responses on the two nerve branches were observed to be near equal. This was also true for d-limonene. In both studies the median discharges to both geraniol and citral were very much smaller on the lateral nerve branch than on the medial nerve branch. The stimulus marker shows only the onset of the stimulus. Vertical time lines occur once every 10 s. Stimulus duration was 3 s and stimulus volume was $0.4\,cm^3$ ($0.4 \times 10^{-6}\,m^3$). (Mozell, 1966, by permission of Rockefeller University Press.)

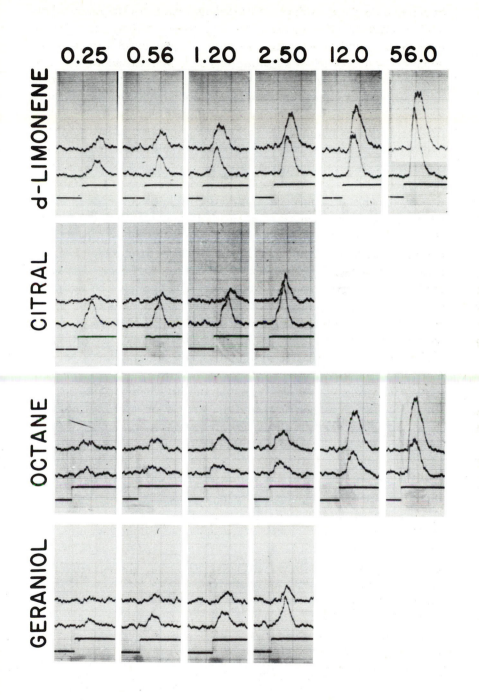

odorants across the mucosa are actually two views of the same under-lying mechanism.

There were at least two mechanisms which could have explained the different mucosal patterns produced by different odorants. First (perhaps more pertinent to the spatial patterns than to temporal ones), the receptor cells particularly selective for some odorants such as geraniol and citral (Figure 1) might simply be more sensitive and/or present in greater numbers around the external naris than around the internal naris. That is, there might be a topographical variation of odorant-selective receptor cells. For other odorants like octane and *d*-limonene (Figure 1) the sensitivity and/or the numbers of the receptor cells might be more evenly distributed. On the other hand, a second mechanism might be that the mucosa attracts and sorbs some molecules (e.g. geraniol and citral) more strongly than it attracts and sorbs other molecules (e.g. *d*-limonene and octane). Thus, in a given sniff, the molecules of the more poorly sorbed odorants would migrate across the mucosa more readily than those of the more strongly sorbed odorants. They would arrive at distant regions along the flow path more rapidly and in relatively greater numbers than the molecules of the more readily sorbed odorants, giving shorter time intervals and large LB/MB ratios.

To choose between these two alternative mechanisms, the flow direction of the odorized air through the olfactory sac was reversed. Flow was introduced through the internal naris towards the external naris rather than in the normal sniff direction of external naris towards the internal naris (Mozell, 1964). The result of this reversed flow was to reverse the relative discharge magnitude of the two nerve branches, i.e., the nerve branch which had yielded the larger response when the ordorant passed from external to internal naris (such as for geraniol and citral) then gave the smaller response when the odorant passed from internal to external naris. When there was little difference in the one direction (such as for octane and *d*-limonene) there was also little difference in the opposite direction. A topographical placement of different selectively-sensitive receptors would have difficulty explaining this discharge reversal since, regardless of the flow direction, the mucosal regions of greater and lesser sensitivity would be expected to remain constant. On the other hand, this reversal is exactly the expectation resulting from a differential sorption of molecules; those most strongly sorbed by the mucosa would be retained at either end, depending upon which naris they entered.

If, as these data suggest, differential sorption does lead to differential migration patterns across the mucosa, an analogy might be drawn between olfaction and gas chromatography. A gas chromatograph has a detecting device at the end of a column packed with a sorbent material (the stationary phase). The chemical to be identified is passed through the column towards the detector in a carrier gas (the moving phase) and, depending upon how the molecules of any given chemical are partitioned between the moving and stationary phases, that chemical will take a longer or shorter time to traverse the column and be detected. The more the partition favors the stationary phase (i.e., the more strongly the molecules are sorbed to the stationary phase), the longer it will take the chemical in question to be detected. The readout, then, is the travel time per column distance which is called that chemical's retention time and which, under a set of specified conditions, is indicative of that particular chemical. The nose could use the identical principle of partitioning, but, because the carrier gas flow is pulsatile rather than continuous, a different readout is needed. This can be accomplished because the olfactory system does not have one detector at the end of the 'column' but millions (the receptor cells) along the entire 'column'. Thus, in the time frame of a given sniff the receptor cells could signal how far and in what relative numbers the molecules move along the column. This molecular migration in turn, as in gas chromatography, depends upon the partitioning of molecules between a moving phase (the sniff of odorized air) and a stationary phase (the olfactory mucosa).

We gained further confidence in this model using non-electrophysiological techniques. After all, the electrophysiological techniques can give only indirect evidence of how the molecules of different odorants migrate across the mucosa since these electrophysiological events are several steps beyond the molecular events presumably giving rise to them. Therefore, a more direct measurement of the molecular migration of different odorants across the mucosa would be useful. In keeping with the chromatographic model, the retention times of different odorants as they were carried across the olfactory mucosa itself were measured by replacing the column of a standard gas chromatograph with the nose of the anesthetized bullfrog (Mozell and Jagodowicz, 1973, 1974). The fifteen tested odorants gave a wide range of demonstrably different retention times representing a 220-fold increase from the shortest to the longest. Therefore, in spite of the bullfrog's rather short flow path from external naris to internal naris, the molecules of different odorants do migrate at demonstrably different rates across the mucosa. Furthermore, there was an excellent correlation between the odorants' retention times and their LB/MB ratios: the longer the retention time, the smaller the LB/MB ratio. This was consistent with the model since in the time frame of a sniff the longer the retention time, the more the molecules will pile up around the external naris and the steeper will be the activity gradient across the mucosa.

As discussed above, one could infer the spatial distribution of the molecules across the mucosa from the electrophysiological and gas chromatographic data. However, a more exact appreciation of how the molecules of different odorants are actually distributed across the mucosa in a sniff required a technique which could provide a more direct display of the molecules themselves. This was provided by radioactive odorants.

Hornung, Lansing and Mozell (1975) used radioactively-labeled odorants to map quantitatively the odorant-specific differential sorption patterns along the mucosa. After presenting bullfrogs with radioactively-labeled odorants, the animals were quick-frozen in liquid nitrogen, their mucosas sectioned antero-posteriorly, and the radioactivity in each section determined by liquid scintillation counting. From these data, the number of sorbed odorant molecules per surface area in each mucosal section was estimated.

Mapping studies have so far been completed using three chemicals: butanol, butyl acetate, and octane (Hornung and Mozell, 1977a, 1981). For butanol there was a significant decrease in the number of molecules per surface area sorbed by the dorsal surface section containing the external naris to that overhanging the internal naris. For butyl acetate this gradient was less steep, and for octane there was a rather even distribution (Figure 2). This isotope work graphically confirmed the prediction from the electrophysiological and chromatographic data that within the time frame of a sniff, a given compound establishes a particular distribution pattern across the olfactory mucosa. It further showed that within a wide range of stimulation parameters (flow rates, concentrations, and times), the distribution patterns were reasonably constant. As expected from the chromatographic model, the gradients for butanol and butyl acetate reversed direction when the stimulus was presented in the reverse direction through the internal naris. Because of its even distribution pattern, reversing the flow path for octane did not significantly affect its mucosal distribution pattern.

The principles of gas chromatography would suggest that these odorant-specific distribution patterns depend to a large extent upon the partitioning of molecules between the air phase and the mucosal phase. To better define these mucosal sorption events, Hornung, Mozell and Serio (1980) used radioisotopes to measure the mucosa/air partition coefficients. Samples of frog mucosa were exposed in a closed environment of humidified air saturated with a radioactive odorant. After allowing sufficient time for equilibrium to occur, the partition coefficient was determined by the ratio of the activity per gram of mucosa to the activity per cubic centimeter of air. When this mucosa/air partition coefficient was compared to the water/air partition coefficient, the mucosa was observed to have a greater ability than water to sorb odorant molecules. Therefore, since the water in the mucosa could not account completely for the mucosa's odorant uptake, a multicompartment model with several partitions (Getchell and Getchell, 1977) was needed to describe the interaction of odorant molecules with the olfactory mucosa. The mucosal distribution seen in Figure 2 was also found to be related to the partition coefficients. The more the partition

Figure 2. Surface area concentration of the antero-posterior sections from the roof of the bullfrog olfactory sac after stimulation with radioactively labeled butanol, butyl acetate, or octane. The 'sniff' parameters of concentration, flow rate, and volume were constant for all odorants. The direction of air flow was from external naris (M1) toward internal naris (M4). (Hornung and Mozell, 1981, by permission of Academic Press.)

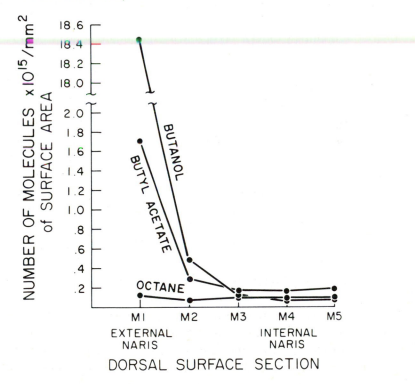

of a given odorant favors the mucosa, the steeper its gradient from the external to the internal naris. Therefore, the physicochemical processes determining mucosa/air partitioning also underly the LB/MB ratios and the mucosal retention times. Thus, as raised in the discussion of the single unit recordings, physicochemical processes are again actually demonstrated to influence peripheral olfactory coding.

The physicochemical processes affecting the mucosa/air partitioning of odorants also surface in the removal of sorbed odorant molecules. To quantify this removal, Hornung and Mozell (1977b) modified the isotope mapping technique to study how desorption into the air, mucus flow, and uptake by the circulatory system are each able to remove odorants from the olfactory sac. For odorants like butanol, in which the mucosa/air partitioning favors the mucosa, these removal mechanisms are not very effective. Thus, even as long as 30 min after a single sniff a large number of sorbed butanol molecules could still be found somewhere in the olfactory mucosa. On the other hand, for an odorant like octane where the mucosa/air partition favors the air phase, odorant removal, especially by desorption into air, was effective and rapid. The importance of these differences in mucosal odorant retention to possible ensuing adaptation effects has yet to be investigated.

Sensitivity differences of mucosal regions

Thus a variety of techniques attest to a very potent chromatographic or sorptive effect across the mucosa which can establish differential mucosal activity patterns. However, within the past eight years Moulton and a number of his students have made observations, mainly in salamanders, which give evidence of yet another mechanism at the level of the olfactory mucosa which could give rise to the differential mucosal activity patterns which we reported for frogs. These authors (Kauer and Moulton, 1974; MacKay-Sim and Kubie, 1982; Kubie, MacKay-Sim and Moulton, 1980) have demonstrated that the sensitivity of the mucosa for a given odorant differs from region to region and that the pattern of this regional shift differs for different odorants.

The basic procedure in these studies was to expose the olfactory mucosa by removing one wall of the olfactory sac and placing an electrode directly upon the surface of different mucosal regions. This electrode recorded a region's electro-olfactogram (EOG) in response to odorants puffed directly onto the exposed mucosa. (The EOG is a slow odorant-produced potential change recorded from the mucosal surface. It is believed to be generated for the most part by excited receptor cells (Getchell, 1974b).) Since the odorant was puffed directly onto the recording site, any possibility that the response would reflect the chromatographic effect due to molecular migration across the mucosal surface was circumvented. Thus, variations in the responses recorded from different sites to the same odorant could be considered the effect of differences in the sensitivities and/or numbers of selective receptors in those different regions. (Yet another possibility is that these variations reflect regional differences in such mucosal characteristics as the composition of the mucus and the proximity of receptor sites to the mucus/air interface. However, there are as yet no definitive data supporting such a possibility. Therefore, following the lead of Moulton and his co-workers, we discuss these variations in terms of differences in the regional sensitivities of the receptor cells.) MacKay-Sim and Kubie (1982) observed that the anterior region of the mucosa is more sensitive to butanol than is the posterior region, whereas the reverse is true for limonene. Several other odorants also shared this anterior-posterior differentiation, whereas still others shared a more or less even sensitivity across the mucosa. Furthermore, within a general region of increased sensitivity for a given odorant, there might be a smaller region of supersensitivity. At any rate, there now seem to be two mechanisms, the regional sensitivity effect and the chromatographic effect, which could both contribute to the spatial activity patterns across the mucosa.

Interplay of chromatographic and regional sensitivity effects

There is an apparent inconsistency between these findings and the findings of the study discussed earlier in which the odorant flow direction was reversed. The earlier study seemed to rule out the possibility of regional differences in sensitivity as a basis for the different LB/MB ratios. Obviously, that conclusion had to be reconsidered in the light of these new data. It is at least possible that for the odorants having a chromatographic effect in the reversed flow experiment, the chromatographic effect was so strong that it masked the effect of regional sensitivity. For instance, in Figure 2, based upon radioactive odorants, almost all of the molecules are sorbed around the external naris with very few reaching the internal naris and, as noted, the reverse is true when the flow of the odorant is in the opposite direction. In such a case, even though the anterior mucosa might be more sensitive and the posterior less sensitive to the odorant, the posterior mucosa could still give the larger response due to the extremely large difference in the numbers of molecules sorbing to the two regions.

In order to parcel out the contribution of the chromatographic effect and the regional sensitivity effect in determining the mucosal activity patterns produced by different odorants, we have derived a new experimental strategy using the reversed flow technique. For each odorant the summated multiunit discharges from both the lateral (LB) and medial (MB) nerve branches will be recorded when the odorized air is presented in the normal sniff direction from external to internal naris (S) and when it is presented in the reverse direction from internal to external naris (R). The LB_S discharge then represents the mucosal activity around the internal naris when the odorant molecules approach that region coming across the mucosal surface from the external naris. Because of the movement across the mucosal surface there is a chance for a chromatographic effect. The LB_R discharge, on the other hand, represents the activity around the internal naris when the odorant reaches that region directly through the internal naris with no travel across the mucosal surface. In this case there is no chance for a chromatographic effect. Furthermore, since LB_S and LB_R both sample the same mucosal region, any difference in the two responses as indexed by the LB_S/LB_R ratio can be considered the result of the chromatographic effect without any contamination by the regional sensitivity effect. The smaller the LB_S/LB_R ratio for a given odorant, the greater is the chromatographic effect upon the mucosal activity pattern.

Continuing the same strategy, the MB_S discharge represents the activity around the external naris when the odorant reaches that region directly through the external naris with no travel across the mucosal surface. This rules out the possibility of a chromatographic effect influencing the MB_S response. Therefore, since LB_R and MB_S are both sampling different regions of the mucosa and each is uninfluenced by the chromatographic effect, the difference in these two responses as indexed by the LB_R/MB_S ratio can be considered the result of the regional sensitivity effect uncontaminated by the chromatographic effect. The smaller the LB_R/MB_S ratio for a given odorant, the more sensitive is the anterior mucosa for that odorant relative to the posterior mucosa. Finally, the LB_S/MB_S ratio is the new terminology for the older LB/MB ratio which includes both the chromatographic effect by virtue of its influence on the LB_S discharge and the regional effect by virtue of the comparison of two different regions. Presumably the activity patterns represented by the LB_S/MB_S ratio are due to the combined influences of the chromatographic effect and the regional sensitivity effect. The above strategy should permit a parceling out of these contributions. It should be noted that to interpret these ratios as suggested, several controls must be initiated. These controls can be found elsewhere (Mozell and Hornung, 1982); this discussion is meant only to outline the strategy.

New experiments using this strategy have not yet been done. However, the data from the earlier reversed-flow experiments (Mozell, 1964), which were based upon six animals, were subjected to the analysis outlined in the above strategy. Notwithstanding the fact that the equipment and technique of that early experiment had little of the finesse and precision of like work done today, the necessary determinations (MB_S, LB_R and LB_S), crude as they may have been, were still available.

The LB_S/LB_R ratios for geraniol and citral were 0.44 and 0.27 respectively demonstrating a rather potent chromatographic effect just as the 1964 reversed-flow experiment showed. However, the LB_R/MB_S ratios for geraniol and citral were both 0.79 showing something not discerned in the earlier work, viz., that for both these odorants there is an effect of regional sensitivity with the anterior region being more sensitive relative to the posterior region. One of these two odorants, geraniol, was also found by MacKay-Sim and Kubie (1982) to have an anterior regional sensitivity and this reanalysis of Mozell's 1964 data confirmed their finding. Although they found a more robust difference between the responses of the two regions, the point is still made that the mucosal activity patterns as measured by the summated multiunit discharges depend upon regional differences in mucosal sensitivity as well as upon differential sorption across the mucosa.

For *d*-limonene the result is considerably less clear. The LB_S/LB_R ratio was 0.95 which if it were not for a more general point to be made later, would be interpreted, considering the variability, as demonstrating no chromatographic effect. However, for the sake of this point it is suggested very tenuously that there is a slight chromatographic effect. The LB_R/MB_S ratio for *d*-limonene was 1.08 which again can be interpreted very tenuously to show a very slight regional sensitivity effect with the posterior mucosa being slightly more sensitive than the anterior mucosa. Although quite tenuous it is tempting to point out that the direction of the regional sensitivity for *d*-limonene is the same as that shown by the MacKay-Sim and Kubie study.

The results for octane, the last odorant used in Mozell's 1964 study, will not be discussed because considerations beyond the intention of this review are required to appreciate fully the octane ratios.

This reanalysis of the earlier reversed-flow data has highlighted the interplay of the regional sensitivity effect and the chromatographic effect in generating the mucosal activity patterns. In a given sniff, the surface concentrations of geraniol and citral decrease from the external naris to the internal naris. At the same time, the decreasing concentration falls upon a decreasing sensitivity from the external naris to the internal naris. Thus, the two effects reinforce each other so that the LB_S/MB_S ratio (the index of the final mucosal activity pattern) was 0.35 for geraniol. This ratio shows a greater drop-off of activity from the external naris to the internal naris than can be accounted for by either the chromatographic effect ($LB_S/LB_R = 0.44$) or the regional sensitivity effect ($LB_R/MB_S = 0.79$) alone. The same reinforcement of the two effects was also true for citral ($LB_R/MB_S = 0.21$; $LB_S/LB_R = 0.27$; $LB_R/MB_S = 0.79$).

On the other hand, for *d*-limonene the chromatographic and regional sensitivity effects seem to oppose each other in determining the mucosal activity pattern. There is a slight chromatographic effect (i.e., a decrease in surface concentration) from the external naris to the internal naris. This falls upon a slight increase in sensitivity from the external naris to the internal naris. Thus, it was that the LB_S/MB_S ratio (1.03) is greater than the LB_S/LB_R ratio (0.95) but less than the LB_R/MB_S ratio (1.08).

Figure 3. A schematic diagram of a heterogeneous distribution of receptor types A, B, C, D in each of four regions of the olfactory epithelium. All receptor types are represented in all regions but to different degrees, thus giving regional differences to the mucosa in its sensitivity to odorants. (Kauer, 1980, by permission Information Retrieval Limited.)

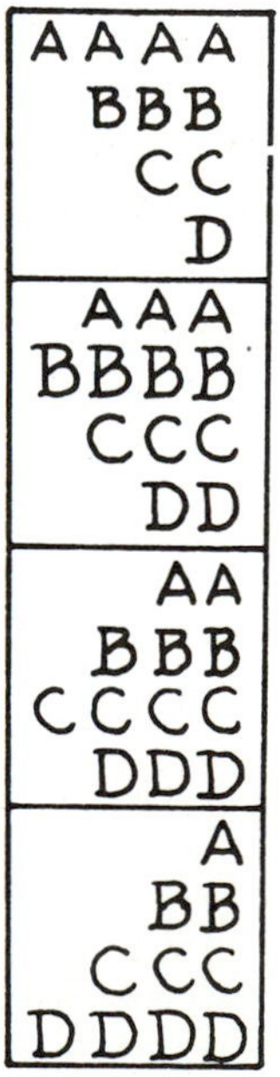

To explore further how these two mechanisms may interplay in establishing different activity patterns across the mucosa and thereby help differentiate odorants, consider Kauer's (1980) model (Figure 3) schematically representing the regions of different sensitivities across the mucosa. In this model each region is responsive to many of the same odorants but to different degrees. Suppose the external naris is at the top of the figure so that a sniff of odorized air travels across the mucosa from top to bottom in the figure. Suppose further that two odorants of the D type are sniffed. If they each have no chromatographic effect, the patterns of regional activity that they will produce will both show an increasing gradient beginning at the external naris and will, therefore, not be differentiated by this mechanism. On the other hand, if one odorant does have a major chromatographic effect, its decreasing concentration along the mucosa will fall upon the increasing sensitivity, producing a less steep, or even a reversed, activity gradient. The two D type odorants would then establish dissimilar activity patterns and might thus be differentiated.

Conclusions

At the peripheral level a number of physicochemical processes have been implicated in the olfactory system's analysis of odorants. We have emphasized how one of these, the partition across the mucosa/air interface, can interplay with the sensitivity organization of the receptor sheet to produce a differential encoding of odorants. Indeed, there is behavioral evidence that topographical activity patterns across the mucosa do play a role in olfactory discrimination (Bennett, 1972). However, even if these activity patterns were not themselves a basic code for olfactory discrimination, the differential distribution of the odorant molecules would still influence any coding process by affecting the access of the odorant molecules to the receptor cells.

Supported by NIH Grant NS03904.

References

Adrian, E. D. (1953). The mechanism of olfactory stimulation in the mammal. *Adv. Sci., Lond.* 9: 417–20.

Adrian, E. D. (1954). The basis of sensation – some recent studies of olfaction. *Br. Med. J. 1:* 287–90.

Beidler, L. M. (1953). Properties of chemoreceptors of tongue of rat. *J. Neurophysiol. 16:* 595–607.

Bennett, M. H. (1972). Effects of asymmetrical mucosal stimulation upon two-odor discrimination in the rat. *Physiol. Behav. 9:* 301–6.

Chastrette, M. (1981). An approach to a classification of odours using physiochemical parameters. *Chem. Senses 6:* 157–63.

Costanzo, R. M., and Mozell, M. M. (1976). Electrophysiological evidence for a topographical projection of the nasal mucosa onto the olfactory bulb of the frog. *J. Gen. Physiol. 68:* 297–312.

Doving, K. B. (1966a). An electrophysiological study of odour similarities of homologous substances. *J. Physiol., Lond. 186:* 97–109.

Doving, K. B. (1966b). Analysis of odour similarities from electrophysiological data. *Acta Physiol. Scand. 68:* 404–18.

Doving, K. B. (1970). Experiments in olfaction. In *Taste and Smell in Vertebrates*, a Ciba Foundation Symposium, ed. G. E. W. Wolstenholme and S. Knight, pp. 197–221. London: Churchill.

Doving, K. B. (1973). Physiological data correlated with physical parameters. In *Transduction Mechanisms in Chemoreception*, ed. T. M. Poynder, pp. 261–73. London: Information Retrieval Limited.

Doving, K. B. (1974). Odorant properties correlated with physiological data. *Ann. NY Acad. Sci. 237:* 184–92.

Doving, K. B., and Pinching, A. J. (1973). Selective degeneration of neurones in the olfactory bulb following prolonged odour exposure. *Brain Res. 52:* 115–29.

Duchamp, A., Revial, M. F., Holley, A., and MacLeod, P. (1974). Odor discrimination by frog olfactory receptors. *Chemical Senses and Flavor 1:* 213–33.

Gesteland, R. C., Lettvin, J. Y., Pitts, W. H., and Rojas, A. (1963). Odor specificities of the frog's olfactory receptors. In *Olfaction and Taste*, ed. Y. Zotterman, pp. 19–44. Oxford: Pergamon.

Gesteland, R. C., Lettvin, J. Y., and Pitts, W. H. (1965). Chemical transmission in the nose of the frog. *J. Physiol., Lond. 181:* 525–59.

Getchell, T. V. (1974a). Unitary responses in frog olfactory epithelium to sterically related molecules at low concentrations. *J. Gen. Physiol. 64:* 241–61.

Getchell, T. V. (1974b). Electrogenic sources of slow voltage transients recorded from frog olfactory epithelium. *J. Neurophysiol. 37:* 1115–30.

Getchell, T. V., and Getchell, M. L. (1977). Early events in vertebrate olfaction. *Chemical Senses and Flavor 2:* 313–26.

Holley, A., Duchamp, A., Revial, M., Juge, A., and MacLeod, P. (1974). Qualitative and quantitative discrimination in the frog olfactory receptors: analysis from electrophysiological data. *Ann. NY Acad. Sci. 237:* 102–14.

Hornung, D. E., Lansing, R. D., and Mozell, M. M. (1975). Distribution of butanol molecules along bullfrog olfactory mucosa. *Nature 254:* 617–18.

Hornung, D. E., and Mozell, M. M. (1977a). Factors influencing the differential sorption of odorant molecules across the olfactory mucosa. *J. Gen. Physiol. 69:* 343–61.

Hornung, D. E., and Mozell, M. M. (1977b). Odorant removal from the frog olfactory mucosa. *Brain Res. 181:* 488–92.

Hornung, D. E., and Mozell, M. M. (1981). Accessibility of odorant molecules to the receptors. In *Biochemistry of Taste and Olfaction*, ed. by R. H. Cagan and M. R. Kare, pp. 33–45. New York: Academic Press.

Hornung, D. E., Mozell, M. M., and Serio, J. A. (1980). Olfactory mucosa/air partitioning of odorants. In *Olfaction and Taste VII*, ed. H. van der Starre, pp. 167–70. London: Information Retrieval Limited.

Kauer, J. S. (1980). Some spatial characteristics of central information processing in the vertebrate olfactory pathway. In *Olfaction and Taste VII*, ed. H. van der Starre, pp. 227–36. London: Information Retrieval Limited.

Kauer, J. S., and Moulton, D. G. (1974). Responses of olfactory bulb neurones to odor stimulation of small nasal areas in the salamander. *J. Physiol., Lond. 243:* 717–37.

Kubie, J. L., MacKay-Sim, A., and Moulton, D. G. (1980). Inherent spatial patterning of response to odorants in the salamander olfactory epithelium. In *Olfaction and Taste VII*, ed. H. van der Starre, pp. 163–6. London: Information Retrieval Limited.

Laing, D. G., and Panhuber, H. (1978). Neural and behavioral changes in rats following continuous exposure to odor. *J. Comp. Physiol. 124:* 259–65.

Land, L. J. (1973). Localized projection of olfactory nerves to rabbit olfactory bulb. *Brain Res. 63:* 153–66.

Land, L. J., and Shepherd, G. M. (1974). Autoradiographic analysis of olfactory receptor projections in rabbit. *Brain Res. 70:* 506–10.

Leveteau, J., and MacLeod, P. (1969). La discrimination des odeurs par les glomérules olfactifs du lapin: influence de la concentration de stimulus. *J. Physiol., Paris 61:* 5–16.

MacKay-Sim, A., and Kubie, J. L. (1981). The salamander nose: a model system for the study of spatial coding of olfactory quality. *Chemical Senses 6:* 249–57.

Mathews, D. F. (1972). Response patterns of single neurones in the tortoise olfactory epithelium and olfactory bulb. *J. Gen. Physiol. 60:* 166–80.

Mathews, D. F., and Tucker, D. (1966). Single unit activity in the tortoise olfactory mucosa. *Fed. Proc. 25:* 329.

Moulton, D. G. (1967). Spatio-temporal patterning of response in the olfactory system. In *Proceedings of the Second International Symposium on Olfaction and Taste*, ed. T. Hayashi, pp. 109–16. New York: Pergamon.

Mozell, M. M. (1964). Evidence for sorption as a mechanism of the olfactory analysis of vapors. *Nature 203:* 1181–2.

Mozell, M. M. (1966). The spatiotemporal analysis of odorants at the level of the olfactory receptor sheet. *J. Gen. Physiol. 50:* 25–41.

Mozell, M. M. (1970). Evidence for a chromatographic model of olfaction. *J. Gen. Physiol. 56:* 46–63.

Mozell, M. M., and Hornung, D. E. (1981). Imposed and inherent olfactory mucosal activity patterns: an experimental design prompted by the work of David Moulton. *Chemical Senses 6:* 267–76.

Mozell, M. M., and Jagodowicz, M. (1973). Chromatographic separation of odorants by the nose: retention times measured across in vivo olfactory mucosa. *Science 181:* 1247–9.

Mozell, M. M., and Jagodowicz, M. (1974). Mechanisms underlying the analysis of odorant quality at the level of the olfactory mucosa Part I, spatiotemporal sorption patterns. *Ann. NY Acad. Sci. 237:* 76–90.

O'Connell, R. J., and Mozell, M. M. (1969). Quantitative stimulation of frog olfactory receptors. *J. Neurophysiol. 32:* 51–63.

Pinching, A. J., and Doving, K. B. (1974). Selective degeneration in the rat olfactory bulb following exposure to different odours. *Brain Res. 82:* 195–204.

Shibuya, T., and Shibuya, S. (1963). Olfactory epithelium: unitary responses in the tortoise. *Science 140:* 495–6.

Shibuya, T., and Tucker, D. (1967). Single unit responses of olfactory receptors in vultures. In *Proceedings of the Second International Symposium on Olfaction and Taste*, ed. T. Hayashi, pp. 219–34. New York: Pergamon.

Stewart, W. B., Kauer, J. S., and Shepherd, G. M. (1979). Functional organization of rat olfactory bulb analyzed by the 2-deoxyglucose method. *J. Comp. Neurol. 185:* 715–34.

Takagi, S. F., and Omura, D. (1963). Responses of the olfactory receptor cells to odors. *Proc. Jap. Acad. 39:* 253–5.

2.2

Neural basis of olfaction in insects

CLAUDINE MASSON

For the neurobiologist the olfactory system of insects seems to be of interest because: on the one hand there are a lot of behavioural responses (mainly in Social Insects) which suggest plasticity of the relevant nervous system (Von Frisch, 1967; Pham and Masson, 1983); on the other hand, this plasticity seems to take place at the level of specific neuronal networks identifiable in position and structure (Menzel, Erber and Masuhr, 1974; Masson, 1977; Erber, 1981).

Nevertheless, before any consideration concerning the plasticity of this system, it is necessary to know its 'normal' morphofunctional organization in the adult.

Neuroanatomical and neurophysiological investigations in different insect species analysed in detail suggest that general rules governing neural connectivity exist for the antennal olfactory system of insects.

An overview of these general features of functional anatomy is given in this paper, by considering (i) the peripheral level, and (ii) the first relay of the afferent olfactory pathway in the brain–respectively equivalent to the olfactory mucosa and to the olfactory bulb in vertebrates.

Interdisciplinary and complementary approaches including studies of behaviour, chemistry and neurophysiology, developed these last ten years lead today to the conclusion that chemical signals of particular importance to insects (intra- and/or interspecific semiochemicals) tend to be complex in structure and are composed of several chemicals.

Consequently, the sensory character of a specific stimulus is determined by a chemical pattern, that is to say by the relative proportions of the different components of the chemical mixture. And these different chemical patterns allow precise identification and discrimination of different chemicals among multiple odorant stimuli by means of a specialized detector system. The detector system translates these chemical patterns into corresponding electrical patterns in the afferent olfactory pathways.

The detection of olfactory signals
Some structural features

The two antennae of an insect are equipped with small cuticular sensory organs, the *sensilla*, which detect different sensory modalities such as chemoreception – olfaction and taste – mechanoreception, proprioception, temperature, CO_2, H_2O...etc. Nevertheless it appears that the olfactory modality is frequently the more developed, due to the decisive role of volatile compounds in the control of insect behaviour. Consequently, in the bulk of insect species, the antennae can be considered as the olfactory organ detector.

The outer cuticular part of the sensilla shows a great variety of shapes (hairs, plates, pegs...). They house the olfactory receptor cells (Figure 1A, B). The walls of the sensilla are screened by pores which are the gateways for the odorant molecules to reach the underlying membranes of the dendrites of the neuroreceptors where the transduction mechanism takes place.

Combined scanning electron microscopy studies and electrophysiological investigations reveal a good correlation between structural types of antennal olfactory sensilla and functional types of the olfactory sensory cells (Altner, 1977). Of course, such a correlation is helpful in perform-

Figure 1. (A) The head of a worker bee with its two antennae (An), main detector organs for the odorant molecules. In (B), the two main types of olfactory sensilla of the antennae, sensilla placodea (s.p.) and sensilla trichodea (s.t.) observed by scanning electron microscopy.

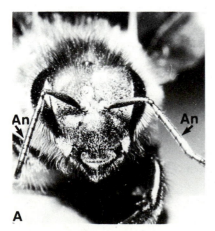
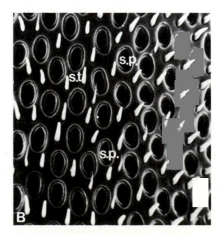

ing electrophysiological recordings to study the functional parameters of the sensory neurons. The number of receptor cells per sensillum varies, but is generally constant for a certain morphological type of sensilla in any one insect species.

The olfactory receptor cells of insects are prototypes of bipolar neuron – as in vertebrates (Holley and MacLeod, 1977). From the soma, a dendrite extends distally inside the cuticular part of the sensilla where it terminates, often by several ramifications in the sensillum liquor (Ernst, 1969; Kaissling and Thorson, 1980). Proximally the receptor cell axon projects to the deutocerebrum in the brain without axon collaterals or synapses. As, in addition, no gap junctions are observed between adjacent neuroreceptors, one can generally consider that the olfactory receptor cells function as true independent sensory units (Masson, 1973; Boeckh, Ernst, Sass and Waldow, 1976; Hilde-brand et al., 1980). These neurons are responsible for the selectivity and for the specificity of detection and for olfactory discriminating mechanisms.

Neural basis of coding at the receptor cell level

General physiological properties. Two general methods are useful tools to investigate extracellularly the functioning of olfactory sensory cells.

The first type is to record the slow monophasic negative change from the antennal nerve generated by populations of olfactory neurons which are simultaneously reacting electrically to the same molecules. It is considered to be an odour-induced summated receptor potential of many sense cells lying in series (more or less). It was originally termed the electro-antennogram (EAG) and first recorded by Schneider (1957). It is very similar to the electro-olfactogram (EOG), recorded in the olfactory mucosa of vertebrates (Ottoson, 1956).

In the second type, the voltage transient is recorded extracellularly as action potentials by micro-electrodes applied close to the sensory cells.

The chemical nature of insect chemoreceptor sites is not clear, but there are theoretical and experimental bases for assuming that most if not all, are proteins (Norris, 1976). A detailed understanding of transduction in insect chemoreception awaits the isolation of receptor and channel protein from the membranes of dendritic outer segments (Klein, 1980). Furthermore, observations on dendritic membranes of olfactory neurons prepared by freeze-fracturing suggest that the densities of receptor channel protein complexes (Menco and Van der Wolk, 1982) are comparable to those of cilia of vertebrate olfactory neurons (Masson, Kouprach, Giachetti and MacLeod, 1977; Masson and Mac-Leod, 1978).

The specificity of olfactory sensory neurons and their discriminatory performances. A discrimination of sensory quality in chemoreception means a discrimination between different compounds, or mixtures of compounds.

As has been said above, each sensory axon is an individual unit which sends an independent input to the brain. Consequently the question arises: are there as many receptor cells as there are pure chemical stimuli?

Such a question can be answered only by using single-cell recordings. It appears that chemoreceptor cells are not tuned to just one compound. With few exceptions they react to series of chemical components, which together form the qualitative olfactory spectrum of the neuron.

If one considers the different possibilities of coding the information concerning the stimulus quality, by comparison with the different data obtained in other animals, mainly vertebrates, in olfaction (Holley and MacLeod, 1977) and taste (Pfaffmann, 1941), the insects seem to possess the same alternatives, either coding of the olfactory quality through 'across-fibre patterns', or through 'labeled lines'.

Very complex stimuli are the numerous allomones and kairomones. Among them the volatile emissions of plant leaves or of flowers are striking attractions – or repellants – for various species (pollinating or pest phytophagous insects).

These mixtures of odorants are extremely complicated to code because they are, on the one hand composed of numerous (up to several hundred!) different effective chemicals with different functions (short-chain aliphatic alcohols, ketones, aldehydes, esters, acids, terpenes...) which are, on the other hand, able to vary in differential proportions according to environmental conditions such as temperature, enzyme degradation...etc. And of course, there is no single compound which represents the complex odour of a food source!

As the same insect is able to detect different, and simultaneously presented, complex chemical sources, and as there is considerable overlap of compounds between these different sources, peripheral coding cannot be assumed to occur by labelled lines, but by a system of neuroreceptors with broad spectra overlapping more or less, as in cockroaches (Sass, 1978; Selzer, 1981) or in the ant (Masson and Friggi, 1974); or by independent broad quality spectra built by groups of cells each with a differential level of sensitivity to the different odours of their common spectra so that there is a difference in the relative level of excitation in the receptor cells of the group considered according to the stimulus, as in the worker bee (Vareschi, 1971).

In other words, these mixtures are coded according to an across-fibre pattern (Figure 2A): each substance evokes a specific profile of relative levels of excitation in the cells (Selzer, 1981; Sass, 1978; Masson and Friggi, 1974; Boeckh, 1980; Masson and Brossut, 1981). The same phenomenon seems to exist in the olfactory neuro-receptors of the amphibians (Holley and MacLeod, 1977). One can term them 'odour generalist cells' and they give a fine-grain olfactory discrimination to the whole system for many complex stimuli present simultaneously in the olfactory environment of the insect.

The second important type of coding of the olfactory signals in insects is well illustrated by the sexual pheromonal receptor cells of the moths where it appears that each component of the pheromonal blend is peripherally coded by different sensory neurons. Moreover a set of sensilla (specific pheromonal sensilla) can be completely tuned solely to detect only the blend; each component in determined proportion is effective only for one receptor cell of the considered sensilla; each cell has a 'key compound' and possesses very particular spectra and dose-response characteristics (Priesner, 1980). Consequently these cells have very narrow and discrete spectra without overlap with those of other neuroreceptors in the antenna (Figure 2B). They are termed 'true specialist cells' and thus work as a labelled line system (Masson and Brossut, 1981).

To summarize and to conclude this section on Detection of olfactory signals, one can assume that the single-cell responses vary according to

Figure 2. Coding of the olfactory messages by the antennal neuroreceptors.

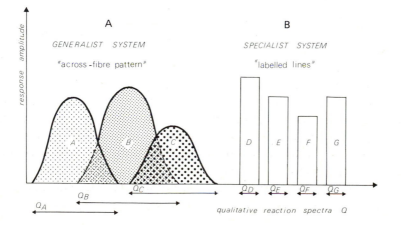

the composition of the odour and there will be a particular profile of response amplitude over the receptor population which is characteristic for each stimulus. Since it is a specific mixture of the compounds – in quality and in intensity – which is the adequate trigger of the behaviour, as the receptor level analyses the chemical pattern of the stimulus, consequently the central nervous system has to integrate these messages to extract and identify the behavioural signal as a whole.

Central olfactory pathways and processing

Compared with the numerous data published concerning the peripheral olfactory system, data related to the central olfactory pathways and processing are still sparse.

Nevertheless papers recently published in this field using combined classical microscopy methods, cobalt staining and electrophysiological recording applied to different insect species (Ernst, Boeckh and Boeckh, 1977; Masson, 1977; Masson and Brossut, 1981: Hildebrand et al., 1980; Arnold and Masson, 1982; Matsumoto and Hildebrand, 1981) allow one now to give a survey of connectivity and functioning of these afferent pathways.

The glomeruli and the spatial organization of afferents

From a comparative point of view it is interesting to note that striking similarities exist between the organization of the insect antennal afferent projections in the brain at the level of the deutocerebrum and that of the vertebrate olfactory bulb (Shepherd, 1972).

In both cases the sensory axons and the second-order neurons (local interneurons and output deutoneurons) organize themselves into spatially distributed discrete neuropile areas: the glomeruli, where all synaptic interactions between these first-order and second-order neurons take place.

The glomeruli are produced by the huge convergence of hundreds of thousands of antennal fibres on to only a few hundred output deutoneurons (ratio circa 1 : 500) (Masson, 1973; Ernest et al., 1977). In cockroaches, histological and computer analysis of their spatial organization has demonstrated that the glomeruli are strictly invariant in number, position and volume, and so are morphologically identifiable (Chambille, Rospars and Masson, 1980; Chambille and Rospars, 1981). This demonstration first done in a cockroach has now been confirmed in other insect species.

Moreover, a sexual dimorphism exists at this level: a male-specific structure is identifiable in the male deutocerebral neuropile, built up by one 'macroglomerulus', or a group of glomeruli 'macroglomerulus complex' (Chambille et al., 1980; Prillinger, 1981; Hildebrand et al., 1980; Arnold, Masson and Budharugsa, 1982).

Furthermore it has been demonstrated that this specific glomerular structure is identifiable as a true functional unit, solely tuned to receive pheromonal inputs and mainly involved in the processing of the female olfactory information (Boeckh et al., 1977; Hildebrand et al., 1980).

All these results strongly support the hypothesis of a non-random organization and of more or less specific spatial projections of the antennal afferents on to the secondary neurons, and suggest that they have specific and reproducible functions as previously proposed on the basis of combined classical histology, histochemistry and electrophysiology in the deutocerebral area of social insects (Masson, 1973; Masson and Strambi, 1977).

It is interesting to note here that in the mammalian olfactory bulb it has been recently demonstrated that among the population of glomeruli some express enhanced neural activity when the olfactory mucosa is specifically stimulated (Orsini, Jourdan and Cooper, 1980).

The cellular organization and functioning

Primary receptor fibres entering the antennal lobe from the ipsilateral sensory parts of the antennal nerve lead to and terminate within the glomeruli which also receive the complex branching dendrites of the output deutoneurons and of the local interneurons.

The glomeruli contain all of the ultrastructurally identifiable chemical synapses in the antennal sensory brain (Masson, 1972, 1973, 1977; Tolbert and Hildebrand, 1981). Their synaptic organization representing the neuronal interactions is complex, involving several types of neuritic profiles and mediated by synapses with different ratios of pre- to post-synaptic elements. Presynaptic elements have been categorized into types containing round clear and dense-cored vesicles (Masson, 1972, 1973; Tolbert and Hildebrand, 1981).

Functional identification of deutoneurons both physiologically by means of extracellular (Waldow 1977; Boeckh and Boeckh, 1979) and intracellular recordings (Matsumoto and Hildebrand, 1981) and morphologically through combined cellular stainings lead to well correlated data. Two major classes of deutoneurons have been identified: local interneurons strictly confined to the deutocerebral neuropile, and output (or relay) deutoneurons projecting to the higher centres in the brain. Moreover, among these second order neurons, those that respond post-synaptically to female sex pheromone have their dendritic arborizations in the sexual area in the male sensory deutocerebrum (Matsumoto and Hildebrand, 1981).

In addition, it appears that the antennal afferent convergence on to the deutoneurons is spatial and multimodal, qualitative and quantitative. In terms of functioning this convergence is very useful, it works on the one hand to amplify the specific signals-to-noise ratio, and on the other hand to integrate as a whole the different parameters of a complex odorant which stimulates the peripheral sensilla (Masson, 1977; Selzer, 1981; Boeckh and Boeckh, 1979; Masson and Brossut, 1981).

One can summarize the different results briefly presented above by considering, firstly the functional organization of the olfactory neuroreceptors in the antennae, and secondly the functional organization of the sensory part (glomerular and cellular areas) of the deutocerebrum. As proposed in the scheme of Figure 3, two olfactory sub-systems exist in insects, one especially implicated in the processing of sex pheromonal messages, the other devoted to integrating the other

Figure 3. General diagram proposed for the morphofunctional organization of the afferent olfactory pathway of an insect. For the peripheral level (sensory neurons) involved in the detection of chemicals as well as for the first central relay (deutocerebrum) involved in the qualitative and/or quantitative integration of the complex natural odorants, two independent and complementary olfactory sub-systems seem to be identified.

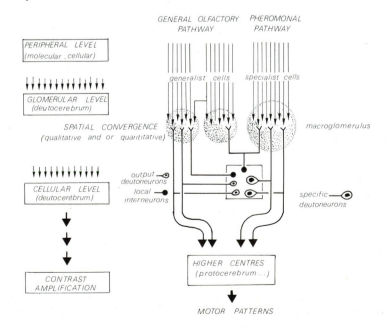

incoming information (as for example the complex naturally occurring stimuli such as food odours, host plant or oviposition locations...). We have proposed terming the two 'the specialist and generalist olfactory sub-systems' (Masson and Brossut, 1981).

References

Altner, H. (1977). Insect sensillum specificity and structure: an approach to a new typology. In *Int. Symp. Olfaction and Taste VI*, ed. J. Le Magnen and P. MacLeod, pp. 295–303. London: IRL.

Arnold, G., and Masson, C. (1983). Mise en place des connexions synaptiques de la voie afférente antennaire au cours du développement nymphal de l'ouvrière d'abeille *Apis mellifica. C. R. Acad. Sci. Paris D, 296:* 131–6.

Arnold, G., Masson, C., and Budharugsa, S. (1983). Organisation spatiale du système nerveux antennaire de l'abeille au moyen d'une technique de marquage aux ions cobalt. *Apidologie 14(2):* 127–35.

Boeckh, J. (1980). Neural basis of coding of chemosensory quality at the receptor level. In *Int. Symp. Olfaction and Taste VII*, ed. H. van der Starre, pp. 113–22. London: IRL.

Boeckh, J., Ernst, K. D., Sass H., and Waldow, U. (1976). Zur nervösen organisation antennaler Sinneseingänge bei Insekten unter besonderer Berücksichtigung der Riechbahn. *Verh. dt. zool. Ges.* 123–9.

Boeckh, J., Boeckh, V., and Kuhn, A. (1977). Further data on the topography and physiology of central olfactory neurons in insects. In *Int. Symp. Olfaction and Taste VI*, ed. J. Le Magnen and P. MacLeod, pp. 315–22. London: IRL.

Boeckh, J., and Boeckh, V. (1979). Threshold and odor specificity of pheromone-sensitive neurons in the deutocerebrum of *Antherea* sp. (Saturnidae). *J. Comp. Physiol. 132:* 235–42.

Chambille, I., Rospars, J. P., and Masson, C. (1980). The deutocerebrum of the cockroach *Blaberus craniifer*. Spatial organization of the sensory glomeruli. *J. Neurobiol. 11(2):* 135–57.

Chambille, I., and Rospars, J. P. (1981). Deutocerebron de la blatte *Blaberus craniifer:* étude qualitative et identification morphologique des glomérules. *Int. J. Insect Morphol. Embryol. 10(2):* 141–65.

Erber, J. (1981). Neural correlates of learning in the honeybee. *Trends Neurosci. 4(11):* 270–3.

Ernst, K. D. (1969). Die Feinstruktur von Riech Sensillen auf der Antenne des Auskäfers *Necrophorus* (Coleoptera). *Z. Zellforsch. mikrosk. Anat. 94(1):* 72–102.

Ernst, K. D., Boeckh, J., and Boeckh, V. (1977). A neuroanatomical study on the organization of the central antennal pathways in insects. *Cell Tiss. Res. 176:* 285–308.

Frisch, K. von (1967). *The Dance Language and Orientation of Bees*, ed. R. Chadwick. Harvard: Belknap Press.

Hildebrand, J., Matsumoto, S. G., Camazine, S. M., Tolbert, L. P., Blank, S., Ferguson, H., and Ecker, V. (1980). Organization and physiology of antennal centres in the brain of the moth *Manduca sexta*. In *Insect Neurobiology and Pesticide Action;* pp. 375–82. London: Society of Chemical Industry.

Holley, A., and MacLeod, P. (1977). Transduction et codage des informations olfactives chez les vertébrés. *J. Physiol., Paris 73:* 725–828.

Kaissling, K. E., and Thorson, J. (1980). Insect olfactory sensilla: structural, chemical and electrical aspects of the functional organization. In *Receptors for Neurotransmitters, Hormones and Pheromones in Insects,* ed. D. B. Satelle et al.; pp. 261–82. New York, London: Elsevier.

Klein, U. (1980). Investigations of proteins from isolated insect olfactory hairs. In *Olfaction and Taste VII,* ed. H. van der Starre, p. 89. London: IRL.

Masson, C. (1972). Le système antennaire chez les fourmis. I. Histologie et ultrastructure du deutocérébron. Etude comparée chez *Camponotus vagus* (Formicinae) et *Mesoponera caffraria* (Ponerinae). *Z. Zellforsch. mikrosk. Anat. 134:* 31–64.

Masson, C. (1973). Contribution à l'étude du système antennaire chez les fourmis. Approche morphologique, ultrastructurale et électrophysiologique. Thèse Doctorat d'Etat Marseille, pp. 1–332.

Masson, C. (1977). Central olfactory pathways and plasticity of responses to odorous stimuli. In *Int. Symp. Olfaction and Taste VI,* ed. J. Le Magnen and P. MacLeod, pp. 315–22. London: IRL.

Masson, C., and Friggi, A. (1974). Coding of information by the olfactory receptor cells of the antenna in *Camponotus vagus* (Hym. Formicidae). *J. Insect Physiol. 20(5):* 763–82.

Masson, C., and Strambi, C. (1977). Sensory antennal organization in an ant and a wasp. *J. Neurobiol. 8:* 537–48.

Masson, C., Kouprach, S., Giachetti, I., and MacLeod P. (1977). Relation between intramembraneous particle density of frog olfactory cilia and EOG responses. In *Olfaction and Taste VI,* ed. J. Le Magnen and P. MacLeod. London: IRL.

Masson, C., and MacLeod, P. (1978). Particules intramembranaires et fonction des cils olfactifs. *J. Physiol., Paris 74(4):* 9A.

Masson, C., and Brossut, R. (1981). La communication chimique chez les insectes. *La Recherche 121:* 406–16.

Matsumoto, S. G., and Hildebrand, J. (1981). Olfactory mechanisms in the moth *Manduca sexta:* response characteristics and morphology of central neurons in the antennal lobes. *R. Soc. Biol. 213:* 249–77.

Menco, B. Ph. M., and van der Wolk, F. M. (1982). Freeze fracture characteristics of insect gustatory and olfactory sensilla. *Cell Tiss. Res. 223:* 1–27.

Menzel, R., Erber, J., and Masuhr, T. (1974). Learning and memory in the honeybee. In *Experimental Analysis of Insect Behaviour,* ed. Barton Brown, pp. 195–217. Berlin, Heidelberg, New York: Springer-Verlag.

Norris, D. M. (1976). Physico-chemical aspects of the effects of certain phytochemicals on insect gustation. In *The Host-plant in Relation to Insect Behaviour and Reproduction,* vol. 16, ed. T. Jermy, pp. 197–201. New York: Plenum Publishing.

Orsini, J. C., Jourdan, F., and Cooper, H. M. (1980). Radioautographic 2-deoxyglucose patterns elicited by female odors in male rat olfactory bulb. In *Olfaction and Taste VII,* ed. H. van der Starre, pp. 323–6. London: IRL.

Ottoson, D. (1956). Analysis of the electrical activity of the olfactory epithelium. *Acta Physiol. Scand. 35,* Suppl. 122, 1–83.

Pfaffman, N. C. (1941). Gustatory afferent impulses. *J. Cell. Comp. Physiol. 17:* 243–58.

Pham, M. H., and Masson, C. (1983). Behavioural attraction thresholds and discrimination power among food scents: a study by associative conditioning in bee. (In preparation.)

Priesner, E. (1980). Sensory encoding of pheromone signals and related stimuli in male moths. In *Insect Neurobiology and Pesticide Action*, pp. 359–66. London: Society of Chemical Industry.

Prillinger L. (1981). Postembryonic development of the antennal lobes in *Periplaneta americana* L. *Cell Tiss. Res. 215:* 563–75.

Sass, H. (1978). Olfactory receptors on the antenna of *Periplaneta americana*. Response constellations that encode food odours. *J. Comp. Physiol. 128:* 227–33.

Schneider, D. (1957). Electrophysiological investigation on the receptors of the silk moth during chemical and mechanical stimulation. *Experientia 13:* 89–91.

Selzer, R. (1981). The processing of a complex food odor by antennal olfactory receptors of *Periplaneta americana*. *J. Comp. Physiol. 144:* 509–19.

Shepherd, G. M. (1972). Synaptic organization of the mammalian olfactory bulb. *Physiol. Rev. 52:* 864–917.

Tolbert, L. P., and Hildebrand, J. (1981). Organization and synaptic ultrastructure of glomeruli in the antennal lobes of the moth *Manduca sexta:* a study using thin sections and freeze fracture. *Proc. R. Soc. B213:* 279–301.

Vareschi, E. (1971). Odor discrimination in the honey bee. Single cell and behavioral responses. *Z. vergl. Physiol. 75:* 143–73.

Waldow, U. (1977). C.N.S. units in cockroach (*Periplaneta americana*): specificity of response to pheromones and other odor stimuli. *J. Comp. Physiol. 116:* 1–17.

2.3

*Olfaction and taste in fish**

JOHN CAPRIO

The most obvious difference between fishes and land vertebrates with respect to the chemical senses is in the stimulus-delivery medium, water and air respectively. Each medium selects for different physicochemical properties of molecules. Volatility is an essential characteristic only for olfactory stimuli of air-breathers, whereas water solubility of the stimulant material or adsorption onto suspended particulate matter is critical for both olfactory and gustatory stimuli in fishes. In both aquatic and terrestrial vertebrates, however, stimulus solubility in the mucus overlying the chemical receptors is necessary. Also, as a result of the aquatic medium, the gustatory sense of fishes is not limited to being a 'contact' sense, but may function additionally as a 'distance' sense due to its relatively high sensitivity to specific compounds.

This chapter will review the organization of the olfactory epithelium and taste bud structure and will provide an overview of salient physiological and behavioral studies to allow for a better understanding of the taste–smell distinctions in fishes. The physiological and behavioral studies presented will focus on the responses to amino acids, which have been identified as an important class of potent chemosensory stimuli in aquatic animals. Although amino acids are ubiquitous in nature, efficient uptake mechanisms, primarily of bacteria and algae, result in low and relatively constant levels ($\leqslant 10^{-7}$ M) of dissolved free amino acids in the water column (Gardner and Lee, 1975). This diminishes the effects of olfactory and gustatory receptor adaptation and provides further evidence that amino acids may serve as excellent water-soluble signal molecules in fishes.

---

* Dedicated to the memory of Dr Don Tucker.

The emphasis placed on amino acids is not to be construed that these compounds are the only significant chemical stimuli to fishes, but only that over the past decade a body of consistent electrophysiological, biochemical and behavioral data has been accruing concerning these stimuli. Other compounds recently indicated as possibly being important stimuli to fishes include bile acids (Selset and Døving, 1980; Døving, Selset and Thommesen, 1980; Hara, Marui and Evans, personal communication) and nucleotides (Mackie and Adron, 1978; Hidaka, Kiyohara and Oda, 1977).

Receptor anatomy
Olfactory
Anatomically, olfactory receptors of all vertebrates are bipolar, primary neurons which send their axonal process to the central nervous system to synapse with mitral cell dendrites within the olfactory bulb. In teleost fishes, both ciliated and microvillous olfactory receptors have been identified and may occur in the same species (Zeiske, Melinkat, Breucker and Kux, 1976; Ichikawa and Ueda, 1977; Yamamoto and Ueda, 1977; Cancalon, 1978); however, only microvillous receptors occur in the olfactory mucosa of the chondrichthyes (Pevzner, 1976). It is in the membrane of the terminal of the receptors and cilia or microvilli where acceptor molecules for olfactory stimuli are assumed to exist.

Olfactory receptor density is quite variable and has been reported by researchers studying different species of fishes to be between 46 000 and 500 000 mm^{-2} (Teichman, 1954; Zeiske et al., 1976; Yamamoto, 1982). The total number of unmyelinated axons (individual diameter, 0.14–0.20 μm) present in a single olfactory nerve of a fish is between 4.2×10^4 and 1.3×10^7 (Gemne and Døving, 1969; Easton, 1971; Kreutzberg and Gross, 1977; Yamamoto, 1982). Cell types other than receptors which have been reported in the olfactory epithelium of fishes include supporting, basal, rod and goblet cells. The goblet cells, which may be distributed in both the sensory and indifferent (non-sensory) epithelia (Schulte, 1972; Bertmar, 1973) or occur only within the indifferent epithelium, along with the supporting cells produce the mucus that covers the olfactory epithelium (Kleerekoper, 1969; Zeiske et al., 1976); this mucous sheet, however, is thinner (Yamamoto, 1982) than that produced in the tetrapods primarily by the subepithelial Bowman's glands, which are lacking in fishes.

The supporting cells, which contain, depending on the species, microvillous and/or ciliated surfaces, also serve to separate the receptor cells (Kleerekoper, 1969; Yamamoto, 1982). Basal cells, progenitor cells of olfactory neurons, differentiate into olfactory receptors during normal receptor turnover or in response to olfactory receptor injury (Holl, 1965; Graziadei and Metcalf, 1971; Moulton, 1975). Rod cells, once thought to be a third receptor cell type (Schulte, 1972; Breipohl, Bijvank and Zippel, 1973) do not undergo retrograde degeneration when the olfactory nerve is transected (Ichikawa and Ueda, 1977) and may not be primary receptors. A recent study indicates that the rod cells observed in the olfactory mucosa of the brown trout were in fact artifacts of conventional aldehyde fixation and could be eliminated by pretreatment of the tissue with osmium (Rowley and Moran, personal communication).

Considerable variation occurs among teleosts in the organization of the olfactory mucosa within the olfactory organ. The olfactory organs consist generally of a pair of blind pits, containing both an incurrent (anterior) and excurrent naris, on the dorsal side of the head (Burne, 1909). In the majority of fishes studied the floor of the nasal cavity is formed into a series of folds, the olfactory lamellae (rosette), in which the sensory epithelium resides. In some species, lamellae do not occur and the sensory and indifferent epithelia are distributed on the relatively flat floor of the organ (Zeiske et al., 1976). The arrangement and number of olfactory lamellae/capsule vary widely (Burne, 1909; Kleerekoper, 1969; Yamamoto and Ueda, 1979). In addition, the organization of sensory and indifferent epithelia within each lamella is variable and has been categorized into three to four types of distribution patterns ranging from a continuous sensory epithelium covering the majority of the lamella to a dispersion of small islets (Burne, 1909; Yamamoto and Ueda, 1979). The indifferent epithelium is characterized by columnar, non-sensory cells with flat and relatively wide free surfaces containing a dense mat of thick cilia (Cancalon, 1978; Caprio and Raderman-Little, 1978; Yamamoto, 1982). In fish with large olfactory rosettes, the action of cilia creates the water current through the organ (isosmates), whereas in other fishes (cyclosmates) the compression and extension of accessory sacs create the water flow (Burne, 1909; Døving, Dubois-Dauphin, Holley and Jourdan, 1977). Each lamella is composed of two layers of epithelium enclosing a thin stromal layer, within which the olfactory receptor axons course towards the olfactory bulb (Caprio and Raderman-Little, 1978; Yamamoto, 1982).

Taste

Taste buds were first discovered in fish by Weber in 1827 (see Herrick, 1901, for a historical review). Generally, taste buds of fishes vary between 30 and 80 μm in length and 20 and 50 μm in width (Hirata, 1966; Crisp, Lowe and Laverack, 1975; Grover-Johnson and Farbman, 1976; Kiyohara, Yamashita and Kitoh, 1980) and contain on the order of 100–150 cells/taste bud (Crisp et al., 1975; Grover-Johnson and Farbman, 1976). Within the taste bud of fishes, generally two types of microvillous cells of ectodermal origin, light and dark (terms based on light-microscopic descriptions of taste buds after formaldehyde fixation), have been described along with the neuroectodermal basal cells (Hirata, 1966; Grover-Johnson and Farbman, 1976; Reutter, 1978). A somewhat similar pattern is repeated in mammals (Farbman, 1965, 1980; Takeda and Hoshino, 1975; Toyoshima and Shimamura, 1981). A clear distinction of which cell type constitutes the receptor is lacking due to the difficulty of identifying synaptic contacts within taste cells. This problem is not peculiar to fish taste buds, as this is a recurring question in mammalian taste bud anatomy. The light cell, interpreted generally as the receptor cell, terminates at the surface in a large (1.5–3 μm) club-shaped microvillus. The dark cell, considered by most investigators to be a supporting cell, contains numerous, small (0.5–1.0 μm) microvilli and encloses the light cell with lobed processes in the distal regions of the taste bud (Hirata, 1966; Crisp et al., 1975; Grover-Johnson and Farbman, 1976; Reutter, 1978). However, taste receptors of elasmobranchs contain 3 to 12 microvilli (Pevzner, 1966). In fish, generally taste pores are lacking and only a thin mucous layer overlays the taste buds. This apparently allows the large microvilli receptor processes of the light cells to penetrate the mucus as SEM observations of freeze-dried specimens indicate (Reutter, 1980). Thus, taste substances may have more direct access to receptor membranes of fish than those of mammals, which are submerged in an apical pore filled with a mucous barrier (Murray, 1973; Takeda and Hoshino, 1975). In both fish (Raderman-Little, 1979) and mammals (Beidler and Smallman, 1965; Farbman, 1980), light and dark cells undergo renewal from post-mitotic daughter cells of epithelial cells surrounding the taste bud. The time course for taste cell renewal (time at which 50% of labeled cells have degenerated) in the catfish at 30°C and rats and mice at 37°C is remarkably similar, taking 10–12 days (Raderman-Little, 1979).

The basal cells which number 2–5/taste bud are located at the base of the bud resting against the basal lamina (Grover-Johnson and Farbman, 1976; Reutter, 1978). Although distinct classical synapses are relatively scarce in vertebrate taste buds, presumed chemical synapses are indicated in catfish between light cells (presynaptic) and afferent nerve processes and basal cells; in turn, basal cells are thought to form synaptic connections with the afferent nerve fibers (Hirata, 1966;

Grover-Johnson and Farbman, 1976; Reutter, 1982). The report (Reutter, 1978) that indicated dark cells also form synaptic connections to both basal cells and afferent nerve terminals in the brown bullhead catfish (*Ictalurus nebulosus*) is the basis to consider the possibility of the dark cell as a second receptor cell type. This, however, was not confirmed in the channel catfish (*Ictalurus punctatus*), as no synapses were found at the basal processes of the dark cells (Grover-Johnson and Farbman, 1976). The basal cell, because of its critical location and synaptic connections, has been proposed to function as a modifier of gustatory receptor activity; also, due to the mechanical responsiveness of peripheral gustatory fibers, the basal cell may possibly function as a mechanoreceptor, similar to Merkel cells (Reutter, 1980, 1982). Although there is recurring speculation concerning efferent connections on to vertebrate taste cells (Paran, Mattern and Henkin, 1975; Outwater and Oakley, 1981), presently there is only agreement for the existence of afferent synapses.

Vertebrate taste cells, secondary receptor cells, are innervated by facial (VII), glossopharyngeal (IX) or vagal (X) nerves. In tetrapods the taste-receptive fields of all these cranial nerves are localized within the oral-pharyngeal cavity. In certain species of fishes, the quantity and distribution of taste buds have increased and the facially innervated extraoral taste buds are found on lips, head, barbels, fins and flank (Herrick, 1901; Atema, 1971; Kiyohara et al., 1980). Facially innervated taste buds also occur within the oral cavity, but are limited to the anterior palate. The glossopharyngeal and vagal nerves innervate only oro-pharyngeal taste buds found on the 'tongue', gill arches, palatal organ and esophagus. Both oral and extra-oral taste bud densities have been estimated as upwards to >130 taste buds mm^{-2} (Kiyohara, Yamashito and Harada, 1981). In some species, such as the Japanese minnow (*Pseudorasbora parva*), the majority (86%) of taste buds are present within the oral cavity (Kiyohara et al., 1980), whereas in other species, the brown bullhead catfish, the extra-oral taste buds predominate (90%) (Atema, 1971). This increase in the number of extra-oral taste buds is thought not to result directly in a sensitivity increase, but in a greater ability of the fish to localize a food source (Bardach, Todd and Crickmer, 1967; Johnsen and Teeter, 1980).

Receptor mechanisms

Introduction

The initial response of an olfactory or taste receptor to a chemical stimulus that is absorbed to a membrane receptor site is a graded depolarization (generally) or hyperpolarization. Both the receptor potential and neural spike activity occur within the olfactory receptor, a primary neuron. Taste cells, however, are secondary sensory receptors in which the receptor potential presumably modulates chemical activity at the synapse between the taste cell and its afferent nerve.

Olfactory receptor

Due to the small size of olfactory receptor cell soma and general mechanical instability of the olfactory lamellae containing the receptors, only a single report exists of intracellular recordings from fish olfactory receptors (Suzuki, 1977; also reviewed in Suzuki, 1982). In this preparation from the lamprey (*Entosphenus japonicus*), the resting membrane potential of olfactory neurons ranged from -37 mV to -60 mV with an input resistance of 75–360 MΩ and membrane time constants averaging 3.5 ms and 0.34 ms. In response to certain olfactory stimuli (10^{-2} M L-arginine), the receptor depolarization, on which spike potentials were superimposed, was accompanied by a decrease in resistance, indicating membrane permeability changes to some ion(s). With other stimuli (10^{-2} M L-glutamic acid), the olfactory receptor hyperpolarized and input resistance increased. Although the reversal potential for the depolarizing response was near zero suggesting that one or more ions carry the generator current, alteration of Na^+, K^+ and Ca^{2+} ion concentration up to 10 mM bathing the olfactory mucosa did not affect significantly the receptor resting potential.

Additional information on olfactory receptor mechanisms comes from the only single-unit recordings obtained from the olfactory receptors of fish (Suzuki, 1978). Single-unit olfactory receptor recordings in fishes have been difficult to obtain due to the instability of the olfactory lamellae mentioned previously and the dense packing of olfactory neurons within the mucosa, making it difficult to resolve individual units clearly. Suzuki (1978) showed that although Na^+ and K^+ ion concentration over the olfactory mucosa of the lamprey had no significant effect on the neural response to L-arginine, the responses were blocked by bathing the receptor surface in a Ca-free solution containing a Ca-chelating agent, such as EGTA. Ca^{2+} and La^{2+} ions in a calcium-free solution bathing the receptors also suppressed the receptor response presumably by binding to membrane receptor sites for Ca^{2+}.

Whether calcium ions serve as the current carrier through the apical membrane of the olfactory receptor is not yet clear as voltage clamp experiments have not been performed. Suzuki (1978, 1982) indicated that the olfactory receptor is capable of functioning even after prolonged bathing of the epithelial surface with deionized water. If it is assumed that the deionized bathing solution prevents the mucus over-lying the receptors from maintaining sufficient ion concentration, then it may be questionable to assume a permeability change to calcium or other ions in the apical olfactory receptor membrane (Suzuki, 1982). Additional data by Suzuki (1980, 1982) indicated that specific binding of labeled L-arginine to lamprey olfactory tissue increased with an increase in Ca^{2+} concentrations over the olfactory epithelial surface between 10^{-7} and 10^{-4} M and decreased at higher Ca^{2+} concentrations. These results suggest that calcium ions act as modifiers of the receptor membrane activity rather than current carriers for receptor depolariza-tion. Thus, the apical membrane of the olfactory receptor may not be involved directly in membrane permeability changes for ions responsi-ble for the receptor depolarization (Suzuki, 1982). The hypothetical model proposed by Suzuki (1982) for the olfactory transduction process assumes functionally and spatially separate receptor membrane zones for stimulus binding on the apical olfactory receptor membrane and electrogenic membrane zones for ionic permeability changes in the dendrite membrane below the apical knob. The coupling between stimulus binding and permeability changes is hypothesized to be en-zymatic in nature.

Taste receptor

Only a single study exists concerning intracellular taste record-ings from fish (Teeter, 1974). The resting membrane potential of 189 presumed taste cells of the brown bullhead catfish averaged -26 mv, whereas input resistance measured in 61 cells averaged 42 MΩ. The membrane time constant estimated from 18 cells was 22 ms. An interesting aspect of the work was that non-taste epithelial cells were also tested for the previously listed membrane parameters and were shown not to be significantly different from those determined for the taste cells. These results suggest that in the catfish both taste and non-taste epithelial cells possess similar ionic mechanisms for respond-ing to taste stimuli (salt, acid, amino acid). Both taste and non-taste cells had linear current–voltage relations, indicating that these cell membranes behave in an ohmic manner. The majority of cells re-sponded to taste stimuli with a depolarization and decreased membrane resistance, although NaCl at less than 1 mM and distilled water evoked a hyperpolarization and increased resistance. The reversal potential for salts ranged from $+4$ mV to $+53$ mV, indicating that in the taste cell, as in the olfactory receptor, there are ionic current carriers, possibly Na^+ for the depolarizing response. However, as hypothesized for the olfac-

Table 1. Olfactory concentration series

Species	Electrophysiological method[a]	Stimulus[b]	Threshold (10^x M)	Highest conc. tested (10^x M)	Saturation[c] (10^x M)	Dose-response function (γ)[d]	References
(A) Olfactory receptors							
Atlantic salmon, *Salmo salar*	MNR	L-Ala	-9	-3	NS	L (~5)	Sutterlin and Sutterlin, 1971
		L-Thr	-6				
White catfish, *Ictalurus catus*	MNR	L-Gln, L-Met	-7 to -8	-2	NS	P (5)	Suzuki and Tucker, 1971; Caprio, 1980
		L-Ala, L-Asn					
Channel catfish, *Ictalurus punctatus*	MNR	L-Cysh, L-Ala	-8 to -9	-2	NS	P (8–11)	Caprio, 1978
	EOG	L-Cysh, L-Met, L-nLeu, L-Ala	-8 to -10	-2	NS to ≥ -2	P (4–5)	Byrd and Caprio, 1982
Spotted bullhead,							
Ictalurus serrancanthus	EOG	L-Cysh	-8	-2	NS	P (5)	Caprio, 1980
Sea catfish, *Arius felis*	EOG	L-Cysh	-8	-2	NS	P (4–5)	Caprio, 1980
Eel, *Anguilla rostrata*	MNR	L-Gln	-8	-2	NS	P (6.5)	Silver, 1979a
	EOG	L-Gln	-7.8	-2		P (5.3)	
	NTR	L-Gln	-9.6	-2		P (10.3)	
Atlantic Stingray, *Dasyatis sabina*	EOG	L-Ala	-7.8	-3	NS	P (2.7)	Silver, 1979b
		L-Met	-7.4	-3		P (3.7)	
Lamprey, *Entosphenus japonicus*	intracell; unit extracell	L-Arg	-5 to -7	-2	NS	P (~4)	Suzuki, 1977, 1978
Hagfish, *Myxine glutinosa*	EOG	L-Ala, L-Gln	-5 to -6	-3	NS	P (~2)	Døving and Holmberg, 1974

(B) Olfactory bulb

Channel catfish, *Ictalurus punctatus*	EEG	L-Cysh, L-Met, L-nLeu, L-Ala	−8 to −10	−2	−2	P (8.2–11.8)	Byrd and Caprio, 1982
Rainbow trout, *Salmo gairdneri*	EEG	L-Ser, L-Cysh,	−7 to −8	−3	≥−3	P (~4–5);S	Hara, 1975, 1982
		L-Gln	−7 to −8	−3	NS	P (~3)	
Brook trout, *Salvelinus fontinalis*	EEG	L-Ser	−7 to −8	−4	−4	P (~3)	Hara et al., 1973
Whitefish, *Coregonus clupeaformis*	EEG	L-Ser	−6 to −7	−4	−4	P (2)	Hara et al., 1973
Red Sea bream, *Chrysophrys major*	EEG	L-Gln	−7	−2	−3	P	Goh et al., 1979; Goh and Tamura, 1980a
Conger eel, *Conger myriaster*	integrated multiunit	L-Gln	−6 to −9	−2	−3	—	Goh et al., 1979
Char, *Salmo alpinus*	EEG	L-Asn, L-Met, L-Gln, L-Ala	−7 to −8	−4	NS	—	Belghaug and Døving, 1977
Mullet, *Mugil cephalus*	EEG	L-Gln	−7	−2	−3	—	Goh and Tamura, 1980a,b

(C) Olfactory tract

Carp, *Cyprinus carpio*	LTR	L-Gln	−6	−2	NS	P	Goh and Tamura, 1978

[a] MNR, Mucosal neural response; EOG, electro-olfactogram; NTR, nerve twig response; EEG, electroencephalogram; LTR, lateral olfactory tract recording.

[b] The compounds used to determine dose-response characteristics were not always the most stimulatory amino acids.

[c] Concentration of stimulus where saturation of response becomes evident, NS, no saturation evident.

[d] Mathematical function that best describes the dose-response data; P, power; L, logarithmic; S, sigmoid; γ, number of log units of stimulus concentration theoretically necessary to produce a one-log-unit change in response magnitude; ~, approximate values not reported, but estimated from published records.

tory receptor, ions are thought not to diffuse into the taste cell through the receptor microvillous membrane (Sato, 1980). Thus, separate sites may also exist in the taste cell membrane for binding taste stimuli (the microvillar membrane surface) and for initiating permeability changes (the taste cell membrane below the apical tight junction). The question of how these different membranes are coupled by additional receptor events, be it electrical, chemical or physical in nature, is currently unknown.

Amino acid chemoreception

Introduction

Olfactory receptors in a wide variety of fishes were shown electrophysiologically to be highly sensitive to amino acids. Thresholds for the more sensitive preparations ranged from between 10^{-7} and 10^{-10} M (Table 1). The results confirmed earlier experimental results implicating the olfactory sense as a 'distance' sense, capable of alerting the fish to minute quantities of food-related or possibly socially-related compounds in the water column (Sheldon, 1909; Parker and Sheldon, 1912; Olmsted, 1918). Although earlier work on the taste sense of fishes indicated that amino acids were stimulatory taste compounds (Bardach and Case, 1965; Fujiya and Bardach, 1966; Bardach et al., 1967), the gustatory sense of fishes was still generally recognized as a 'contact' sense having relatively low sensitivity to the classical taste compounds (NaCl, sucrose, quinine and HCl), much like the gustatory sense of the terrestrial vertebrates. Sutterlin and Sutterlin's (1970) electrophysiological work on the taste sense of the Atlantic salmon (*Salmo salar*) appeared to confirm the idea of the taste system being far less sensitive than olfaction even in a fish. Where the olfactory receptors of the Atlantic salmon were highly excited by amino acids at low concentration, the gustatory sense was generally insensitive to these compounds. It was not until taste responses to extremely dilute concentrations of amino acids (10^{-9}–10^{-11} M) were obtained from the channel catfish (Caprio, 1975), the same genus for which Bardach and colleagues had presented preliminary evidence of amino acid taste acuity, that a resurgence of effort into fish taste physiology began. Concurrent with the report in the catfish, the lip taste system of the Japanese puffer (*Fugu pardalis*), although not as sensitive as the catfish, was also shown to respond to amino acid stimuli (Kiyohara, Hidaka and Tamura, 1975; Hidaka, Nyu and Kiyohara, 1976). Recently, the taste sensitivities of the Japanese eel (*Anguilla japonica*; Yoshii, Kamo, Kurihara and Kobataki, 1979) and minnow (*Pseudorasbora parva*; Kiyohara et al.,

1981) were shown to parallel that of the catfish. Other species showing relatively high taste sensitivity to amino acids include the Japanese sea bream (*Chrysophrys major*), mullet (*Mugil cephalas*; Goh and Tamura, 1980a), rainbow trout (*Salmo gairdneri*; Hara and Marui, personal communication) and carp (*Cyprinus carpio*; Marui, personal communication) (Table 2). As the eel, sea bream, mullet and rainbow trout indicate, the presence of a large number of extraoral taste buds as found in ictalurid catfish (Atema, 1971) and minnow (Kiyohara et al., 1980) is not a prerequisite for high taste sensitivity to amino acids.

Recording methods and dose-response functions

Olfactory receptor responses in fishes (Table 1) are generally exponential functions of the logarithm of amino acid stimulus concentration. The electrophysiological threshold is determined by extrapolating a double-log plot of response versus stimulus concentration to the control level. When the data are plotted with log–log coordinates and fitted with a straight line, the slope is γ^{-1}. Thus, γ is the number of log units of stimulus concentration necessary to produce a one-log-unit change in response magnitude. From the values listed in Table 1, olfactory receptors of the majority of fishes tested are capable of responding to a 100 000- to million-fold change in amino acid stimulus concentrations. The linear relation between the log of the stimulus concentration and the log response over such a wide concentration range may be explained either by amino acid binding to several populations of receptor sites each with different binding constants or as the result of negative cooperativity between receptor sites (Yoshii et al., 1979; Caprio, 1982).

Electro-olfactogram (EOG), mucosal neural (NR) and olfactory nerve twig (NTR) responses are obtained from recording olfactory receptor activity from within the olfactory capsule proper (Silver, 1979a, Table 1). The EOG is a slow (d.c.) potential change recorded in the water above the surface of the olfactory mucosa with non-polarizable electrodes in response to chemical stimulation (Silver, Caprio, Blackwell and Tucker, 1976). It is thought to consist primarily of the population average of receptor potentials responsible for the initiation of the neural impulses (Ottoson, 1971; Getchell, 1974). The MNR is obtained by contacting metal-filled glass capillary electrodes tip-plated with platinum black (Gesteland, Howland, Lettvin and Pitts, 1959) with the surface of the sensory region of an olfactory lamella; the resulting neural activity is then integrated. The NTR is obtained by recording olfactory receptor neural activity at some distance from the olfactory capsule. This multiunit activity recorded from dissected bundles of olfactory nerve axons with bipolar metal hook electrodes is then integrated.

Induced waves from the olfactory bulb (EEG), thought to arise from the excitatory–inhibitory dendrodendritic interactions between mitral and granule cells, have been described in salmonids as being typical sigmoidal response functions of log stimulus concentration (Hara, 1982). However, published dose-response curves (Hara, Law and Hobden, 1973; Hara, 1982) indicate that for the more highly stimulatory amino acids, the integrated EEG response rises exponentially with logarithmic increase in stimulus concentration until approximately 10^{-4}–10^{-3} M, similar to both EEG recordings in channel catfish (Byrd and Caprio, 1982) and American eel (Silver, 1979a) and receptor responses listed above. Similarly, integrated neural recordings from the olfactory tract of the carp (*Cyprinus carpio*) rose exponentially as a function of log stimulus concentration (Goh and Tamura, 1978).

Dose-response functions in fish taste to amino acids are best described by power (catfish, minnow, rainbow trout), logarithmic (eel, sea bream) or sigmoid (rainbow trout) functions depending on the species and amino acid tested (Table 2). However, in catfish (Caprio, 1978), minnow (Kiyohara et al., 1981) and eel (Yoshii et al., 1979) taste, the dose-response functions for different amino acids of varying stimulating efficacy are shifted approximately in parallel along the concentration axis. This same relationship is indicated for olfactory responses in catfish (Caprio, 1978), eel (Silver, 1979a), and hagfish (Døving and Holmberg, 1974); interestingly this was also shown for amino acid responses of dactyl receptors of the crayfish (*Orconectes limosus*), a freshwater crustacean (Bauer, Dudel and Hatt, 1981). Therefore, thresholds could be deduced by geometry from responses to different amino acid stimuli tested at a single concentration. This, in fact, was indicated for olfactory bulbar responses (EEG) in the char (*Salmo alpinus*), where a high correlation between the ranking of the olfactory stimuli obtained by threshold determinations and by measuring the size of the responses to the same compounds applied at 10^{-4} M (Belghaug and Døving, 1977). This relationship among dose-response curves gives credence to the reports comparing the relative stimulatory effectiveness of amino acid stimuli tested at a single concentration.

The question of whether olfactory or taste differences observed within Tables 1–3 were due to differences in the respective responses at various anatomical levels, to the heterogeneity of the recording techniques, or to real species or system differences needs to be addressed. Although a

Table 2. Gustatory concentration series

Species	Stimulus	Threshold (10^X M)	Highest conc. tested (10^X M)	Saturation[a] (10^X M)	Dose-response[b] function (γ)	Reference(s)
(A) Taste (VII)[c]						
Catfish, *Ictalurus punctatus*						
barbel nerve	L-Ala, L-Arg	−9 to −11	−2	≥−2	P (5.3)	Caprio, 1978, 1982
recurrent nerve	L-Ala, L-Arg	−8 to −9	−3	≥−4	P (6.9)	Davenport and Caprio, 1982
Puffer, *Fugu pardalis*	Gly	−5 to −6	−2	NS	P (~3)	Hidaka et al., 1976
	L-Pro, betaine	−5	−2	NS	P (~3)	Hidaka, 1982
	L-Ala	−4	−2	NS	P (~3)	
Eel, *Anguilla japonica*	Gly, L-Ala, L-Arg	−8 to −9	−2	NS	L (~4)	Yoshii et al., 1979
Minnow, *Pseudorasbora parva*	L-Pro	−10 to −11	−1	−5	P (5.9)	Kiyohara et al., 1981
	L-Ala	−9 to −10	−1	−3	P (8.3)	
	L-Ser	−8 to −9	−1	NS	P (8.3)	
Red sea bream, *Chrysophrys major*	L-Ala	−6	−2	NS	L (~4)	Goh and Tamura, 1980a
Mullet, *Mugil cephalus*	L-Ala	−6	−2	NS	P (~5)	Goh and Tamura, 1980a
Rainbow trout, *Salmo gairdneri*	L-Pro	−7 to −8	−2	variable	—	Hara and Marui, personal communication
	L-Hypro	−6				
Carp, *Cyprinus carpio*	L-Pro, L-Ala, L-Ser	−6 to −7	−2	≥−2	—	Marui, personal communication
(B) Taste (IX–X)[d]						
Catfish, *Ictalurus punctatus*	L-Ala, L-Arg	−5.5 to −7.5	−1	−3 to >−1	P (5.0)	Kanwal and Caprio, 1983
	L-Pro	−4.5 to −5.5	−1	NS	P (3.2)	

[a] Concentration of stimulus where saturation of response becomes evident; NS, no saturation evident.
[b] Mathematical function that best describes the dose-response data; P, power; L, logarithmic; γ, number of log units of stimulus concentration theoretically necessary to produce a one-log-unit change in response magnitude, is in parentheses; ~, approximate values not reported, but estimated from published records.
[c],[d] Integrated multiunit recordings from teased bundles of facial (c) and glossopharyngeal and vagal (d) nerves.

variety of multiunit techniques were used in the olfactory research, a high correlation has been indicated between some of the various methods applied in the same species. For threshold estimates and chemospecificity rankings, there were no significant differences in the MNR and EOG responses recorded in the channel catfish (Caprio, 1978) and American eel (*Anguilla rostrata*) (Silver, 1979a). Similarly, for chemospecificity measurements, the olfactory capsule recording techniques (EOG and MNR) and NTR were significantly correlated; there was, however, a lowering of the electrophysiological threshold estimated from NTR by 1.5 log units (Silver, 1979a), which is relatively minor considering the multi-log unit responding range of fish olfactory receptors (Table 1). Further, olfactory receptor EOG and bulbar EEG activity were similar in both threshold and chemospecificity measurements in the catfish (Byrd and Caprio, 1982). All taste recordings listed in Table 2 were integrated responses from peripheral nerve in *in vivo* preparations. Thus, the data indicate that any differences observed in Tables 1 and 2 or in the succeeding section (Table 3) on the chemospecificity of olfactory and gustatory responses, respectively, are most likely due to species rather than experimental differences.

Structure-activity relations

An advantage of olfactory and gustatory receptors of fish being highly responsive to amino acids is that a multitude of amino acids, analogs and derivatives are commercially available in relatively high purity that allows for the determination of the molecular characteristics required for stimulatory effectiveness. Extensive structure-activity studies were performed on olfactory and gustatory receptors in the channel catfish (Caprio, 1978) and olfactory receptors in rainbow trout (Hara, 1977, 1982). For both olfaction and taste in these and other studies listed in Tables 1–3, the L-isomer of an amino acid was more effective than its enantiomer, indicating that the receptors involved possessed a corresponding chirality. Further, amino acids with an amino group in the alpha position (i.e., those derived from proteins) were the more stimulatory forms; a single exception to this finding occurs for palatal taste responses in Japanese eel, where there was no appreciable difference in the effectiveness of α- and β-alanine (Yoshii et al., 1979).

Alterations of the α-amino or α-hydrogen or amide substitution at the primary carboxyl group of an amino acid, including peptide bond formation or replacement of the carboxylic group with alcoholic or sulfonic groups resulted in compounds that were relatively poor olfactory and gustatory stimuli. Peptides were less stimulatory than the most effective amino acid residue in the molecule (Hara, 1977; Caprio, 1978; Silver, 1979a; Kiyohara et al., 1981). However, primary esters of certain amino acids produced varying results depending on the system and species tested. In the Japanese minnow (Kiyohara et al., 1981), L-alanine methyl and ethyl esters were more stimulatory taste stimuli than L-alanine, while for olfactory receptors of the eel (Silver, 1979a), alanine esters were just as stimulatory as the free amino acid; for certain other amino acid esters in catfish olfaction (Caprio, 1978) and all amino acid esters tested at $<10^{-4}$M in the rainbow trout olfactory system (Hara, 1977, 1982), esters were generally less stimulatory than their parent compound. Thus, amino acid receptor sites may involve at least one anionic charged subsite to bind with the ionized amino group of an amino acid, whereas a cationic charged subsite may be essential for certain stimuli; this latter subsite would not be required for receptors that bind esterified amino acids. An additional membrane subsite is assumed to interact with the amino acid side chain, and, depending on the molecular constituents and configuration of this subsite, different olfactory and gustatory receptor specificities would result.

Taste–smell distinctions

One of the more important findings of the last decade in fish chemoreception research is that although olfactory and gustatory receptors in a particular species are both highly sensitive to amino acid stimuli, neither system is redundant, as the population of receptors in each system is 'tuned' maximally to a different portion of the amino acid spectrum (Table 3). For example, olfactory receptors of the channel catfish are highly responsive to cysteine and methionine, whereas taste receptors respond best to alanine and arginine (Caprio, 1977, 1978). The finding of different amino acid chemospecificities between olfaction and taste is supported by subsequent electrophysiological evidence obtained from red sea bream, mullet (Goh and Tamura, 1980a) and rainbow trout (Hara, 1973; Hara and Marui, personal communication). It is important to emphasize, however, that the above data were obtained primarily from multiunit recordings and are only indicative of the responsiveness of the entire population of receptor cells that are stimulated by a particular amino acid. This does not negate the probability that olfactory and gustatory receptor cells exist that have a somewhat different specificity than that indicated from the population response.

Although olfactory and gustatory specificities of an individual species for amino acids are different, the variability of respective olfactory and gustatory specificities across species needs to be considered. Are profound species-specific differences clearly evident or do the data indicate a high degree of similarity across species? A recent hypothesis is that the olfactory spectrum of amino acids among different fishes is similar, whereas the taste spectrum is species specific and related directly to different feeding substances among the different species; olfaction is hypothesized to have a general species non-specific chemoreceptive function (Goh, Tamura and Kobayashi, 1979; Goh and Tamura, 1980a). Supportive evidence exists for olfactory responses to amino acids being generally non-specific across salmonids (Hara et al., 1973; Belghaug and Døving, 1977; Goh and Tamura, 1980a). For the salmonids and the majority of other fishes tested (Table 1 references), unsubstituted L-α-amino acids and derivatives containing 3–6 carbons and consisting of linear, unbranched and uncharged side chains (e.g. methionine, ethionine, glutamine, norvaline, norleucine, alanine, serine, cysteine; not all compounds were tested on each species) were highly effective stimuli. Basic and acidic amino acids were not stimulatory except in the carp (*Cyprinus carpio*; Goh and Tamura, 1978) where they were highly effective compounds. In the majority of the studies, the pH levels of the solutions of acidic and basic amino acids were adjusted as a control to that of the neutral amino acid solutions; however, for the carp this was not indicated and the large responses to glutamic acid and lysine might possibly be compounded by a pH effect. The imino acids, proline and hydroxyproline, were exceptionally poor olfactory stimuli in all species studied. Thus, although species specificities exist, the present evidence supports the hypothesis that olfactory responses to amino acids are generally similar across freshwater and marine fishes and that the population of olfactory receptors in general are 'tuned' primarily to the neutral portion of the amino acid spectrum.

Electrophysiological recordings from the taste system of fishes do not support the contention (Goh et al., 1979; Goh and Tamura, 1980a) that the amino acid spectrum is highly species specific across closely related genera. Recent comparisons between the gustatory specificities of the channel (*Ictalurus punctatus*) and bullhead (*Ictalurus natalis*) catfishes, thought to be the most typical example of gustatory species specificity (Goh et al., 1979), are highly similar (Caprio, 1982; unpublished). Taste recordings from four species of bullheads and the channel catfish indicate that all ictalurid catfishes tested were stimulated best by L-alanine and L-arginine and that the taste responses were described by similar dose-response functions; amino acids that were relatively poor taste stimuli in one species were also poor stimuli in the other catfish species (Caprio, unpublished). Currently, only nine species of fishes (not including the bullhead catfishes) have been systematically tested electrophysiologically for taste responses to amino acids. In eight of these species (Table 2), amino acid taste sensitivity was identified. In the only exception, the Atlantic salmon, a general insensitivity to these compounds was reported (Sutterlin and Sutterlin, 1970). An analysis of the stimulatory amino acids indicates a general pattern of taste specificity across species. The taste systems of the majority of fishes tested responded best to 2–3 carbon, neutral amino acids (glycine, alanine, serine), basic (arginine and/or lysine) amino acids and an imino acid (proline). Electrophysiological cross-adaptation (competition) studies in the channel catfish indicated relatively independent receptor mechanisms for imino, basic and neutral amino acids, respectively (Kanwal and Caprio, 1983; Caprio, 1982; Davenport and Caprio, 1982). In addition, enzymatic treatment with papain and pronase E of palatine taste buds in the Japanese eel provided further evidence for the independence of the proline receptor (Yoshii et al., 1979). Thus, taste recordings in a number of species (catfish, eel, minnow, sea bream and mullet; Tables 2 and 3) indicate at least three 'types' of amino acid taste receptor sites present. However, species specificities can still occur, for in two species, puffer and carp, the basic system is absent; also, in the rainbow trout, arginine and lysine are non-stimulatory, but an arginine derivative, L-α-amino beta-guanidino-propionic acid, is highly effective (Table 3). These results also confirm that a significantly different gustatory spectrum for amino acids exists compared to that determined for the olfactory receptors.

Although chemical information is transmitted centrally by olfactory axons making up a single cranial nerve (I), gustatory neural activity is carried centrally by facial (VII), glossopharyngeal (IX) and vagal (X) cranial nerves which innervate taste cells at different anatomical locations (see p. 261). With but one exception (Kanwal and Caprio, 1983) all extracellular electrophysiological reports on the peripheral taste system of fishes that were responsive to amino acids have consisted solely of facial nerve recordings (Table 2). Since facially innervated taste buds may be widely separated in space (e.g. tip of maxillary barbel and caudal fin in ictalurid catfish), it was questioned whether the taste cells innervated by different branches of the facial nerve might have different response properties. From a number of reports, the electrophysiological data indicate that taste cells innervated by facial nerves have a similar sensitivity and chemospecificity irrespective of their anatomical location (Goh and Tamura, 1980a; Kawamura and Yama-

shita, 1981; Hidaka, 1982; Davenport and Caprio, 1982). The importance for a large number of external body taste buds as found in catfish is
thought to allow for a more effective means to localize a food source
(Atema, 1971) both by temporal (klinotaxis) and instantaneous spatial
(tropotaxis) comparisons of a chemical gradient across the body surface
(Johnsen and Teeter, 1980).

The single report of IX–X amino acid taste response in a fish indicate
that oro-pharyngeal taste buds of the channel catfish have a similar
amino acid response spectrum as that determined from VII recordings
(Kanwal and Caprio, 1983); however, there was a decrease in the
sensitivity as the dose-response curves for alanine and arginine, the
more stimulatory amino acids of oral or extra-oral taste buds, were
shifted by 2 log units towards the high concentration end of the stimulus
concentration axis. This is consistent with high concentrations of food
materials being in direct contact with oro-pharyngeal taste buds during
feeding. Oro-pharyngeal taste buds act as guardians of the gastro-
intestinal tract and are implicated in initiating the swallowing or
rejection reflexes (Finger, 1981).

Receptor-binding studies

An independent more direct method than electrophysiology in
obtaining information concerning the initial events in chemoreception
and the effectiveness of various stimuli is through binding experiments
of olfactory and gustatory tissue with radioactive amino acids. These
studies can provide an indication of whether different stimuli share or
have independent receptor sites; this method can be used in conjunction
with electrophysiological competition studies (cross-adaptation) for
further confirming evidence concerning receptor site 'types'. Binding
activities of tritiated amino acids have been measured in sedimentable
fractions of olfactory mucosa of the rainbow trout (Cagan and Zeiger,
1978; Rhein and Cagan, 1980; Brown and Hara, 1981; Hara, 1982),
brook trout (Brown and Hara, 1982), channel catfish (Cancalon, 1978),
Japanese lamprey (Suzuki, 1980) and skate (Novoselov, Krapivinskaya
and Fesenko, 1980) and in gustatory tissue from the channel catfish
(Krueger and Cagan, 1976; Cagan, 1981). For the olfactory experiments, a significant correlation resulted between the amino acid relative
effectiveness for the trout, catfish and lamprey determined electrophysiologically and biochemically; no electrophysiological data were
available for the species of skate (*Dasyatis pastinacea*). Additionally,
this correlation was restricted to the sensory tissue in a series of control
experiments and specific binding was shown to decrease upon denerva-

tion of the receptors which resulted in olfactory receptor degeneration. The correlation between the relative effectiveness of amino acid stimuli determined electrophysiologically and by binding studies for the taste system of the catfish was not as good as that determined for the olfactory experiments in other species listed above. However, both the electrophysiological (Caprio, 1980; Kanwal and Caprio, 1983; Davenport and Caprio, 1982) and binding (Cagan, 1980) studies were consistent in demonstrating at least two populations of relatively independent receptor sites for alanine (neutral) and arginine (basic), respectively, in the facial taste system of the catfish. Electrophysiological data have indicated further that there are at least two taste fiber types that innervate taste cells that have predominantly alanine and arginine receptor sites, respectively (Caprio and Tucker, 1976; Davenport and Caprio, 1982).

Behavior

A number of studies since the 1960s have shown conclusively that amino acids acting singly and in combinations stimulate feeding behavior in fishes (for reviews see Hidaka, 1982; Carr, 1982; Mackie, 1982; Sutterlin, Solemdal and Tilseth, 1982). Although given the extreme paucity of chemosensory information concerning all but a few species of fishes, a correlation between the electrophysiologically potent amino acids and those that are behaviorally effective is indicated for some species. Table 3 is a summary of this information on five species in which behavioral and electrophysiological results (olfactory and/or gustatory) are available for comparison. There is considerable overlap between the effective behavioral and electrophysiologically determined gustatory stimuli for the sea bream, eel and puffer. In the sea bream a correlation of 0.78 was found between the amino acids that were effective in initiating feeding behavior and those stimulating gustatory neural activity; a correlation of only 0.01 occurred between the behavioral and olfactory neural responsiveness (Goh and Tamura, 1980b). Additionally, in the sea bream, all amino acids that were effective behaviorally were also electrophysiologically potent; however, the reverse was not indicated. In the Japanese eel (*Anguilla japonica*), the identical three amino acids shown to evoke exploratory and feeding behavior (Hashimoto, Konosu, Fusetani and Nose, 1968) were determined electrophysiologically to be the most effective taste stimuli tested (Yoshii et al., 1979). Although olfactory neural data are not available for the Japanese eel, the amino acids that stimulate best the olfactory receptors of the American eel (*Anguilla rostrata*, Silver, 1979a), were similar to the amino acid spectrum determined generally for the

Table 3. *Electrophysiologically (EI′) and behaviorally potent amino acids*

Species	Olfactory EI′	Gustatory EI′	Feeding Behavior
Channel catfish, *Ictalurus punctatus*	Cysh, Met, Gln, nVal, nLeu[a]	Ala, Arg,[a] Pro[b]	Arg, Cysh, Met, Ala, Glu[c]
Eel, *Anguilla japonica*, *Anguilla rostrata*	—	Arg, Gly, Ala, Pro[d]	Arg, Ala, Gly[e] —
Puffer, *Fugu pardalis*	Cysh, Gln, Met, Ala[f]	—	—
Rainbow trout, *Salmo gairdneri*	Gln, Met, Leu, Asn, Ala[i]	Gly, Pro, betaine, Ala[g] αAβGPA, Pro, OHPro, Leu, Ala, Phe[j]	Pro, betaine, Ala, Gly[h] (Tyr, Phe and His) or (Tyr, Phe and Lys)[k]
Sea bream, *Chrysophyrys major*	Gln, Met, Ala[l]	Ala, Gly, Arg, Ser, Lys, betaine, Pro[l]	Ala, Gly, Ser, Pro, Arg[m]

(a) Caprio, 1978.
(b) Kanwal and Caprio, 1983; Pro highly stimulatory at 10^{-3}–10^{-1} M.
(c) Holland and Teeter, 1981; for normal and anosmic catfish.
(d) Yoshii et al., 1979.
(e) Hashimoto et al., 1968.
(f) Silver, 1979a.
(g) Hidaka et al., 1976.
(h) Hidaka et al., 1978.
(i) Hara, 1973.
(j) Hara and Marui, personal communication; αAβGPA, α-amino-β-guanidino-propionic acid.
(k) Adron and Mackie, 1978; 2 different stimulatory mixtures.
(l) Goh and Tamura, 1980a.
(m) Goh and Tamura, 1980b.

olfactory system in other species and different from the behaviorally effective amino acids.

In the puffer, the amino acids effective electrophysiologically on the lip receptors were effective in stimulating feeding behavior, but the amino acid concentration necessary to produce a behavioral response was greater by two to three orders of magnitude than that eliciting gustatory neural activity (Hidaka, Ohsugi and Kubomatsu, 1978). Also, certain electrophysiologically potent stimuli (e.g. nucleotides) had no effect on feeding behavior. Olfactory recordings have not been reported in this species. In the channel catfish, however, both the electrophysiological taste ($10^{-8.6}$–10^{-11} M; Caprio, 1978; Davenport and Caprio, 1982) and behavioral (10^{-8}–10^{-9} M; Holland and Teeter, 1981) thresholds for the more stimulatory amino acids are in fair agreement. Three of the six amino acids (CysH, Met, Glu) most effective in eliciting a conditioned feeding response in normal and anosomic catfish would not be predicted from the peripheral gustatory neural response to these compounds; however, all six of the potent behavioral stimuli would be detected by the taste system at the reported behavioral threshold concentrations. Similar results were obtained using a conditioned cardiac reflex assay as an index of the gustatory detection threshold for amino acids in the catfish (Holland and Teeter, 1981); however, the olfactory sense may also serve as the afferent limb of the conditioned cardiac response (Little, 1981). Olfactory detection thresholds in the channel catfish reported by Little were identical to the olfactory electrophysiological thresholds in the same species (10^{-7}–10^{-9} M; Caprio, 1978). In this latter study, the amino acids that produced a large reduction in heart rate were not highly correlated with those amino acids that evoked a large population neural response.

In the rainbow trout, the results are more confusing (Adron and Mackie, 1978). Tyr, Phe and either Lys or His were the constituents of the simplest mixture tested that stimulated feeding activity. When this mixture was subdivided into two fractions, neither of the fractions was active. When these same compounds were omitted from the effective mixture of L-amino acids based on squid extract concentrations, the resulting mixture was not reduced in stimulatory activity. Of four amino acids identified, in the simplest effective mixture, histidine is an effective electrophysiological olfactory stimulus (Hara, 1973) and phenylalanine is a relatively stimulatory gustatory stimulus (Hara and Marui, personal communication). Proline, which was in highest concentration in the squid synthetic extract, was inactive as a feeding stimulus (Adron and Mackie, 1978), but was highly stimulatory to the taste system when tested electrophysiologically (Hara and Marui, personal communication); lysine, tyrosine and histidine were inactive physiological stimuli.

Numerous other species need to be tested with both behavioral and physiological methods before a definitive statement can be made concerning the correlation of electrophysiological and behavioral results in fishes. It does appear, however, that in some species there is a stronger relation between the sense of taste and feeding behavior than that found for olfaction. This is consistent with behavioral evidence obtained from bullhead catfish in which the gustatory sense was involved primarily in stimulus localization and swallowing or rejection reflexes during feeding (Atema, 1971), whereas the olfactory system served as a general alerting sense involved in social interactions (Todd, Atema and Bardach, 1967). Further experiments are required to determine if this functional distinction between olfaction and taste indicated for catfish is common among other species.

Portions of the work performed by J. Caprio and colleagues reported in this chapter were supported by NIH Grant NS14819. I thank Ms Lynnda Halbrook for secretarial assistance.

References

Adron, S. W., and Mackie, A. M. (1978). Studies in the chemical nature of feeding stimulants for rainbow trout, *Salmo gairdneri* Richardson. *J. Fish. Biol. 12:* 303–10.

Atema, J. (1971). Structures and functions of the sense of taste in catfish (*Ictalurus natalis*). *Brain Behav. Evolut. 4:* 273–94.

Bardach, J. E., and Case, J. (1965). Sensory capabilities of the modified fins of squirrel hake (*Urophycis chuss*) and searobins (*Prionotus carolinsus*). *Copeia 2:* 194–206.

Bardach, J. E., Todd, J. H., and Crickmer, R. (1967). Orientation by taste in fish of the genus *Ictalurus*. *Science 155:* 1276–8.

Bauer, U., Dudel, J., and Hatt, H. (1981). Characteristics of single chemoreceptive units sensitive to amino acids and related substances in the crayfish leg. *J. Comp. Physiol. 144:* 67–74.

Beidler, L. M., and Smallman, R. L. (1965). Renewal of cells within taste buds. *J. Cell Biol. 27:* 263–72.

Belghaug, R., and Døving, K. B. (1977). Odour threshold determined by studies of the induced waves in the olfactory bulb of the char (*Salmo alpinus* L.). *Comp. Biochem. Physiol. 57A:* 327–30.

Bertmar, G. (1973). Ultrastructure of the homing Baltic sea trout *Salmo trutta trutta. Mar. Biol. 19:* 74–88.

Breipohl, W., Bijvank, G. J., and Zippel, H. P. (1973). Rastermikroskopische Untersuchungen der olfactorischen Rezeptoren im Riechepithel des Goldfisches (*Carassius auratus*). *Z. Zellforsch. mikrosk. Anat. 138:* 439–54.

Brown, S. B., and Hara, T. J. (1981). Accumulation of chemostimulatory amino acids by a sedimentable fraction isolated from olfactory rosettes of rainbow trout (*Salmo gairdneri*). *Biochim. Biophys. Acta 675:* 149–62.

Brown, S. B., and Hara, T. J. (1982). Biochemical aspects of amino acid receptors in olfaction and taste. In *Chemoreception in Fishes*, ed. T. J. Hara, pp. 159–80. New York: Elsevier.

Burne, R. H. (1909). The anatomy of the olfactory organ of teleostean fishes. *Proc. Zool. Soc. Lond.* No. 2, 610–37.

Byrd, R. P., and Caprio, J. (1982) Comparison of olfactory receptor (EOG) and bulbar (EEG) responses to amino acids in the catfish, *Ictalurus punctatus*. *Brain Res. 249:* 73–80.

Cagan, R. H. (1981). Recognition of taste stimuli at the initial binding interaction. In *Biochemistry of Taste and Olfaction*, ed. R. H. Cagan and M. R. Kare, pp. 175–203. New York: Academic Press.

Cagan, R. H., and Zeiger, W. N. (1978). Biochemical studies of olfaction: binding specificity of radioactivity labeled stimuli to an isolated olfactory preparation from rainbow trout (*Salmo gairdneri*). *Proc. Natn. Acad. Sci., USA 75:* 4679–83.

Cancalon, P. (1978). Isolation and characterization of the olfactory epithelial cells of the catfish. *Chem. Senses Flav. 3:* 381–96.

Caprio, J. (1975). High sensitivity of catfish taste receptors to amino acids. *Comp. Biochem. Physiol. 52A:* 247–51.

Caprio, J. (1977). Electrophysiological distinctions between the taste and smell of amino acids in catfish. *Nature 266:* 850–1.

Caprio, J. (1978). Olfaction and taste in the channel catfish: an electrophysiological study of the responses to amino acids and derivatives. *J. Comp. Physiol. 123:* 357–71.

Caprio, J. (1980). Similarity of olfactory receptor responses (EOG) of freshwater and marine catfish to amino acids. *Can. J. Zool. 58:* 1778–84.

Caprio, J. (1982). High sensitivity and specificity of olfactory and gustatory receptors of catfish to amino acids. In *Chemoreception in Fishes*, ed. T. J. Hara, pp. 109–34. New York: Elsevier.

Caprio, J., and Raderman-Little, R. (1978). Scanning electron microscopy of the channel catfish olfactory lamellae. *Tissue & Cell 10:* 1–9.

Caprio, J., and Tucker, D. (1976). Specialist and generalist taste fibers in the catfish. *Soc. Neurosci. Abstr. 2:* 152.

Carr, W. E. S. (1982). Chemical stimulation of feeding behavior. In *Chemoreception in Fishes*, ed. T. J. Hara, pp. 259–74. New York: Elsevier.

Crisp, M., Lowe, G. A., and Laverack, M. S. (1975). On the ultrastructure and permeability of taste buds of the marine teleost *Ciliata mustela*. *Tissue & Cell 7:* 191–202.

Davenport, C. J., and Caprio, J. (1982). Taste and tactile recordings from the ramus recurrens facialis innervating flank taste buds in the catfish. *J. Comp. Physiol. 147:* 217–29.

Døving, K. B., Dubois-Dauphin, M., Holley, A., and Jourdan, F. (1977). Functional anatomy of the olfactory organ of fish and the ciliary mechanism of water transport. *Acta Zool. 58:* 245–55.

Døving, K. B., and Holmberg, K. (1974). A note on the function of the olfactory organ of the hagfish *Myxine glutinosa*. *Acta Physiol. Scand. 91:* 430–2.

Døving, K. B., Selset, R., and Thommesen, G. (1980). Olfactory sensitivity to bile acids in salmonid fishes. *Acta Physiol. Scand. 108:* 123–31.

Easton, D. M. (1971). Garfish olfactory nerve: easily accessible source of numerous long, homogeneous nonmyelinated axons. *Science 72:* 952–5.

Farbman, A. I. (1965). Fine structure of the taste bud. *J. Ultrastruct. Res. 12:* 328–50.

Farbman, A. I. (1980). Renewal of taste bud cells in rat circumvallate papillae. *Cell Tiss. Kinet. 13:* 349–57.

Finger, T. E. (1981). Laminar and columnar organization of the vagal lobe in goldfish: possible neural substrate for sorting food from gravel. *Soc. Neurosci. Abstr. 7:* 665.

Fujiya, M., and Bardach, J. E. (1966). A comparison between the external taste sense of marine and freshwater fishes. *Bull. Jap. Soc. Sci. Fish. 32:* 45–56.

Gardner, W. S., and Lee, G. F. (1975). The role of amino acids in the nitrogen cycle of Lake Mendota. *Limnol. Oceanog. 20:* 379–88.

Gemne, G., and Døving, K. B. (1969). Ultrastructural properties of primary olfactory neurons in fish (*Lota lota* L.). *Am. J. Anat. 126:* 457–76.

Gesteland, R. C., Howland, B., Lettvin, T. Y., and Pitts, W. H. (1959). Comments on microelectrodes. *Proc. Inst. Radio Eng. 47:* 1856–62.

Getchell, T. V. (1974). Electrogenic sources of slow voltage transients recorded from frog olfactory epithelium. *J. Neurophysiol. 37:* 1115–30.

Goh, Y., and Tamura, T. (1978). The electrical responses of the olfactory tract to amino acids in carp. *Bull. Jap. Soc. Sci. Fish. 44:* 341–4.

Goh, Y., and Tamura, T. (1980a). Olfactory and gustatory responses to amino acids in two marine teleosts – red sea bream and mullet. *Comp. Biochem. Physiol. 66C:* 217–24.

Goh, Y., and Tamura, T. (1980b). Effect of amino acids on the feeding behavior in red sea bream. *Comp. Biochem. Physiol. 66C:* 225–9.

Goh, Y., Tamura, T., and Kobayashi, H. (1979). Olfactory responses to amino acids in marine teleosts. *Comp. Biochem. Physiol. 62A:* 863–8.

Graziadei, P. P. C., and Metcalf, J. F. (1971). Autoradiographic and ultrastructural observations on the frog's olfactory mucosa. *Z. Zellforsch. mikrosk. Anat. 116:* 305–18.

Grover-Johnson, N., and Farbman, A. I. (1976). Fine structure of taste buds in the barbel of the catfish, *Ictalurus punctatus. Cell Tiss. Res. 169:* 395–403.

Hara, T. J. (1973). Olfactory responses to amino acids in rainbow trout, *Salmo gairdneri. Comp. Biochem. Physiol. 44A:* 407–16.

Hara, T. J. (1975). Olfaction in fish. In *Progress and Neurobiology*, vol. 5, ed. G. A. Kerkut and J. W. Phillips, pp. 271–335. Oxford: Pergamon.

Hara, T. J. (1977). Further structure-activity relationships of amino acids in fish olfaction. *Comp. Biochem. Physiol. 56A:* 559–65.

Hara, T. J. (1982). Structure-activity relationships of amino acids as olfactory stimuli. In *Chemoreception in Fishes*, ed. T. J. Hara, pp. 135–57. New York: Elsevier.

Hara, T. J., Law, Y. M. C., and Hobden, B. R. (1973). Comparison of the olfactory response to amino acids in rainbow trout brook and whitefish. *Comp. Biochem. Physiol. 45A:* 969–77.

Hashimoto, Y., Konosu, S., Fusetani, N., and Nose, T. (1968). Attractants for eels in the extracts of short-necked clam. I. Survey of constituents eliciting feeding behavior of the omission test. *Bull. Jap. Soc. Sci. Fish. 34:* 39–48.

Herrick, C. J. (1901). The cranial nerves and cutaneous sense organs of the North American siluroid fishes. *J. Comp. Neurol. 11:* 177–249.

Hidaka, I. (1982). Taste receptor stimulation and feeding behavior in the puffer. In *Chemoreception in Fishes*, ed. T. J. Hara, pp. 243–57. New York: Elsevier.

Hidaka, I., Kiyohara, S., and Oda, S. (1977). Gustatory response in the puffer – III.

Stimulatory effectiveness of nucleotides and their derivatives. *Bull. Jap. Soc. Sci. Fish.* *43:* 423–8.

Hidaka, I., Nyu, N., and Kiyohara, S. (1976). Gustatory response in the puffer – IV. Effects of mixtures of amino acids and betaine. *Bull. Fac. Fish., Mie. Univ. 3:* 17–28.

Hidaka, I., Oshugi, T., and Kubomatsu, T. (1978). Taste receptor stimulation and feeding behavior in the puffer, *Fugu pardalis.* I. Effect of single chemicals. *Chem. Senses Flav. 3:* 341–54.

Hirata, Y. (1966). Fine structure of the terminal buds on the barbels of some fishes. *Arch. Histol. Jap. 26:* 507–23.

Holl, A. (1965). Vergleichende morphologische und histologische Untersuchungen am Geruchsorgan der Knochenfirsche. *Z. Morphol. Ökol. Tiere 54:* 707–82.

Holland, K. N., and Teeter, J. H. (1981). Behavioral and cardiac reflex assays of the chemosensory acuity of channel catfish to amino acids. *Physiol. Behav. 27:* 699–707.

Ichikawa, M., and Ueda, K. (1977). Fine structure of the olfactory epithelium in the goldfish, *Carassius auratus.* A study of retrograde degeneration. *Cell Tiss. Res. 183:* 445–55.

Johnsen, P. B., and Teeter, J. H. (1980). Spatial gradient detection of chemical cues by catfish. *J. Comp. Physiol. 140:* 95–9.

Kanwal, J. S., and Caprio, J. (1983). An electrophysiological investigation of the oro-pharyngeal (IX–X) taste system in the channel catfish, *Ictalurus punctatus.* *J. Comp. Physiol. 150:* 345–57.

Kawamura, T., and Yamashita, S. (1981). Chemical and thermal responses from buccal and maxillary nerves in the minnow, *Pseudorasbora parva. Comp. Biochem. Physiol. 69A:* 187–95.

Kiyohara, S., Hidaka, I., and Tamura, T. (1975). Gustatory response in the puffer – II. Single fiber analyses. *Bull. Jap. Soc. Sci. Fish. 41:* 383–91.

Kiyohara, S., Yamashita, S., and Harada, S. (1981). High sensitivity of minnow gustatory receptors to amino acids. *Physiol. Behav. 26:* 1103–8.

Kiyohara, S., Yamashita, S., and Kitoh, J. (1980). Distribution of taste buds on the lips and inside the mouth in the minnow, *Pseudorasbora parva. Physiol. Behav. 24:* 1143–7.

Kleerekoper, H. (1969). *Olfaction in Fishes.* Bloomington, Indiana: Indiana University Press.

Kreutzberg, G. W., and Gross, G. W. (1977). General morphology and axonal ultrastructure of the olfactory nerve of the pike, *Esox lucius. Cell Tiss. Res. 181:* 443–57.

Krueger, J. M., and Cagan, R. H. (1976). Biochemical studies of taste sensation. Binding of L-[^{3}H]alanine to a sedimentable fraction from catfish barbel epithelium. *J. Biol. Chem. 251:* 88–97.

Little, E. E. (1981). Conditioned cardiac response to the olfactory stimuli of amino acids in channel catfish, *Ictalurus punctatus. Physiol. Behav. 27:* 691–7.

Mackie, A. M. (1982). Identification of the gustatory feeding stimulants. In *Chemoreception in Fishes,* ed. T. J. Hara, pp. 275–291. New York: Elsevier.

Mackie, A. M., and Adron, J. W. (1978). Identification of inosine and inosine-5′-monophosphate as the gustatory feeding stimulants for the turbot, *Scophthalamus maximus. Comp. Biochem. Physiol. 60A:* 79–83.

Moulton, D. (1975). Cell renewal in the olfactory epithelium of the mouse. In *Olfaction and Taste V,* ed. D. A. Denton and J. P. Coghlan, pp. 111–14. New York: Academic Press.

Murray, R. G. (1973). The ultrastructure of taste buds. In *The Ultrastructure of Sensory Organs*, ed. I. Friedmann, pp. 1–81. Amsterdam, London: North-Holland Publishing Co.

Novoselov, V. I., Krapivinskaya, L. D., and Fesenko, E. E. (1980). Molecular mechanisms of odor sensing. V. Some biochemical characteristics of the alanineous receptor from the olfactory epithelium of the skate *Dasyatis pastinaca*. *Chem. Senses* 5: 195–203.

Olmsted, J. M. D. (1918). Experiments on the nature of the sense of smell in common catfish, *Amiurus nebulosus* (LeSueur). *Am. J. Physiol. 46:* 443–58.

Ottoson, D. (1971). The electro-olfactogram. In *Handbook of Sensory Physiology*, IV, Part 1, ed. L. M. Beidler, pp. 95–131. Berlin, Heidelberg, New York: Springer-Verlag.

Outwater, E., and Oakley, B. (1981). Inhibition of IXth nerve taste responses involves cholinergic efferent fibers. *Soc. Neurosci. Abstr. 7:* 664.

Paran, N., Mattern, C. F. T., and Henkin, R. I. (1975). Ultrastructure of the taste bud of the human fungiform papilla. *Cell Tiss. Res. 161:* 1–10.

Parker, G. H., and Sheldon, R. E. (1912). The sense of smell in fishes. *Bull. U.S. Bur. Fish. 32:* 33–46.

Pevzner, R. A. (1976). Electron microscope study of the taste buds of elasmobranchs, *Trigon pastinaca* and *Raja clavata*. *Tsitologiya 18:* 560–6.

Raderman-Little, R. (1979). The effect of temperature on the turnover of taste bud cells in catfish. *Cell Tiss. Kinet. 12:* 269–80.

Reutter, K. (1978). Taste organ in the bullhead (Teleostei). *Adv. Anat. Embryol. Cell Biol. 55:* 1–98.

Reutter, K. (1980). SEM-study of the mucus layer on the receptor field of fish taste buds. In *Olfaction and Taste VII*, ed. H. van der Starre, p. 107. London, Washington D.C.: IRL Press.

Reutter, K. (1982). Taste organ in the barbel of the bullhead. In *Chemoreception in Fishes*, ed. T. J. Hara, pp. 77–91. New York: Elsevier.

Rhein, L. D., and Cagan, R. H. (1980). Biochemical studies of olfaction: isolation, characterization, and odorant binding activity of cilia from rainbow trout olfactory rosettes. *Proc. Natn. Acad. Sci., USA 77:* 4412–16.

Sato, T. (1980). Recent advances in the physiology of taste cells. *Progr. Neurobiol., Psychol. 19:* 273–311.

Schulte, E. (1972). Untersuchungen an der Regio olfactoria des Aals, *Anguilla anguilla* L. I. Feinstruktur des Riechepithels. *Z. Zellforsch. mikrosk. Anat. 125:* 210–28.

Selset, R., and Døving, K. B. (1980). Behavior of mature anadromous char (*Salmo alpinus* L.) towards odorants produced by smolts of their own population. *Acta Physiol. Scand. 108:* 113–22.

Sheldon, R. E. (1909). The reactions of the dogfish to chemical stimuli. *J. Comp. Neurol. Psychol. 19:* 273–311.

Silver, W. L. (1979a). Electrophysiological responses from the olfactory system of the American eel. Ph.D. Thesis, Florida State University, Tallahassee, Florida, USA.

Silver, W. L. (1979b). Olfactory responses from a marine elasmobranch, the Atlantic stingray, *Dasyatus sabina*. *Mar. Behav. Physiol. 6:* 297–305.

Silver, W. L., Caprio, J., Blackwell, J. F., and Tucker, D. (1976). The underwater electro-olfactogram: a tool for the study of the sense of smell of marine fishes. *Experientia 32:* 1216–17.

Sutterlin, A. M., Solemdal, P., and Tilseth, S. (1982). Baits in fisheries with emphasis on the North Atlantic cod fishing. In *Chemoreception in Fishes*, ed. T. J. Hara, pp. 293–305. New York: Elsevier.

Sutterlin, A. M., and Sutterlin, N. (1970). Taste responses in Atlantic salmon (*Salmo salar*) parr. *J. Fish. Res. Bd Can. 27:* 1927–42.

Sutterlin, A. M., and Sutterlin, N. (1971). Electrical responses of the olfactory epithelium of Atlantic salmon (*Salmo salar*). *J. Fish. Res. Bd Can. 28:* 565–72.

Suzuki, N. (1977). Intracellular responses of lamprey olfactory receptors to current and chemical stimulation. In *Food Intake and Chemical Senses*, ed. Y. Katsuki, M. Sato, S. F. Takagi and Y. Oomura, pp. 13–22. Tokyo: University of Tokyo Press.

Suzuki, N. (1978). Effects of different ionic environments on the responses of single olfactory receptors in the lamprey. *Comp. Biochem. Physiol. 61A:* 461–7.

Suzuki, N. (1980). Binding activities of radioactively labeled amino acids to the lamprey olfactory tissue and its fractions. In *Proceedings of the 14th Japanese Symposium on Taste and Smell*, ed. H. Tomita, pp. 33–6.

Suzuki, N. (1982). Responses of olfactory receptor cells to electrical and chemical stimulation. In *Chemoreception in Fishes*, ed. T. J. Hara, pp. 93–108. New York: Elsevier.

Suzuki, N., and Tucker, D. (1971). Amino acids as olfactory stimuli in freshwater catfish, *Ictalurus catus* (Linn.). *Comp. Biochem. Physiol. 40A:* 399–404.

Takeda, M., and Hoshino, T. (1975). Fine structure of taste buds in the rat. *Arch. Histol. Jap. 37:* 395–413.

Teeter, J. (1974). Electrical properties of taste bud cells and surrounding epithelial cells in catfish and mudpuppies. Ph.D. Thesis, University of Pennsylvania, Philadelphia, Pennsylvania, USA.

Teichman, H. (1954). Vergleichende Untersuchungen an der Nase der Fische. *Z. Morphol. Ökol. Tiere 43:* 171–212.

Todd, J. H., Atema, J., and Bardach, J. E. (1967). Chemical communication in social behavior of a fish, the yellow bullhead (*Ictalurus natalis*). *Science 158:* 672–3.

Toyoshima, K., and Shimamura, A. (1981). A scanning electron microscopic study of taste buds in the rabbit. *Biomed. Res.*, Suppl. 2, 459–63.

Yamamoto, M. (1982). Comparative morphology of the peripheral olfactory organ in teleosts. In *Chemoreception in Fishes*. ed. T. J. Hara, pp. 39–59. New York: Elsevier.

Yamamoto, M., and Ueda, K. (1977). Comparative morphology of fish olfactory epithelium I. Salmoniformes. *Bull. Jap. Soc. Sci. Fish. 43:* 1163–74.

Yamamoto, M., and Ueda, K. (1979). Comparative morphology of fish olfactory epithelium. X. Perciformes, Beryciformes, Scorpaeniformes, and Pleuronectiformes. *J. Fac. Sci., Univ. Tokyo*, Sect. 4, *14:* 273–97.

Yoshii, K., Kamo, N., Kurihara, K., and Kobatake, Y. (1979). Gustatory responses of eel palatine receptors to amino acids and carboxylic acids. *J. Gen. Physiol. 74:* 301–17.

Zeiske, E., Melinkat, R., Breucker, H., and Kux, J. (1976). Ultrastructural studies on the epithelia of the olfactory organ of cyprinodonts (Teleostei, Cyprinodontoidea). *Cell Tiss. Res. 172:* 245–67.

2.4

Biochemical studies of physiological function: olfactory recognition in rainbow trout

ROBERT H. CAGAN

Of central importance in olfaction is the initial input of information. How the recognition of an odorant occurs is a question that has fascinated generations of scientists. Ideas about possible mechanisms have been discussed (see Beets, 1978) but until recently they have had no experimental biochemical basis.

The analogy with a specific 'lock and key' relationship for enzyme-substrate interactions was proposed by Emil Fischer near the end of the nineteenth century (Dixon and Webb, 1964). This idea relies upon a strict steric complementarity between the two molecules, and has been used to describe odorant interactions with olfactory receptors (Amoore, 1970). Cooperative interactions in proteins, including allosteric effects, although sometimes discussed in connection with olfactory receptors, have not been studied experimentally in the olfactory system. These conceptual developments have greatly affected our understanding of the biochemistry of enzymes, and more recently of receptors for neurotransmitters and hormones, but have not been incorporated into our understanding of olfactory receptors. Relatively little experimental biochemistry has been reported so the data base is small, but during the past four years progress has been made. This paper focuses on an experimental model found to be exceptionally useful for biochemical studies of olfaction, the rainbow trout *Salmo gairdneri*.

Knowledge about receptors for hormones and neurotransmitters (Cuatrecasas and Hollenberg, 1976; Kahn, 1976) has expanded greatly in recent years. Generally such a receptor is membrane-bound and interacts with relatively high affinity and specificity for a particular hormone or neurotransmitter. Technical advances in methodology, both preparative and analytical, for isolating receptors and measuring binding interactions (Yamamura, Enna and Kuhar, 1978) have under-lain the significant progress made. The approach to measure binding to receptors directly was applied to olfaction in an investigation of interactions of odorant amino acids with olfactory receptors from the rainbow trout *Salmo gairdneri* (Zeiger and Cagan, 1975; Cagan and Zeiger, 1978), an experimental model upon which this paper focuses. A brief introduction to the experimental rationale is first presented, followed by descriptions of specific findings that have emerged from its application.

Recognition of odorants by receptors

The initial step in odor sensing appears to be a reversible binding interaction between an odorant molecule and a receptor site. The number of such events necessary, at the molecular level, to depolarize a receptor cell or to evoke a perceptible odor sensation or a behavioral response is not known. It is commonly assumed, however, that the sensitivity of an organism to an odorant is directly related to the affinity of the binding interaction at the periphery.

A long-standing question concerns the array of different receptors that exist at the molecular level. Intimately related to this question is the range of specificity of a particular receptor site. Is a receptor site narrowly tuned for only one compound or a limited range of its structural variants, such as a receptor for a neurotransmitter or hormone? Or is a receptor broadly tuned to interact with a wider range of stimuli? Must a stimulus interact with only a single receptor type, or can it interact with several sites in addition to one which preferentially recognizes that compound? These are questions that can be answered by a biochemical approach with an animal model that enables measurement of binding of olfactory stimuli.

The approach to measure stimulus-receptor interactions directly in chemical sensory receptors using radioactively-labeled stimulus compounds as ligands was begun in 1971, when we studied interactions of sweet taste stimuli with mammalian taste papillae homogenates (Cagan, 1971). Although that system was not optimal for more detailed investigation because of the weak binding interactions (Cagan, 1974, 1981), it enabled demonstration of the approach and encouraged the search for better experimental models for both taste and olfaction. Progress has been made in studies on taste receptors of both mammals and fish (see Cagan, 1981), and has been applied successfully to olfactory receptors.

Where the olfactory receptors are located in the cell is another long-standing question. Although the cilia at the apical surface of receptor cells are seemingly a likely location of receptor sites, this hypothesis has had a controversial history. This question also can be approached biochemically.

We have learned something about these important aspects of olfaction at the receptor level from biochemical experiments with the rainbow trout, that are described in greater detail below. The utility of the approach using radiolabeled ligands is not limited to trout, as it has been extended to olfactory receptors of catfish (Cancalon, 1978), skate (Novoselov, Krapivinskaya and Fesenko, 1980), rat (Fesenko, Novoselov and Krapivinskaya, 1979), sow (Gennings, Gower and Bannister, 1977; but see also Dodd and Persaud, 1981; Gower, Hancock and Bannister, 1981; Pelosi, Baldaccini and Pisanelli, 1982; Persaud, Pelosi and Dodd, 1980), sheep (Dodd and Persaud, 1981), bovine and rabbit (Pelosi et al., 1982).

Biochemical measurement of odorant recognition

It is perhaps surprising that the common biochemical approach to determining receptor specificity, by measuring binding of radiolabeled ligands, has not been more widely used in olfaction. Electrophysiological, psychophysical and behavioral methods are the predominant means by which investigators attempt to learn how the olfactory system responds to and processes this information. The biochemical approach, however, is able to assess receptor specificity directly and is beginning to be used more widely in olfaction studies.

In the taste system, the generally weak interactions of most taste stimuli with mammalian taste receptors led us to search for an experimental animal with a more sensitive taste system. We developed a biochemical model using the cutaneous taste receptors of the channel catfish (Krueger and Cagan, 1976; Cagan, 1979), from which a receptor-enriched preparation was derived in a highly reproducible manner. Binding of relevant taste-stimulus compounds, amino acids, is readily measured with this isolated preparation. The approach seemed directly applicable to the olfactory system because the studies of Sutterlin and Sutterlin (1971) had shown the olfactory responsiveness of salmonid fishes to amino acids as odorants.

The essential feature of our biochemical approach is to measure the direct interaction of a stimulus compound with a receptor site by employing compounds that are known to be odorants to the species being investigated. These radioactively-labeled compounds are used as ligands for binding measurements.

Many amino acids are stimulatory to the olfactory receptors of the rainbow trout, which provided us with an opportunity to establish the biochemical approach. Responsiveness of salmon (Sutterlin and Sutterlin, 1971) and rainbow trout (Hara, 1973) had been assessed by electrophysiological recordings in response to amino acid solutions flowed over the olfactory rosettes of the fish. The responses of rainbow trout to a series of amino acids (10^{-4} M) enabled them to be rank-ordered as to their stimulatory effectiveness (Hara, 1973). From that series we selected odorants of relatively high, intermediate, and low effectiveness, with the condition that they be available in radiolabeled form.

The data in Figure 1 show binding of ten amino acids to Fraction P2. This sedimentable fraction is obtained by differential centrifugation of a homogenate of trout olfactory rosettes. The results in Figure 1 are a compilation of data from four experiments, in each of which binding was measured to all ten compounds at a fixed concentration (6μM). This design controls for variability among preparations, but sufficient material was available (from 50 fish per preparation) to assess binding at only a single ligand concentration. The correlation coefficient between binding and electrophysiological responses was $+0.80$ (Cagan and Zeiger, 1978). This correspondence is especially good considering the different experimental measures and conditions under which the two experiments were carried out, and the fact that they were done independently. In further experiments, we determined binding over a concentration range, thereby demonstrating binding to be saturable as

Figure 1. Binding of odorant amino acids compared with electrophysiological responsiveness in the rainbow trout. (Figure taken from Cagan and Zeiger, 1978.)

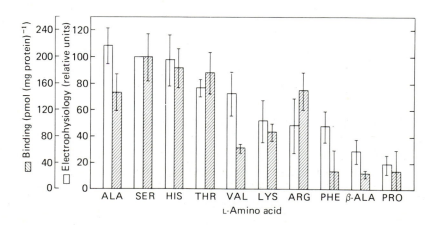

the concentration of ligand increased (Figure 2). Binding is reversible as well as saturable.

Binding occurs to only a small extent to the sedimentable fraction from non-olfactory tissues (brain and gill) of the trout (Cagan and Zeiger, 1978; Brown and Hara, 1981). Furthermore, recent data (Brown and Hara, 1981) show that denervation of the olfactory rosettes results in a marked decrease in binding activity of Fraction P2, similar to the decrease in taste-ligand binding following denervation of catfish taste receptors (Krueger and Cagan, 1976).

The biochemical approach also allows assessment of effects of potential toxicants to fish. Chemicals that might affect the olfactory acuity of fish, but are not toxic to an individual, could affect a population by interfering with home-stream migration to their spawning waters; olfaction is involved in the later stages of homing by salmonids (Hasler, 1960; Hasler, Scholz and Horrall, 1978). In a relatively limited series of experiments (Cagan and Zeiger, 1978), we examined the effects on binding of odorant amino acids by some metal ions and by sulfhydryl group-reactive reagents. The effects of Hg^{2+}, Cu^{2+}, and Cd^{2+} on binding are shown in Figure 3; at low concentrations only Hg^{2+} was strongly

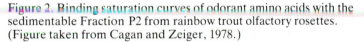

Figure 2. Binding saturation curves of odorant amino acids with the sedimentable Fraction P2 from rainbow trout olfactory rosettes. (Figure taken from Cagan and Zeiger, 1978.)

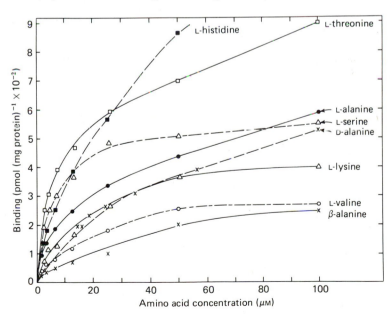

inhibitory. A brief survey also showed 1 mM Ag^+ and Pb^{2+} to be inhibitory, but not Zn^{2+}. At 0.1 mM, *p*-hydroxymercuribenzoate was inhibitory. The inhibition by Hg^+ and by the organic mercurial appeared to be irreversible.

Inhibition of electro-olfactogram responses in frogs by 4 mM *N*-ethyl-maleimide had suggested the possible involvement of sulfhydryl groups in odorant (ethyl *n*-butyrate) stimulation of olfactory receptors (Getchell and Gesteland, 1972). Our results in trout, however, suggested the effects of mercurials to be irreversible, which did not support sulfhydryl involvement. Moreover, Kleene and Gesteland (1981) recently showed that 2–8 mM *N*-ethylmaleimide causes disruption of the olfactory epithelium. With Fraction P2 from rainbow trout, neither 1 mM iodoacetate nor 0.1 mM *N*-ethylmaleimide inhibited binding, thus not supporting the idea of an essential sulfhydryl group in odorant binding in the trout. From the results of binding inhibition studies, however, it appears that assessment of toxicant effects on olfactory receptors is possible using binding assays.

Odorant binding in other species

Only a handful of studies have employed the approach described above, in which radiolabeled ligand binding is determined with preparations derived from olfactory tissue. Our binding technique

Figure 3. Effects of Hg^{2+}, Cu^{2+}, and Cd^{2+} on binding of L-[³H]alanine to the sedimentable Fraction P2 from rainbow trout olfactory rosettes. (Figure taken from Cagan and Zeiger, 1978.)

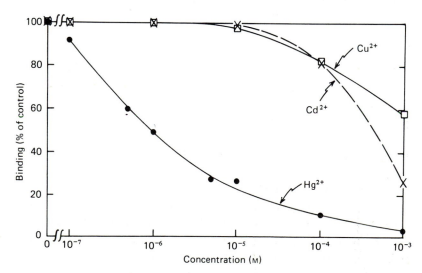

(Krueger and Cagan, 1976) was used to measure interactions of radiolabeled amino acid odorants to cells isolated from the catfish olfactory epithelium (Cancalon, 1978). A high correlation was shown between binding and reported electrophysiological responses measured *in vivo*. Because binding was measured with whole cells, the extent to which transport into the cells occurred remains a question. Even with an isolated subcellular fraction, the possibility of transport (Cagan, 1979; Brown and Hara, 1981) cannot easily be discounted.

Binding activity for L-[^{3}H]alanine was recently reported to occur in a sedimentable fraction isolated from a homogenate of skate olfactory rosettes (Novoselov et al., 1980). The binding activity was solubilized by treatment of the preparation with 0.3% Triton X-100 and found to be in a macromolecular fraction upon electrophoresis. Binding of [^{3}H]camphor to a preparation from rat olfactory epithelium was reported (Fesenko et al., 1979). The rat tissue was homogenized in the presence of [^{3}H]camphor and then fractionated to obtain a sedimentable fraction. This was solubilized with 0.3% Triton X-100. Following these treatments, radioactivity was found in a macromolecular fraction.

An earlier study by Gennings et al. (1977) reported specific binding of the steroid pheromones [5α-^{3}H]-androst-16-en-3-one and [5α-^{3}H]-androst-16-en-3α-ol to a homogenate of sow olfactory epithelium. These results with respect to an olfactory receptor appear to be in doubt, as noted recently by Gower et al. (1981) and by other authors (Dodd and Persaud, 1981; Pelosi et al., 1982; Persaud et al., 1980).

Recent work by Pelosi et al. (1982) demonstrated binding of [^{3}H]2-isobutyl-3-methoxypyrazine to supernatant extracts of homogenates of bovine and rabbit olfactory epithelium and to a lesser extent to that of rat. This compound has an odor of bell pepper to humans, and is thought by Pelosi et al. (1982) to stimulate similar olfactory receptors in other mammalian species. Competition for binding by 2-isopropyl-3-methoxypyrazine and 4-butyl-5-propylthiazole, both of which possess a bell pepper odor quality, provided further support for the hypothesis that binding of the labeled compound measures odorant recognition by receptors. In no case, however, has a well defined, characterized olfactory receptor macromolecule (receptor protein) been described.

Localization of olfactory receptor sites

Subcellular fractionation is a well established approach in biochemistry, by which it is possible to separate subcellular components after disrupting a tissue. Based upon differences in sedimentation properties under a centrifugal force, various organelles can be separ-

Table 1. *Distribution of* L-*[³H]alanine binding activity following fractionation of trout olfactory rosettes*

Fraction	Protein (mg)	Amount bound (pmol)	Specific binding (pmol mg^{-1})
Homogenate	34.4 (28.7)	695 (1024)	20.2
Low-speed pellet	16.0	217	13.5
High-speed pellet (Fraction P2)	3.0	742	246
Supernatant	9.5	295	30.9
Recovery (%)	99	122	

Olfactory rosettes from 50 rainbow trout were homogenized and fractionated. The values in parentheses are for the sum of the low-speed pellet + initial supernatant (which represents the initial division of homogenate); recoveries are based on those values. Taken from a more extensive table in Cagan and Zeiger (1978).

ated. It has thereby been possible to study functional characteristics in various tissues of many of these organelles, including mitochondria, Golgi apparatus, microsomal membranes, and plasma membranes. Despite possible problems with cross-contamination, significant knowledge has been gained of the functions of the major components of cells.

In our initial studies on the olfactory system of the rainbow trout (Cagan and Zeiger, 1978) we demonstrated that the binding activity for odorant amino acids was enriched in a sedimentable Fraction P2 (Table 1). The fractionation scheme was similar to that we had used with taste receptor tissue from the channel catfish (Krueger and Cagan, 1976). The results with the catfish showed the binding activity for taste stimuli (amino acids) to be localized to this sedimentable fraction. Marker enzymes showed Fraction P2 to be enriched in plasma membranes, with significant mitochondrial but little microsomal contamination. Virtually exact replication of these assays recently with the rainbow trout olfactory Fraction P2 (Brown and Hara, 1981) showed similar results.

The important functional criterion relevant to olfaction is specific binding of odorant amino acids. Under the separation conditions we used (Cagan and Zeiger, 1978), the sedimentation of binding activity for amino acids indicated a membrane localization for the olfactory receptors. Using more highly purified plasma membranes, the specific localization of taste receptors to the plasma membranes has been demonstrated in the catfish (Cagan and Boyle, 1978; Cagan, 1981). The surface of olfactory receptor cells, however, contains cilia (Bannister, 1965; Bertmar, 1973; Gemne and Døving, 1969; Ichikawa and Ueda, 1977; Lowe and MacLeod, 1975; Rhein, Cagan, Orkand and Dolack,

Table 2. *Enrichment of markers in cilia preparation from trout olfactory rosettes*

Sample	Mg^{2+}-ATPase (nmol min^{-1} (mg protein)$^{-1}$)	Nucleotide base content Guanine Adenine Ratio, G : A (μg (mg protein)$^{-1}$)		
Whole rosettes	73.9	0.99	1.50	0.66
Deciliated rosettes	65.5	0.12	1.55	0.08
Supernatant	44.4	—	—	—
Cilia	275	1.31	0.76	1.73

Cilia were isolated from olfactory rosettes of 300 and 385 rainbow trout, respectively, for the assays of ATPase and nucleotides. Taken from Rhein and Cagan (1980).

1981; Yamamoto and Ueda, 1977). A question of fundamental import-ance in olfaction, and one with a controversial history, is the role of the cilia in olfaction. A widely cited preliminary report (Tucker, 1967) claimed that the olfactory cilia are not necessary for stimulation by odorants, but other studies suggest that cilia are involved. Bronshtein and Minor (1977) found that after removing the cilia from frog olfactory epithelium with the detergent Triton X-100, the electro-olfactogram response declined. Upon regeneration of the cilia the electrophysiolo-gical response was restored. The subject is further discussed in a recent review (Rhein and Cagan, 1981).

We sought to answer the question of involvement of cilia using a classical biochemical approach to isolate and characterize the cilia, and to determine whether or not they bind odorant amino acids. They do. The cilia were removed from intact rosettes by calcium-ethanol treat-ment (Watson and Hopkins, 1962; Linck, 1973). The data in Table 2 show enrichment, in an isolated preparation, of two biochemical markers for cilia components (Rhein and Cagan, 1980). Furthermore, electron microscopy revealed the presence of cilia, and the presence of tubulin in the preparation was demonstrated by polyacrylamide gel electrophoresis. Although no markers are available that are both characteristic and unique to cilia, the data on the markers used indicates enrichment of cilia in the preparation.

Importantly, binding of several odorant amino acids was demon-strable, and the binding characteristics (Figure 4) were similar to those for binding to Fraction P2. This evidence supports the hypothesis that the cilia contain odorant-receptor sites. Further, preliminary evidence suggests that the receptors are in the membranes covering the cilia (Rhein and Cagan, 1981). Questions still remain, however, about the specific receptor localization along a cilium and the amount of a cilium actually needed for a response to occur. It is worth noting species differences. For example, cilia in frogs are considerably longer (30–200 μm) than in fish (2–30 μm), and comparisons based upon a percentage of mature length would therefore have little meaning.

The possibility of transport occurring during the binding assay is a question considered in our earlier work on catfish taste receptor Fraction P2 (Cagan, 1979). The same experiments as we reported were repeated on trout Fraction P2 (rather than cilia), and the authors (Brown and Hara, 1981) proposed some degree of transport being involved. Brown and Hara's data suggest that if transport occurs, it is a small component of the measured values. Specifically, the effect of Na^+ was small, and the effect in the preloading (countertransport) experiment appears to be an artifact stemming from addition of unlabeled L-alanine (0.5 μM) to the medium of the two comparison samples; this would dilute the specific radioactivity of the ligand being measured. The transport inhibitors were ineffective with nearly all of the ligands tested. Similar to our findings with the taste tissue Fraction P2 (Cagan, 1979), a

Figure 4. Binding saturation curves of odorant amino acids to cilia preparation from rainbow trout olfactory rosettes. (Figure taken from Rhein and Cagan, 1980.)

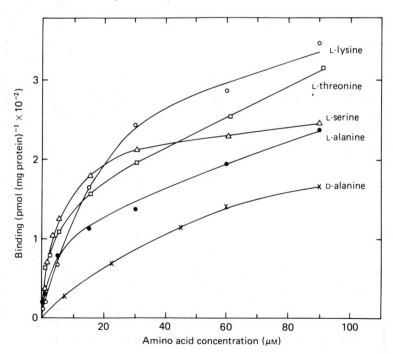

large osmotic effect was observed with trout Fraction P2 (Brown and Hara, 1981), suggestive of a vesicular compartment.

A microvillous cell type is often present in fish olfactory epithelium (Bannister, 1965; Bertmar, 1973; Ichikawa and Ueda, 1977; Lowe and MacLeod, 1975), including that of salmonids (Rhein et al., 1981; Yamamoto and Ueda, 1977). Based on a degeneration study, the microvillous cell has been suggested (Ichikawa and Ueda, 1977) to be an additional type of receptor cell in goldfish. Receptor cells in both the taste and vomeronasal systems have microvilli on their surface. Although no physiological evidence currently exists for the hypothesis that microvillous cells in the olfactory epithelium are receptors, it will be interesting when neurophysiologists are able to provide recordings of responses of these cell types.

Specificity of olfactory receptor sites

Of fundamental interest is the question of how narrowly or broadly tuned a receptor is. Generally this has been approached by indirect methods, principally by cross-adaptation using either psychophysical or electrophysiological methods to assess responses. Because neither technique is able to measure receptor interactions, such results are at best only suggestive. Direct binding of odorants to receptors offers a means to assess the specificity of a particular receptor site, in the same way that neurotransmitter-receptor interactions, hormone-receptor interactions and drug-receptor interactions have been so rewardingly studied.

Our approach is to measure binding of a radiolabeled ligand and to determine the recognition of other odorants by the same receptor site using competition experiments. In these studies the unlabeled competitor is present in the binding assay with the radiolabeled odorant. In an initial survey of competitive interactions with trout Fraction P2, we obtained evidence (Cagan and Zeiger, 1978) for several types of receptor sites: site TSA, which binds L-threonine, L-serine and L-alanine, site L, which binds L-lysine, and site A_B, which binds β-alanine. Tentative assignments were made for site V, which binds L-valine, site H, which binds L-histidine, and site A_D, which binds D-alanine. Some overlap in specificity was observed; for example, L-valine appeared to bind to site TSA, and there were other examples also. Two clearly distinguishable sites appeared to be TSA and L, as there was no competition by the relevant ligands for binding to these sites.

Sites TSA and L were therefore examined in our studies with isolated cilia; we confirmed their presence in the isolated cilia preparation

(Rhein and Cagan, 1980). Furthermore, L-threonine, L-serine and L-alanine are all mutually inhibitory, but L-lysine does not compete for binding of these ligands. Similarly, the former three amino acids do not inhibit L-lysine binding (Rhein and Cagan, 1983). Our studies therefore show the presence of at least two clearly distinguishable odorant-binding sites, which disproves the single-site hypothesis of Hara (1976). Detailed analysis of the competitive interactions has been carried out (Rhein and Cagan, 1983).

Summary

The mechanisms underlying initial recognition of odor stimuli by olfactory receptors have been of theoretical interest for many years, but relatively little experimental work has been done at the biochemical level. A major impediment has been the difficulty of identifying and establishing an experimental model with which to investigate the biochemical basis of odorant recognition.

Our approach has focused on the initial interaction by measuring binding of odorant compounds utilizing radiolabeled ligands. Our choice of the rainbow trout *Salmo gairdneri* as the experimental animal was predicated upon reports of its responsiveness to amino acids as olfactory stimuli. With terrestrial vertebrates, volatility is necessary for a compound to reach the olfactory organ. With fish, however, water solubility of the stimulus is to be expected. This confers a significant advantage for biochemical studies.

Binding assays are carried out *in vitro* by incubating the labeled ligand, under defined conditions, with the isolated receptor-containing preparation from the olfactory epithelium. We measured binding of a series of odorant amino acids to an isolated membrane-containing fraction prepared by differential centrifugation of a homogenate of the olfactory rosettes of the rainbow trout. The extent of binding parallels the reported stimulatory effectiveness measured electrophysiologically. More recently, we isolated cilia from the intact rosettes without homogenizing the tissue. We characterized the cilia biochemically and demonstrated that they bind odorant amino acids. Specific binding of odorant amino acids is saturable and reversible. Our evidence supports the hypothesis that the initial recognition of odor stimuli occurs upon binding to sites located on the cilia.

References

Amoore, J. E. (1970). *Molecular Basis of Odor.* Springfield, Ill.: Charles C. Thomas.

Bannister, L. H. (1965). The fine structure of the olfactory surface of teleostean fishes. *Q. Jl Microsc. Sci. 106:* 333–42.

Beets, M. G. J. (1978). *Structure–Activity Relationships in Human Chemoreception.* London: Applied Science Publishers, Ltd.

Bertmar, G. (1973). Ultrastructure of the olfactory mucosa in the homing Baltic sea trout *Salmo trutta trutta. Marine Biol. 19:* 74–88.

Bronshtein, A. A., and Minor, A. V. (1977). The regeneration of olfactory flagella and restoration of electroolfactogram after treatment of the olfactory mucosa with Triton X-100. *Tsitologiya USSR 19:* 33–9.

Brown, S. B., and Hara, T. J. (1981). Accumulation of chemostimulatory amino acids by a sedimentable fraction isolated from olfactory rosettes of rainbow trout (*Salmo gairdneri*). *Biochim. Biophys. Acta 675:* 149–62.

Cagan, R. H. (1971). Biochemical studies of taste sensation. I. Binding of ^{14}C-labeled sugars to bovine taste papillae. *Biochim. Biophys. Acta 252:* 199–206.

Cagan, R. H. (1974). Biochemistry of sweet sensation. In *Sugars in Nutrition*, ed. H. L. Sipple and K. W. McNutt, pp. 19–36. New York: Academic Press.

Cagan, R. H. (1979). Biochemical studies of taste sensation. VII. Enhancement of taste stimulus binding to a catfish taste receptor preparation by prior exposure to the stimulus. *J. Neurobiol. 10:* 207–20.

Cagan, R. H. (1981). Recognition of taste stimuli at the initial binding interaction. In *Biochemistry of Taste and Olfaction*, ed. R. H. Cagan and M. R. Kare, pp. 175–203. New York: Academic Press.

Cagan, R. H., and Boyle, A. G. (1978). Plasma membranes from taste receptor tissue: Isolation and binding activity. *Fedn. Proc. 37:* 1818 (Abstract).

Cagan, R. H., and Zeiger, W. N. (1978). Biochemical studies of olfaction: I. Binding specificity of radioactively labeled stimuli to an isolated olfactory preparation from rainbow trout (*Salmo gairdneri*). *Proc. Natn. Acad. Sci. USA 75:* 4679–83.

Cancalon, P. (1978). Isolation and characterization of the olfactory epithelial cells of the catfish. *Chem. Senses Flav. 3:* 381–96.

Cuatrecasas, P., and Hollenberg, M. D. (1976). Membrane receptors and hormone action. *Adv. Protein Chem. 30:* 251–451.

Dixon, M., and Webb, E. C. (1964). *Enzymes.* New York: Academic Press.

Dodd, G., and Persaud, K. (1981). Biochemical mechanisms in vertebrate primary olfactory neurons. In *Biochemistry of Taste and Olfaction*, ed. R. H. Cagan and M. R. Kare, pp. 333–57. New York: Academic Press.

Fesenko, E. E., Novoselov, V. I., and Krapivinskaya, L. D. (1979). Molecular mechanisms of olfactory reception. IV. Some biochemical characteristics of the camphor receptor from rat olfactory epithelium. *Biochim. Biophys. Acta 587:* 424–33.

Gemne, G., and Døving, K. B. (1969). Ultrastructural properties of primary olfactory neurons in fish (*Lota lota* L.). *Am. J. Anat. 126:* 457–75.

Gennings, J. N., Gower, D. B., and Bannister, L. H. (1977). Studies on the receptors to 5α-androst-16-en-3-one and 5α-androst-16-en-3α-ol in sow nasal mucosa. *Biochim. Biophys. Acta 496:* 547–56.

Getchell, M. L., and Gesteland, R. C. (1972). The chemistry of olfactory reception: stimulus-specific protection from sulfhydryl reagent inhibition. *Proc. Natn. Acad. Sci. USA 69:* 1494–8.

Gower, D. B., Hancock, M. R., and Bannister, L. H. (1981). Biochemical studies on the boar pheromones, 5α-androst-16-en-3-one and 5α-androst-16-en-3α-ol, and their metabolism by olfactory tissue. In *Biochemistry of Taste and Olfaction*, ed. R. H. Cagan and M. R. Kare, pp. 7–31. New York: Academic Press.

Hara, T. J. (1973). Olfactory responses to amino acids in rainbow trout, *Salmo gairdneri*. *Comp. Biochem. Physiol. 44A:* 407–16.

Hara, T. J. (1976). Structure-activity relationships of amino acids in fish olfaction. *Comp. Biochem. Physiol. 54A:* 31–6.

Hasler, A. D. (1960). Guideposts of migrating fishes. *Science 132:* 785–92.

Hasler, A. D., Scholz, A. T., and Horrall, R. M. (1978). Olfactory imprinting and homing in salmon. *Am. Sci. 66:* 347–55.

Ichikawa, M., and Ueda, K. (1977). Fine structure of the olfactory epithelium in the goldfish, *Carassius auratus*. A study of retrograde degeneration. *Cell & Tiss. Res. 183:* 445–55.

Kahn, C. R. (1976). Membrane receptors for hormones and neurotransmitters. *J. Cell Biol. 70:* 261–86.

Kleene, S. J., and Gesteland, R. C. (1981). Dissociation of frog olfactory epithelium with *N*-ethylmaleimide. *Brain Res. 229:* 536–40.

Krueger, J. M., and Cagan, R. H. (1976). Biochemical studies of taste sensation. IV. Binding of L-[^{3}H]alanine to a sedimentable fraction from catfish barbel epithelium. *J. Biol. Chem. 251:* 88–97.

Lowe, G. A., and MacLeod, N. K. (1975). The ultrastructural organization of olfactory epithelium of two species of gadoid fish. *J. Fish Biol. 7:* 529–32.

Linck, R. W. (1973). Comparative isolation of cilia and flagella from the lamellibranch mollusc, *Aequipecten irradians. J. Cell Sci. 12:* 345–67.

Novoselov, V. I., Krapivinskaya, L. D., and Fesenko, E. E. (1980). Molecular mechanisms of odor sensing. V. Some biochemical characteristics of the alanineous receptor from the olfactory epithelium of the skate *Dasyatis pastinaca. Chemical Senses 5:* 195–203.

Pelosi, P., Baldaccini, N. E., and Pisanelli, A. M. (1982). Identification of a specific olfactory receptor for 2-isobutyl-3-methoxypyrazine. *Biochem. J. 201:* 245–8.

Persaud, K., Pelosi, P., and Dodd, G. (1980). Binding of 5α-androstan-3-one to sheep olfactory mucosa. In *Olfaction and Taste VII*, ed. H. van der Starre, p. 101. Washington, D.C.: IRL Press, Ltd. (Abstract).

Rhein, L. D., and Cagan, R. H. (1980). Biochemical studies of olfaction: II. Isolation, characterization, and odorant binding activity of cilia from rainbow trout olfactory rosettes. *Proc. Natn. Acad. Sci. USA 77:* 4412–16.

Rhein, L. D., and Cagan, R. H. (1981). Role of cilia in olfactory recognition. In *Biochemistry of Taste and Olfaction*, ed. R. H. Cagan and M. R. Kare, pp. 47–68. New York: Academic Press.

Rhein, L. D., and Cagan, R. H. (1983). Biochemical studies of olfaction: III. Binding specificity of odorants to a cilia preparation from rainbow trout olfactory rosettes. *J. Neurochem. 41:* 569–77.

Rhein, L. D., Cagan, R. H., Orkand, P. M., and Dolack, M. K. (1981). Surface specializations of the olfactory epithelium of rainbow trout, *Salmo gairdneri. Tissue & Cell 13:* 577–87.

Sutterlin, A. M., and Sutterlin, N. (1971). Electrical responses of the olfactory epithelium of Atlantic salmon (*Salmo salar*). *J. Fish. Res. Bd Can. 28:* 565–72.

Tucker, D. (1967). Olfactory cilia are not required for olfactory function. *Fedn Proc. 26:* 544 (Abstract).

Watson, M. R., and Hopkins, J. M. (1962). Isolated cilia from *Tetrahymena pyriformis*. *Expl Cell Res. 28:* 280–95.

Yamamoto, M., and Ueda, K. (1977). Comparative morphology of fish olfactory epithelium. I. Salmoniformes. *Bull. Jap. Soc. Sci. Fish. 43:* 1163–74.

Yamamura, H. I., Enna, S. J., and Kuhar, M. J., eds (1978). *Neurotransmitter Receptor Binding*. New York: Raven Press.

Zeiger, W. N., and Cagan, R. H. (1975). Biochemistry of olfactory specificity. Binding of labeled stimuli to a preparation from olfactory epithelium. *Am. Chem. Soc., 169th Natn. Meet., Philadelphia*, Abstr. no. 8.

2.5

Pheromone biology in the Lepidoptera: overview, some recent findings and some generalizations

DIETRICH SCHNEIDER

Pheromones are defined as odorous intraspecific communication signals, which are produced by one or both sexes (Karlson and Lüscher, 1959). The different types of pheromones are named according to their biological functions: sexual attractants, aphrodisiacs, assembly scents, alarm substances, trail substances, etc. The first pheromone, which was chemically identified, was the sexual attractant of the silkworm moth *Bombyx mori* (Butenandt, Beckmann, Stamm and Hecker, 1959). In the meantime, numerous female moth attractants have been identified, mainly under the assumption that they may be useful as elements of a biological pest control (for some more recent insect-pheromone overviews see: Birch, 1974; Priesner, 1973; Schneider, 1980, 1984; Shorey, 1977; Silverstein and Young, 1977; Steinbrecht and Schneider, 1980; Tamaki, 1977; Brand, Young and Silverstein, 1979).

The presently available information on the pheromone biology in the butterflies and moths allows one to distinguish between the *female pheromones* of most moth (and perhaps some butterfly) species and of *male odour* signals which may, or may not, be pheromones. The biological meaning of the female signals is mainly the longer-distance attraction of the males, where the odour signal is in reality the basic 'behaviour command' for the male to approach the odour source by a visually controlled anemotaxis (Kramer, 1975, 1978; Preiss and Kramer, 1982). The pheromone biology of the Lepidoptera is displayed in condensed form in Table 1.

Female moth lure odour and male responses

The scent-producing organs of female moths are mostly specialized glandular areas of the epidermis under the cuticle between the 8th

301

Table 1. *Pheromones of Lepidoptera:*
biological meaning, production, dissipation,
reception, and processing

	♀ Lepidoptera pheromones ♂	
Meaning	reproduction and reproductive isolation	seduction, attraction, competition
glands at	abdominal tip	all body parts
chemistry	lipoids	no rule
components	(1) 2–5	(1) – many
weight/gland	< μg	> μg
production	mostly when calling	before use; one charge only (?)
biosynthesis	*de novo*	*de novo* and precursors
exposure	long hours	short or long
receptors on	♂ antenna only	♀ and ♂ antennae
receptor cells for	each component	?
molecular catch-capacity, threshold	extreme to moderate	moderate
CNS-processing	via macroglomerulus	via 'normal' glomeruli in olfactory brain

and the 9th abdominal segments (Barth, 1960). These organs – typical in *Bombyx* – can be expanded into 'calling' position by hemolymph pressure (Steinbrecht, 1964). Some arctiid moths possess tubular lure glands which reach deeply into the female body but cannot be evaginated. These females call by a pumping ventilation of such tubes (Conner et al., 1980).

The one, two or more components of the female attracting scents function in an additive way. In some cases, the anemotactic behaviour is elicited only if the components are emitted in a rather exact ratio, such as 80/20 (Minks, Roelofs, Ritter and Persoons, 1973). Originally, when the *Bombyx* attractant alcohol (E-10, Z-12-hexadecadien-1-ol = Bombykol) was the only identified pheromone, one assumed that the females of each species would only produce their single, private, attracting compound and that, consequently, all moth species would have different attractants. In the following years, more and more species with two-to-three component attractants became known and different, often closely related species were found to share lure substances, e.g. species A with components a, b, c, and species B with components a, c, d. By this, cross-attraction of sympatric species can in principle be avoided, particularly if the components elicit the male up-wind flight only if they are presented in the proper ratio. In quite a number of moth species, one now even finds components in the female emanation which play no rôle in the attraction of the males of this species, but which inhibit males of 'neighbouring' species which may without this inhibiting component mistake the first species' lure odour for that of his own female (Priesner, 1977, 1980; Silverstein and Young, 1977). Even in *Bombyx* a second component (Bombykal) was found, which might also serve such a function (Kaissling et al., 1978; Kasang, Kaissling, Vostrowsky and Bestmann, 1978).

A particularly striking and now partially understood case of attraction and inhibition between closely related species has now been studied in my laboratory. The gypsy- and the nun-moth (*Lymantria dispar* and *L. monacha*) live with overlapping diel activity rhythms sympatrically in parts of Europe. Both share the female attractant 'disparlure' (2-methyl-(Z)-7,8-epoxy-octadecan). This substance may occur in two different chiral (optically active) or enantiomeric forms (here now called: (+)- and (−)-disparlure) which are available in 98% optically-pure synthetic form (Iwaki et al., 1974; Mori, Takigawa and Matsu, 1976). Nobody, so far, knows which optical form of disparlure these two female moth species produce. Our approach to this problem made use of the recording technique from single pheromone-odour receptor cells which are located on the male antennae. Already in earlier experiments, I found in collaboration with M. Boppré (unpublished, see also Schneider, 1980) that males of both species possess odour-receptor cells with a specific affinity for the (+)-disparlure. Recently, Kurt Hansen (unpublished) continued this work and has now nearly clarified this puzzle. He found that the gypsy-moth male possesses two types of disparlure-receptor cells, one for the (+)- and one for the (−)-enantiomer. However, on the male nun-moth antenna, he only found receptors for the (+)-disparlure. This explains to some extent the results of field trapping experiments with these two important forest defoliating species: gypsy-moths' attraction is maximal with (+)-disparlure alone and progressively less effective with (−)-disparlure added; trapping of nun-moths is also only possible with (+)-disparlure, but here, the addition of the (−)-enantiomer is without effect (for literature see Schneider, 1984). The reason why the chirality of the gland products of the females is unknown is that the presently available analytical (polarimetric) chemical methods are inadequate for the tiny amounts of substances produced by even reasonable numbers of *Lymantria* females. However, as in other cases, our recordings allow predictions as to which enantiomer a female moth produces. Here, Hansen (1984) compared the excitatory effects of the female gland extracts of the two species with those of the synthetic enantiomers. These recordings indicate that the female nun-moth produces approximately 90% (−)-

and 10% (+)-disparlure, while the female gypsy-moth only (or mainly) produces (+)-disparlure. These observations can explain why the male gypsy-moths do not care for the calling female nun-moth (too much inhibitor involved!), but the male nun-moths, which only care for the (+)-enantiomer, should also approach a calling female gypsy-moth. This, however, has never been observed in nature and even in captivity, the nun-moth males care very little for the gypsy females. Part of the answer to this remaining mystery might be the partial difference of the diel activity rhythms of the two species (see Schröter, 1976). As always in such cases, we try with our recordings to predict further pheromone components in the female glands, which the chemists have not yet found, but in these two species so far we have been unsuccessful.

Generally speaking, the chemistry of the female moths' lure substances is somewhat monotonous. Standard attractants have between 7 and 21 carbon atoms, are straight-chain compounds, and usually have between one and three (sometimes conjugated) double bonds and some epoxides. The polarity of the substances varies: there are alcohols, aldehydes and esters (acetates).

In 1953, the nearly unknown function of odour receptors was the challenge which led me to try my electrophysiological techniques on the male *Bombyx* antenna, really not knowing that this was the beginning of a long-lasting occupation. The 1982 facit of some of the studies on female moth pheromone biology done in my laboratory and also elsewhere, is this: female moths produce their lure odour bouquet in pico- and nanogram amounts, barely reaching microgram-contents in some species. The males in some groups (striking examples are the Lymantriidae, Saturniidae, Bombycidae) have rather large, comb-structured antennae with up to 50 000 receptor hairs for the attractant. These hairs are supplied by the dendritic receptorial endings of the pheromone-component-specific receptor cells (Schneider and Kaissling, 1957; Boeckh, Kaissling and Schneider, 1960; Schneider and Steinbrecht, 1968; Steinbrecht, 1970). The antennae are built to catch up to one-third of the odour molecules from the air which passes through these organs. The molecules are adsorbed on the hair surface, then diffuse from here through cuticular pores and tubules of the hair wall into the hair lumen and then, presumably, to the membranous receptors of the dendrite (Steinbrecht and Kasang, 1972). This causes the generation of local receptor potentials and consequent nerve impulses (summaries by Kaissling, 1971; Schneider, 1980, 1984).

Each receptor cell neurite independently sends its impulse message to the olfactory lobe in the deuto-cerebrum (Steinbrecht, 1969). The

Bombyx male has approximately 15000 receptors for bombykol (the attractant) and an equal number of receptors for the corresponding bombykal (a substance which inhibits the male moth if presented in more than natural concentrations) (Steinbrecht, 1970, 1973; Kaissling, 1979). The fibres of these receptor nerve cells end in a male-specific macroglomerular complex in the olfactory brain (M. Koontz, unpublished). A few hundred secondary fibres (interneurons or relay-neurons) respond in a complex manner to bombykol and bombykal, some in addition also respond to air currents and light (R. M. Olberg; D. M. Light, unpublished). – Descending neurons in the thoracic nerve cord show activity when the animals are stimulated with odour currents and/or light. This activity can be related to behavioural reactions such as antennal movements and turns of the animal (R. M. Olberg, 1983).

The single 'dark-adapted' receptor cells for bombykol respond to impacts of single bombykol molecules with an elementary receptor potential and a nerve impulse (Kaissling and Priesner, 1970; Kaissling, 1974, 1979). We have little doubt that many or most pheromone receptor cells in other moth species can also be activated by the hit of single adequate molecules, although this has never been proven. In *Bombyx*, the activation of several hundred bombykol receptor cells per second suffices to elicit the first behaviour reactions. In this threshold situation, the air which passes through the antenna with its branches and many hairs contains approximately 1000 bombykol molecules cm^{-3} (Kaissling and Priesner, 1970).

Although the individual receptor cells in most moths may be as sensitive as the *Bombyx* cells, the majority of moths with their rod- or whip-shaped antennae and the now necessarily reduced molecule-catching capacity (Boeckh et al., 1965; Kaissling, 1971) will need many more than just 1000 pheromone cm^{-3} of air to eventually overcome the receptor noise (Kaissling and Priesner, 1970), in order to convey a meaningful message to the 'behaviour-controlling centre' in the brain.

One would now expect that those species which developed slender antennae overcome this reduced catching capacity by higher pheromone production rates in the female, but this seems not to be the case. Consequently, these females are able to lure their partner only over a distance much shorter than the hundreds of metres or even a kilometre claimed for saturniids and some other groups.

The system of female moth lure and male moth response is in my view characterized by the relatively small amounts of attractant pheromone produced. In some cases (*Bombyx*, *Lymantria*, saturniids) the males developed large antennae, seemingly to improve the sensitivity and by this the effective range of the plume of the female odour. If the females were 'interested' to expand this range, one wonders, why do they not produce more attractant? That this can in principle be done is apparent from the male scent glands. What then is the adaptive value of this female 'coyness', or are they selecting their male partners for their ability to track them? But it could, of course, be that we badly underestimate the productivity of the female lure glands. New measurements of the glandular emanations of calling gypsy-moths indicate a rather high productivity. A rough estimate shows that such females evaporate during one daily calling period as much attractant as the total amount eluted by the chemists during the analysis of glands (see Richerson and Cameron, 1974; Charlton and Cardé, 1982).

A final comment to this system: female moths' attractants are odourless to the human nose – and to the female moth herself (Schneider, 1957)! This is a nuisance for the experimenter and looks like an expression of 'arrogance' by the female moth, since she seems to say: 'I have no need for a sensory control of my attractivity!'

Male scent production and responses by both sexes

In many species of butterflies and moths, the males possess a great variety of structures with a proven or at least very probable scent-producing function. Many of these are complex, eversible organs (Barth, 1960; Birch, 1970, 1974, 1979) of sometimes spectacular size and in some species they are even brightly coloured. One finds such organs on nearly all parts of the male body: antennae, legs, wings, thorax and abdomen. The mechanisms of eversion are either mechanical (by leverage or connected to wing-movements) or hydraulic/pneumatic in the cases of tubular organs, which are evaginated when used. Less-spectacular scent-producing scales are found in bands, patches, pouches or even covering large parts of the wing. The glandular function and odour production of such scales can only be ascertained by microscopic and chemical analysis and the corresponding behavioural tests.

The function of the male scents is understood in only a few cases. The males of some noctuid and arctiid moths and of the danaine butterflies display their hairbrushes to the female to initiate the final courtship phase. In these cases, the male odour can be understood as an aphrodisiac which also serves for the identification of the conspecific male. Since in some female moths one finds that they would fly off unless the male displays, these pheromones have also been called arresting scents.

In quite a number of cases, one finds not only the normal odour transfer, but in addition pheromone transfer-particles (hair or scale fragments) which are disseminated when the male 'hair-pencils' his female. In the danaine butterflies such particles stick to the female antennae because they are impregnated not only with pheromone but also with a sticky diol which keeps the aphrodisiac odour on the female's nose, even after the end of the male's display (Pliske and Eisner, 1969; Schneider and Seibt, 1969; Boppré, 1978, 1979).

In these relatively well studied danaines (the milkweed butterflies) males of many species contained one and/or several types of dihydropyrrolizines (heterocyclic, N-containing substances) as key elements of the male scent bouquet (Meinwald et al., 1966, 1974; Meinwald, Meinwald and Mazzocchi, 1969; Petty, Boppré, Schneider and Meinwald, 1977). These compounds – one of which was also found in the two arctiid genera *Utetheisa* and *Creatonotos* (Culvenor and Edgar, 1972; Conner et al., 1981; Schneider et al., 1982) – cannot be biosynthesized *de novo* in the insect body. It was found that they are made from pyrrolizidine alkaloids (esters) which occur in some plant groups, where they seem to be an element of chemical protection against herbivores. A number of arctiid moth larvae overcome the toxicity of such plants and feed on them. They are now themselves protected against predators and seem not to metabolize the substances but to store them and even pass them on to the pupa and the moth. From this stock of alkaloids, the male moths then synthesize their dihydropyrrolizine pheromone. The uptake of this pheromone precursor is much more complicated in the danaines. They find dry alkaloid plants, guided by their olfactory system, then wet the plant surface by a fluid through their proboscis and suck the alkaloid solution up (Schneider et al., 1975; Edgar, Boppré and Schneider, 1979; Boppré, 1981). Unless this access to alkaloids is allowed either through the larval food or to the adult, no dihydropyrrolizine pheromone is produced. In some danaines (genera *Danaus* and probably also *Amauris*) one more requirement for the pheromone biosynthesis must be fulfilled: the male insects have to contact glandular scale patches or pouches on their hindwings with their abdominal hairbrushes to 'complete' the pheromone biosynthesis. Details of this process are not yet known (Boppré, Petty, Schneider and Meinwald, 1978; Boppré, 1979).

In general, little is known of the chemistry of male moth and butterfly odours. There are reports on quite a number of fatty acids and 'aromatic' compounds in male moth's hairbrushes (see Birch, 1974; Priesner, 1973). Recently (Schäfer and Schneider, unpublished) we found alpha-keto-butyric acid in microgram amounts in the hairpencils of the freshly emerged noctuid *Bene fagana* L., a penetrating 'soup-spice' odour for the human nose. As always with the male odours, there are receptors for this compound on the antennae of both sexes, but so far nothing is known of the biological meaning in this case. Interestingly, the odour reminds us of that of the umbelliferous plant 'lovage' (*Levisticum officinale* L.), but this plant is not the larval foodplant of *Bene*.

With respect to just this question of the 'meaning' of male lepidopteran scents, evidence is now slowly accumulating that these odours in many cases do not simply function as aphrodisiacs (typically in *Danaus gilippus* and *Utetheisa* spp., see Pliske and Eisner, 1969; Conner et al., 1981) but are elements of much more complicated communication systems. Recently a most striking report on the behaviour of the arctiid moth *Estigmene acrea* (Willis and Birch, 1982) illustrated what I mean. The males of this species possess abdominal hairy tubes (coremata) which presumably produce an odorant. After sunset, the males evaginate these structures when sitting on the tips of vegetation. Soon (by odorous attraction??) a number of males assemble and all of them start 'calling'. Now also females fly in, crawl up to the males, which now pull their coremata in, and mating begins. Such male assembly and female attraction to them is called lekking (for reference see Willis and Birch, 1982). Later at night, when the described male-induced assembling is over, those females which are still virgins begin calling and now *Estigmene* males fly in and mate without any coremata display, as in most other species of moths.

In two arctiid species which we study (*Creatonotos gangis* and *C. transiens*) the giant pneumatic coremata contain also the same pyrrolizine as *Utetheisa* and, again, its production depends upon the uptake of precursor by the larva. To our surprise – and this was totally unknown before in any other insect – the formation of the coremata, the morphogenesis, was quantitatively dependent on the amount of alkaloid precursor consumed by the last instar larva: tiny, barely visible coremata without alkaloid and coremata as big as the moth after plenty of alkaloid in the larval diet (Schneider et al., 1982). The preference of the larva for alkaloid plants and even pure alkaloid in crystal form was striking.

Until recently, we were uncertain about the biological meaning of this male odour system in *Creatonotos*, although the antennae of both species and sexes do have receptor cells for the odour of the coremata. Our still incomplete recent behaviour studies in the laboratory, however, indicate similarities to *Estigmene* because the males do also display their odour-dissipating organs after sunset with or without calling females in their neighbourhood (unpublished observations by Boppré, Hansen, Schneider and H. Wunderer). Possibly, this is also a lek. If male corema odour is blown to isolated females, they are activated and start an upwind flight as the males do to females unless they are just themselves calling in a lek. There are quite a number of still-unknown essentials in this system, particularly also with respect to the meaning of the morphogenesis. Males with small coremata and without their odour might join a lek, but would not attract other males or females, but later, they mate as effectively as their odour-producing brothers. Odourless males are also 'fertile'. Nothing is known about the field behaviour of this tropical forest species, except that field-caught males also show a variety of coremata sizes. With respect to mate selection it has been proposed by Eisner (1980) (see also Rutowsky, 1981) that the smell of the male coremata might indicate to the females whether they are dealing with a chemically well-protected or not so well-protected male. In a way, such proposed female behaviour would in the sense of natural selection operate in parallel to predation: selection favours the content of the pheromone and/or its precursor. So far, it has not yet been shown whether the female moths prefer to mate with the best stinkers (incidentally, these pyrrolizines are odourless to the human nose).

Odours of the less-spectacular male butterfly scent scales have been chemically identified in only a few cases. In *Colias*, closely related sympatric species have different scale scents on the male wings and seem to use this for reproductive isolation (Grula, McChesney and Taylor, 1980).

Generalizing, one may say that some odours of the male Lepidoptera are known so far to be aphrodisiacs, some serve for species recognition, others facilitate the forming of leks and are then also attracting signals for the females and males; and I think male odours might also act as signals for such male–male interaction as competition or even territorial display.

The amount of odour produced by male Lepidoptera seems to be between 100 and 1000 times more than in the female moths. Danaines and *Creatonotos* scent-producing organs contain about 0.5 mg, and microgram amounts are found in other cases. Further, male odours can be detected by specific receptors in both sexes of a given species which is, of course, necessary in the case of male–male signals and in the case of leks. But why so much odour, particularly since often (but not so in leks?) these odours are used only for short-distance communication? It is difficult to speculate on this question. If – in the case of the calling female moth – one argues that they dissipate minute amounts of odour in order to reach only the best-performing males, one may by the same token also say that minute amounts of a given aphrodisiac should make sure that the males seduce only the most sensitive females. Although such contemplations on the biological meaning of these fascinating communication mechanisms are probably helpful, one must be careful with too simplistic explanations. One should also never forget that this chemical communication behaviour, particularly in the case of the male Lepidoptera, is often intricately combined with stimuli of other sensory modalities, particularly vision. Therefore, while (gladly) speculating, we should never forget how far we mostly are from an understanding of the adaptive values of the respective structures and functions.

References

Barth, R. (1960). *Órgãos odoríferos dos Lepidópteros*. Boletin Número 7, Parque Nacional do Itataia, Rio de Janeiro: Ministério da Agricultura Serviço Florestal.

Birch, M. C. (1970). Pre-courtship use of abdominal brushes by males of the nocturnal moth, *Phlogophora meticulosa* (Lepidoptera: Noctuidae). *Anim. Behav. 18:* 310–16.

Birch, M. C., ed. (1974). *Pheromones*. Amsterdam, London, New York: Elsevier/North-Holland.

Birch, M. C. (1979). Eversible structures. In *Moths and Butterflies of Great Britain and Ireland*, vol. *9*, Sphingidae-Noctuidae, ed. J. Heath and A. M. Emmet, pp. 9–18. London: Curwen Books.

Boeckh, J., Kaissling, K. -E., and Schneider, D. (1960). Sensillen und Bau der Antennengeissel von *Telea polyphemus* (Vergleiche mit weiteren Saturniiden: *Antheraea, Platysamia* und *Philosamia*). *Zool. Jb. (Anat.). 78:* 559–84.

Boeckh, J., Kaissling, K.-E., and Schneider, D. (1965). *Insect Olfactory Receptors. Cold Spring Harb. Symp. Quant. Biol. 30:* 263–80.

Boppré, M. (1978). Chemical communication, plant relationships, and mimicry in the evolution of danaid butterflies. *Entomologia Exp. Appl. 24:* 264–77.

Boppré, M. (1979). *Untersuchungen zur Pheromonbiologie bei Monarchfaltern (Danaidae)*. Dissertation Universität München, Fakultät Biologie.

Boppré, M. (1981). Adult Lepidoptera feeding at withered *Heliotropium* plants (Boraginaceae) in East Africa. *Ecol. Entomol. 6:* 449–52.

Boppré, M., Petty, R. L., Schneider, D., and Meinwald, J. (1978). Behaviorally mediated contacts between scent organs: another prerequisite for pheromone production in *Danaus chrysippus* males (Lepidoptera). *J. Comp. Physiol. 126:* 97–103.

Brand, J. M., Young, J. C., and Silverstein, R. M. (1979). Insect pheromones: a critical review of recent advances in their chemistry, biology, and application. *Prog. Chem. Org. Nat. Prod. 37:* 1–190.

Butenandt, A., Beckmann, R., Stamm, D., and Hecker, E. (1959). Über den Sexuallockstoff des Seidenspinners *Bombyx mori*. Reindarstellung und Konstitution. *Z. Naturf. 14b:* 283–4.

Charlton, R. E., and Cardé, R. T. (1982). Rate and diel periodicity of pheromone emission from female gypsy moths (*Lymantria dispar*) determined with a glass-adsorption collection system. *J. Insect Physiol. 28:* 423–30.

Conner, W. E., Eisner, T., Van der Meer, R. K., Guerrero, A., Ghiringelli, D., and Meinwald, J. (1980). Sex attractant of an arctiid moth (*Utetheisa ornatrix*): a pulsed chemical signal. *Behav. Ecol. Sociobiol. 7:* 55–63.

Conner, W. E., Eisner, T., Van der Meer, A., Guerrero, A., and Meinwald, J. (1981). Precopulatory sexual interaction in an arctiid moth (*Utetheisa ornatrix*): role of a pheromone derived from dietary alkaloids. *Behav. Ecol. Sociobiol. 9:* 227.

Culvenor, C. C. J., and Edgar, J. A. (1972). Dihydropyrrolizidine secretion associated with coremata of *Utetheisa* moths (family Arctiidae). *Experientia 28:* 627–8.

Edgar, J. A., Boppré, M., and Schneider, D. (1979). Pyrrolizidine alkaloid storage in African and Australian danaid butterflies. *Experientia 35:* 1447–8.

Eisner, T. (1980). Chemistry, defense and survival: case studies and selected topics. In *Insect Biology of the Future*, ed. D. Smith and M. Locke, pp. 847–78. London and New York: Academic Press.

Grula, J. W., McChesney, J. D., and Taylor Jr., O. R. (1980). Aphrodisiac pheromones of the sulfur butterfly *Colias eurytheme* and *C. philodice* (Lepidoptera, Pieridae). *J. Chem. Ecol. 6:* 241–56.

Hansen, K. (1984). Discrimination and production of disparlure enantiomers by the gypsy moth and nun moth. *Physiol. Entomol.*, in press.

Iwaki, S., Marumo, S., Saito, T., Yamada, M., and Katagiri, K. (1974). Synthesis and activity of optically active disparlure. *J. Am. Chem. Soc. 96:* 7842–4.

Kaissling, K.-E. (1971). Insect olfaction. In *Handbook of Sensory Physiology*, vol. IV, Chemical Senses, part 1, Olfaction and Taste, ed. L. M. Beidler, pp. 351–431. Berlin, Heidelberg, New York: Springer-Verlag.

Kaissling, K.-E. (1974). Sensory transduction in insect olfactory receptors. In *Biochemistry of Sensory Functions*, ed. L. Jaenicke, 25. Moosbacher Colloquium der Gesellschaft für Biologische Chemie, pp. 243–73. Berlin, Heidelberg, New York: Springer-Verlag.

Kaissling, K.-E. (1979). Recognition of pheromones by moths, especially in saturniids and *Bombyx mori*. In *Chemical Ecology: Odour Communication in Animals*, ed. F. J. Ritter, pp. 43–56. Amsterdam: Elsevier/North-Holland Biomedical Press.

Kaissling, K.-E., Kasang, G., Bestmann, H. J., Stansky, W., and Vostrowsky, O. (1978). A new pheromone of the silkworm moth *Bombyx mori*. Sensory pathway and behavioral effect. *Naturwissenschaften 65:* 382–4.

Kaissling, K.-E., and Priesner, E. (1970). Die Riechschwelle des Seidenspinners. *Naturwissenschaften 57:* 23–8.

Karlson, P., and Lüscher, M. (1959). 'Pheromones', a new term for a class of biologically active substances. *Nature 183:* 55–6.

Kasang, G., Kaissling, K.-E., Vostrowsky, O., and Bestmann, H. J. (1978). Bombykal, eine zweite Pheromonkomponente des Seidenspinners *Bombyx mori*. *Angew. Chem. 90:* 74–5.

Kramer, E. (1975). Orientation of the male silkmoth to the sex attractant bombykol. In *Olfaction and Taste V*, ed. D. A. Denton and J. P. Coghlan, pp. 329–35. New York, San Francisco, London: Academic Press.

Kramer, E. (1978). Insect pheromones. In *Taxis and Behaviour* (Receptors and Recognition, ser. B, vol. 5), ed. G. L. Hazelbauer, pp. 207–29. London: Chapman and Hall.

Meinwald, J., Boriack, C. J., Schneider, D., Boppré, M., Wood, W. F., and Eisner, T. (1974). Volatile ketones in the hairpencil secretion of danaid butterflies (*Amauris* and *Danaus*). *Experientia 30:* 721–2.

Meinwald, J., Meinwald, Y. C., and Mazzocchi, P. H. (1969). Sex pheromone of the queen butterfly: chemistry. *Science 164:* 1174–5.

Meinwald, J., Meinwald, Y. C., Wheeler, J. W., Eisner, T., and Brower, L. P. (1966). Major component in the exocrine secretion of a male butterfly (*Lycorea*). *Science 151:* 583–5.

Minks, A. K., Roelofs, W. L., Ritter, F. J. and Persoons, C. J. (1973). Reproductive isolation of two tortricid moth species by different ratios of a two-component sex attractant. *Science 180:* 1073–4.

Mori, K., Takigawa, T., and Matsu, M. (1976). Stereoselective synthesis of optically active disparlure, the pheromone of the gypsy moth (*Porthetria dispar*). *Tetrahedron Lett. 44:* 3953–6.

Olberg, R. M. (1983). Pheromone-triggered flip-flopping interneurons in the ventral nerve cord of the silkworm moth, *Bombyx mori*. *J. Comp. Physiol. 152:* 297–307.

Petty, R. L., Boppré, M., Schneider, D., and Meinwald, J. (1977). Identification of volatile hairpencil components in male *Amauris ochlea* butterflies (Danaidae). *Experientia 33:* 1324–6.

Pliske, T. E., and Eisner, T. (1969). Sex pheromone of the queen butterfly: biology. *Science 164:* 1170–2.

Preiss, R., and Kramer, E. (1982). Stabilization of altitude and speed in tethered flying gypsy moth males: influence of (+)- and (−)-dispature. *Physiol. Entomol.* (in press).

Priesner, E. (1973). Artspezifität und Funktion einiger Insektenpheromone. *Fortschr. Zool. 22:* 49–135.

Priesner, E. (1977). Evolutionary potential of specialized olfactory receptors. In *Olfaction and Taste VI*, ed. J. Le Magnen and P. MacLeod, pp. 333–41. London, Washington D. C.: Information Retrieval.

Priesner, E. (1980). Sensory encoding of pheromone signals and related stimuli in male moths. In *Insect Neurobiology and Insecticide Action* (Neurotox 79), pp. 359–66. London: Society of Chemical Industry.

Richerson, J. V., and Cameron, E. A. (1974). Differences in pheromone release and sexual behaviour between laboratory-reared and wild gypsy moth adults. *Environ. Entomol. 3:* 475–81.

Rutowsky, R. (1981). Mate choice and lepidopteran mating behaviour. *Florida Entomologist 65:* 72–81.

Schneider, D. (1957). Elektrophysiologische Untersuchungen von Chemo- und Mechanorezeptoren der Antenne des Seidenspinners *Bombyx mori* L. *Z. vergl. Physiol. 40:* 8–41.

Schneider, D. (1980). Pheromone von Insekten: Produktion – Rezeption – Inaktivierung. *Nova Acta Leopoldina*, N.F. *51:* No. 237, 249–78.

Schneider, D. (1984). Insect olfaction – our research endeavour. In *Foundations of the Sensory Sciences*, ed. W. Dawson and E. J. Enoch (in press). Heidelberg: Springer-Verlag.

Schneider, D., Boppré, M., Schneider, H., Thompson, W. R., Boriack, C. J., Petty, R. L., and Meinwald, J. (1975). A pheromone precursor and its uptake in male *Danaus* butterflies. *J. Comp. physiol. 97:* 245–56.

Schneider, D., Boppré, M., Zweig, J., Horsley, S. B., Bell, T. W., Meinwald, J., Hansen, K., and Diehl, E. W. (1982). Scent organ development in *Creatonotos* moths: regulation by pyrrolizidine alkaloids. *Science 215:* 1264–5.

Schneider, D., and Kaissling, K.-E. (1957). Der Bau der Antenne des Seidenspinners *Bombyx mori* L. II. Sensillen, cuticulare Bildungen und innerer Bau. *Zool. Jb. (Anat.)* 76: 223–50.

Schneider, D., and Seibt, U. (1969). Sex pheromone of the queen butterfly: electroantennogram responses. *Science 164:* 1173–4.

Schneider, D., Steinbrecht, R. A. (1968). Checklist of insect olfactory sensilla. *Symp. Zool. Soc. Lond. 23:* 279–97.

Schröter, H. (1976). *Lymantria (Porthetria): Isolationsmechanismen im Paarungsverhalten von Nonne und Schwammspinner.* Dissertation Universität Freiburg/Breisgau, Forstwissenschaftliche Fakultät.

Shorey, H. H. (1971). *Animal Communication by Pheromones.* New York, London: Academic Press.

Silverstein, R. M., and Young, J. C. (1977). Insects generally use multicomponent pheromones. In *Pest Management with Insect Sex Attractants and other Behavior-Controlling Chemicals,* ed. M. Beroza, pp. 1–29. Washington: *Am. Chem. Soc. Symp., Ser. 23.*

Steinbrecht, R. A. (1964). Feinstruktur und Histochemie der Sexualduftdrüse des Seidenspinners *Bombyx mori* L. *Z. Zellforsch. mikrosk. Anat. 64:* 227–61.

Steinbrecht, R. A. (1969). On the question of nervous syncytia: lack of axon fusion in two insect sensory nerves, *J. Cell Sci. 4:* 39–53.

Steinbrecht, R. A. (1970). Zur Morphometrie der Antennen des Seidenspinners *Bombyx mori* L.: Zahl und Verteilung der Riechsensillen (Insecta, Lepidoptera). *Z. Morphol. Tiere, 68:* 93–126.

Steinbrecht, R. A. (1973). Der Feinbau olfaktorischer Sensillen des Seidenspinners (Insecta, Lepidoptera). *Z. Zellforsch. mikrosk. Anat. 139:* 533–65.

Steinbrecht, R. A., and Kasang, G. (1972). Capture and conveyance of odour molecules in an insect olfactory receptor. In *Olfaction and Taste IV*, ed. D. Schneider, pp. 193–9. Stuttgart: Wissenschaftliche Verlagsgesellschaft.

Steinbrecht, R. A., and Schneider, D. (1980). Pheromone communication in moths: sensory physiology and behaviour. In *Insect Biology of the Future*, ed. M. Locke and D. Smith, pp. 685–703. London: Academic Press.

Tamaki, Y. (1977). Complexity, diversity, and specificity of behaviour-modifying chemicals in Lepidoptera and Diptera. In *Chemical Control of Insect Behavior*, ed. H. H. Shorey and J. J. McKelvey Jr, pp. 253–86. New York: Wiley & Sons – Interscience.

Willis, M. A., and Birch, M. C. (1982). Male lekking and female calling in the same population of the arctiid moth, *Estigmene acraea. Science 216* (in press).

This chapter is dedicated to my colleague, Martin C. Birch, of Oxford University.

2.6

Comparative study of electrophysiological phenomena in the olfactory bulb of some South American marsupials and edentates

JORGE MARIO AFFANNI and LORENZO GARCIA SAMARTINO

The olfactory bulb (OB) has an obvious importance in olfactory sensation and discrimination: for this reason the study of its physiological features is an excellent way of acquiring knowledge about them.

The study of the electrical activity of the OB is one of the most direct and powerful means of obtaining information about it. Three kinds of electrical activities have been described in the mammalian OB, namely: (i) Slow potentials (Ottoson, 1954, 1959a,b), (ii) intrinsic activity (Adrian, 1950); and (iii) sinusoidal activity (Adrian, 1950). These three kinds of activity become particularly interesting in all sorts of experimental conditions in which the OB is used as an experimental model. The same happens when the physiological basis of olfactory sensation and discrimination, or when the 'non-olfactory' functions (Alberts and Friedman, 1972; Murphy, 1976) are investigated.

The study of the influence of peripheral and central inputs to the OB reveal that the three activities are modified in different ways by the suppression of bulbar peripheral and central connections. Thus, slow activity is suppressed by destruction of the olfactory mucosa (OM) (Vaccarezza, Santamarina and García Medina, 1975). Section of the olfactory peduncle (OP) has produced no clear results, the existence of a central influence on the slow waves being still controversial (Vaccarezza et al., 1975). On the other hand, the generation of 'intrinsic' activity needs neither peripheral nor central connections (Adrian, 1950; Gerard and Young, 1937).

Sinusoidal activity disappears in chronic and wakeful preparations after destruction of the OM. This fact was interpreted as proof that peripheral input was essential for its generation. Contrarily, interruption of central connections in chronic and wakeful preparations do not

315

abolish it, but only modify it (Affanni, Morita and García Samartino, 1968). Again, this was interpreted as proof that central input is not essential for its generation.

Both marsupials and edentates are particularly suitable for studying the electrical activity of the olfactory bulb because of the great development of that structure and others related to olfaction which represent a relatively large proportion of the total brain volume. They combine admirably a large brain size with considerably primitive and 'schematic' brain features (Loo, 1930, 1931; Howe, 1933).

Comparative studies often reveal new aspects of physiological problems. As will be seen in this paper, the use of the edentate and marsupial OB as an experimental model has allowed us to add new facts that modify some current views on the role played by the peripheral and central inputs to the OB. Thus, in addition to the three already well-known electrical activities we could observe a fourth one, namely an electrical rhythm of 8–12 Hz in both the opossum and in the armadillo, which needs the convergence of peripheral and central inputs. Furthermore, we could observe in the armadillo the existence of sinusoidal waves which do not need peripheral input to the bulb being centrally determined.

Methods

One-hundred-and-seventy-four male armadillos (*Chaetophractus villosus*, 2.350–3.500 kg) and one-hundred-and-seventy-four male opossums (*Didelphis albiventris*, 3.000–3.500 kg) were used. They were all chronically implanted with stainless steel electrodes insulated except at the tips. The electrodes were placed over the surface of the main olfactory bulbs. Recording of the electrical activity was made on a NIHON-KHODEN Poligraph.

The OM was destroyed in some animals by using zinc sulphate (ZS) perfusion (Winans and Powers, 1977) and in others by surgical removal aided by topical application of silver nitrate. Tracheal tubes were of two different designs according to the method of Gault and Coustan (1965). In both cases the tubes permitted the animals either to (1) breathe normally through the nose ('nose position'), or (2) breathe directly through the trachea with little or no air flowing through the nose ('throat position'). Nasal insufflation in curarized animals was made through a plastic tube inserted into the nose. *The experiments of part I were* performed on armadillos and opossums. Both kinds of animals were divided into groups of six submitted to the following procedures five days after the chronic implantation of electrodes:

Group I. Chronic implantation exclusively. This group will later on be referred to as 'normal'.

Group II. Tubocurarine administration ($0.5\,mg\,kg^{-1}$).

Group III. Destruction of the OM by means of ZS.

Group IV. Perfusion of the nasal cavities with saline (Sham operation – SO – of group III).

Group V. Xylocaine on the OM.

Group VI. Surgical closure of one nostril.

Group VII. Surgical closure of both nostrils.

Group VIII. Tracheotomy and insertion of a two-way tracheal tube which could be adjusted to either 'nose' or 'throat' position.

Groups IX and X. Section of one OP and its SO respectively.

Groups XI and XII. Section of both olfactory peduncles and the SO respectively.

Group XIII. Surgical extirpation of the tongue muscles.

Group XIV. Surgical extirpation of the eyes and extraocular muscles.

Groups XV and XVI. Bilateral section of the trigeminal nerve and its SO.

Groups XVII and XVIII. Bilateral destruction of the vomeronasal organ (VNO) and its SO.

The experiments of part II were performed on armadillos and opossums. Both kinds of animal were divided into groups of six submitted to the following procedures in addition to the chronic implantation of electrodes.

Group I–II. Destruction of the OM with ZS and SO respectively.

Groups III and IV respectively: (a) nasal perfusion with ZS immediately followed by an additional surgical destruction of OM and the VNO plus bilateral retrogasserian section of the trigeminal nerves; (b) SO of the procedures described in (a).

Groups V–VI. Destruction of the VNO and SO respectively.

Groups VII and VIII. Combined destruction of the OM and VNO and its SO.

Groups IX and X. Bilateral retrogasserian section of the trigeminal nerves and SO.

Group XI. Insertion of a tracheal tube left in 'nose' position, which could be adjusted either to 'nose' or 'throat' position. After five days from the performance of all these procedures groups I, III, VII, IX and XI were submitted to section of one OP. We allowed them to survive for another five days. Three animals of Group I were submitted to a second perfusion four days after the first one and one day before the section of the OP. The extent and distribution of the destruction of the OM or of the other nasal receptors after ZS was studied in coronal sections of the nasal cavities. These sections were done with the method described by Winans and Powers (1977). Ten days after the different procedures the animals were killed under ether. The section of the OP was controlled in serial sections stained with the Luxol fast-blue technique (Klüver and Barrera, 1953).

Results

Here we shall restrict ourselves merely to report: (1) the presence or absence of the 8–12 Hz rhythm in different experimental conditions; and (2) the presence or absence of centrally induced sinusoidal waves, which do not need peripheral participation for their generation, in different experimental conditions.

Part I: Armadillos

Normal animals (Group I). During wakefulness, the olfactory bulb of 153 animals showed a very conspicuous rhythm of 8–12 Hz (Figure 1). When the animals were in relaxed wakefulness the rhythm clearly dominated the tracings; when they became excited or engaged in very intense exploratory activity with sniffing, Adrian's sinusoidal waves and Ottoson's slow waves dominated. However, the rhythm sometimes coexisted with both kinds of waves (Figure 1). If the animals became excited or engaged in very intense exploratory activity, the rhythm was not observable and Adrian's sinusoidal waves dominated the tracing. The rhythm continued to be present even after: (1) extirpation of the tongue muscles (group XIII); (2) extirpation of the eyes and extraocular muscles (group XIV); (3) extirpation of the VNO and its SO (groups XVII and XVIII); (4) bilateral section of the trigeminal nerve and its SO (groups XV and XVI); or (5) section of the contralateral OP.

During slow sleep (SS), the rhythm was never observed.

During paradoxical sleep (PS), the rhythm was never observed.

Curarized animals (Group II). In order to estimate the possible importance of muscular movement we tried to verify the existence of the rhythm in curarized animals. In these animals, the rhythm could always be observed provided that olfactory stimuli were applied (Figure 2).

Effect of destruction of the OM and of the SO (Groups III and IV). There was complete disappearance of the rhythm (Figure 3). The disappearance still persisted at the time of killing the animals. The SO did not produce any effect on the rhythm.

Effect of local anesthesia of the OM (Group V). Application of xylocaine produced an effect comparable to that of destruction of the OM, the only difference being that it lasted for approximately 30 min and that it was completely reversible.

Figure 1. Wakefulness. 1, neocortex; 2, 3, right olfactory bulb (ROB); 4, 5, left olfactory bulb (LOB); 6, EKG. Vertical bar, 50 μV; horizontal bar, 1 s.

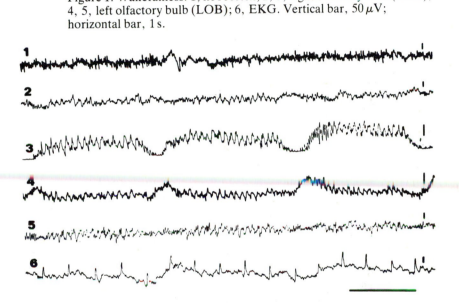

2.6   Figure 2. Electrical activity of OB of curarized animals. Arrow indicates the application of an olfactory stimulus. 1, 2, ROB and LOB; 3, neocortex. Vertical bar, 50 μV; horizontal bar, 1 s.

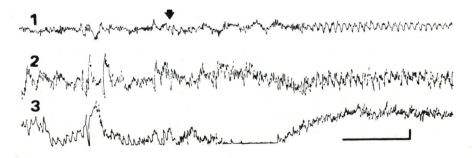

Effect of disturbance of the air flow passing through the nose (Groups VI, VII, and VIII). If one nostril was chronically sutured (Groups VI and VII), the rhythm disappeared in the homolateral olfactory bulb (Figure 4B). If both nostrils were sutured, the rhythm disappeared from both OB (Figure 4C).

If a tracheal tube (Group VIII) was in the 'nose' position the rhythm was observable (Figure 5A). This disappeared if the tube was in the 'throat' position (Figure 5B). This effect was reversible depending on the two possible positions of the tube.

Figure 3. Destruction of OM. A, before; B, after nasal perfusion. 1, neocortex; 2, 3, ROB; 4, 5, LOB. Vertical bar, 50 μV; horizontal bar, 1 s.

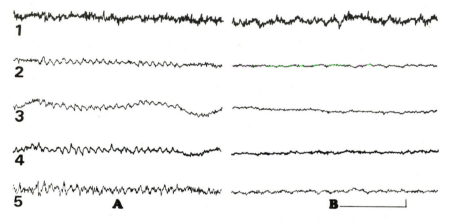

Figure 4. Closure of one or both nostrils. A, before closure; B, after closure of left nostril. C, after closure of both nostrils. 1, neocortex; 2, 3, ROB; 4, 5, LOB. Vertical bar, 50 μV; horizontal bar, 1 s.

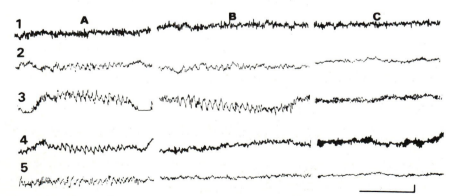

Effect of section of one olfactory peduncle and its SO (Groups IX and X). The section of one OP produced complete disappearance of the rhythm in the homolateral OB. The disappearance lasted until the animals were killed. On the contralateral side the rhythm was still observable (Figure 6). Contrarily, after the SO the rhythm was clearly observable on both hemispheres.

Effects of section of both olfactory peduncles and its SO (Groups XI and XII respectively). Section of both OP produced complete bilateral disappearance of rhythm which lasted until the animals were killed. Contrarily, after SO rhythm was clearly observable on both OB.

Figure 5. Tracheal tube. A, 'nose position'; B, 'throat position'; C, 'nose position' again. 1, neocortex; 2, 3, ROB; 4, 5, LOB. Vertical bar, $50\,\mu V$; horizontal bar, 1 s.

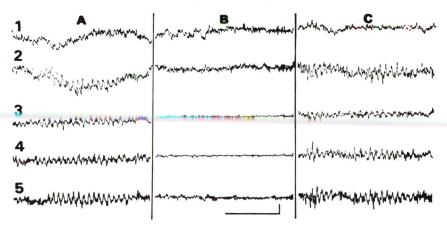

Figure 6. Section of one OP. A, before; B, after section of LOP. 1, neocortex; 2, 3, ROB; 4, 5, LOB. Vertical bar, $50\,\mu V$; horizontal bar, 1 s.

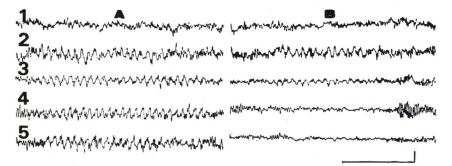

Part I: Opossums

The OB of 142 animals showed an 8–12 Hz rhythm very similar to that of the armadillos. The repetition in *Didelphis* of all the experiments performed in the armadillo gave essentially similar results.

Part II: Armadillos

Effects of destruction of the OM (Groups I–II). During wakefulness, sinusoidal activity was completely absent even during intense sniffing (Figure 7). Only low-voltage irregular activity remained.

During slow sleep (SS), very conspicuous bursts of sinusoidal activity appeared (30–39 Hz). They were not continuous and always showed greater amplitude than the sinusoidal waves seen in the animals with intact mucosa during wakefulness (Figure 7). They were clearly seen as soon as the first neocortical slow waves were noticed (Figure 7). If an arousing stimulus, for instance a sound, was applied, the sinusoidal waves immediately disappeared (Figure 8). (The sinusoidal waves of SS and PS will subsequently be referred to as 'High amplitude sinusoidal waves of sleep' (H.A.S.W.S.).

During paradoxical sleep (PS), the sinusoidal waves were even

Figure 7. Destruction of OM. A, before destruction: 1, neocortex; 2, 3, ROB; 4, 5, LOB. B, after destruction: 1, 2, ROB; 3, 4, LOB. Vertical bar, 50 μV; horizontal bar, 1 s.

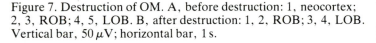

greater, taking up much more time of the tracings and being more continuous although their frequency was similar to those seen in SS sinusoidal waves (Figure 7). Here again if an arousing stimulus was applied, the sinusoidal waves were immediately interrupted. The animals with SO did not differ from normal animals.

When a second perfusion was applied, the H.A.S.W.S. did not change.

Effect of destruction of the VNO (Group III–IV). The tracings did not differ from normal ones. The same happened with SO.

Effects of combined destruction of OM and VNO (Groups V–VI). After destruction of the olfactory epithelium the typical results described above were obtained. When these animals were later submitted (three days later) to destruction of the VNO, a sinusoidal activity could be observed, much greater in amplitude and slower in frequency (24–30 Hz) than that seen after destruction of the OM only. This activity was present during both SS (Figure 9) and PS (Figure 10). Destruction of the OM combined with the sham extirpation of the VNO produced the same results as destruction of the OM alone.

Figure 8. Effects of a sound stimulus after destruction of OM. 1, neocortex; 2, 3, ROB; 4, 5, LOB. Vertical bar, $50\,\mu$V; horizontal bar, 1 s.

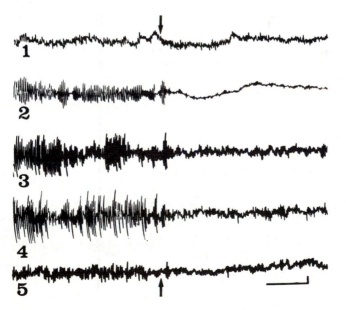

Figure 9. Combined destruction of OM and VNO during SS. A, before destruction of OM; B, after destruction of OM; C, after combined destruction of OM and VNO. 1, 2, ROB; 3, 4, LOB; 5, neocortex. Vertical bar, 50 μV; horizontal bar, 1 s.

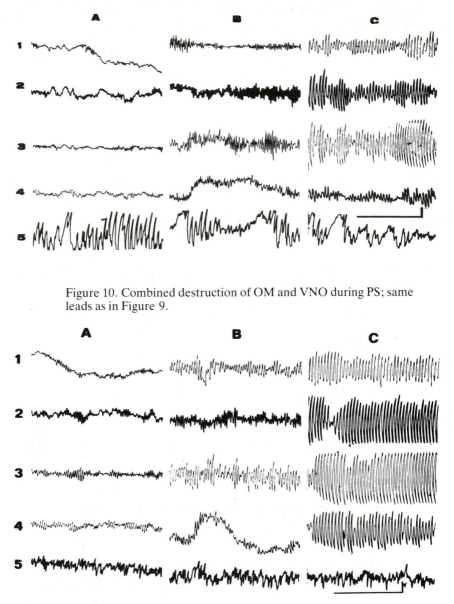

Figure 10. Combined destruction of OM and VNO during PS; same leads as in Figure 9.

Effects of bilateral retrogasserian section of the trigeminal nerves (Groups VII–VIII). Continuous sinusoidal waves (28–33 Hz) appeared during SS and PS (Figures 11, 12). They were seen only during the first four or six days after the operation, then disappeared. They were not seen after SO.

Figure 11. Effects of trigeminal section during SS. 1, neocortex; 2, 3, ROB; 4, 5, LOB. Vertical bar, 50 μV; horizontal bar, 1 s.

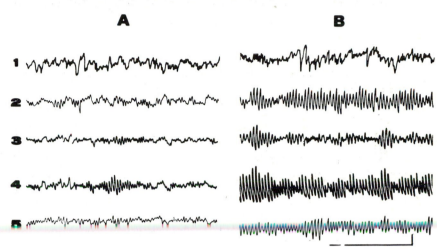

Figure 12. Effects of trigeminal section during PS; same leads as in Figure 11.

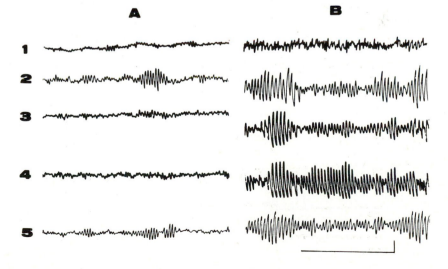

*Effects of interfering with nasal air-flow through the insertion of a
tracheal tube.* If the tube was in the 'throat' position (Group X) the
animals showed electrical activity quite similar to that which appeared in
the animals with destruction of the OM (Group I), i.e. the sinusoidal
waves were seen only during SS and PS, being absent during wakefulness. If the tube was in 'nose' position the electrical activity was quite
similar to that of normal animals (Group IX).

*Effect of the section of one OP in each one of the groups which showed
H.A.S.W.S.* H.A.S.W.S. disappeared (Figure 13).

Part II: Opossum

When the animals were submitted to the procedures described
in Part II: Armadillos, no bursts of sinusoidal activity were seen during
SS and PS.

Discussion

Our results clearly show two interesting findings, namely (a) the
existence of a fourth kind of activity constituting a rhythm which ought

Figure 13. Section of LOP after destruction of OM. A, before
destruction of olfactory mucosa; B, after destruction of olfactory
mucosa and with section of LOP (3, 4). Compare Figure 7.

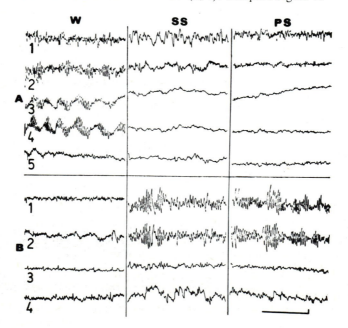

to be added to the three kinds of electrical activity already known in the mammalian olfactory bulb, and (b) the existence of bulbar sinusoidal waves which can be generated in the absence of peripheral olfactory input during sleep.

Regarding (a), our results indicate that the rhythm is a genuine one originating in brain structures and that it is not an artifact. Several of our experimental findings provide the evidence for this assertion: it is not a vascular pulsation because the heart frequency differs greatly from the frequency of the rhythm as the simultaneous record of the electrocardiogram (Figure 1) clearly shows. The rhythm cannot be due to a muscular artifact because even curarized animals continue to show it provided that olfactory stimulation is supplied. There is also some other evidence proving that the rhythm is not caused by muscular action: it is present after extirpation of the eyes and extraocular muscles, and after extirpation of the muscles of the tongue. The presence of the rhythm after this last operation is particularly pertinent because the tongue was shown to be the source and seat of a very powerful rhythmic activity (Megirian et al., 1978). Finally, the series of experiments with unilateral occlusions of the narines together with those of extirpation of the OM or section of the OP allows one to rule out the possibility of the rhythm being an artifact. As the rhythm is present after destruction of the VNO it is clear that the latter is not necessary for its generation.

We want to stress that the rhythm was observed only during W. It was never seen during SS or PS. On this ground, we suggest that the mechanisms responsible for its generation are counteracted or not operating during both phases of sleep. The rhythm may have practical importance during the course of neurophysiological experiments because it provides a rapid and simple means of discriminating between quiet W and PS; this is useful when observation of the peripheral signs of PS (muscular twitches, irregular respiration, ocular movement) is impossible or difficult. Such may be the case with curarized animals, or with animals submitted to brainstem sectioning.

Future investigations will probably clear up the biological meaning of the rhythm and its role in olfactory sensation and discrimination. It may thus be helpful in developing new trends in olfactory research.

Regarding generation of the rhythm, the experiments with chronic insertion of a tracheal tube in 'throat' position or those with occlusion of the nostrils are particularly instructive. After any of these experimental procedures the rhythm disappears, while the 'nose' position or the opening of the nostrils provokes its immediate return. This shows clearly that at least a certain flow of air through the nasal cavity is essential for generation of the rhythm. It is also clear that the OM must be intact: if it is destroyed by means of ZS the rhythm disappears even in the presence of the respiratory or sniffing current. It is therefore probable that the odoriferous particles conveyed by air flowing through the nostrils excite the olfactory receptors, thus initiating the events responsible for generation of the rhythm.

Regarding the importance of the central connections of the OB, our results indicate: (a) the rhythm in one OB is not due to the influence of the contralateral OB because section of the contralateral OP does not abolish it; and (b) they are essential for generation of the rhythm since section of the OP completely abolishes it. Its absence cannot be ascribed to faulty circulation of the OB produced by section of the OP, because the other activities (slow waves, sinusoidal waves, rapid irregular waves) were still present. On the other hand, direct observation of the circulation before killing the animals showed intact blood vessels.

From the fact that the rhythm needs peripheral influences coming from the nose and central influences coming from the brain we suggest calling it 'rhino-central rhythm'.

We also want to stress the fact that the rhythm was seen both in armadillos and opossums and that in both species it appears to have similar characteristics: in both of them its generation needs the presence of the OM and the integrity of the OB connections with the rest of the brain. It is probable that similar generative mechanisms exist in those primitive mammals.

Regarding (b), above, we must consider several important points:

(1) The finding that during sleep there are sinusoidal waves which do not need peripheral input for their generation indicates that sleep can be used as an experimental variable allowing us to disclose an unexpected feature of the functional organization of the olfactory system. It was only when deciding to continue our observation of the electrical activity of the OB through the different stages of sleep that the new fact was discovered. However, it seems probable that there are important differences between species. In fact, Peñaloza Rojas and Alcocer-Cuaron (1967) reported bursts of sinusoidal activity in alert tracheotomized cats.

(2) It is necessary to discuss whether our experiments prove the absence of peripheral input. We think we have achieved this condition only in the experiments combining nasal perfusion using ZS with the additional surgical destruction of the mucosa, and with the destruction of the VNO. Anatomical study of the serial sections showed that the

mucosa was completely destroyed and that no fragments of VNO remained. Our combined experiments (destruction of OM + destruction of VNO + bilateral section of trigeminal nerves) show that the sinusoidal waves of sleep are generated even in the absence of peripheral input to the bulb and of trigeminal input to the brain. However, we think that complete absence of peripheral input is not necessary for the appearance of sinusoidal waves during sleep. In fact, they appear after disturbance of the nasal air-flow or after nasal perfusion.

In the latter case anatomical study showed that approximately 85% of the mucosa had been destroyed. The question arises whether the H.A.S.W.S. are the product of stimuli coming from the remnants of mucosa or whether they have a central origin. The idea that they are of central origin is strongly supported by their disappearance after section of the OP. The central origin is also supported by the observation that these waves are very conspicuous when the mucosa is almost completely destroyed but are not to be seen at all, or are hardly observable, when the mucosa is intact, during sleep.

(3) The animals could be wakeful or asleep; in either case our results show that nasal respiration is very important for the control of the electrical activity of the OB. While they are awake, nasal respiratory flow is necessary to maintain the 8–12-Hz rhythm; while they remain asleep it is necessary in order to prevent production of H.A.S.W.S. If we take into account that these waves are not restricted to the OB – we have found them in the prepiriform cortex and olfactory tubercle (Affanni, unpublished) – we must admit that nasal respiration, at least in these animals, exerts a powerful influence on the electrical activity of a rather considerable proportion of the total brain surface. If we accept the importance of nasal respiration we must also admit that activity of the medullary and pontile respiratory centres influences indirectly through the upper airways the electrical activity of the OB and other olfactory regions of the brain.

(4) As we have seen before, the H.A.S.W.S. appear after olfactory deafferentation or disturbance of the nasal air-flow and disappear after section of the OP; thus they are probably the product of a certain kind of interaction between intrinsic neural systems of the OB and brain influences moving along centrifugal pathways to the bulb. Therefore, the study of H.A.S.W.S. may be important for investigating the so-called non-olfactory functions of the OB, since those waves are a significant part of the electrical activity of the bulb deprived of its peripheral connections. One important issue in the comparative physiology of the OB might be the assessment of the relative degrees of

importance of olfactory and non-olfactory functions throughout the evolutionary tree. The verification of H.A.S.W.S. after olfactory deafferentation might contribute to that assessment for which the presence of the above-mentioned waves in the armadillo and their absence in the opossum might be different functional organizations of the olfactory systems during sleep.

(5) Although the centrally induced H.A.S.W.S. are of much higher amplitude than the sinusoidal waves evoked by peripheral stimulation their frequency is quite similar. So we suggest that this phenomenon characteristic of armadillos might be useful for the study of the physiological basis of olfactory hallucinations. Armadillos are therefore excellent experimental models for olfactory physiology studies.

(6) A further consequence of our research is the finding that either destruction of the OM or bilateral section of the trigeminal nerve induces production of H.A.S.W.S. although the effects of the latter are very transient. Regarding the effect of trigeminal section we might think that trigeminal afference normally prevents the appearance of H.A.S.W.S. But as it is an effect of short duration compared to the effect of the destruction of OM one could argue that the production of H.A.S.W.S. is not due to lack of afference but to irritation of the proximal end of the trigeminal nerve. One thing remains clear: no matter whether its cause is the absence of impulses through the trigeminal pathways or the presence of irritation, section induces the production of H.A.S.W.S. This means that the traffic of impulses through trigeminal pathways exerts a powerful influence on the OB. This poses the interesting question whether the OB might play some role in integration of smell sensations produced not via olfactory pathways but via trigeminal ones. The lack of effect on the production of H.A.S.W.S. after destruction of the VNO and the extraordinary increase of those waves after the combined destruction of both the OM and the VNO indicate that their prevention is the result of some kind of interaction between the two systems. We cannot avoid comparing these results with those of Winans et al. (1977), in which they found that some animals showed no disturbance in their sexual behaviour, after either destruction of the OM or section of the vomeronasal nerves, but the animals became very handicapped after combination of the two operations.

(7) Last but not least, we can affirm that the H.A.S.W.S. cannot be due to the remarkable capacity for neurogenesis that persists in the olfactory nares epithelium of adult mammals (Graziadei and Monti Graziadei, 1978) because the H.A.S.W.S. were seen from the very first

moment of the post-perfusion period and persisted unchanged until the animals were killed. There are three further facts which lead us to reject that interpretation, namely: (1) the H.A.S.W.S. were maintained after a second perfusion; (2) they disappeared after section of the OP; and (3) there were no Adrian's sinusoidal waves during wakefulness through the whole period of observation.

This work was supported by grants from National Research Council (CONICET) and Albert J. Roemmers Foundation.

References

Adrian, E. D. (1950). The electrical activity of the mammalian olfactory bulb. *Electroencephalog. Clin. Neurophysiol. 2:* 377–88.

Affanni, J. M. Unpublished results.

Affanni, J. M., Morita, E., and García Samartino, L. (1968). Efectos de la sección de los pedúnculos olfatorios y de la comisura anterior sobre la actividad del bulbo olfatorio del marsupial *Didelphis azarae. Rvta Soc. Argent. Biol. 44:* 183–8.

Alberts, J. R., Friedman, M. I. (1972). Olfactory bulb removal but not anosmia increases emotionality and mouse-killing. *Nature 238:* 454–5.

Gault, F. P., and Coustan, D. R. (1965). Nasal air flow and rhinenphalic activity. *Electroenceph. Clin. Neurophysiol. 18:* 617–24.

Gerard, R. W., and Young, J. Z. (1937). Electrical activity in the central nervous system of the frog. *Proc. Roy. Soc., London, B122:* 343–51.

Graziadei, P. P. C., and Monti Graziadei, G. A. (1978). The olfactory system: a model for the study of neurogenesis and axon regeneration in mammals. In *Neuronal Plasticity*, ed. C. W. Cotman, pp. 131–53. New York: Raven Press.

Howe, H. A. (1933). The basal diencephalon of the armadillo. *J. Comp. Neurol. 58:* 311–75.

Klüver, H., and Barrera, E. (1953). A method for the combined staining of cells and fibers in the nervous system. *J. Neuropath. Exp. Neurol. 12:* 400–3.

Loo, Y. T. (1930). The forebrain of the opossum, *Didelphis virginiana. J. Comp. Neurol. 51:* 13–64.

Loo, Y. T. (1931). The forebrain of the opossum, *Didelphis virginiana. J. Comp. Neurol. 52:* 1–148.

Megirian, D., Cespuglio, R., and Jouvet, M. (1978). Rhythmical activity of the rat's tongue in sleep and wakefulness. *Electroenceph. Clin. Neurophysiol. 44:* 8–13.

Murphy, M. R. (1976). Olfactory impairment, olfactory bulb removal, and mammalian reproduction. In *Mammalian Olfaction, Reproductive Processes, and Behavior*, ed. R. L. Doty, pp. 95–117. New York: Academic Press.

Ottoson, D. (1954). Sustained potentials evoked by olfactory stimulation. *Acta Physiol. Scand. 32:* 384–6.

Ottoson, D. (1959a). Studies on slow potentials in the rabbit's olfactory bulb and nasal mucosa. *Acta Physiol. Scand. 47:* 136–48.

Ottoson, D. (1959b). Comparison of slow potentials evoked in the frog's nasal mucosa and olfactory bulb by natural stimulation. *Acta Physiol. Scand. 47:* 149–59.

Peñaloza-Rojas, J. H., and Alcocer-Cuarón, C. (1967). The electrical activity of the olfactory bulb in cats with nasal and tracheal breathing. *Electroenceph. Clin. Neurophysiol. 22:* 468–72.

Vaccarezza, O. L., Santamarina, A., and García Medina, M. R. (1975). Electrical activity of the olfactory bulb. Changes induced by lesions of contralateral olfactory areas. *Acta Physiol. Latinoam. 25:* 365–70.

Winans, S. S., and Powers, J. B. (1977). Olfactory and vomeronasal deafferentation of male hamsters: histological and behavioral analyses. *Brain Res. 126:* 325–44.

3
Visual systems

3.1

Visual systems of cephalopods

PETER H. HARTLINE and G. DAVID LANGE

The simple camera eye, the variable pupil, the eye movements, and the complex visual behavior of squid, octopus, and cuttlefish invite a search for similarities and differences between the ways that the nervous systems of cephalopods and vertebrates are organized to analyse the visual world. The sophistication of octopus visual behavior has been extensively documented using discrimination learning paradigms similar to those applied to mammals (Review: Young, 1961). Cuttlefish are capable of fine visual discrimination while searching for and capturing their prey (Boulet, 1958). Squid have complex visual displays during mating (Hurley, 1977) and form schools partly on the basis of visual cues (Hurley, 1976). In these cases, the evolutionary convergence of the more intricate visual capabilities of vertebrates and cephalopods stands out clearly. Even in the most primitive of living cephalopods, the chambered nautilus, pupillary control of light falling on the retina, (Hurley, Lange and Hartline, 1978) and vestibular stabilization of images against body movement (Hartline, Hurley and Lange, 1979) are in evidence (Figure 1). There are evidently profound similarities between the operational solutions evolved by vertebrates and cephalopods to cope with the information available through visual experience.

Paralleling the work on visual behavior, substantial progress has been made in describing the anatomy of cephalopod visual systems (Cajal, 1917; Young, 1971, 1974). But, compared to what we know about anatomy and behavior, we know little about the physiology of cephalopod visual systems. Judging from the few published studies since MacNichol and Love (1960) first reported visual responses in squid, these animals are relatively difficult subjects for the neurophysiologist; the modest state of our progress toward understanding cephalopod visual neurophysiology is not due to lack of interesting questions. In this review, we summarize the findings from a physiologist's point of view, but attempt to call attention to points at which anatomy can be seen to have important impact on the physiology. We also call attention to some

Figure 1. (A) Pupil of chambered nautilus closing and opening in response to light (dark bar). (From Hurley, Lange and Hartline, *J. Exp. Zool. 205:* 37–43 (1978). Reprinted with permission of publisher.) (B) Orientation of *Nautilus* eye relative to gravity (dots) during rocking motion mimicking swimming motion (solid curve). No trace of oscillation of eye orientation is seen even though the amplitude of imposed motion is about 30 degrees peak to peak. Vestibular compensation of eye position is in evidence. (From Hartline, Lange and Hurley, *J. Comp. Physiol. 132:* 117–26 (1979). Reprinted with permission of publisher.)

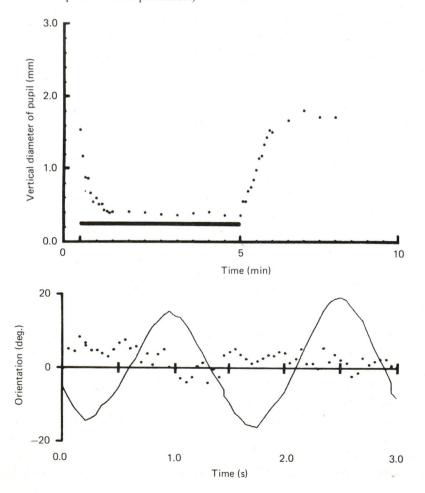

questions that we find particularly intriguing or important, and, though they seem within reach, are as yet unanswered.

The retina

The most distal layer of the retina consists of photoreceptors whose microvillar outer segments face the light directly. No neural cells are recognized in the retina besides the receptors (although there are glial and pigment cells); this has led to the cephalopod retina's reputation for simplicity, and stands in contrast to the five or six major cell types in the vertebrate retina. There is a prominent layer of lateral processes near where the photoreceptor axons form. It contains inter-receptor contacts as well as synapses involving centrifugal axons.

In cephalopods, as in other invertebrates, absorption of light by the rhodopsin-bearing microvilli leads to a local increase in membrane current (Hagins, Zonana and Adams, 1962). The current, carried largely by Na^+, depolarizes the receptor cell. The intracellular responses to moderately bright sustained light (Duncan and Weeks, 1973; Pinto and Brown, 1977; Duncan and Pynsent, 1979) are similar to those of other invertebrates, having transient and sustained components. It is widely held that the waveform of the invertebrate photoresponse is largely a reflection of the time course of the conductance change induced in microvillar membrane. We previously advanced a kinetic scheme that could account for the time course of the cephalopod photoresponse for small intensity changes (squid and octopus: Hartline and Lange, 1977; nautilus: Lange, Hartline and Hurley, 1979). It was a variant of the Fuortes and Hodgkin (1964) model in which a cascade or chain of simple chemical decay reactions generates a messenger molecule that opens ionic channels in the membrane.

However, this model (applied in Figure 2A to the electroretinogram of *Nautilus*), and all others like it, assume that the membrane whose conductance is increased by light is electrically accessible to the soma and extracellular fluids. Odette and Hartline (1981, 1983a) have challenged this assumption. Their calculations indicate that the tight packing of microvilli and narrow extracellular spaces of the rhabdom (see Cohen, 1973a, and Figure 5 below) may slow the photoresponse substantially compared to the time course of the conductance change. If this is so, then the time scale of chemical reactions that control conductance may be substantially faster than the observed photoresponses.

Odette and Hartline (1981, 1983a) modeled current flow in rhabdomal regions tightly packed with microvilli. Such regions have passive electrical behavior like that of a core conductor or simple decrementally conducting cable as in Figure 3. Such a cable would slow and attenuate any signal passing through it. The time and space constants of the rhabdomal cable depend on transmembrane resistivity, the dimensions and resistivity of extracellular space, and the capacitance and area of microvillar membrane. These parameters are not known for cephalopods and are not securely known for any invertebrate photoreceptor. But one can make reasonable estimates by taking parameters from electrical studies and electron micrographs published for various invertebrates (see Odette and Hartline, 1983a). They lead to an unexpected result, illustrated in Figures 2B and 4. Assume that each

Figure 2. Electroretinogram of *Nautilus* in response to moderately bright flash occurring at the beginning of the two second traces, fitted by two different models. (A) Model curve (F) for a chain of four filters or chemical decay reactions having time constants 160 ms, 53 ms, 45 ms, and 28 ms, but with an additional simple delay of 120 ms. The delay could be replaced by a combination of additional filters with short time constants. (Reprinted from Lange, Hartline and Hurley, *J. Comp. Physiol. 134:* 281–5 (1979).) (B) Model curve (C) for a rhabdomal cable having a membrane time constant of 80 ms and absorbing light at a depth 9.1 times the cable's characteristic length. No delay term is required for this two-parameter model. Both models generate good fits to the response waveform, except for deviations in the tail of the response.

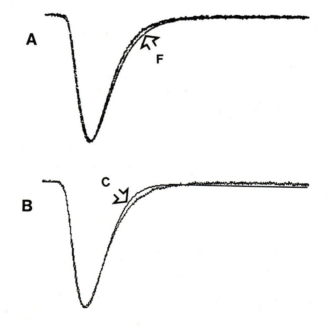

photon generates a very brief transmembrane current, much faster than the photoresponse. This current must charge up microvillar membranes on the way through the extracellular spaces to the retinal surface where one might insert a microelectrode, or measure ERG. The path is therefore electrically much longer than the geometric distance. The current waveform, and thus the voltage waveform measured at the soma (Figure 4), could be slowed sufficiently to match the response dynamics

Figure 3. Schematic diagram of a section of the receptor layer of cephalopod retina indicating how microvillar regions can be treated as a set of cables (if illumination is uniform and all currents can be assumed to traverse the retina radially). The inner conductor of the cable corresponds to the extracellular space around the microvilli. Because of the large membrane area per unit rhabdomal depth and the restricted (high resistance) extracellular space, the rhabdomal cable's space constant is short, leading to slowing and attenuation of the electrical cable over relatively short intra-rhabdomal distances; a relatively long length of conventional axon would be required to generate similar delay and attenuation (schematized at right).

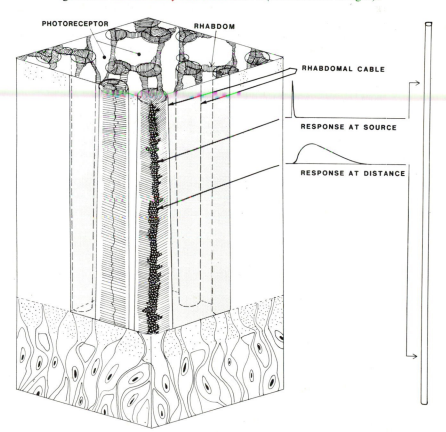

that have been measured (Odette and Hartline, 1983b). Thus, the anatomy of the microvillar rhabdomal cylinders may be a potent determinant of the ability of cephalopod photoreceptors (and indeed those of other invertebrates) to respond to changing visual stimuli.

There is another notable feature of microvillar organization, which most likely determines capability of cephalopod visual systems to detect and analyse patterns of polarization of incident light. Figure 5 is a tangential section through a sheet of receptors. The microvilli of any one receptor are parallel to each other. The retina consists of an array of receptors having one of two perpendicular orientations of their micro-villi (Figure 5). Two lines of evidence (besides the anatomy and the behavioral capability to discriminate polarization (Moodey and Parriss, 1961) indicate that the receptors can analyse polarization patterns. Tasaki and Karita (1966) adapted an octopus retina to polarized light. They then found that the ERG evoked by a subsequent polarized flash was maximum for an *E* vector perpendicular to that of the adapting light (a result later extended to squid, Ito, Karita, Tsukahara and Tasaki, 1973). More recently, Saidel, Lettvin and MacNichol (1983) found that optic nerve units exhibit polarization preference. The degree to which one plane of polarization is preferred depends on the state of light

Figure 4. Transfer function from light to ERG of squid retina measured by sinusoidal modulation of light intensity and measurement of amplitude and phase of resultant ERG (triangles). A rhabdomal cable model transfer function (curve) fits the empirical data very well. The depth at which illumination was assumed was 2.97 times the characteristic length, and the membrane time constant was 200 ms. The same empirical transfer function was fitted by a chain of five filters plus a 35-ms delay, or a chain of 10 filters with no delay by Hartline and Lange (1977).

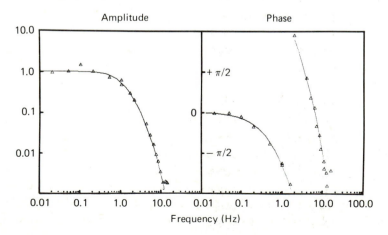

Figure 5. Electron micrograph of cross-section of squid retinal receptors. Note the two approximately perpendicular orientations of the microvilli. The short dimension of the plate is about 23 μm. (Reprinted from A. I. Cohen, 1973, *J. Comp. Neurol. 147:* 351–78, with permission of author and publisher.)

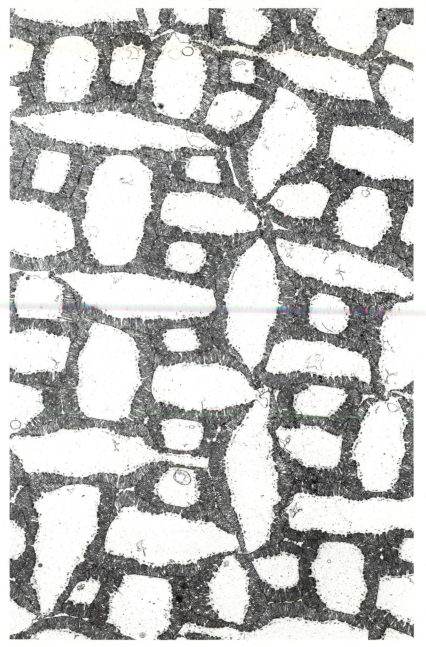

adaptation of the eye (Figure 6). Dark-adapted eyes are less selective than light-adapted ones. It is tempting to conjecture that there is an interaction between horizontally and vertically polarized receptors that can be altered by the state of adaptation.

Searching the vertebrate repertoire for an analogous function, the retinal mosaic of cones having different spectral sensitivities comes to mind (Bernard and Wehner, 1977). The key to the analogy is the fine-grained intermixture of at least two populations of receptor types (necessary to distinguish intensity contrast from polarization or color contrast). Thus an interesting question for future research is whether there is an opponent-polarization mechanism in the cephalopod retina or optic lobe. An obvious advantage to the animal of such a mechanism would be to allow objects to be seen by polarization-contrast borders even when intensity contrast is undetectable.

Plexiform layer in the retina

The plexiform layer contains lateral processes of receptors and also the terminal fields of centrifugal axons originating in the optic lobe. The lateral spread of intra-retinal potentials, the action of centrifugal

Figure 6. Responses of a squid optic nerve afferent fiber to polarized light. Zero degrees was approximately the optimum angle of polarization. In the dark-adapted case, the response is reduced to about 19% by changing the plane of polarization so that it is perpendicular to the optimum angle. In light-adapted preparations, the response is reduced to about 45% of the optimum by the same shift of polarization. (Comparisons are made to the optimum response at each adaptation level.) (From Saidel, Lettvin and MacNichol, *Nature 304:* 534–6. Reprinted with permission of author and publisher.)

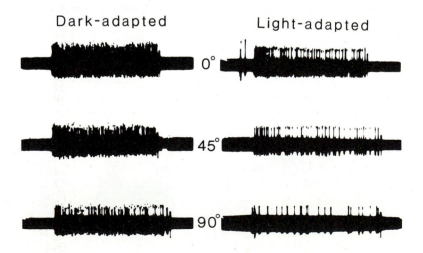

input to the retina, and the generation of complex temporal response patterns are among them. Electron-microscopic examination of octopus sections has been interpreted as suggesting inter-receptoral chemical synapses (Tonosaki, 1965; Gray, 1970). Cohen (1973b), examining the squid plexiform, identified gap junctions between receptors, but was not convinced that receptors make classical chemical synapses. Thus, at this point the evidence for receptor–receptor chemical synapses must be regarded as uncertain. Proximal to the zone of receptor processes, large-diameter profiles appear that run long distances and make some chemical synapses onto receptors. According to Cohen, these are candidates for the main elements of the plexus of fibers that staining with silver has revealed. Most of these fibers are thought to be branches of centrifugal axons.

Both chemical and electrical interactions among receptors could affect extracellularly recorded electrical activity of the retina. Clark (1975), Pynsent and Duncan (1977), and Duncan and Pynsent (1979) observed a waveform difference between surface and deep intra-retinal extracellular potentials that might be due to deep current generators in the hypothetical synaptic regions. Synaptic currents would be likely to have different dynamics from the receptor potential, thus accounting for differences between waveforms recorded at the surface and in deeper regions. Tasaki and his collaborators (Tasaki, Norton and Fukuda, 1963; Tasaki, Oikawa and Norton, 1963; Ito et al., 1973), measuring spatial spread of extracellular potentials, concluded that at the surface, a negative potential was distributed symmetrically about an illuminated spot. A deeper positive potential spread further toward the retina's center than away from it. If the positive potential is due to a deep current source such as might be set up by synaptic activity, one might expect to find some anisotropy of the underlying synaptic connections. It would be interesting to know whether potassium release and retinal glia have important effects on retinal potentials, as seems highly likely in the case of vertebrates (Miller and Dowling, 1970). The slow potentials of cephalopod retina would be better understood after a study using current source density analysis, such as that recently applied to the frog retina (Newman, 1980).

Transient or steady illumination can lead to large-amplitude oscillatory retinal potentials. Tsukahara, Makoto and Tasaki (1973) attributed these potentials to synchronous activity in the receptors and their axons, finding them to be abolished by tetrodotoxin. One immediately suspects that lateral interactions must play a role, otherwise the observed spatial coherence is difficult to explain. Lange, Hartline and Hurley (1976) pointed out that if appropriate lateral inhibitory feedback were present, oscillatory behavior might result. If each receptor is itself oscillatory, lateral spread of excitation could also result in oscillations synchronized over broad regions of the network. Such excitation might spread via the electrotonic connections suggested by the inter-receptoral gap junctions.

We previously described two other complex retinal phenomena that may have related origins, and may involve lateral interconnection of receptors. If a flash of low or moderate intensity was superimposed on weak background illumination, we frequently observed enhancement of the flash response. This 'background enhancement' is the opposite of what one usually expects from light adaptation; it is illustrated for a squid optic nerve in Figure 7, but also occurs in ERG (Lange and Hartline, 1974). Probably related to this is the facilitation of the spike or ERG response to a dim or moderate flash due to a preceding conditioning flash. Neither background enhancement nor facilitation has a demonstrated origin in lateral interaction in the plexus but both are intrinsic to the retina. They persist even if all optic nerve connections to the CNS are cut. One can imagine a mechanism requiring either lateral

Figure 7. Responses of squid optic nerve afferent fiber to identical flashes superimposed on (1) no background, (2)–(5) progressively brighter background illumination. Lines (2) and (3) show progressively greater enhancement by greater background illumination. Latency also shortens as background illumination increases. Sweep time, 0.5 s. (From Hartline and Lange, *J. Comp. Physiol. 93:* 37–54 (1974). Reprinted with permission of publisher.)

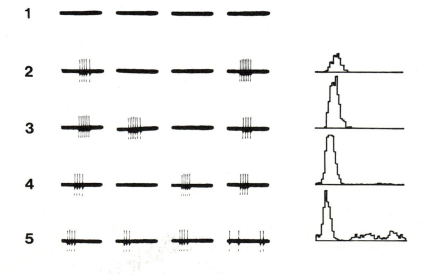

excitatory or inhibitory synaptic activity that would account for these phenomena (Lange et al., 1976). Of course, the individual receptors could have intrinsic mechanisms that by themselves would be sufficient, as appears true under some conditions for *Limulus* ventral photo-receptors (Fein and Charlton, 1977). An experiment that tests for mutual facilitation of responses to spatially distinct stimuli would go a long way toward settling this question.

Optic nerve responses, first recorded by MacNichol and Love (1960) have in our hands (Hartline and Lange, 1974) shown very complex response behaviors. Figure 8 illustrates a phenomenon that could be a manifestation of an inhibitory network in the retina (Lange et al., 1976). Transient and sustained increases of the firing frequency are seen when the stimulus brightens; transient and sustained decrements of spike frequency are seen after it dims. However, if the intensity of the stimulus (both lower level and step magnitude) are increased several-fold, under some circumstances, one immediately sees a response that is inverted in sign; the action potentials are at first silenced following the increment step, and return during the decrement step. An *on* burst gradually appears as the unit adapts to the stimulus regime, and the

Figure 8. Response changing sign during adaptation. Square wave intensity modulation at low level (B) for trace A, at high level (G) for traces C–F (shown to proper scale). Tonic and phasic excitation visible in A becomes tonic *off* response in C and evolves to a transient *on* response in F. Square wave was 0.1 Hz; C was taken immediately after changing to brighter stimulation; F was after 5 min at the brighter levels. (From Hartline and Lange, *J. Comp. Physiol. 93:* 37–54 (1974). Reprinted with permission of publisher.)

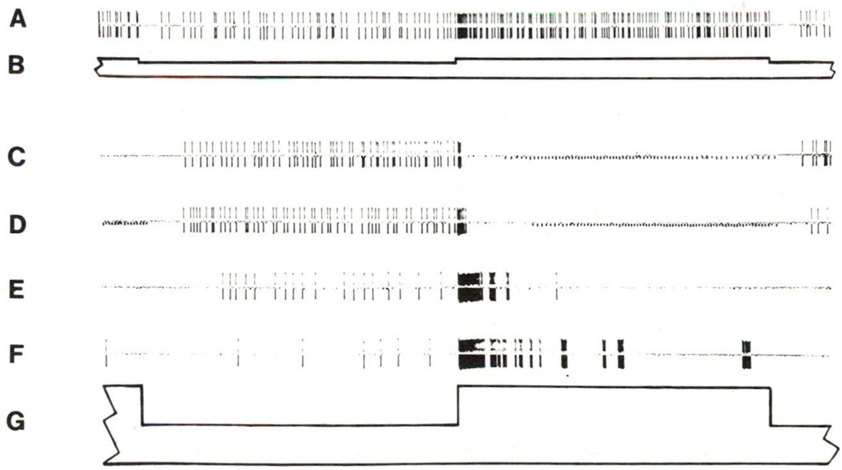

tonic firing during the decrement step becomes weaker. Eventually, the transient bursts at the increment step dominate the response. Ratliff and Mueller (1957) demonstrated experimentally that the lateral inhibitory network in *Limulus* could generate *on*, *off*, and *on–off* responses, although light only excites any single receptor in the network. Intuitively, we might hypothesize that, at the beginning of the bright stimulus regime, inhibitory activity of neighbors of the recorded squid receptor is strong and rapid enough to stifle even the strong initial direct excitation. As the neighbors become light adapted and as their inhibitory synapses perhaps fatigue, the magnitude of direct excitation transiently exceeds the summed inhibition, leaving a brief burst at the increment step. Further adaptation and fatigue eventually lead to an almost pure excitatory response, as appears in the bottom trace of the figure.

Several types of experiments might help evaluate the above conjecture that an inhibitory network exists in the retina. One would be a direct demonstration of lateral inhibition requiring spatially controlled stimuli to the retina, and an exploration of the time course of adaptation of the excitatory and inhibitory processes. A second would be to compare the responses evoked by a point light source (presumably illuminating a very small number of receptors) with that evoked by intermediate and wide-field illumination. A different approach is suggested by Lam, Wiesel and Kaneko's (1974) identification of synthetic enzymes for acetylcholine in the optic nerves and retina. This would be to test the effects of blocking acetylcholine pharmacologically. If ACh is the transmitter for lateral interaction, the complex behaviors of optic nerve fibers might be reduced to simple tonic *on* responses, and background enhancement might disappear.

Besides the 'fast' optic nerve afferents, whose dynamics are typified by the top trace of Figure 8, we have remarked upon a class of centripetally conducting optic nerve fibers with slow dynamics, usually responding only to bright lights. One such is barely visible in the second and third traces of Figure 8. It is tonically responsive, and fires regularly. Such units were not encountered frequently, but we believe they are not simply sick fibers. They generally have very large and ill-defined receptive fields (15° to the whole field). To our knowledge, no anatomical class of receptors is recognized in the retina that might account for them. But besides a spectrum of sizes and the two orientations of microvilli, anatomists do recognize three classes of receptors by their differing terminal morphology in the optic lobe. The rarest of those (which penetrate the lobe deeply before branching see Figure 9B) might turn out to be our 'slow' category. We would be left with a puzzle even so, since in the plexiform layer of the retina, fibers that travel long distances have been associated with centrifugal axons in the optic nerves, not with receptors or interneurons (Young, 1971).

Retinal centrifugal fibers

A prominent and intriguing feature of cephalopod retinas is the presence of axons in the optic nerves whose somata lie in the cortex of the optic lobe, or deeper. Silver stains reveal that these enter the extensive network of tangential fibers in the proximal retinal plexiform layer. These efferent or centrifugal fibers are probably seen in EM sections as large-diameter processes that contain open synaptic vesicles plus a few large, dense-core vesicles. Cohen (1973b) has shown that they synapse with receptors along their paths. In the same layer, at least in squid, there are other finer processes packed with small dense-core vesicles. Cohen did not trace them to cells or fibers of origin. If all centrifugal influences are mediated by the tangential network of large fibers, one would expect the effects of efferents to be distributed over large retinal areas. Golgi material has revealed retinal arborizations of several hundred micrometers, corresponding to fields as large as 4.5° (Patterson and Silver, 1983); whether there are efferents with larger terminal fields is not known.

That optic nerve bundles carry some centrifugally conducted impulses has been demonstrated. In a few cases, we have recorded from two loci on the same optic nerve bundle and demonstrated the direction of travel of an action potential by a relative delay of the spikes recorded peripherally compared to the spike recorded centrally. More routinely, we and others cut the nerve bundle proximal or distal to the recording site. A persistent action potential in the central stump indicates centrifugal conditions.

Many centrifugal fibers in squid and octopus can be excited by visual stimulation (Boycott, Lettvin, Maturana and Wall, 1965; Lange and Hartline, 1974; Patterson and Silver, 1983). In our study, most of them responded sluggishly (long latency, slow changes of firing frequency) to relatively bright lights. These units have broad receptive fields (15° to entire field) similar to those of the slow afferents. However, on at least one occasion, we observed a multi-unit response in a central optic nerve stump that showed relatively rapid dynamics; Patterson and Silver (1983) recorded similar efferent activity. They also found prominent *off* or *on–off* bursting activity in multi-unit recordings from the central ends of several optic nerve bundles. Thus, there are probably at least two classes of visually driven centrifugals: those with slow dynamics and those with rapid dynamics. The difference in dynamics probably signals differences in function. In addition to visually excited efferents, Boycott et al. (1965) reported that, in octopus, some could be activated by tactile stimulation or without any overt cause.

The function of retinal centrifugals is not known. The complex electroretinogram and receptor spike responses (facilitation, enhancement, oscillations, change from *on* to *on–off* to *off* behavior, etc.) do not require central connections of the retina. Tasaki and Suzuki (1980) state in an abstract that optic nerve responses are depressed and the electroretinogram is enhanced by stimulating the optic nerve. Thus, control of receptor responsiveness or sensitivity is a candidate function for the efferents.

The realm of function of optic nerve efferents is replete with

Figure 9. A, B, C: Cell types found in cortex and superficial medulla of the optic lobe of squid. o.gr., outer granule layer; o.pl., outer plexiform layer; i.gr., inner granule layer; i.pl., inner plexiform layer; p., palisade layer. Note optic nerve centrifugal (n.f.cent.) and several different types of amacrines and visual neurons in various layers of the cortex. Note three types of retinal inputs to the cortex in B (n. ret. 1, 2, 3). The deeply-penetrating type is uncommon. Visual neurons with long initial segments bearing dendrites within the plexiform layers are common (e.g. ce. vis.2, out. center of A). Calibration bars: 0.1 mm approx. (From J. Z. Young (1974), *Phil. Trans. R. Soc. Lond. B267:* 263–302. Reprinted with permission of author and publisher.)

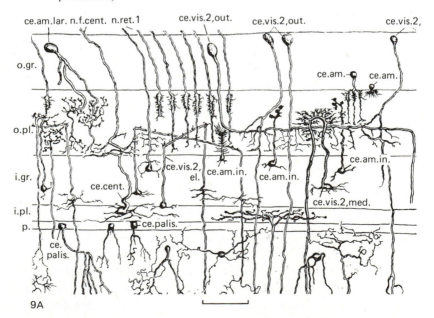

9A

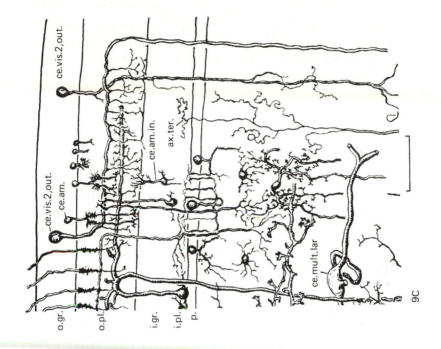

o.gr. o.pl. i.gr. i.pl. p.

n.ret.3

n.ret.2

n.ret.1

ce.am.lar.

ce.bi.

ce.palis.

ce.mult.sm.

ce.mult.lar.

9B

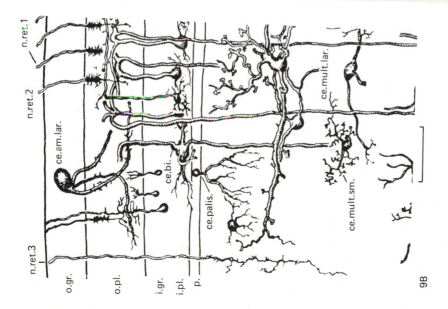

o.gr. o.pl. i.gr. i.pl. p.

ce.vis.2.out.

ce.vis.2.out.

ce.am.

ce.am.in.

ax.ter.

ce.mult.lar.

9C

unanswered questions. If, as in *Limulus* (Barlow, Bolanowski and Brachman, 1977), and as is suggested by Tasaki and Suzuki (1980), efferents to the retina control sensitivity or responsiveness, one very important question is whether different retinal regions are separately controlled. If they are, then this could be a mechanism for spatially selective visual attention. It is also clearly of interest to look for effects of centrifugals on receptive fields and other response properties of visual afferents. Such effects have been found in the visual efferent system of birds (Pearlman and Hughes, 1976). Since there are several distinct classes of centrifugals (visually driven, sluggish and rapid dynamics, non-visual), the question immediately arises of whether different aspects of retinal function are affected by each different class. Do all retinal receptors receive essentially the same functional contacts, or do different subsets receive different central input?

Optic nerve centrifugals in the optic lobe

The somata of some centrifugals lie deep in the optic lobe or possibly elsewhere in the brain. These presumably account for the touch-sensitive and spontaneous centrifugals recorded in the optic nerves. But most of the somata are in the lobe's inner granule cell layer. Dendritic fields, figured by Young (1971, 1974) as having spreads of not much more than $100\,\mu m$, are in the plexiform layer (outer plexiform in squid). We have usually found that centrifugals with slow dynamics have large receptive fields. Thus, it seems that horizontal elements in the plexiform layer that spread several millimeters must channel retinal input from broad areas of the lobe to at least one class of centrifugals. Whether centrifugals with rapid dynamics also have very large receptive fields remains to be determined. Saidel (1979) has shown, by iontophoresis of cobalt into optic nerve bundles, that the centrifugals and centripetal fibers of each optic nerve bundle at the chiasm map in close proximity to each other in the lobe. One suspects that the precision of spatial organization of centrifugals has functional significance; thus, some spatially specific efferent functions are likely to be found in future research.

After their exit from the retina, receptor axons from thin vertically elongated patches of retina aggregate into bundles, interweave in a dorso-ventral chiasm, and end in the superficial layers of the optic lobe. There they array themselves in an exquisitely precise manner, forming a spatial map of the world analogous to visual spatiotopic maps evident in central visual structures of vertebrates (Young, 1971). The outer surface of the squid optic lobe, the cortex, has three cellular layers and two major plexiform layers (Young, 1974). In *Octopus*, there is one plexiform layer separating two cellular layers (Young, 1971). Cajal called the cortex the 'retina profunda'. From the time of Lenhossek (1896) and Cajal (1917), the layering of the superficial optic lobe and the diverse cell types found therein have attracted attention. With the monumental work of J. Z. Young (1971, 1974), we now have a catalog of many cell types all of which are still waiting to be characterized by physiologists (Figure 9). Several classes of amacrine cells having distinct morphologies participate in the plexiform neuropil regions; their cell bodies are in the granule layers. There are several types of axon-bearing neurons whose somata are in the granule layers as well. Most send large processes into the plexiform (outer, in squid); there the processes branch extensively, and the main axonal process turns inward toward the medulla of the lobe (Figure 9). The outer plexiform layer is recognizably divided into alternating radial and tangential zones, based on light microscopy. Amacrines and axon-bearing neurons reside in either of the two granule layers; they may be categorized by soma size, by morphology of their major processes, by their dendritic fields, and by destination. Dendrites may be confined to one or several of the zones of the plexiform layer. In the literature, there is not the slightest physiological clue to the function of such anatomical features.

Some predictions of physiological properties have been based on known anatomy. Young found cells with very long horizontal branches (several millimeters) in the plexiform layer. These will certainly have large receptive fields. Young also suggested that some classes of amacrines may function like vertebrate horizontal cells. He further identified a class of axon-bearing neuron whose major (presumably dendritic) process travels within the plexiform layer in a straight path that can be several hundred micrometers long, then plunges (presumably as an axon) toward the lobe's depths. This type of cell makes an impressive network of fibers, with horizontal and vertical paths occurring most frequently. Young suggests that these are detectors of oriented contours. Surely, many physiologists, armed with Lucifer or HRP-filled microelectrodes can spend productive lives unraveling the structure–function relationships of cells in the cortex of the optic lobe.

Medulla of the optic lobe

In the medulla of the lobe, visual axons are organized into radial columns that receive broad lateral interconnections as they proceed deeper. Young (1973, 1974) has suggested that this organization might provide a substrate for feature-detecting neurons similar to those of the visual cortex of mammals. The medulla receives inputs from not only the retina and retina profunda, but also other sensory modalities and other brain regions. It has a broad integrative function: there is not a clear boundary between 'visual system' and higher brain function. Saidel's (1982) HRP study indicates that the deeper lobe receives input from a large number of regions within the rest of the brain. Many of them, Saidel points out, are those associated (through behavioral and lesion studies) with learning, attack/retreat decisions, and other functions that require initiation of coordinated acts.

Several features of the optic lobes are reminiscent of the vertebrate optic tectum (in mammals, called the superior colliculus). The precise spatiotopic organization of the surface of the lobe is also a feature of the vertebrate optic tectum. By itself, this argument is weak, since other visual centers of vertebrates are spatiotopically organized. But the presence of non-visual sensory modalities in both structures strengthens the argument. One would like to know if non-visual modalities are topographically arranged in the optic lobe, as they are in the optic tectum (see Hartline, 1983; Konishi, 1983). Electrical stimulation of deep optic lobe neuropil can elicit a wide variety of behavioral responses in octopus and cuttlefish. Many sequences resemble vertebrate-orienting responses (Chichery and Chanelet, 1976), and include coordinated movements of eyes, arms and locomotor activity. Stimulation of the superior colliculus of mammals evokes orienting responses. Initiation of orientation behavior is widely held to be a major function of the optic tectum.

That important features of both the mammalian visual cortex and superior colliculus are shared by the optic lobes suggests that an organizational principle of the cephalopod visual system may be quite different from its counterpart in mammals. In mammalian cortex, there are many complete two-dimensional copies of the retina in distinct regions (the superior colliculus is yet another). Each region is seemingly concerned with its own specialized set of functions. Among brain structures receiving visual projections (Saidel, 1982) spatiotopic organization has been found only in the basal lobe and peduncle lobe complex (Young, 1976; Messenger, 1979). In the peduncle lobe only one axis of the spatial mapping is well defined (Saidel, 1981) and because of their analogous structure and function, this is likely to be the case in the basal lobes as well. This leaves the optic lobe as the only fully space-mapped central visual structure, and consequently, many more functions must be subsumed within the lobe's single two-dimensional map. It is a matter for future investigation to determine whether this suggested organizational dissimilarity between vertebrates and cephalopods is real or is due to gaps in our knowledge of the cephalopod visual system.

References

Barlow, R. B., Jr., Bolanowski, S. J., Jr., and Brachman, M. (1977). Efferent optic nerve fibers mediate circadian rhythms in the *Limulus* eye. *Science 197:* 86–9.

Bernard, G. D., and Wehner, R. (1977). Functional similarities between polarization vision and color vision. *Vision Res. 17:* 1019–28.

Boulet, P. C. (1958). Contribution à l'étude expérimentale de la perception visuelle du mouvement chez la perche et la seiche. *Mém. Mus. Natn. Hist. Nat. Paris* (A), *17:* 1–132.

Boycott, B. B., Lettvin, J. Y., Maturana, H. R., and Wall, P. D. (1965). Octopus optic responses. *Expl. Neurol. 12:* 247–56.

Cajal, S. Ramon y (1917). Contribucion al conocimiento de la retina y centros opticos de los cefalopodos. *Trab. Lab. Invest. Biol. Univ. Madr. 15:* 1–82.

Chichery, R., and Chanelet, J. (1976). Motor and behavioral responses obtained by stimulation with chronic electrodes of the optic lobe of *Sepia officinalis. Brain Res. 105:* 525–32.

Clark, R. B. (1975). Components of the cephalopod electroretinogram. *Expl. Eye Res. 20:* 499–504.

Cohen, A. I. (1973a). An ultrastructural analysis of the photoreceptors of the squid and their synaptic connections. I. Photoreceptive and non-synaptic regions of the retina. *J. Comp. Neurol. 147:* 351–78.

Cohen, A. I. (1973b). An ultrastructural analysis of the photoreceptors of the squid and their synaptic connections. II. Intraretinal synapses and plexus. *J. Comp. Neurol. 147:* 379–98.

Duncan, G., and Pynsent, P. B. (1979). An analysis of the waveforms of photoreceptor potentials in the retina of the cephalopod *Sepiola atlantica. J. Physiol., Lond. 288:* 171–88.

Duncan, G., and Weeks, F. I. (1973). Photoreception by a cephalopod retina *in vitro. Expl. Eye Res. 17:* 183–91.

Fein, A., and Charlton, J. S. (1977). Enhancement and phototransduction in the ventral eye of *Limulus. J. Gen. Physiol. 69:* 553–69.

Fuortes, M. G. F., and Hodgkin, A. L. (1964). Changes in time scale and sensitivity in the ommatidia of *Limulus. J. Physiol., Lond. 172:* 239–63.

Gray, E. G. (1970). A note on synaptic structures of the retina of *Octopus vulgaris. J. Cell Sci. 7:* 203–15.

Hagins, W. A., Zonana, H. V., and Adams, R. G. (1962). Local membrane current in the outer segments of squid photoreceptors. *Nature 194:* 844–7.

Hartline, P. H. (1983). Infrared and visual senses in snake optic tectum. In *Comparative Physiology of Sensory Systems*, ed. L. Bolis, R. D. Keynes and S. H. P. Maddrell, chapter 3.4. Cambridge: Cambridge University Press.

Hartline, P. H., Hurley, A. C., and Lange, G. D. (1979). Eye stabilization by statocyst mediated oculomotor reflex in *Nautilus. J. Comp. Physiol. 132:* 117–26.

Hartline, P. H., and Lange, G. D. (1974). Optic nerve responses to visual stimuli in squid. *J. Comp. Physiol. 93:* 37–54.

Hartline, P. H., and Lange, G. D. (1977). Sinusoidal analysis of electroretinogram of squid and octopus. *J. Neurophysiol. 40:* 174–87.

Hurley, A. C. (1976). School structure of the squid *Loligo opalescens. U.S. Natl Mar. Fish. Serv. Fish. Bull. 76(2):* 433–42. *–c132:* 117–26.

Hurley, A. C. (1977). Mating behavior of the squid *Loligo opalescens. Mar. Behav. Physiol. 4:* 195–205.

Hurley, A. C., Lange, G. D., and Hartline, P. H. (1978). The adjustable 'pinhole camera' eye of *Nautilus. J. Exp. Zool. 205:* 37–44.

Ito, S., Karita, K., Tsukahara, Y., and Tasaki, K. (1973). Electrical activity of perfused and freely swimming squids as compared with *in vitro* responses. *Tohoku J. Exp. Med. 109:* 223–33.

Konishi, M. (1983). Spatial receptive fields in the auditory system. In *Comparative Physiology of Sensory Systems*, ed. L. Bolis, R. D. Keynes and S. H. P. Maddrell, chapter 1.5. Cambridge: Cambridge University Press.

Lam, D. M. K., Wiesel, T. N., and Kaneko, A. (1974). Neurotransmitter synthesis in cephalopod retina. *Brain Res. 82:* 365–8.

Lange, G. D., and Hartline, P. H. (1974). Retinal responses in squid and octopus. *J. Comp. Physiol. 93:* 19–36.

Lange, G. D., Hartline, P. H., and Hurley, A. C. (1976). The question of lateral interactions in the retinas of cephalopods. In *Neural Principles in Vision*, ed. F. Zettler and R. Weiler, pp. 389–93. New York: Springer-Verlag.

Lange, G. D., Hartline, P. H., and Hurley, A. C. (1979). Retinal responses in *Nautilus. J. Comp. Physiol. 134:* 281–5.

Lenhossek, M. von (1896). Histologische Untersuchungen am Sehlappen der Cephalopoden. *Arch. Mikrosk. Anat. 47:* 45–120.

MacNichol, E. F.Jr., and Love, W. E. (1960). Electrical responses of the retinal neural and optic ganglion of the squid. *Science 132:* 737–8.

Messenger, J. B. (1979). The nervous system of *Loligo* sp. IV. The peduncle and olfactory lobes. *Phil. Trans. R. Soc. Lond. B285:* 275–309.

Miller, R. F., and Dowling, J. E. (1970). Intracellular responses of the Muller (glial) cells of mudpuppy retina: their relation to b-wave of the electroretinogram. *J. Neurophysiol. 33:* 323–41.

Moody, M. F., and Parriss, J. R. (1961). The discrimination of polarized light by *Octopus:* a behavioral morphological study. *Z. vergl. Physiol. 49:* 268–91.

Newman, E. A. (1980). Current source density analysis of the b-wave of the frog retina. *J. Neurophysiol. 43:* 1355–66.

Odette, L. O., and Hartline, P. H. (1981). Electrical cable model of the invertebrate rhabdom. *Invest. Ophthal.*, Suppl. *20:* 232.

Odette, L. O., and Hartline, P. H. (1983a). Electrical cable model of the invertebrate rhabdom: consequences for voltage clamp and photoresponse measurement (in preparation).

Odette, L. O., and Hartline, P. H. (1983b). Electrical cable and diffusion models of invertebrate photoresponse dynamics (in preparation).

Patterson, J. S., and Silver, S. C. (1983). Afferent and efferent components of *Octopus* retina. *J. Comp. Physiol.* (in press).

Pearlman, A. L., and Hughes, C. P. (1976). Functional role of efferents to the avian retina I. Analysis of retinal ganglion cell receptive fields. *J. Comp. Neurol. 166:* 111–22.

Pinto, L., and Brown, J. E. (1977). Intracellular recording from photoreceptors of the squid (*Loligo pealii*). *J. Comp. Physiol. 122:* 241–50.

Pynsent, P. B., and Duncan, G. (1977). Reconstruction of photoreceptor membrane potentials from simultaneous intracellular and extracellular recordings. *Nature 269:* 257–9.

Ratliffe, F., and Mueller, C. G. (1957). Synthesis of 'on–off' and 'off' responses in a visual nervous system. *Science 126:* 840–1.

Saidel, W. M. (1979). Relationship between photoreceptor terminations and centrifugal neurons in the optic lobe of octopus. *Cell Tiss. Res. 204:* 463–72.

Saidel, W. M. (1981). Evidence for visual mapping in the peduncle lobe of octopus. *Neurosci. Lett. 24:* 7–11.

Saidel, W. M. (1982). Connections of the octopus optic lobe: an HRP study. *J. Comp. Neurol. 206:* 346–58.

Saidel, W. M., Lettvin, J. Y., and MacNichol, E. F. Jr (1983). Processing of polarized light by squid receptors. *Nature 304:* 534–6.

Tasaki, K., and Karita, K. (1966). Discrimination of horizontal and vertical planes of polarized light by the cephalopod retina. *Jap. J. Physiol. 16:* 205–16.

Tasaki, K., Norton, T., and Fukuda, Y. (1963). Regional and directional differences in the lateral spread of retinal potentials in the octopus. *Nature 198:* 1206–8.

Tasaki, K., Oikawa, J., and Norton, A. C. (1963). The dual nature of the octopus electroretinogram. *Vision Res. 3:* 61–73.

Tasaki, K., and Suzuki, H. (1980). Efferent inhibitory system in the octopus retina. 3rd Annual Meeting of the Japan Neuroscience Society, Tokyo, Japan. *Neurosci. Lett.* (Suppl. 4): S63.

Tonosaki, A. (1965). The fine structure of the retinal plexus in *Octopus vulgaris*. *Z. Zellforsch. mikrosk. Anat. 67:* 521–35.

Tsukahara, Y., Makoto, T., and Tasaki, K. (1973). Oscillatory potentials of the octopus retina. *Proc. Jap. Acad. 49(1):* 57–62.

Young, J. Z. (1961). Learning and discrimination in the octopus. *Biol. Rev. 36:* 32–96.

Young, J. Z. (1971). The anatomy of the nervous system of *Octopus vulgaris*. Oxford: Oxford University Press. 690 pp.

Young, J. Z. (1973). Receptive fields of the visual system of the squid. *Nature 241:* 469–70.

Young, J. Z. (1974). The central nervous system of *Loligo* I. The optic lobe. *Phil. Trans. R. Soc. Lond. B267:* 263–302.

Young, J. Z. (1976). The 'cerebellum' and control of eye movements in cephalopods. *Nature 264:* 572–4.

3.2

Relative movement and figure–ground discrimination by the visual system of the fly (towards a neuronal circuitry)

WERNER REICHARDT

Motion of an animal in the visual world generates a distribution of apparent velocities on its eyes. Discontinuities in this optical flow field are a good indication of object boundaries and can be used to segment images into regions that correspond to different objects (Helmholtz, 1896). In particular, the relative movement of an object against a background can be used to reveal its presence and to delineate its boundaries. The human visual system is very efficient at exploiting this fact (Julesz, 1971). Quite similarly, a fly is able to detect and to discriminate an object or a figure that moves relative to a background (ground) texture (Virsik and Reichardt, 1974; Hausen, 1976; Reichardt and Poggio, 1979).

Before turning to the experimental facts, it might be useful to speculate about possible evaluation principles for relative movement discrimination. To this end let us designate the motion fields of ground and figure with $\vec{x}$ and $\vec{y}$ respectively. A rather trivial solution of the problem could lead to a behavioural response $\vec{R}$ of a fly that depends only on a linear combination of $\vec{x}$ and $\vec{y}$. In a more powerful solution $\vec{R}$ could in addition depend on a non-linear interaction or 'interference' of the two motion fields so that the computation of relative movement may be described by the expression

$$\vec{R} = \vec{x} + \vec{y} + J(\vec{x}, \vec{y}) \tag{1}$$

with J a non-linear interference term.

The experimental paradigm

In the experiments reported here, the tests were carried out by means of a highly sensitive and fast mechanoelectric servotransducer,

357

which fixes a fly in space and senses the flight torque generated by its wings. When a contrasted optical environment is presented to a fixed flying test-fly, it is operating under 'open loop' conditions. Since the head of the test-fly is fixed to the thorax, a steady pattern represents a stabilized retinal image for the fly. Contrasted environments (ground and figure) were provided by statistical patterns with pixels (either black or white) by 3° * 3° (Julesz patterns), mounted on two concentric cylinders. In Figure 1 the technique used in the experiments is shown in a schematic diagram.

Figure 1. Schematic drawing of the experimental set-up used in the behavioural experiments described in the paper. A test-fly TF is suspended from a torque compensator TC which is connected to the compensator electronics CE. The voltage output of CE is proportional to the torque signal generated by the fly under compensation. The CE output is evaluated by a data evaluation device DE. For on-line data evaluation an Intertechnique DIDAC 800 computer and a Princeton Signal Averager Model 4202 are used. The motion of two cylinders C1 and C2 is controlled by two 400-Hz servomotors SM1 and SM2 whose shafts carry ring potentiometers RP1, RP2 and gears G1 and G2. The inner cylinder is connected with the servomotor SM1 whereas the outer cylinder is driven by a transmission belt TB from servomotor SM2. The ring potentiometer voltages are fed back to the inputs of the servomotor electronics SE1 and SE2, so that SM1 and SM2 are operated under position control from the inputs S1 and S2, respectively. Under these conditions an angular displacement of a cylinder is strictly proportional to the voltage S applied to an input of the SE electronics. The two cylinders are illuminated by four d.c. driven fluorescent ring bulbs (not shown). The average brightness at the surface of the cylinders amounts to about $700\,\mathrm{cd\,m^{-2}}$. (From Reichardt and Poggio, 1979.)

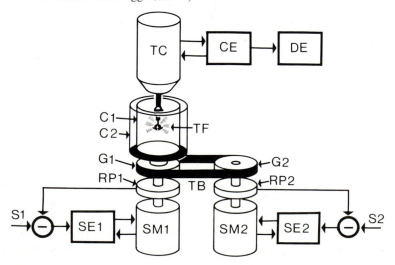

In the figure–ground behavioural experiments described in this paper, the figure (either a black or random-dot textured, vertically oriented stripe) was oscillated around a position $\psi = +30°$, where ψ is the horizontal angle in the equatorial plane of a fly; $\psi = 0°$ designates the symmetry direction between the two compound eyes. Figure and ground were oscillated sinusoidally. The oscillation frequencies of figure and ground amounted to 2.5 Hz and the oscillation amplitudes to $\pm 5°$. The torque response generated by a test-fly was stored in an averager and plotted after the test. Computer simulations were carried out with an HP 9826 computer. The behavioural experiments were performed on female, wild type *Musca domestica* from our laboratory stock.

A key experiment

As has been stated before, flies can detect an object against a textured background, provided the latter move relative to each other. The same behaviour can be observed when the object is replaced by a textured figure even if the textures of figure and ground are statistically equivalent.

In the experiment reported in this section, we restricted ourselves to time-averaged behavioural responses. A typical figure–ground test where the time-averaged response is plotted as a function of the phase between oscillating figure and oscillating ground is shown in Figure 2. The fly optimally detects the figure for phase 90° and 270°; detection decays from 90° (270°) to 180° (0°) where it is negligible in the time-averaged reaction. The outcome of the experiment suggests that figure and ground are discriminated by relative movement. The discrimination depends on the phase difference between oscillatory motions of figure and ground which indicates that the discrimination is non-trivial as otherwise the time-averaged response characteristic would not depend on the phase angle (Reichardt and Poggio, 1979).

Neuronal circuitry

A model of the neuronal circuit for figure–ground discrimination via relative movement by the visual system of the fly *Musca domestica* was suggested by Poggio, Reichardt and Hausen (1981). This circuitry may be located in the lobula complex whose anatomy and physiology are suggestive of the major aspects of the theory. The design of the theory is based on the analysis of time-averaged behaviour and on registrations of the torque response at the onset and in the stationary phase of relative movement. Some of these registrations are shown in the next section. Two main results have been obtained:

(1) The figure–ground discrimination effect exists not only under binocular but also under monocular stimulation by the ground texture.

(2) The torque response of the fly follows the oscillation of a given pattern, as is well known from studies of the optomotor behaviour. Experiments clearly show that the amplitude of the response increases with the movement amplitude whereas it is almost independent of the dimensions of the pattern, suggesting a quite specific gain control mechanism. Consequently the effect of a small figure in determining the phase of the optomotor response is as large as the ground's despite their different areas. These findings have prompted us to consider a model for the neuronal circuit obeying the following constraints: The circuit should contain a gain control mechanism for the overall optomotor reaction. The interaction between movement detectors is not realized through a lateral inhibitory network but rather through large-field

Figure 2. Phase dependence of the figure–ground discrimination effect. Average torque responses of ten flies to sinusoidally-oscillating figure and ground patterns. The figure consists of a black, vertically oriented stripe, 3° wide, oscillated around the mean position $\psi = \pm30°$. The ground pattern consists of a random-dot texture which can be moved independently from the stripe. A white, stationary screen (12° wide) is mounted between the stripe and the ground pattern in order to avoid mixed stimulations of receptors by the stripe and by the ground. The oscillation frequency amounted to 2.5 Hz and the oscillation amplitude to $\pm1°$. The vertical bars denote standard errors of the mean. The continuous line is the component $K_4 \cdot \cos(2\varphi)$ derived from a Fourier analysis of the data plotted in the Figure. The inset of the figure indicates the stimulus conditions. Each point is an average from ten flies. (From Reichardt and Poggio, 1979.)

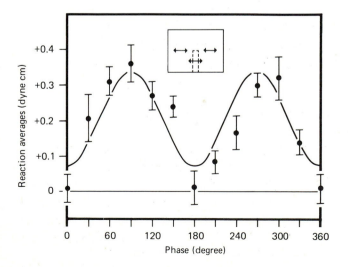

movement-selective neurons inhibiting elementary movement detectors. The neuronal theory should reproduce the characteristic dynamics of the response for all phases between figure and ground and for binocular and monocular stimulations.

A model for the neuronal circuit satisfying these constraints is outlined in Figure 3. The circuit receives channels from a retinotopic

Figure 3. The outline of a neuronal circuit for the right (R) and for the left (L) eye. Considering the right eye as example, two retinotopic arrays of elementary movement detectors, responding selectively to progressive ($\rightarrow$) and regressive ($\leftarrow$) motion, serve as input channels to the neuronal circuitry. The two arrays share the same field of view. For convenience they are drawn apart from each other. A pool neuron (S_R) summates the detector outputs ($\blacktriangleleft\!\!-\!\!$ indicates excitatory synapses) as well as the input from its contralateral homologue (S_L). Its output is assumed to undergo a saturation effect (modelled by taking the square root of its overall excitation) and to shunt each elementary movement detector output via presynaptic inhibition. The synapses involved ($\triangleright\!\!-\!\!$) should therefore inhibit (opening ionic channels with an equilibrium potential close to the resting potential) the output terminal of each elementary detector channel. The output cell X summates the progressive (excitatory, ↥). and the regressive detectors (inhibitory, ↧). Progressive channels have a higher amplification than regressive ones, possibly because of the different ionic batteries involved. The synapses on the X cell are assumed to operate with a non-linear input–output characteristic, leading to postsynaptic signals that are approximately the square of the inputs. The motor output is controlled by the X-cell via a direct channel and a channel T computing the running average of the X-cell's output. (Adapted from Poggio, Reichardt and Hausen, 1981.)

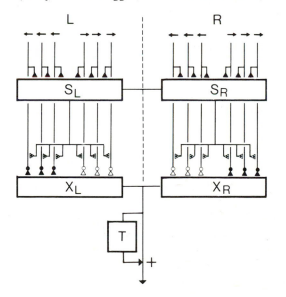

array of elementary movement detectors as its input. Each channel carries output signals from one and only one movement detector. The usual assumption is made that all cells carry only positive signals: in particular, detectors for progressive movement are separate from detectors for regressive movement. Large field cells (S_L and S_R) summate the signals from the elementary movement detectors over a large part of the visual field of the two compound eyes and receive a corresponding contralateral input. They inhibit the signals provided by the individual detectors through shunting inhibition, irrespective of their preferred direction. After shunting inhibition of each detector channel all signals are summated by other large-field cells (X_L and X_R). Before summation, each synaptic input to the (X_L and X_R) cells undergoes a non-linear transformation – like a squaring operation – representing either the non-linear presynaptic–postsynaptic characteristic at the synapse or local active properties of the postsynaptic membrane. It is further assumed that the behavioural response is given by adding the running-time integral of the cells X_L and X_R to the output.

Figure 4a. Oscillation amplitude of the torque response as function of the angular extent of an oscillating figure (0° to 48° wide). Parameter is the oscillating amplitude of the figure (0° to 10°). In the experiments the ground is not oscillated. For a given amplitude of the oscillating figure, the amplitude of the response increases with increasing figure width but reaches a fairly constant level as soon as the figure's extent amounts to more than 12°. Each point derived from 100 sweep averages.

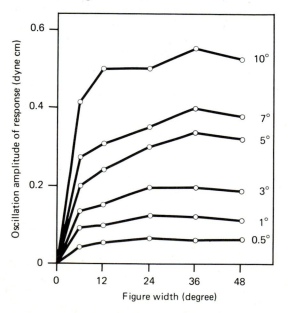

Experiments and predictions

The theory outlined in the preceding section has been tested in a series of relative-movement (figure–ground) experiments. Only a few tests are shown here; they are compared with the computed results.

Gain control for overall optomotor response

When only a figure is oscillated in front of one of the two compound eyes and the ground is at rest, we observe an oscillatory response of the fly with the same frequency. The outcome of these experiments is shown in Figure 4a; parameter is the amplitude of the oscillating figure. The experiments indicate that response amplitudes are relatively independent of the width of the oscillating figure, but increase when the amplitude of the oscillating figure is increased.

Testing the specific gain control mechanism with the neuronal model leads to the plots shown in Figure 4b. The response amplitude increases

Figure 4b. Computer plot demonstrating the gain control mechanism that operates on the angular extent of the oscillating figure. As pointed out in the discussion, the model outlined in Figure 3 relates the detector channel output x to the response R through the relation $R = Nx^n/(\beta + (Nx)^q)^n$. N is the number of excited detectors; n the exponent describing the non-linear property of the synaptic links between detector channels and X_L, X_R cells and $q = \frac{1}{2}$ the exponent describing the saturation of the pool cells S_L, S_R; β designates the shunting inhibition coefficient. In the simulations the settings are $n = 2.0$, $q = 0.5$ and $\beta = 0.05$. The diagram shows the response as function of N with x the parameter. The different curves represent different x values. With increasing x, the level of the response plateau increases.

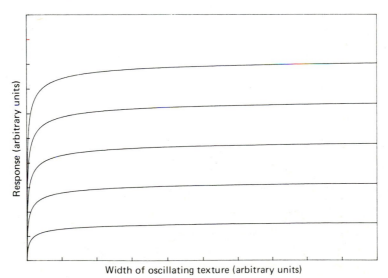

Width of oscillating texture (arbitrary units)

Response (arbitrary units)

with an increase of the figure's angular extent and reaches a constant level. However, it depends strongly on the detector channel output. With increasing output, i.e. with increasing oscillation amplitude of the figure, one gets response curves of different levels. The computer simulation is quite in accordance with the experimental data plotted in Figure 4a.

A typical figure–ground test

A test animal is stimulated by a small figure (a vertically oriented and textured stripe of 12° width) sinusoidally oscillated in front of one of the two compound eyes. A random-dot textured ground (of the same texture as the figure) is also oscillated with the same frequency, amplitude and phase ϕ, relative to the oscillating figure. The

Figure 5a. Typical response of a test-fly in a bilateral figure–ground experiment. A textured stripe of 12° angular width is sinusoidally oscillated in front of a 360°-textured background which oscillates with the same amplitude and the same frequency (2.5 Hz). The stripe oscillates around the mean position $\psi = +30°$ that is in front of the right eye. Oscillation amplitudes amount to $\pm5°$. The time courses of the figure and the ground oscillations (in terms of positions) are plotted in the lower part of the figure. With regard to the right compound eye, movements from $-5°$ to $+5°$ are progressive movements, whereas movements from $+5°$ to $-5°$ are regressive movements. At time 0.4 s the relative phase between figure and ground switches from 0° to 90°. The response (torque) of the fly increases after the phase has shifted and oscillates around a positive average response level with 2.5 Hz frequency. The increase of the response means that the fly is attracted by the oscillating figure. The response plotted is an average of 100 sweeps.

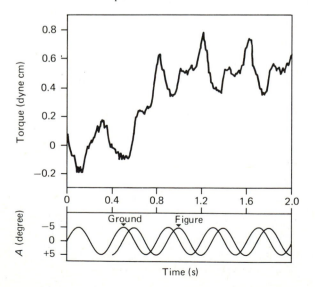

Time (s)

response plotted in Figure 5a consists of an initial part in which the phase between figure and ground oscillation is 0°, followed by a part in which the phase has been switched to 90°. The oscillatory response of the fly increases after the phase ϕ is switched to 90° and reaches a positive level around which it oscillates in a rather complicated fashion. In the $\phi = 90°$ region, the time average of the response is positive; the fly is attracted by the oscillating figure. This finding agrees with the earlier result (shown in Figure 2) when the time average of the response was measured.

The result of the computer test, based on the neuronal circuitry is plotted in Figure 5b. The response at phase 0° is a sinusoid that changes drastically when the phase changes. Since the running average time amounts to 0.4 s, the transition phase ends at 0.8 s. From 0.8 s on the response is stationary, quite similar to the torque response plotted in Figure 5a.

Similar experimental and computational tests of the model have been carried out for other phase differences including 180° and 270°. They will be published elsewhere.

A contralateral figure–ground experiment

Interestingly, figure–ground discrimination is not only confined to conditions where the figure moves in front of the ground texture.

Figure 5b. Computer simulation of the figure–ground experiment reported in Figure 5a. Parameters of the simulation (n, q, β) are the same as specified in Figure 4b. The figure–ground phase changes from 0° to 90° at 0.4 s. The transition phase is completed at 0.8 s since the running average time is one period of response or 0.4 s.

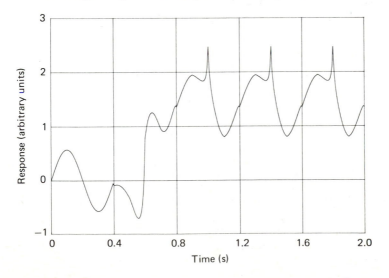

Figure 6a. A contralateral figure–ground experiment. All parameters are as specified in the legend of Figure 5a, except for the angular extension of the ground. The textured ground covers only 180° and extends from $\varphi = 0°$ to $\varphi = -180°$. It therefore stimulates the left compound eye whereas the figure oscillating around $\varphi = +30°$ stimulates the right compound eye. The edges of the oscillating ground are covered by 10°-wide screens. The response of the fly is oscillatory and increases when the phase of the oscillating figure and ground changes from 0° to 90°. That is to say, even under these conditions, the figure is discriminated and the fly attracted by the figure when the phase is 90°. Note that the average response levels are negative. This is due to the fact that the ground texture stimulates only one of the compound eyes. The plot is an average from 100 sweeps.

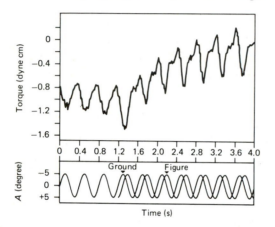

Figure 6b. Computer simulation of the contralateral figure–ground experiment reported in Figure 6a. Parameters of the simulation (n, q, β) are the same as specified in Figure 4b. The phase between figure and half-ground changes from $\varphi = 0°$ to $\varphi = 90°$ at 0.4 s. The response to both phases is negative. The running average time amounts to 0.4 s.

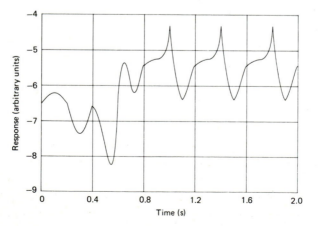

'Discrimination' is even observed when the figure oscillates in front of one compound eye and a half-ground (180° wide texture) in front of the other compound eye. An example of a contralateral figure–ground experiment is presented in Figure 6a. Figure and half-ground oscillate in synchrony initially, then the phase shifts to 90° at time 1.2 s. Throughout the experiment the response is negative since a much larger area in the left eye is stimulated than in the right eye. The observation shown in Figure 6a leads to the conclusion that figure–ground discrimination is a binocular phenomenon in the sense that interactions between the two compound eyes are critically involved.

The contralateral figure–ground situation has also been tested by the computer program verifying the neuronal theory. The result of the computation is shown in Figure 6b. Deviations between the experiment and the theoretical predictions are confined solely to the transition period which in the computer program is set to one cycle of oscillation.

A figure–figure experiment

So far I have dealt with stimulus conditions where the ground consisted of either a 360° or a 180° texture. In the last experiment reported here the ground was replaced by a textured figure of 12° width, positioned at $\psi = -40°$, whereas another textured figure of equal width was mounted in the contralateral position, $\psi = +40°$. The two figures were oscillated in two different phase conditions: in synchrony (phase 0°) up to 0.4 s, then the figure in front of the right compound eye was switched to 90° phase relative to the figure in front of the left compound eye. A typical response of a test-fly is shown in Figure 7a. After the initial transients in the response have decayed, the reaction is periodic, with different rising and falling phases. The amplitude of the response during phase-90° condition amounts to about twice the amplitude during synchronous oscillation.

The corresponding simulation, presented in Figure 7b, is quite in accordance with the experimental tests, indicating that the theory also explains this unusual stimulus condition.

Discussion

This short paper contains only a few relative motion or figure–ground experiments together with computer simulations that are based on the neuronal circuitry sketched on p. 361. Many more test experiments with different figure–ground oscillations (amplitudes, phases, and frequencies) have been carried out and were compared with predictions

Figure 7a. A bilateral figure–figure experiment. A textured stripe of 12° angular width is sinusoidally oscillated in front of the right eye around the mean position $\varphi = +40°$. Another textured stripe of the same width is oscillated in front of the left eye around the mean position $\varphi = -40°$. Oscillation amplitudes amount to $\pm5°$, oscillation frequencies to 2.5 Hz. At time 0.4 s the relative phase between figure (1) and figure (2) switches from 0° to 90°. The fly's response is oscillatory around zero torque and increases in amplitude after the phase has shifted from 0° to 90°. Note that the response oscillates around zero. The response plotted is an average of 100 sweeps.

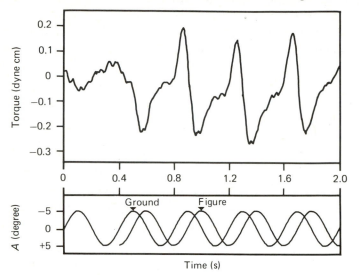

Figure 7b. Computer simulation of the figure–figure experiment reported in Figure 7a. The phase between the oscillations of the two figures changes from 0° to 90° at time 0.4 s. The transition phase is completed at 0.8 s. All parameter setting (n, q, β) as specified in the legend of Figure 4b.

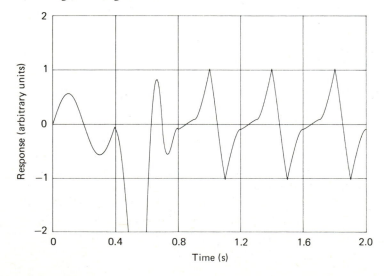

of the theory. So far the theory is in full agreement with all the behavioural data, including the characteristic dynamics of the responses.

Let us now come back to the speculations raised in the introduction. The key experiment described on p. 360 has already shown that the movement fields x of the ground and y of the figure (vector notations are dropped since figure and ground are oscillated here in one direction only) interact in a non-linear fashion. The nature of this interaction should now be derived from the neuronal circuitry.

Except for the running average at the output of the model, the behavioural response of the fly is, according to the circuitry, given by the relation

$$R = \frac{Nx^n}{(\beta + (Nx)^q)^n} \tag{2}$$

provided that all channels N are equally excited by a moving pattern. x designates the output of each of the N movement detectors, β the shunting inhibition coefficient, n the presynaptic-postsynaptic characteristic of the synapses at the inputs to the X-cells, and q a possible saturation of the S-cells. The gain control experiment described on p. 362 requires that, for increasing N, the response R should become independent of N, which means that $n \cdot q$ has to be unity, neglecting β for $(Nx)^q \gg \beta$. Since the response under phase $0°$ conditions is sinusoidal, $n = 2$ so that $q = 1/2$. In order to simplify the argument, I consider here now only the case that figure and ground both excite N channels and designate with y the output of each of the movement detectors which receive their inputs from the oscillating figure. Under these conditions equation (2) becomes

$$R = \frac{Nx^n + Ny^n}{(\beta + (Nx + Ny)^q)^n} \tag{3}$$

Under normal conditions $(Nx = Ny)^q \gg \beta$, and with $n = 2$, $q = 1/2$ one arrives at

$$R = \frac{x^2 + y^2}{x + y} = x + y - \frac{2xy}{x + y} \tag{4}$$

That is to say, the response of the fly depends linearly on the movement fields x and y which are inhibited (minus sign) by the weighted correlation of x and y. Equation (4) immediately tells us that the contributions from the figure (y) and the ground (x) to the response become independent when figure and ground move in statistical independence, a prediction which has been tested experimentally and confirmed.

Interestingly, equation (4) has a striking similarity to the formation of a hologram where x and y denote the squares of the light-wave amplitudes of reference and object beams respectively and xy the interference between the two waves of coherent light. This finding should not be interpreted as suggesting that the fly's visual system computes a short-term hologram of the optical environment since the overlap of the receptor fields is small and not wide. The conclusion is that the evaluation of relative movement by the visual system of the fly makes use of computations analogous to those that take place during the process of hologram formation, without leading, however, to a holographic pattern of the fly's optical environment. The only important point is the experimentally established fact that the fly is equipped with neuronal components whose functions could be implemented for the processing of information if the nervous system were to process and possibly store data in holographic fashion (Reichardt, 1980).

Electrophysiological experiments are under way to clarify the open aspects of the theory.

I would like to thank Dr Roger Hardie for correcting the English text and Mrs Inge Geiss for typing and correcting the manuscript.

References

Hausen, K. (1976). Functional characterization and anatomical identification of motion sensitive neurons in the lobula plate of the Blowfly *Calliphora erythrocephala. Z. Naturforsch. 31c:* 629–33.

Helmholtz, H. von (1856–1896). *Handbuch der Physiologischen Optik*. Hamburg: Voss.

Julesz, B. (1971). *Foundations of Cyclopean Perception*. Chicago: University of Chicago Press.

Poggio, T., Reichardt, W., and Hausen, K. (1981). A neuronal circuitry for relative movement discrimination by the visual system of the fly. *Naturwissenschaften 68:* 443–6.

Reichardt, W. (1980). Analogy between hologram formation and computation of relative movement by the visual system of the fly. *Naturwissenschaften 67:* 411–12.

Reichardt, W., and Poggio, T. (1979). Figure–ground discrimination by relative movement in the visual system of the fly. Part I: Experimental results. *Biol. Cybernetics 35:* 81–100.

Virsik, R., and Reichardt, W. (1974). Tracking of moving objects by the fly *Musca domestica. Naturwissenschaften 61:* 132–3.

Note added in proof. A detailed account has recently been published: Reichardt, W., Poggio, T., and Hausen, K. (1983). Figure–ground discrimination by relative movement in the visual system of the fly. Part II. *Biol. Cybernetics 46:* 1–30.

3.3

Local circuits in the distal retina of vertebrates

MARCO PICCOLINO and PAUL WITKOVSKY

In recent years morphological and functional study of the nervous system has revealed aspects of the neural organization which depart from the classical conceptual framework of the 'neuron doctrine', as it was formulated during the epoch of Cajal and later developed with the application of sophisticated techniques for visualizing nerve cells and recording their electrical activity.

According to the classical view the morphological and functional unit of the nervous system is the neuron, whose characteristic feature is its 'dynamic polarization' along the dendro-axonic direction. This model neuron receives the input at the dendro-somatic region and, by way of the action potential, which propagates centrifugally and non-decrementally along the axon, influences other neurons through specialized synaptic contacts situated at the axon terminal. The mechanism of synaptic action is, typically, the phasic release of the chemical transmitter, stored in vesicular form at the axon terminal, triggered by the impulsive depolarization associated with the action potential.

Nerve cells have been now described which have output synapses localized on the dendrites, or receive input at the axon. In some cells there is no axon at all. In others, in which a dendritic and axonal compartment have been identified on morphological grounds, the two compartments are functionally independent: electrical signals generated in one of them do not spread effectively to the other, each compartment having private input–output connections with other cells and thus functioning as a separated cell (see Shepherd, 1979, and Schmitt and Worden, 1979, for reviews).

Moreover, nerve cells can be coupled electrically to one another through junctions (gap junctions) which allow for the direct passage of

371

ions, in such a way that distinct cells do not work as separate units, but realize a sort of functional network, reminiscent of the syncytium of the 'reticular theory'.

Nerve cells have also been identified which do not discharge action potentials: the electrical signalling occurs only through graded potentials, and the release of chemical transmitter is modulated in a tonic way by these non-impulsive potentials (see Roberts and Bush, 1981, for review).

Many of these unusual aspects of neural organization occur in the distal region of vertebrate retina. Here different classes of nerve cells establish synaptic contacts which are the sites of the initial processing of visual information.

The purpose of this article is to review some recent morphological and physiological data on the synaptic interactions taking place at this level, with particular reference to those involving the horizontal cells (HC), which illustrate many of the operational mechanisms discussed. Our approach will be to draw particularly from studies performed in turtle retina, where these interactions have been more thoroughly investigated, with the caveat to the reader that not all conclusions will be applicable to all retinas.

General organization of the distal retina

Figure 1 illustrates schematically the morphology of nerve cells (A) and the functional pathways (B) of the distal retina, and Figure 2 shows typical examples of light responses recorded at this level in the turtle.

In the outer plexiform layer (OPL) photoreceptors make synaptic contacts with two classes of second-order neurons, bipolar and horizontal cells. A third category of retinal neuron is the interplexiform cell whose processes also contribute to the contacts of the OPL, but, in contrast to bipolar and horizontal cells, the interplexiform cell does not make direct connections with photoreceptors.

Photoreceptors absorb light and generate electrical responses at their outermost segment, and provide synaptic input to second-order neurons, through chemical synapses situated at their proximal ending. Functionally these synapses can be either of the sign-preserving or of the sign-inverting type, depending on the post-synaptic cell. Photoreceptors are subdivided into two main classes, rods and cones, on the basis of morphological and functional differences. In each class different subtypes can be distinguished according to their spectral characteristics. In lower vertebrates photoreceptors can exist as pairs, consisting of two

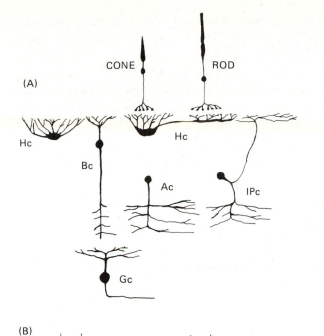

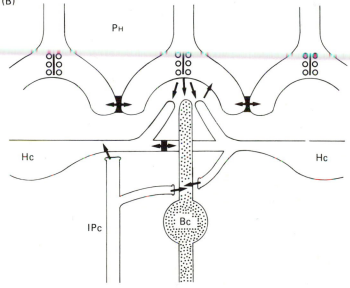

Figure 1. Schematic representation of neuronal elements of the vertebrate retina (A) and synaptic pathways of the outer plexiform layer (B). Hc, horizontal cell; Bc, bipolar cell; Ac, amacrine cell; IPc, interplexiform cell; Gc, ganglion cell; Pн, photoreceptor. In (B) the electrical junctions are represented as heavy-black double-arrow contacts.

similar or dissimilar members (twin or double photoreceptors, respectively) partially fused together. Electrical contacts can exist between photoreceptors, most commonly between elements of the same functional type.

Bipolar cells are part of the main line of transmission of visual information, receiving input from photoreceptors at their distal dendritic arborization and making output synapses onto amacrine ganglion cells at their proximal axonal endings.

Horizontal cells are tangentially stratified interneurons whose pro-

Figure 2. Intracellular recording of the responses induced by white-light stimuli in different retinal neurons, as indicated at the left of each row of tracings. CDB, center-depolarizing bipolar; CHB, center-hyperpolarizing bipolar; HC, horizontal cell. The light stimulus is monitored above the recordings in (a)–(g), and the stimulus traces in (e)–(g) also refer to the underlying recordings. Numbers above the stimulus traces in (a)–(d) indicate the attenuation of the light stimuli in log units with respect to the maximum available flux density (of about $3 \times 10^{-5}\ \mu W\ \mu m^{-2}$ for all the responses illustrated in this article). The light was attenuated by 3.6 log units in (e)–(n). Stimulus dimensions: (a)–(d) spot, 250 μm diameter; annulus (Ann), 3700 μm outer diameter (O.D.), 430 μm inner diameter (I.D.). (e)–(n): spot, 870 μm diameter, annulus, 3700 μm O.D., 870 μm I.D.

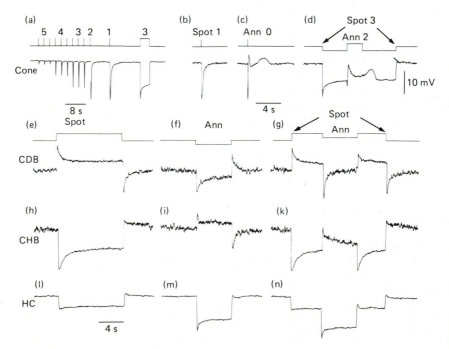

cesses contact photoreceptors at junctions which can be sites of two-way synaptic transmission. In the forward pathway (photoreceptors-HC) the transmission is of the sign-preserving type, while in the feedback pathway it involves a sign-inverting synapse. Adjacent HC can be electrically coupled to each other, and in some instances HC can have an output synapse onto bipolar cells (supposed to be of the sign-inverting type).

Interplexiform cells have cell bodies situated at a proximal level of the retina and dendrites which ascend toward the OPL to make synapse onto bipolar, horizontal or other interplexiform cells. The functional characteristics of these synapses are unknown.

The responses elicited in cones by small light spots (Figure 2*a*) are graded hyperpolarizations whose amplitudes and time course depend on the intensity and duration of the stimulus. Illumination of the receptive field surround can elicit complex responses showing a late depolarizing component, which is the result of the recurrent action of HC (Figure 2*c*). These feedback depolarizations are better seen when surround illumination is applied in the presence of a steady central stimulus, to attenuate the effects of scattered light (Figure 2*d*). The light responses of rods are also graded hyperpolarizations which differ from those of cones with respect to their sensitivity, time course and absence of feedback surround influence.

Bipolar cells, which also respond to light with graded potential changes, show a clear center-surround antagonistic organization of the receptive field. According to the polarity of the response elicited by center illumination, bipolar cells are divisible into center-depolarizing (CDB, Figure 2*e–g*) and center-hyperpolarizing types (CHB, Figure 2*h–k*). Opposite polarity responses are elicited in both types by light annuli either flashed alone or in the presence of a central background. As illustrated in Figure 2 the membrane potential of bipolar cells is characterized by the presence, in darkness, of large-amplitude fluctuations (dark noise) which are decreased by central illumination and can be increased by peripheral illumination (Figure 2*e,h* and *g,k*).

Horizontal cells also give graded responses to illumination of their receptive field. In many cases these responses are hyperpolarizing in sign and require large area illumination to attain large amplitudes (Figure 2*l,n*).

There is no documented recording of the light responses of interplexiform cells and hypotheses concerning their functional role are based mainly on anatomical and biochemical evidence.

Morphology of HC

This subject has been studied intensively since the days of Cajal (Cajal, 1893), and many reviews of the literature exist (Stell, 1972; Gallego, 1976; Stell, Kretz and Lightfoot, 1983). We confine ourselves to a few general remarks, describing in some detail only the HC of the turtle.

Every vertebrate retina appears to have several varieties of HC distinguished by the presence or absence of axons, types of photo-receptors contacted, cell body size and position, length of dendrites, etc. Axon-bearing HC have been demonstrated in representatives of all vertebrate classes with the exception of elasmobranch fish. As illus-trated in Figure 3*a–i*, these cells vary considerably in form and size, but a common characteristic is that the perikaryon and the axon terminal are joined by a slender fiber running horizontally for relatively long distances. The axon ending is poorly developed in teleosts (Figure 3*a*) whereas it ramifies more or less extensively in other species and bears a particularly rich arborization in some mammals (Figure 3*f* and *g*). The pattern of dendritic branching radiating from the perikaryon also exhibits considerable variability.

As a general rule both the cell body and axon terminal regions are connected with photoreceptors, and the types of photoreceptors con-tacted can be different, with many possible variations among species and, sometimes, among subtypes in the same species. In the cat, for instance, and in one type of monkey the perikaryal dendrites contact only cones whereas the axonal arborization is connected exclusively to rods (Kolb, 1970, 1974; Gallego, 1971, 1976; Boycott, Peichl and Wässle, 1978). In pigeons and turtles the perikaryon is similarly connected only to cones, but the axon terminal contacts both rods and cones (Mariani and Leure-du Pree, 1977; Leeper, 1978*b*). In the gray squirrel and in a second type of the monkey this HC type contacts exclusively cones at both cell body and axon terminal (West, 1978; Kolb, Mariani and Gallego, 1980). In the salamander and frog both perikaryon and axon terminal are connected with a mixture of both cone and rods (Lasansky, 1978; Stephan and Weiler, 1981). Finally in goldfish and carp the axon seems not to contact any photoreceptor at all, whereas the perikaryon is connected exclusively with cones (Stell, 1975; Weiler, 1978). In fact, three different axon-bearing HC can be distin-guished in the goldfish according to the spectral type of cones contacted by the perikaryal dendrites (Stell and Lightfoot, 1975).

Axonless HC have been described in many vertebrates with the notable exception of primates. As illustrated in Figure 3*k–r*, these cells also show considerable morphological variations. Moreover, their contacts with photoreceptors can be different among species and subtypes. In cat, pigeon and turtles, axonless HC are connected exclusively with cones (Kolb, 1974; Wässle, Boycott and Peichl, 1978; Gallego, 1976; Mariani and Leure-du Pree, 1977; Leeper, 1978b). In frogs they are connected with a mixture of both cones and rods (Stephan and Weiler,

Figure 3. Golgi-stained HC of different animals. (*a*)–(*i*): axon-bearing types. (*k*)–(*r*) axonless types. Animals and references:
(*a*), (*m*) goldfish, Stell (1975); (*b*), (*n*), (*o*) turtle, Leeper (1978*a*); (*c*), (*p*) pigeon, Mariani and Leure-du Pree (1977); (*d*) chicken, Cajal (1893); (*e*), (*q*) gray squirrel, West (1978); (*f*), (*r*) cat, Fisher and Boycott (1974); (*g*) calf, Marenghi (1901); (*h*) monkey, Kolb, Mariani and Gallego (1980); (*i*) monkey, Ogden (1974); (*k*), (*l*) dogfish, Stell and Witkovsky (1973).

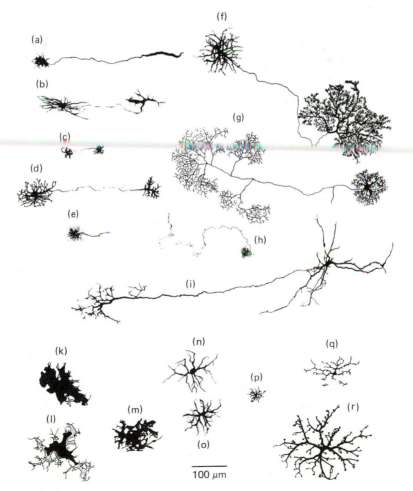

1981) while in goldfish and carp they contact only rods (Stell, 1975; Weiler, 1978). In stingray fish, axonless HC can contact a mixture of both cones and rods (Toyoda, Saito and Kondo, 1978), whereas in dogfish different subtypes contact either rods or cones (Stell and Witkovsky, 1973).

In goldfish and turtles a careful morphological investigation has permitted identification of the spectral types of photoreceptors contacted by the different HC types (Stell and Lightfoot, 1975; Leeper, 1978*b*). In the turtle, one type of axon-bearing HC (indicated as H1) and three axonless HC (H2, H3 and H4) have been distinguished on these grounds. The cell body region of the H1 (H1CB) contacts both red-sensitive cones (red single cones and red members of double cones) and green-sensitive cones (green single cones and green members of double cones), while the axon terminal (H1AT) is connected with red-sensitive cones and rods. The H2 type contacts both green- and blue-sensitive cones, the H3 only blue cones and finally the H4-type contacts only the green member of double cones.

These studies show a great variety of morphological types of HC and of their connections with photoreceptors and predict a similar great variety of functional type of HC. The results of these morphological investigations are of great importance for understanding the mechanism of generation of the HC light responses. However, due to the complexity and intricacy of neural interactions in the distal retina, all the morphological data concerning the connections between HC and photoreceptors must be evaluated critically before drawing any positive conclusion on the functional meaning of the anatomical contacts. We will see later in this article that a given HC type can be influenced by photoreceptors not directly contacted by it, and on the other hand, that a HC may not receive input from photoreceptors which have a direct connection with it.

Morphology of the contacts in the OPL

The forward photoreceptor–HC synapse

The ultrastructural evidence reveals great structural complexity of the synaptic contacts at the photoreceptor endings. The processes of HC penetrate more or less deeply in the photoreceptor base terminating in close proximity to the junctional specializations of the photoreceptor (Dowling and Boycott, 1966; Lasansky, 1971, 1973; Stell, 1972). In these 'invaginated junctions', the processes of HC are usually in contiguity with the dendrites of some bipolar cells, the actual spatial arrangement of the different processes varies considerably according to the subtype of photoreceptors and second-order neurons participating to the contacts and between retinas (Stell et al., 1983).

The specializations on the photoreceptor side are remarkably constant and such as to favor the idea of a chemical mechanism of transmission in the forward pathway (photoreceptors–second-order neurons). The photoreceptor surface membrane forms a ridge (synaptic ridge) whose subjacent cytoplasm contains a proteinaceous mass, the arciform density, toward which a lamellar formation (the 'synaptic ribbon') points (Chen and Witkovsky, 1978). The ribbon itself is a protein structure (Bunt, 1971) bearing short side arms which may bind, or at any rate are associated with, synaptic vesicles (Gray and Pease, 1971; McLaughlin and Boykins, 1977). By reference to other well-studied chemical synapses (Akert, 1973) the arciform density conforms to the presynaptic grid whose dual function is to orient vesicles toward sites of exocytosis, and to cross-link membrane proteins (presumed membrane channels) so as to maintain them in high concentration in the presynaptic active zone (Couteaux and Pecot-Dechavassine, 1970; Heuser and Reese, 1973). Freeze-fracture studies of photo-receptor-active zones show that the protoplasmic or P-face of the membrane at the synaptic ridge bears an array of particles in high concentration (Raviola and Gilula, 1975; McLaughlin and Reese, 1981; Nagy and Witkovsky, 1981).

There is no functional counterpart of the synaptic ribbon in conventional chemical synapses. Presumably the ribbon plays a role in directing vesicles towards the synaptic ridge, but the mechanism by which this occurs is not yet understood.

The photoreceptor synaptic vesicles are mainly agranular, 30–50 nm in diameter and are distributed more or less homogeneously throughout the receptor base, only being clustered around the ribbon. Although they do not tend to pile up adjacent to the active zone, their arrangement is clearly non-random (Gray and Pease, 1971). Studies using HRP as a tracer indicate that the photoreceptor vesicular membrane is cycled (Ripps, Shakib and MacDonald, 1976; Schacher, Holtzman and Hood, 1976) in general accord with the Heuser-Reese scheme (Heuser and Reese, 1973), i.e., exocytotic vesicles fuse with the surface membrane, the fused membrane material is displaced laterally and is recaptured as coated vesicles.

The membrane specializations of the HC processes at their synapse with photoreceptors consist of paramembranous cytoplasmic 'fuzz' or undercoating that lies opposite the synaptic ridge, but may well extend beyond it laterally (Lasansky, 1971, 1973).

Freeze-fracture replicas reveal a broad area of P-face particles corresponding to the region of HC membrane undercoating (Raviola and Gilula, 1975; Nagy and Witkovsky, 1981). By analogy with neuro-muscular junction (Heuser, Reese and Landis, 1974) one might suppose that the HC P-face particles correspond to the post-synaptic, trans-mitter-gated, ion channels. However, it should be noted that some HC processes also contain external (E)-face particle arrays, although these are small and linear, compared to the P-face cluster. Studies of other known chemical synapses reveal both P to P-face arrays (e.g., neuro-muscular junction) and P to E-face arrays (e.g., cerebellar cortex: Landis and Reese, 1974) in pre- and post-synaptic membranes, respec-tively, so it is not yet clear whether HC conform always to one or another of these patterns.

The HC-cone feedback synapse

In spite of compelling physiological evidence in favour of a feedback synapse between HC and cones, clear morphological evidence in support of such a synapse is lacking. Lasansky (1971) has speculated that some junctions situated on the HC processes penetrating in the cone base, away from the ridge ('distal junctions') could be the site of the feedback transmission. There is no cluster of vesicles opposite to these junctions (and indeed HC possess only a few sparse agranular vesicles). Freeze-fracture replicas fail to reveal either pre- or post-synaptic particle arrays that could correspond to the feedback synapse.

We will discuss later the possibility that the feedback involves mechanisms other than the classical chemical transmission, which could account for the lack of typical synaptic specializations at this level. It must be noted, however, that indirect morphological evidence in support of the feedback synapse exists in the retina of the goldfish. Here the position of HC processes in the invaginated junctions varies systematically depending on the HC and cone subtypes involved. These differences are correlated with the presumed polarity of the synaptic transmission: HC processes occupy a central position with respect to the synaptic ridge at sites of supposed forward transmission, and a lateral position where the transmission is supposed to occur in the feedback direction (Stell, Lightfoot, Wheeler and Leeper, 1975).

Gap junctions between HC

It is generally accepted that gap junctions mediate the electrical transmission between nervous (and non-nervous) cells (reviewed in Bennett, 1977; Lowenstein, 1981).

Gap junctions have been found between HC of the same functional type in a variety of animal species (Yamada and Ishikawa, 1965; Kolb, 1977; Witkowsky, Burkhardt and Nagy, 1979; Schaeffer, Raviola and Heuser, 1982). The structure of the gap junction is quite uniform. In tissue stained *en bloc* with uranyl acetate, gap junctions appear septalaminar in thin section: two-unit membranes separated by a 1–3-nm gap which is accessible to extracellular space (Brightman and Reese, 1969). In freeze-fracture replicas gap junctions are characterized by a P-face array of closely grouped particles together with corresponding E-face pits in both the participating membranes. Thus, the junction is symmetrical.

What can vary from gap junction to gap junction is the area of the participating membrane, and the frequency of the junctions themselves.

Large and numerous gap junctions are found in the turtle between the membrane of the axon terminals of the H1 cells. In contrast the perikarya of the same cell type are joined by smaller, and perhaps fewer, gap junctions, and, moreover, no junction is found in the area of apposition between the membrane of the axon and the membrane of perikaryal dendrites (Witkovsky, Owen and Woodworth, 1983). A similar pattern is found in the retina of some amphibians and fish (Yamada and Ishikawa, 1965; Stell, 1972; Lasansky, 1976, 1980; Stell et al., 1983). In the retina of the cat, however, gap junctions are found only between HC of the axonless type, while they are absent between axon-bearing HC (Sobrino and Gallego, 1970; Kolb, 1977).

These differences in the characteristics of the gap junctions between HC anticipate differences in the characteristics of the electrical coupling between HC types.

HC–bipolar cell synapse

There is evidence in some amphibia that HC contact bipolar cells via conventional chemical synapses, i.e. ones characterized on the presynaptic side by a cluster of vesicles adjacent to the membrane, and paramembranous subsynaptic densities in both pre- and post-synaptic membranes (Dowling and Werblin, 1969; Witkovsky and Powell, 1981). Freeze-fracture characterization of these synapses is lacking. The identity of pre- and post-synaptic neurons had to be established through serial sections or some other unequivocal method, because other conventional synapses are also found in the OPL, for example those of interplexiform cells (see below). Most importantly, in certain well-studied fish retinas, where horizontal–bipolar cell interactions are well-documented (Naka, 1982; Toyoda and Kujiraoka, 1982) there is no evidence for direct horizontal-to-bipolar cells synapses. Finally, it has been claimed that in salamander retina, bipolar cells are presynaptic to horizontal cells and not the reverse (Lasansky, 1980).

Other synapses in the OPL

Bipolar cells make dendritic connections with photoreceptors in the OPL and axonal connections with amacrine and ganglion cells in the inner plexiform layer (Stell, 1972). With regard to photoreceptors, bipolars may contact only rods or cones, as in mammalian retina (Kolb, 1970), a mixture of both rods and cones as seen in amphibian retina (Lasansky, 1973; Witkovsky and Powell, 1981), or be dominated by rods with a small cone input, as observed in certain bipolars of fish retina (Stell, 1978). The photoreceptor-to-bipolar cell junction varies in structure. A commonly observed configuration is the basal junction (also called 'flat') in which the bipolar dendrite indents the photo-receptor base to varying degree (Kolb, 1970; Lasansky, 1971, 1973). No photoreceptor ribbon is seen at this site although both pre- and post-synaptic elements exhibit prominent paramembranous undercoatings. The synaptic cleft also contains proteinaceous material. Freeze-fracture replicas reveal P-face particles in the photoreceptor and E-face particles in the bipolar cell membrane (Raviola and Gilula, 1975; Nagy and Witkovsky, 1981). This is the particle aggregate pattern seen at some excitatory synapses in CNS (Landis and Ree, 1974). At another sort of photoreceptor–bipolar junction (invaginated or ribbon junctions), the bipolar dendrite penetrates more or less deeply into the receptor base and is aligned, together with flanking HC processes, opposite to the synaptic ridge (Dowling and Boycott, 1966; Raviola and Gilula, 1975). The bipolar cell membrane lacks obvious terminal specializations; freeze-fracture study does not provide any clear evidence for particle aggregation in the bipolar cell membrane (Raviola and Gilula, 1975). The main reason for calling this a synapse is that in primates such invaginating bipolars apparently make no other contact with the photoreceptors.

The ascending dendrite of interplexiform cells also contributes to the synaptic contacts of the OPL (Ehinger, Falk and Laties, 1969; Boycott et al., 1975). At this level the interplexiform cell may synapse on bipolar, horizontal or other interplexiform cells (Dowling and Ehinger, 1975; Kolb and West, 1977). These synapses have the classical features of conventional chemical synapse and according to the Dowling's view, most, if not all, the conventional synapses seen in the OPL involve interplexiform cell dendrites as presynaptic elements. Interplexiform

cells have been identified in representative retinas of numerous vertebrate classes and must therefore be considered as generally present.
Pharmacologically they have been found to be dopaminergic or glycinergic in teleosts (Ehinger et al., 1969; Marc and Lam, 1981) and
dopaminergic in mammals (Boycott et al., 1975; Nguyen-Legros, Berger, Vigny and Alvarez, 1981; Frederick et al., 1982).

As indicated earlier, gap junctions are also present at the level of
photoreceptors. In most cases, they are found between photoreceptors
of the same sort. In many retinas, rod photoreceptors form a spatial
network through extensive gap junctions among neighboring rods
(Gold, 1979). Cones tend to be coupled via gap junctions (Raviola and
Gilula, 1973) to other cones bearing the same visual pigment (Detwiler
and Hodgkin, 1979). However, in some instances, gap junctions are also
present between rods and cones (Kolb, 1977). In general, photoreceptor
gap junctions are found among basal processes (telodendria) that
extend laterally from photoreceptor synaptic base and enter the OPL,
although in the toad and catfish retinas they are noted at the level of
photoreceptor inner segment. There is also considerable variation as to
area of membrane involved in these junctions. For instance, in the cat,
the cone–cone gap junctions are large, whereas those between rods and
cones are extremely restricted (Kolb, 1977). Similar minute gap junctions are also present between photoreceptors of the monkey and turtle
(Raviola and Gilula, 1973; Schaeffer et al., 1982).

The existence of crossed rod to cone gap junctions, as in the cat
retina, is functionally important since through these junctions a rod
input can be provided to cells, or regions of a cell, directly connected
only to cones (Nelson, Lutzow, Kolb and Gouras, 1975; Nelson, 1977)
and vice versa.

Physiology of HC
General remarks
The aim of the physiological study of HC has been directed to: (i)
identify and analyse their light responses and to correlate these responses with the results of the morphological observations; (ii) establish
the mechanisms of generation of the HC responses; and (iii) ascertain
the functional role of HC in the neural operations of the distal retina.

These different aspects of the HC physiology are difficult to separate
because of the complexity and interdependency of the neural interactions involving these neurons. For instance, the feedback onto cones,
which represents an output for the HC, allowing these cells to intervene
in the elaboration of the visual message (point (iii) above), must be

taken into account also when considering the generation mechanism of the HC light responses (point (ii)), since HC receive input from cones and can be thus influenced by electrical signals reverberating along the feedback loop.

Functional classification and morpho-functional correlations

In almost all the retinas so far investigated different types of HC light responses have been identified (see Laufer and Drujan, 1983). In the turtle HC responses have been differentiated according to their spectral characteristics and receptive field properties (Simon, 1973; Fuortes and Simon, 1974; Saito, Miller and Tomita, 1974). One type is the luminosity HC (L–HC, Figure 4a) in which receptive field illumination with light spots always evokes hyperpolarizing responses irrespective of the spectral characteristics of the stimulus. These units have maximal responsiveness for stimulus wavelengths between 600 and 650 nm and can be differentiated into two subtypes according to their receptive field profile: a large field type (L1–HC) having optimal summation areas of more than three-millimeters diameter, and a small

Figure 4. (a)–(c). Intracellular recordings of the light responses induced by monochromatic light of different wavelengths in respectively a luminosity horizontal cell (L-HC), red–green chromaticity horizontal cells (RG-HC), and green–blue chromaticity horizontal cells (GB-HC). Numbers near the stimulus traces in (a) give the stimulus wavelength in nanometers. The stimulus was a spot of 3700 μm diameter delivering about 1.7×10^5 quanta $\mu m^{-2} s^{-1}$.
(d), (e). Intracellular recordings of the light responses of respectively a large-field (L1-HC) and a small-field (L2-HC) luminosity horizontal cell, elicited by white-light stimuli covering different areas of their receptive fields as indicated. Annulus, 3700 μm O.D., 870 μm I.D. The diameter of the spots is indicated in μm near the stimulus traces. The light was attenuated by 2.7 log units.

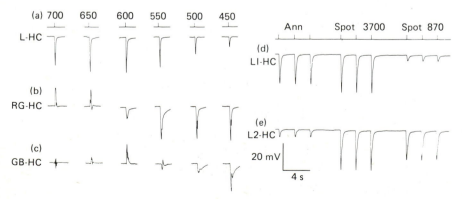

field type (L2–HC) whose optimal summation area has a diameter of about one millimeter. As illustrated in Figure 4d,e these two L–HC can be differentiated by comparing the amplitude of their response to small light spots (about one millimeter in diameter) with the amplitude of their response to large light annuli.

A different type of HC response is the chromaticity type (C-HC). In these units the response polarity depends on the stimulus wavelength. In the turtle two different C-HC have been identified. In one of these, the RG-HC, the response is hyperpolarizing for short wavelengths and depolarizing for long wavelengths (Figure 4b). In the second subtype (GB-HC), the response is also a hyperpolarization for short wavelengths and a depolarization for longer ones, but the maximal responsiveness for both response polarities is displaced toward the short wavelength side of the spectrum as compared to the RG-HC (Figure 4c). Deep-red stimuli can elicit biphasic responses in GB-HC.

The intracellular injection of dyes through the recording electrode has permitted identification of the origin of many of the HC responses in turtle, as well in other animals. Simon (1973) and Saito et al. (1974) injected Procion yellow dye into the cellular elements responsible for the origin of, respectively, the L1-, L2- and RG-HC responses in turtle. By comparing their observations with the morphology of Golgi-impregnated HC, Leeper (1978*a*) concluded that the site of origin of the L1- and the L2-HC responses were respectively the axon terminal and the perikaryon of the H1 type cell, whereas the H2 gave rise to the RG-HC light responses. These conclusions were confirmed by Stewart (1978) and ourselves (Piccolino, Neyton, Witkovsky and Gerschenfeld, 1982, and unpublished observations) using Lucifer yellow, a fluorescent dye which not only diffuses through the injected cell, but also permeates the gap junctions, thus revealing the possible existence of functional coupling between neighboring cells. When the dye was injected through electrodes recording either L2- or L1-HC responses the whole H1 cell was stained, that is both perikaryon and axon terminal. However, the most fluorescent cellular element, corresponding to the injection site, was the perikaryon when recording L2-HC responses and the axon terminal when recording L1-HC responses. When the dye was injected through electrodes recording RG-HC responses, axonless cells were stained similarly to the H2 types. Figure 5 compares the Lucifer yellow staining profiles obtained when recording respectively L2-HC and RG-HC responses, with the H1 and H2 cells impregnated by the Golgi method and illustrates the close correspondence of the data obtained with the two techniques.

The results concerning the origin of the L-HC response are interesting also in that they show that the H1 cell is not a functional unit according to the principles of the 'neuron doctrine'. The differences between the two responses recorded from the perikaryon and the axon terminal region of the H1 indicate that the fiber joining the two regions must be unable to support effective electrical conduction between them. This is not unexpected if one considers that this fiber is very thin (<0.5 μm) and rather long (200–300 μm) and that its membrane expands at both ends.

The ineffectiveness of the transmission along the joining fiber is of course a necessary but not sufficient condition for the differences in the light responses between H1 perikaryon and axon terminal. We will discuss later the probable reasons for these differences. It is worth noting here that a functional separation has been found also between the axon terminal and the perikaryon in the HC of salamander, catfish

Figure 5. Comparison between intracellular staining profiles and Golgi-impregnated HC of the turtle retina. (a), (b) were obtained by injecting Lucifer yellow dye through electrodes recording respectively L2- and RG-HC-type responses. (From Piccolino, Neyton, Witkovsky and Gerschenfeld, 1982, and unpublished.) (c), (d) are respectively H1 and H2 cells visualized with the Golgi technique by Leeper (1978a). To allow for a better comparison the Lucifer dye profiles have been photographically inverted. Notice the difference in scale between respectively (a), (c) and (b), (d). The arrows in (a) indicate the perikarya of two adjacent H1 faintly stained by the dye diffused from the injection site across the gap junctions.

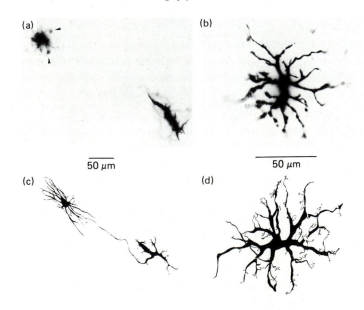

(a)   (b)

50 μm   50 μm

(c)   (d)

and cat (Lasansky and Vallerga, 1975; Chan and Naka, 1980; Nelson et al., 1975). Interestingly, in catfish and salamander, the responses recorded from the two regions show receptive field differences similar to those recorded from the turtle.

In the axon-bearing HC of the carp the situation is at variance with this scheme. The responses recorded from the axon terminal do not differ from those recorded from the perikaryon of the same cell type (Weiler and Zettler, 1979). This is surprising also since, as previously noted, the axon terminal apparently does not contact photoreceptors. It has been supposed (Weiler and Zettler, 1979) that the axon fiber has, in this case, some active membrane mechanism allowing for non-decremental conduction from perikaryon to axon terminal, in spite of the limitations imposed by the cable properties of the fiber. If this is the case, this conduction would represent an unusual instance of active transmission of graded electrical signals.

Electrical coupling and receptive field of L-HC

The identification of the origin of the different HC responses permits a correlation between the response properties of a given HC type and its shape and connectivity as revealed by morphological study. A first point concerns the comparison between the size of the anatomical arborization and the spatial extent of the receptive field. As first reported by Tomita, Tosaka, Watanabe and Sato (1958) for the fish HC, the receptive field of many HC types is much larger than their dendritic field. In the turtle, for instance, the diameter of the receptive field of the L1-HC can be several millimeters, whereas the anatomical arborization of the cellular elements originating these responses (H1AT) has a diameter of less than 200 μm. In these units a light spot equivalent in size to the cell anatomical arborization elicits a response which is only a small fraction of the maximum responses to diffuse illumination. Naka and Rushton (1967) provided evidence that the large spatial integration area of HC is the consequence of a lateral current spread in the HC network, and Kaneko (1971) demonstrated directly the existence of electrical coupling between homologous HC of the dogfish retina. Demonstration of the existence of gap junctions between HC in many animals (see above) provided the morphological basis for this coupling.

In the retina of the turtle, Simon (1973) and Byzov (1975) demonstrated the existence of a strong electrical coupling between the sites of origin of the L1-HC responses (H1AT), of a loose coupling between the sites of origin of the L2-HC responses (H1CB), and, moreover, the absence of a significant cross-coupling between the L1- and L2-HC recording sites. It appeared therefore that the strong coupling was responsible for the large field properties of the L1-HC, while the loose coupling accounted for the small receptive field properties of the L2-HC. This hypothesis was later confirmed by the EM observation of turtle HC referred to above, and by the results of the intracellular injection of Lucifer yellow to be discussed now in detail. Figure 5a, which illustrates the staining profile obtained while recording a L2-HC response, shows around the injection site (the perikaryon of a H1 cell) faintly stained round spots which could be identified as the perikarya of adjacent H1 cells. The dye had diffused to these structures via the gap junctions from the injected perikaryon. A very different staining was obtained when the dye was injected through an electrode recording L1-HC responses (Figure 6a). Around the injected axon terminal an extensive network of adjacent axon terminals appears well-stained. Moreover, structures corresponding to the H1CB are also stained. The dye had diffused from the injection site to the neighboring axon terminals via the gap junctions, and to the perikarya by backfilling through the axon fibers, which are in some cases visible, at least partially. It appears confirmed therefore that the differences of the spatial extensions of the receptive field profile between L2- and L1-HC are the consequence of the difference in the coupling.

In a more general context these results are at further variance with the neuron doctrine, since it appears that in the L-HC the functional units

Figure 6. Lucifer yellow staining profiles obtained by injecting the dye in the axon terminal of the H1 cell: (a), in control conditions; (b), in the presence of 100 μM bicuculline; (c), in the presence of 100 μM picrotoxin; and (d), in the presence of 10 μM dopamine. Scale bar, 100 μm.

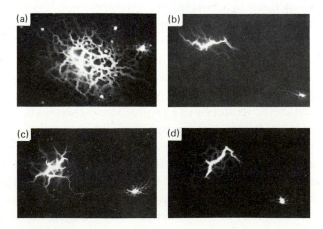

do not correspond to the neurons as visualized by the Golgi technique, but are more akin to the syncytia, of either the perikarya or the axon terminals, as they appear following injection of Lucifer yellow. It is difficult at present to discover the rationale of this unusual organization which, on one hand, separates a cell into two functional parts and, on the other hand, groups together each of these parts with corresponding parts of adjacent cells into functional ensembles. One could speculate on the advantage of having numerous cellular elements joined by gap junctions instead of a single cell possessing a rich dendritic arborization covering the same spatial extent. Experiments to be described later suggest that the permeability of the HC gap junctions is under the physiological control of a neurotransmitter mechanism. If this is so then the networks of coupled elements would be dynamic ensembles whose functional extent could be varied according to the physiological requirements of the visual processing. It would be more difficult to conceive how a similar physiological plasticity could be realized with a single extended cell.

On the other hand, the existence of morphological continuity between perikarya and axon terminals could permit metabolic cooperation between these elements and could also assure a flow of cellular messages other than by electrical signals.

The forward cone–HC synapse

As discussed earlier in this article, morphological features of the contacts between photoreceptors and HC are consistent with a chemical transmission type in the forward pathway (from photoreceptors to HC). This was confirmed in experiments employing ionic manipulation of the extracellular medium, aimed to interfere with the entry of calcium ions at the presynaptic ending of the photoreceptors (Dowling and Ripps, 1973; Cervetto and Piccolino, 1974; Kaneko and Shimazaki, 1976). The light responses of HC were blocked by these ionic changes while the responses of photoreceptors were scarcely affected.

Interestingly, the dark potential of the HC hyperpolarized and eventually reached the level obtained in control conditions with saturating lights. These results gave support to the hypothesis, first advanced by Trifonov (1968), according to which photoreceptors in darkness release the synaptic transmitter in a continuous tonic way. The action of this transmitter on HC would be to keep their membrane depolarized in the dark. The light, by hyperpolarizing the photoreceptor, would reduce in a tonic, graded way the transmitter release, leading to the hyperpolarization of the HC. According to this view, the light-induced hyperpolarization of HC should not be considered as an IPSP, but as the reduction of a tonic EPSP.

Feedforward versus feedback synapse HC–cone

As discussed above, morphological investigations have permitted in some retinas identification of the types of photoreceptor contacted by the different subtypes of HC. In principle these contacts could be the site of either a forward or feedback transmission between photoreceptor and HC. Regarding contacts between rods and the axon terminal of the H1 type of the turtle, there is little doubt that they are sites of exclusive forward transmission since (i) turtle rods do not show any feedback effect (Owen and Copenhagen, 1977), and (ii) the responses recorded from the axon terminal in the dark-adapted state show a significant rod component, which is lacking in the response recorded from the perikaryon (Leeper and Copenhagen, 1979). Moreover, the transmission must be, at least in part, in the forward direction also at the contacts between red-sensitive cones and both axon terminals and perikarya of the H1, since, as noted above, the responses recorded from these two regions (L1 and L2-HC, respectively) are dominated by a red input. On the other hand, at the contacts between green-sensitive cones and perikaryon the transmission is probably not in the forward direction, since the responses recorded from this cellular region do not exhibit a green input significantly greater than that of H1AT, which does not contact any green cones (Fuortes and Simon, 1974). The possibility remains therefore that the transmission at these sites would be toward cones. As we will show the electrophysiological data are consistent with this hypothesis. Moreover, by comparing electrophysiological and morphological observations it is also possible to infer the direction of the transmission between photoreceptors and other HC types.

Functional characteristics of the feedback synapse

Baylor, Fuortes and O'Bryan (1971) first demonstrated the feedback action of L-HC on cones in turtle retina. They showed that the response of turtle cones to large-diameter light spots exhibited a late depolarization whose time course coincided with the peak of the L-HC light-induced hyperpolarization. More direct proof that L-HC initiated this cone depolarization came from passing hyperpolarizing current pulses into a L-H and noting a depolarizing response in red cones (Baylor et al., 1971; Gerschenfeld, Piccolino and Neyton, 1980). Further experiments showed that red, green and blue cones all exhibited feedback depolarizations (Fuortes, Schwartz and Simon, 1973; Piccolino, Neyton and Gerschenfeld, 1980). In green cones, it was possible to evoke pure depolarizing responses with red light stimuli. Red light is poorly absorbed by green-cone photopigment, whereas it evokes large responses in LHC (which are driven mainly by red cones): therefore red stimuli selectively activate the feedback circuit impinging on green cones.

The feedback was shown to involve activation of a voltage-dependent calcium conductance in cone membrane (Piccolino and Gerschenfeld, 1978, 1980; Gerschenfeld and Piccolino, 1980). Since transmission from cone to second-order neurons occurs through a chemical synapse, and is therefore dependent on the entry of calcium ions into the cone presynaptic membrane, it was suggested that the feedback signal could act as a pre-synaptic modulation mechanism (Gerschenfeld et al., 1980). In further experiments it was reported that modification of the chloride permeability is also associated with feedback depolarization (Lasansky, 1981). It is conceivable that the two membrane events are causally related: for instance the entry of calcium ions could activate a Ca-dependent chloride conductance (such as that recently described in the inner segment of salamander rods by Bader, Bertrand and Schwartz, 1982).

Question remains concerning the synaptic mechanism of the feedback mainly because as described earlier, there is no morphological evidence for a chemical synapse between HC and cones, which could account for the sign-inverting features and synaptic conductance changes associated with the feedback transmission. Recently it has been reported that HC can release a chemical transmitter in a non-vesicular and non-calcium-dependent way (Schwartz, 1982): possibly these data could explain the lack of morphological evidence for chemical feedback synapse, but it remains to be seen whether the feedback effect is mediated by this non-vesicular release. As an alternative to a chemical synaptic mechanism, it has been proposed (Byzov, Golubtzov and Trifonov, 1977) that the feedback could work through an electrical field effect, such as that operating in the fish medulla between the Mauthner cells and some small adjacent neurons (Korn and Faber, 1975): the current generated by the HC membrane during the light-induced hyperpolarization would be constrained to flow across a particular area of the cone membrane, thus evoking a localized depolarization there. This depolarization would in turn produce a conductance change in cones by activating voltage-gated channels. The invaginated position of the HC processes at the cone base and the existence of voltage-dependent calcium channels in the cone membrane are consistent with this model. It remains to be seen whether the resistance of the extracellular space in the invaginated junction is sufficiently high to avoid a significant shunt, through extracellular paths, of the current generated by the HC membrane.

Specificity of the feedback connection H1–cone

In turtle retina red cones make direct synapses only with cell bodies and axon terminals of the H1 horizontal cell. Are both parts of the cell involved in feedback? This question can be approached by comparing the feedback effect of small-centered spots with those of annular stimuli. As shown earlier the former stimulus is highly effective for the H1CB (originating L2-HC responses), and rather ineffective for the AT (originating L1-HC responses), whereas the latter has the reverse efficacy. In experiments in which the response of a red cone to such stimuli was compared to that recorded from a H1AT and H1CB, it appeared that the feedback depolarization of the red cone correlated well with the amplitude of the H1AT hyperpolarization and was not correlated with the light-induced hyperpolarization of H1CB (Piccolino, Neyton and Gerschenfeld, 1981, and unpublished observations). This therefore suggested that the H1AT is primarily responsible for the feedback on red cones.

Figure 7. Depolarizing response elicited in a small-field luminosity horizontal cell by peripheral illumination in the presence of central background illumination. The receptive field was stimulated with a white light annulus (Ann, 3700 μm O.D., 870 μm I.D.) attenuated by 3.6 log units in (A), by a spot of white light (870 μm in diameter) of the same light intensity in (B), and by a temporal combination of both stimuli in (C), as monitored by the stimulus traces. (From Piccolino, Neyton and Gerschenfeld, unpublished.)

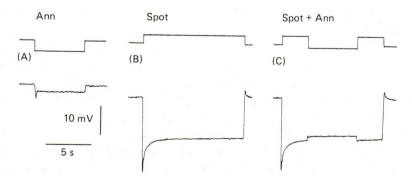

Similar experiments performed on green cones using red light to elicit pure feedback depolarization gave opposite results. Depolarizing responses were better elicited by red-light spots than by red annuli (Neyton, Piccolino and Gerschenfeld, 1981). It appears, therefore, that the H1CB is primarily responsible for the feedback depolarization in green cones. This is consistent with the anatomical data presented earlier which show that H1CB, but not H1AT, contacts green cones. It should be noted also that the H2, which also contact green cones, can be excluded as sources of feedback input to green cones, since they are depolarized by red light, and it is the HC hyperpolarization which initiates the feedback response.

In experiments using different spatial stimuli to investigate the receptive field of L2-HC, it appeared that peripheral illumination could result, in some cases, in depolarization rather than hyperpolarization of these units (Piccolino, Neyton and Gerschenfeld, 1981). This is illustrated in Figure 7C, where an annulus of light was presented during a background illumination of the receptive center, to reduce the effect of scattered light. No similar responses could be obtained from the L1-HC, which, on the contrary, were always hyperpolarized by surround illumination. Experimental analysis of the peripheral depolarizing responses of L2-HC indicated that they were the consequence of the feedback depolarization of the red cones situated in the center of their receptive field. Since the feedback depolarization of red cones depends, in turn, on the recurrent action of the H1AT, it appears that the axon terminals of the H1 cell can influence the perikarya of the same cell type through the red cones. Thus, the feedback loop establishes a functional connection between axon terminals and cell bodies of the H1 cell in the absence of an effective direct communication (Piccolino et al., 1981; Piccolino and Neyton, 1983).

Figure 8 summarizes the feedback circuitry between the H1 cells and red and green cones. From this figure, it appears that the difference in coupling between H1CB and H1AT is primarily responsible for the difference of their receptive field. This difference, and the specificity of the feedback connections between the two regions of the H1 and the red and green cones, account for the difference in the spatial properties of feedback responses in the two cone types, and, moreover, for the peripheral depolarizing responses of the L2-HC.

According to this scheme the H1AT could influence green cones, through a polysynaptic path, even in the absence of direct connections. In fact, it was observed that red-light annuli could reduce the feedback depolarization evoked in green cones by optimal-size red spots, and that this effect was consistent with a polysynaptic action of the H1AT (Neyton et al., 1981).

How chromatic HC-responses are built up

The prevailing idea on the genesis of the C-type responses was first proposed by Gouras (1972) and later developed experimentally by Fuortes and Simon (1974), and it assumes that these cells receive input only from cones responsible for their primary hyperpolarizing response through sign-preserving synapses. Leeper (1978a) surmised from a comparison of anatomical and physiological data that the H2 horizontal cells generated the RG-HC whereas the H3 horizontal cell gave rise to

Figure 8. Diagram of the input–output relationships between cones and the cell body (CB) and axon terminal (AT) regions of the H1 cell. (+) and (−) indicate the sites of sign-preserving and sign-inverting transmission, respectively. Differences in the electrical coupling are symbolized by the difference in the surface of the contacts. The fiber joining H1CB with H1AT is represented by a broken line to emphasize the relative ineffectiveness of the electrical communication between the two regions. The elements at the left are supposed to be central with respect to both recording and stimulation sites. A centered light spot would induce in (CB) a response larger than in (AT) since relatively less synaptic current would be shunted through the lateral electrical contacts joining (CB) than those joining (AT). This stimulus will therefore be powerful in activating the feedback on the green cone (G), but ineffective in inducing feedback responses in the central red cone. A light annulus would have the reverse effects in driving both (CB) and (AT), and in inducing the feedback response in cones. Through the feedback influence on central cones the peripheral stimulus could result in a depolarizing influence on (CB) and this, in turn, could reduce the feedback on the green cone. The notations L2 and L1 indicate the functional networks of respectively the H1-CB and H1-AT.

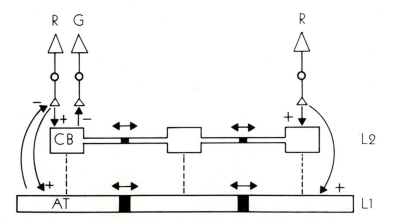

the GB-HC. As schematized in Figure 9, H2 would receive input from green cones and H3 from blue cones: the hyperpolarization of these cones by, respectively, green and blue light would be responsible for the hyperpolarizing responses of these cells to short-wavelength light. The depolarizing responses of the H2 cell to long-wavelength light would involve the feedback loop: red cone (hyperpolarization) → H1CB (hyperpolarization) → green cone (depolarization) → H2 (depolarization). A comparable polysynaptic path would generate the depolarizing responses of the H3 to intermediate-wavelength light, whereas the response of the H3 cell to deep-red light would involve a hyperpolarizing component resulting from a two-stage sequential activation of the feedback loop.

This scheme is oversimplified in that, for example, it does not consider the possibility that the connection between H3 and blue cones will be also the site of a feedback transmission (otherwise the H3 would be without output). Nevertheless, this scheme has the advantages that it is consistent with the anatomy of the HC-cone connections, and with the known properties of the feedback synapse, and it is capable of explaining chromatic responses of particular HC types without evoking other, as yet unidentified, chemical synapses.

Figure 9. Diagram of the synaptic relation between cones and horizontal cells responsible for the generation of the chromaticity type responses. Symbols as in Figure 8. H1, H2 and H3 are the three HC types according to the morphological classification of Leeper (1979a); L2-HC, small-field luminosity horizontal cell; RG-HC red–green chromaticity horizontal cells; GB-HC, green–blue chromaticity horizontal cell. (Modified from Leeper, 1978b.)

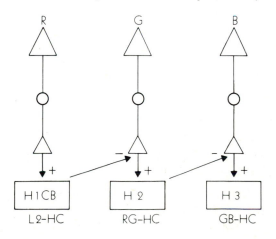

HC–bipolar cell synapse

Maksimova (1969) was the first to show that extrinsic polarization of the HC led to ganglion cell discharge. Her finding established clearly that HC have a functional role in the elaboration of visual message. Naka's extensive studies (Naka, 1982) demonstrated clearly that hyperpolarization of LHC elicited in ganglion cells the discharge characteristic of the surround responses, thus suggesting that HC could mediate for these responses. On anatomical grounds the HC-ganglion cell link must be joined through bipolar cells and it was proposed that L-HC could mediate the surround responses of bipolar cells. In fact, hyperpolarization of the L-HC by extrinsic current was shown to mimic the surround responses of center depolarizing and center hyperpolarizing bipolar cells in both turtle (Marchiafava, 1978) and fish retina (Toyoda and Kujiraoka, 1982). This surround response of bipolar cells was supposed to be the consequence of the activation of a direct chemical synapse HC–bipolar cells (Werblin and Dowling, 1969). As previously discussed there is, however, no evidence in many retinas for such a direct chemical synapse between HC and bipolar cells. It was later suggested that the surround responses of the bipolar cells could result, at least in part, from the feedback action of HC on cones (Richter and Simon, 1975). Studies of the ionic mechanisms of the responses elicited in bipolar cells by either surround illumination (Saito, Kondo and Toyoda, 1981) or HC hyperpolarization (Toyoda and Kujiraoka, 1982), are consistent with the feedback hypothesis, but do not exclude the possibility of a direct action HC–bipolars. It is possible that, in the future, noise-analysis studies of the light response of the bipolar cells (Ashmore and Copenhagen, 1980, 1981) could help in identification of the neural circuit (or circuits) originating these responses. It must also be considered that cells other than HC could intervene in the generation of surround responses of bipolar cells, since there is anatomical evidence that bipolar cells receive synaptic input also from interplexiform cells, in the OPL, and from amacrine cells in the inner plexiform layer.

Is the permeability of HC gap junctions under chemical control?

As previously discussed the large receptive field properties of L-HC are the consequence of electrical coupling among adjacent cells mediated by gap junctions joining their membranes. Several studies have reported that the receptive field profile of L-HC in different animals is narrowed by application to the retina of drugs known to affect chemical transmission processes elsewhere in the nervous system. In fish retina this narrowing followed application of dopamine agonists (Negishi and Drujan, 1978; Laufer, Negishi and Drujan, 1981; Laufer and Salas, 1981) and in turtle retina a similar effect was observed with dopamine and its agonists (Neyton, Piccolino and Gerschenfeld, 1982), and antagonists of GABA (Piccolino et al., 1982). At micromolar concentration these drugs resulted in an increase of L-HC responses to small central light spots, and in a decrease of responses to annuli of light, whereas response to diffuse illumination was scarcely affected. Current injection experiments indicated that this effect was due to a decrease of the electrical coupling, consequent upon decreased permeability of the gap junctions. This hypothesis was confirmed in experiments with turtle retina in which Lucifer yellow was injected into the L1-HC units. As illustrated in Figure 6, in the presence of either bicuculline and picrotoxin, powerful GABA antagonists, or following the application of dopamine, the dye-stained profile appeared significantly restricted compared to the control. Instead of an extensive network of well-stained axon terminals and surrounding perikarya, only the injected cell appeared densely stained.

The possible mechanism of this effect will be discussed elsewhere (Gerschenfeld, Neyton, Piccolino and Witkovsky, 1982; Neyton, Piccolino and Gerschenfeld, in preparation). It is worth noting here that there are other pieces of evidence suggesting a possible physiological role for a GABA-ergic and a dopaminergic system at this level of the retina. In many species it has been shown that GABA is associated with HC. These cells take up GABA in fish (Marc, Stell, Bok and Lam, 1978), are endowed with GABA-synthesizing enzyme in both fish (Lam et al., 1979) and turtle (Eldred, Karten and Oertel, unpublished), and are also closely associated with GABA receptors in the chicken (Yazulla and Brecha, 1981). Moreover, isolated HC of goldfish (Yazulla and Kleinschmidt, 1982) and of toad (Schwartz, 1982) are able to release GABA in a voltage-dependent, but calcium-independent way, probably via a carrier-mediated process.

As to the dopaminergic system, there is evidence that dopamine receptors of the D1 type are present in the retina (Brown and Macmann, 1972; Watling and Dowling, 1981) and associated with HC (Van Buskirk and Dowling, 1981). Moreover, as previously mentioned, the interplexiform cells in many species contain dopamine (Dowling and Ehinger, 1975; Nguyen-Legros et al., 1981; Frederick et al., 1982).

If future work will show clearly the presence in the distal retina of a control system allowing for chemical modulation of the permeability of the gap junctions between HC, then the study of this part of the nervous system will have revealed another interesting aspect of the functional complexity attained by a local circuit involving only a few neuronal elements.

The authors would like to thank Piero Taccini for help in the preparation of the illustrations and for photographic work, and Bernard Lacaisse for the technical assistance in the experimental work performed at the Ecole Normale Supérieure.

References

Akert, K. (1973). Dynamic aspects of synaptic ultrastructure. *Brain Res. 49:* 511–18.

Ashmore, J. F., and Copenhagen, D. R. (1980). Different postsynaptic events in two types of retinal bipolar cells. *Nature 288:* 84–6.

Ashmore, J. F., and Copenhagen, D. R. (1981). Surround mechanism of cone-bipolar cells in the turtle retina. *J. Physiol., Lond. 317:* 73–74P.

Bader, C. R., Bertrand, D., and Schwartz, E. A. (1982). Voltage-activated and calcium-activated currents studied in solitary rod inner segments in the salamander retina. *J. Physiol., Lond. 331:*253–84.

Baylor, D. A., Fuortes, M. G. F., and O'Bryan, P. M. (1971). Receptive field of cones in the retina of the turtle. *J. Physiol., Lond. 214:* 265–94.

Bennett, M. V. L. (1977). Electrical transmission: a functional analysis and comparison to chemical transmission. In *Cellular Biology of Neurons; Handbook of Physiology, Section 2: The Nervous system*, ed. E. R. Kandel, vol. 1, pp. 357–416. Baltimore: Williams and Wilkins.

Boycott, B. B., and Dowling, J. E. (1969). Organization of the primate retina: light microscopy. *Phil. Trans. Roy. Soc. Lond. B255:* 109–84.

Boycott, B. B., Dowling, J. E., Fisher, S. K., Kolb, H., and Laties, A. M. (1975). Interplexiform cells of the mammalian retina and their comparison with catecholamine-containing retinal cells. *Proc. Roy. Soc. Lond. B191:* 353–68.

Boycott, B. B., Peichl, L., and Wässle, H. (1978). Morphological types of horizontal cells in the retina of the domestic cat. *Proc. Roy. Soc. Lond. B203:* 229–45.

Brightmann, M. W., and Reese, T. T. (1969). Junctions between intimately apposed cell membranes in the vertebrate brain. *J. Cell Biol. 40:* 648–77.

Brown, J. H., and Makmann, M. H. (1972). Stimulation by dopamine of adenylate cyclase in retinal homogenate and of adenosine 3′,5′-cyclic monophosphate formation in intact retina. *Proc. Natn. Acad. Sci. USA 69:* 539–43.

Bunt, A. H. (1971). Enzymatic digestion of synaptic ribbons in amphibian retinal photoreceptors. *Brain Res. 25:* 571–7.

Byzov, A. L. (1975). Interaction between horizontal cells in the turtle retina. *Neurofiziologia* (in Russian), 7: 279–86.

Byzov, A. L., Golubtzov, A. W., and Trifonov, Yu. A. (1977). The model of feed-back between horizontal cells and photoreceptors in vertebrate retina. In *Vertebrate Photoreception*, ed. H. P. Barlow and P. Fatt, pp. 265–74. London: Academic Press.

Cajal, Ramon y, S. (1893). La rétine des vértebrés, *La Cellule 9:* 17–257.

Cervetto, L., and Piccolino, M. (1974). Synaptic transmission between photoreceptors and horizontal cells in the turtle retina. *Science 183:* 417–19.

Chan, R. Y., and Naka, K-I. (1980). Spatial organization of catfish retinal neurons. II. Circular stimulus. *J. Neurophysiol. 43:* 832–50.

Chen, F., and Witkovsky, P. (1978). The formation of photoreceptor synapses in the retina of the larval *Xenopus. J. Neurocytol. 7:* 721–40.

Couteaux, R., and Pecot-Dechavassine, M. (1970). Vesicules synaptiques et poches au niveau des zones activés de la jonction neuromusculaire. *Comp. Rend. Hebd. Séanc. Acad. Sci., Paris 271:* 2346–9.

Detwiler, P. B., and Hodgkin, A. L. (1979). Electrical coupling between cones in turtle retina. *J. Physiol., Lond. 291:* 75–100.

Dowling, J. E., and Boycott, B. B. (1966). Organization of the primate retina: electron microscopy. *Proc. Roy. Soc. Lond. B166:* 80–111.

Dowling, J. E., and Ehinger, B. (1975). Synaptic organization of the amine-containing interplexiform cells of the goldfish and cebus monkey retinas. *Science 188:* 270–3.

Dowling, J. E., and Ripps, J. H. (1973). Effects of magnesium on horizontal cell activity in the skate retina. *Nature 242:* 101–3.

Dowling, J. E., and Werblin, F. S. (1969). Organization of the retina of the mudpuppy *Necturus maculosus:* I. Synaptic structure. *J. Neurophysiol. 32:* 315–38.

Ehinger, B., Falck, B., and Laties, A. M. (1969). Adrenergic neurons in teleost retina. *Z. Zellforsch. mikrosk. Anat. 97:* 295–7.

Fisher, S. K., and Boycott, B. B. (1974). Synaptic connexions made by horizontal cells within the outer plexiform layer of the retina of the cat and the rabbit. *Proc. Roy. Soc. Lond. B186:* 317–31.

Frederick J. M., Rayborn, M. E., Laties, A. M., Lam, D. M. K., and Hollyfield, J. G. (1982). Dopaminergic neurons in the human retina. *J. Comp. Neurol. 210:* 65–79.

Fuortes, M. G. F., Schwartz, E. A., and Simon, E. J. (1973). Colour dependence of cone responses in the turtle retina. *J. Physiol., Lond. 234:* 199–216.

Fuortes, M. G. F., and Simon, E. J. (1974). Interaction leading to horizontal cells response in the turtle retina. *J. Physiol., Lond. 240:* 177–80.

Gallego, A. (1971). Horizontal and amacrine cells in the mammals retina. *Vision Res. 11:* 33–50.

Gallego, A. (1976). Comparative study of the horizontal cells in the vertebrate retina: mammals and birds. In *Neuronal Principles in Vision*, ed. F. Zettler and R. Weiler, pp. 26–62. Berlin: Springer-Verlag.

Gerschenfeld, H. M., Neyton, J., Piccolino, M., and Witkovsky, P. (1982). L-horizontal cells of the turtle: network organization and coupling modulation. *Biomedical Res.*, Suppl. *3:* 21–32.

Gerschenfeld, H. M., and Piccolino, M. (1980). Sustained feedback effects of L-horizontal cells on turtle cones. *Proc. Roy. Soc. Lond. B206:* 465–80.

Gerschenfeld, H. M., Piccolino, M., and Neyton, J. (1980). Feedback modulation of cone synapses by L-horizontal cells of turtle retina. In *Neurotransmission, Neurotransmitters, and Neuromodulators*, ed. E. A. Kravitz and J. E. Treherne, pp. 177–92. Cambridge, England: Cambridge University Press.

Gold, G. H. (1979). Photoreceptor coupling in the retina of the toad, *Bufo marinus.* II. Physiology. *J. Neurophysiol. 42:* 311–28.

Gouras, P. (1972). S-Potentials. In *Handbook of Sensory Physiology*, vol. VII/2, ed. M. G. F. Fuortes, pp. 513–30. Berlin: Springer-Verlag.

Gray, E. G., and Pease, H. L. (1971). On understanding the organization of the retinal receptor synapses. *Brain Res. 35:* 1–15.

Heuser, J. E., and Reese, T. S. (1973). Evidence for recycling of synaptic vesicles membrane transmitter released at the frog neuromuscular region. *J. Cell Biol. 57:* 315–44.

Heuser, J. K., and Reese, T. (1979). Structure of the synapse. In *Cellular Biology of Neurons; Handbook of Physiology, Section 2: The Nervous System*, ed. E. R. Kandel, vol. 1, pp. 261–94. Baltimore: Williams & Wilkins.

Heuser, J. E., Reese, T. S., and Landis, D. M. D. (1974). Functional changes in frog neuromuscular junctions studied with freeze-fracture. *J. Neurophysiol. 3:* 109–31.

Kaneko, A. (1971). Electrical connexions between horizontal cells of the dogfish retina. *J. Physiol., Lond. 213:* 95–105.

Kaneko, A., and Shimazaki, H. (1976). Effects of external ions on the synaptic transmission from photoreceptors to horizontal cells in carp retina. *J. Physiol., Lond. 252:* 509–22.

Kolb, H. (1970). Organization of the outer plexiform layer of the cat: electron microscopy of Golgi impregnated cells. *Phil. Trans. Roy. Soc. Lond. B255:* 177–84.

Kolb, H. (1974). The connections between horizontal cells and photoreceptors in the retina of the cat: electron microscopy of Golgi preparations. *J. Comp. Neurol. 155:* 1–14.

Kolb, H. (1977). The organization of the outer plexiform layer in the retina of the cat: electron microscopic observations. *J. Neurocytol. 6:* 131–53.

Kolb, H., Mariani, A., and Gallego, A. (1980). A second type of horizontal cell in the monkey retina. *J. Comp. Neurol. 180:* 31–44.

Kolb, H., and West, R. W. (1977). Synaptic connections of the interplexiform cell in the retina of the cat. *J. Neurocytol. 6:* 155–70.

Korn, H., and Faber, D. S. (1975). An electrically mediated inhibition in goldfish medulla. *J. Neurophysiol. 38:* 452–71.

Lam, D. M. K., Su, Y. Y. T., Swain, L., Marc, R. E., Brandon, C., and Wu, J. K. (1979). Immunocytochemical localization of L-glutamic acid decarboxylase in the goldfish retina. *Nature 278:* 565–7.

Landis, D. M. D., and Reese, T. S. (1974). Differences in membrane structure between excitatory and inhibitory synapses in the cerebellar cortex. *J. Comp. Neurol. 155:* 93–126.

Lasansky, A. (1971). Synaptic organization of cone cells in the turtle retina. *Phil. Trans. Roy. Soc. Lond. B262:* 365–81.

Lasansky, A. (1973). Organization of the outer synaptic layer in the retina of the larval tiger salamander. *Phil. Trans. Roy. Soc. Lond. B265:* 471–89.

Lasansky, A. (1976). Interactions between horizontal cells of the salamander retina. *Investve Ophthalmol. 15:* 909–16.

Lasansky, A. (1978). Contacts between receptors and electrophysiologically identified neurons in the retina of the tiger salamander. *J. Physiol., Lond. 285:* 531–42.

Lasansky, A. (1980). Lateral contacts and interactions of horizontal cells in the retina of the larval tiger salamander. *J. Physiol., Lond. 301:* 59–68.

Lasansky, A. (1981). Synaptic action mediating cone responses to annular illumination in the retina of the larval tiger salamander. *J. Physiol., Lond. 310:* 205–14.

Lasansky, A., and Vallerga, S. (1975). Horizontal cell responses in the retina of the larval tiger salamander. *J. Physiol., Lond. 251:* 145–65.

Laufer, M., and Drujan, B., eds (1983). *The S-potential*. New York: A. R. Liss.

Laufer, M., Negishi, K., and Drujan, D. (1981). Pharmacological manipulation of spatial properties of S-potentials. *Vision Res. 21:* 1657–60.

Laufer, M., and Salas, R. (1981). Intercellular coupling and retinal horizontal cell receptive field. *Neurosci. Lett.*, Suppl. *7:* 338.

Leeper, H. F. (1978*a*). Horizontal cells of the turtle retina: I. Light microscopy of Golgi preparations. *J. Comp. Neurol. 182:* 777–94.

Leeper, H. F. (1978*b*). Horizontal cells of the turtle retina: II. Analysis of interconnections between photoreceptor cells and horizontal cells by light microscopy. *J. Comp. Neurol. 182:* 795–810.

Leeper, H. F., and Copenhagen, D. R. (1979). Mixed rod-cone responses in horizontal cells of snapping turtle retina. *Vision Res. 19:* 407–11.

Lowenstein, W. R. (1981). Junctional intercellular communications: the cell-to-cell membrane channel. *Physiol. Rev. 61:* 829–913.

Maksimova, Ye. M. (1969). Effect of intracellular polarization of horizontal cells on the activity of the ganglionic cells of the retina of the fish. *Biofizika* (in Russian) *14:* 537–44.

Marc, R. E., and Lam, D. M. K. (1981). Glycinergic pathways in the goldfish retina. *J. Neurosci. 1:* 152–65.

Marc, R. E., Stell, W. E., Bok, D. C., and Lam, D. M. K. (1978). GABA-ergic pathways in the goldfish retina. *J. Comp. Neurol. 182:* 221–6.

Marchiafava, P. L. (1978). Horizontal cells influence membrane potential of bipolar cells in the retina of the turtle. *Nature 275:* 141–2.

Marenghi, G. (1901). Contributo alla fina organizzazione della retina. *Boll. Soc. Med. Chir. Pavia* 1–33.

Mariani, A. P., and Leure-du Pree, A. E. (1977). Horizontal cells of the pigeon retina. *J. Comp. Neurol. 175:* 13–26.

McLaughlin, B. J., and Boykins, L. (1977). Ultrastructure of E-PTA stained synaptic ribbons in the chicken retina. *J. Neurobiol. 8:* 91–6.

McLaughlin, B. J., and Reese, T. S. (1981). A freeze-fracture study of photoreceptor presynaptic membranes during ribbon synapses formation. *J. Neurocytol. 10:* 183–99.

Nagy, A. R., and Witkovsky, P. (1981). A freeze-fracture of synaptogenesis in the distal retina of the larval *Xenopus. J. Neurocytol. 10:* 897–919.

Naka, K-I. (1982). The cells horizontal cells talk to. *Vision Res. 22:* 653–60.

Naka, K-I., and Rushton, W. A. H. (1967). The generation and spread of S-potentials in the retina of the fish (*Cyprinidae*). *J. Physiol., Lond. 192:* 437–61.

Negishi, K., and Drujan, B. D. (1979). Effect of catecholamines and related compounds on horizontal cells in the fish retina. *J. Neurosci. Res. 4:* 311–34.

Nelson, R. (1977). Cat cones have rod input: a comparison of the response properties of cones and horizontal cell bodies in the retina of the cat. *J. Comp. Neurol. 172:* 109–36.

Nelson, R., Lutzov, A. V., Kolb, H., and Gouras, P. (1975). Horizontal cells in the cat retina with independent dendritic systems. *Science 189:* 137–9.

Neyton, J., Piccolino, M., and Gerschenfeld, H. M. (1981). Involvement of small field horizontal cells in feedback effects on green cones of turtle retina. *Proc. Natn. Acad. Sci. USA 78:* 4616–19.

Neyton, J., Piccolino, M., and Gerschenfeld, H. M. (1982). Dopamine and drugs that increase intracellular cyclic AMP decrease junctional communication between L-horizontal cells. *Neurosci. Abstr. 8:* 37.6.

Nguyen-Legros, J., Berger, B., Vigny, A., and Alvarez, C. (1981). Tyrosine hydroxylase-like immunoreactive interplexiform cells in the rat retina. *Neurosci. Lett. 27:* 255–9.

Ogden, T. E. (1974). The morphology of retinal neurons of the owl monkey *Aotes. J. Comp. Neurol. 153:* 399–428.

Owen, G. W., and Copenhagen, D. R. (1977). Characteristics of the electrical coupling between rods in the turtle retina. In *Vertebrate Photoreception*, ed. H. B. Barlow and P. Fatt, pp. 169–92. London: Academic Press.

Piccolino, M., and Gerschenfeld, H. M. (1978). Activation of a regenerative calcium conductance in turtle cones by peripheral stimulation. *Proc. Roy. Soc. Lond. B201:* 309–15.

Piccolino, M., and Gerschenfeld, H. M. (1980). Characteristics and ionic processes involved in feed-back spikes of turtle cones. *Proc. Roy. Soc. Lond. B206:* 439–63.

Piccolino, M., and Neyton, J. (1982). The feedback from luminosity horizontal cells to cones in the turtle retina: a key to understanding the response properties of horizontal cells. In *The S-Potential*, ed. M. Laufer and B. Drujan, pp. 161–79. New York: A. R. Liss.

Piccolino, M., Neyton, J., and Gerschenfeld, H. M. (1980). Synaptic mechanisms involved in the responses of chromaticity horizontal cells of the turtle retina. *Nature 284:* 58–60.

Piccolino, M., Neyton, J., and Gerschenfeld, H. M. (1981). Center surround antagonistic organization in the small field L-horizontal cells of the turtle retina. *J. Neurophysiol. 45:* 361–73.

Piccolino, M., Neyton, J., Witkovsky, P., and Gerschenfeld, H. M. (1982). γ-Aminobutyric acid antagonists decrease junctional communication between horizontal cells of the retina. *Proc. Natn. Acad. Sci. USA 79:* 3671–5.

Raviola, E., and Gilula, N. B. (1973). Gap junctions between photoreceptor cells in the vertebrate retina. *Proc. Natn. Acad. Sci. USA 70:* 1677–81.

Raviola, E., and Gilula, N. B. (1975). Intramembrane organization of specialized contacts in the outer plexiform layer of the retina. A freeze-fracture study in monkeys and rabbits. *J. Cell Biol. 65:* 192–222.

Richter, A., and Simon, E. J. (1975). Properties of centre-hyperpolarizing bipolar cells in the turtle retina. *J. Physiol., Lond. 248:* 317–34.

Ripps, H., Shakib, M., and MacDonald, E. D. (1976). Peroxidase uptake by photoreceptor terminals of the skate retina. *J. Cell Biol. 70:* 86–96.

Roberts, A., and Bush, B. M. H., eds (1981). *Neurons Without Impulses*. Cambridge, U.K.: Cambridge University Press.

Saito, T., Kondo, H., and Toyoda, J. (1981). Ionic mechanisms of on-center bipolar cells in the carp retina. II. The response to annular illumination. *J. Gen. Physiol. 78:* 569–89.

Saito, T., Miller, W. H., and Tomita, T. C. (1974). C- and L-type horizontal cells in the turtle retina. *Vision Res. 14:* 119–23.

Schacher, S., Holtzmann, E., and Hood, D. C. (1976). Synaptic activity of frog retinal photoreceptors. A peroxidase study. *J. Cell Biol. 70:* 178–92.

Schaeffer, S. F., Raviola, E., and Heuser, J. E. (1982). Membrane specializations in the outer plexiform layer of the turtle retina. *J. Comp. Neurol. 204:* 253–67.

Schmitt, F. O., and Worden, F. G., eds (1979). *The Neurosciences: Fourth Study Program. Cambridge, Mass.: MIT Press.*

Schwartz, E. S. (1982). Calcium-independent release of GABA from isolated horizontal cells of the toad retina. *J. Physiol., Lond. 323:* 211–27.

Shepherd, G. M. (1979). *The Synaptic Organization of the Brain*, 2nd edn. New York, Oxford: Oxford University Press.

Simon, E. J. (1973). Two types of luminosity horizontal cells in the retina of the turtle. *J. Physiol., Lond. 230:* 199, 211.

Sobrino, J. A., and Gallego, A. (1970). Células amacrinas de la capa plexiforme de la retina. *Acta Soc. Esp. Cienc. Fisiol. 12:* 373–5.

Stell, W. K. (1972). The morphological organization of the vertebrate retina. In *Handbook of Sensory Physiology*, vol. VII/2, ed. M. G. F. Fuortes, pp. 111–213. Berlin: Springer-Verlag.

Stell, W. K. (1975). Horizontal cells axons and axon terminals in goldfish retina. *J. Comp. Neurol. 159:* 503–20.

Stell, W. K. (1978). Inputs to bipolar cell dendrites in goldfish retina. *Sensory Processes 2:* 329–49.

Stell, W. K., Kretz, R., and Lightfoot, D. O. (1983). Horizontal cell connectivity in goldfish. In *The S-potential*, ed. M. Laufer and B. Drujan, pp. 51–75. New York: A. R. Liss.

Stell, W. K., and Lightfoot, D. O. (1975). Color specific interconnections of cones and horizontal cells in the retina of the goldfish. *J. Comp. Neurol. 159:* 143–502.

Stell, W. K., Lightfoot, D. O., Wheeler, T. G., and Leeper, H. F. (1975). Goldfish retina: functional polarization of cone horizontal cell dendrites and synapses. *Science 190:* 989–90.

Stell, W. K., and Witkovsky, P. (1973). Retinal structure in the smooth dogfish *Mustelus canis*: light microscopy of photoreceptors and horizontal cells. *J. Comp. Neurol. 148:* 33–46.

Stephan, P., and Weiler, R. (1981). Morphology of horizontal cells in the frog retina. *Cell Tiss. Res. 221:* 443–9.

Stewart, W. W. (1978). Functional connections between cells revealed by dye coupling with a highly fluorescent naphthalmide tracer. *Cell 14:* 741–59.

Tomita, T., Tosaka, T., Watanabe, K., and Sato, Y. (1958). The fish EIRG in response to different types of illumination. *Japan J. Physiol. 8:* 41–50.

Toyoda, J-I., and Kujiraoka, T. (1982). Analysis of bipolar cell responses elicited by polarization of horizontal cells. *J. Gen. Physiol. 79:* 131–45.

Toyoda, J-I., Saito, T., and Kondo, H. (1978). Three types of horizontal cells in the stingray retina: their morphology and physiology. *J. Comp. Neurol. 179:* 569–80.

Trifonov, Y. A. (1968). Study of synaptic transmission between photoreceptors and horizontal cells by means of electrical stimulation of the retina. *Biofizica 13:* 809–17 (in Russian).

Van Buskirk, R., and Dowling, J. E. (1981). Isolated horizontal cells from carp retina demonstrate dopamine-dependent accumulation of cAMP. *Proc. Natn. Acad. Sci. USA 78:* 7825–9.

Wässle, H., Boycott, B. B., and Peichl, L. (1978). Receptor contacts of horizontal cells in the retina of the domestic cat. *Proc. Roy. Soc. Lond. B203:* 247–67.

Watling, K. J., and Dowling, J. E. (1981). Dopaminergic mechanisms in the teleost retina. *J. Neurochem. 36:* 559–68.

Weiler, R. (1978). Horizontal cells in the carp retina: Golgi impregnation and procion-yellow injection. *Cell Tiss. Res. 195:* 515–26.

Weiler, R., and Zettler, F. (1979). The axon-bearing horizontal cells in the teleost retina are functional as well as structural units. *Vision Res. 19:* 1261–8.

Werblin, F. S., and Dowling, J. E. (1969). Organization of the retina of the mudpuppy *Necturus maculosus*: II. Intracellular recording. *J. Neurophysiol. 32:* 339–55.

West, R. W. (1978). Bipolar and horizontal cells of the gray squirrel retina: Golgi morphology and receptor connections. *Vision Res. 18:* 129–36.

Witkovsky, P., Burkhardt, D. A., and Nagy, A. R. (1979). Synaptic connections linking cones and horizontal cells in the retina of the pikeperch (*Stizostedion vitreum*). *J. Comp. Neurol. 186:* 541–50.

Witkovsky, P., Owen, W. G., and Woodworth, M. (1983). Gap junctions among the perikarya, dendrites and axon terminals of the luminosity-type horizontal cells of the turtle retina. *J. Comp. Neurol. 216:* 359–68.

Witkovsky, P., and Powell, C. C. (1981). Synapse formation and modification between distal retinal neurons in the larval juvenile *Xenopus. Proc. Roy. Soc. Lond. B211:* 373–89.

Yamada, E., and Ishikawa, I. (1965). The fine structure of the horizontal cells in some vertebrate retinae. *Cold Spring Harb. Symp. Quant. Biol. 30:* 383–92.

Yazulla, S., and Brecha, N. (1981). Localized binding of [^{3}H]muscimol to synapses in chicken retina. *Proc. Natn. Acad. Sci. USA 78:* 643–7.

Yazulla, S., and Kleinschmidt, J. (1982). Dopamine blocks carrier-mediated release of GABA from retinal horizontal cells. *Brain Res. 233:* 211–15.

3.4

Infrared and visual senses in snake optic tectum

PETER H. HARTLINE

Pit vipers (*Crotalinae*) such as American rattlesnakes, and pythons (*Boidae*) have evolved the ability to use infrared radiation to localize and perhaps to identify remote objects such as their warm blooded prey. The infrared sense is served by the trigeminal nerve (Bullock and Cowles, 1952; Bullock and Diecke, 1956; Bullock and Barrett, 1968), and is thus apparently derived from a somatic modality. In these two groups of snakes, the original somatic modality has evolved into one that reports location and movements of objects that are remote from the snake. On the basis of the new modality, snakes can orient toward their prey in the absence of light. The infrared sense has become very much like a second form of vision.

In the past decade, there has been increasing recognition that the optic tectum, homolog of the mammalian superior colliculus, is concerned with spatial localization of visual stimuli, and has an important role in orienting behaviors such as looking toward, or lunging at appropriate objects (Schneider, 1969; Ingle, 1970; Ewart, 1970; reviews: Sprague, Berlucci and Rissolatti, 1973; Wurtz and Albano, 1980). Sensory modalities, other than vision, that give information about the location of objects are often represented in the tectum or superior colliculus. Examples are auditory (Wickelgren, 1971) and tactile (Stein, Magalhaes-Castro and Kruger, 1976) senses in cat, auditory and tactile senses in mice (Drager and Hubel, 1975, 1976), the tactile sense in lizards (Stein and Gaither, 1981), in salamanders (Gruberg, 1969) and in fish (Fish and Voneida, 1979), the electrolocation sense in fish (Bastian, 1981) and the auditory sense in birds (Knudsen, 1982).

It is not surprising, then, that the snake's infrared modality is

405

prominently represented in the tectum (Goris and Terashima, 1973; Hartline, 1974). In both the Boidae (Haseltine, 1978) and Crotolinae (Kass, Loop and Hartline, 1978), infrared neurons lie below the superficial layer of visual cells (Figure 1). I will concentrate in this review on spatial and functional aspects of the infrared modality in the optic tectum, and on its relationship and integration with vision.

Spatial organization of rattlesnake infrared and visual systems

Since the spatiotopic mapping of the visual field onto the optic tectum is a feature shared by all vertebrates, one might anticipate that the infrared sense is similarly arranged. This expectation has been

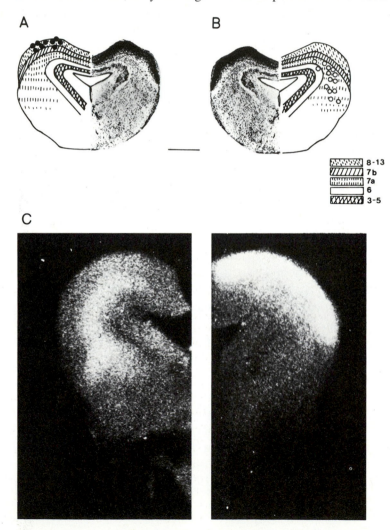

proven correct (Hartline, 1974; Terashima and Goris, 1975; Hartline, Kass and Loop, 1978). Figure 2 shows results from a rattlesnake tectal mapping experiment illustrating that, in both visual and infrared modalities, there is an orderly progression of receptive fields from the rostral pole to the caudal pole of the rectum. At more rostral tectal locations, the receptive field centers are located more nasally (or anteriorly). Similar medio-lateral penetration series show that progressively more medial locations are associated with progressively elevated or superior receptive fields.

An important feature of the evolution of the infrared sensory system emerges from considering the infrared tectal map, the optics of the pit organ, and the somatic origin of the infrared sense. Tactile systems map to the tectum or superior colliculus in a spatially organized fashion, so that anterior receptive fields are located in the rostral tectum, and dorsal fields are represented medially. I refer to this axis system as the conventional vertebrate somatic map. It has been found in mammals (Stein et al., 1976; Drager and Hubel, 1976) and salamanders (Gruberg, 1969). Thus, the rostral part of the tectum represents the more anterior part of both tactile and visual space. The visual and tactile axes are apparently rotated about 90 degrees in the lizard, *Iguana*; but nonetheless, anterior visual fields and anterior skin are represented in the same part of the tectum (Stein and Gaither, 1981).

The rattlesnake's infrared-sensitive pit organ is an image-inverting optical system (Otto, 1972). Infrared radiation in the nasal portion of the pit's 'field of view' illuminates (and thus excites) heat-sensitive endings located towards the caudal edge of the sensory membrane

Figure 1. (A) Diagram and section of optic tectum of *Crotalus viridis* illustrating superficial locations of recording sites of visual neurons. (B) The same, but illustrating deeper locations of recording sites of neurons excited by infrared stimulation. Scale bar, 1.0 mm. The layering system is from Ramon (1896); A and B are reprinted with permission from *J. Comp. Neurol.* Kass et al. (1978).
(C) Autoradiographs of two hemitecta taken from different snakes after labeled 2-deoxyglucose (2-DG) injections. Left: the right pit was stimulated with an intermittent infrared stimulus. A band in the middle tectal layers contralateral to the stimulated pit organ shows 2-DG labeling, indicating high metabolic activity, from which high electrical activity is inferred. Right: the left eye of a different snake was stimulated. The 2-DG label is concentrated over the superficial tectal layer contralateral to the visually-stimulated eye. The unstimulated eye(s) and pit(s) were intact, but covered with opaque blinders. (These autoradiographs are from Gruberg, Newman and Hartline, 1982.)

(Figure 3). If the map between the sensory endings in the pit organ and the tectum had retained the orientation of the conventional vertebrate somatic map, the caudal sensory endings would project to posterior tectum; thus one would find nasal infrared-receptive fields in the caudal tectum, not the rostral tectum. Evidently during the course of evolution, the map of somatic-tectal connections from the pit has been rotated 180 degrees.

Spatial organization of python infrared system

Boid snakes, particularly pythons, have many infrared-sensitive pits along their lips. Is there nonetheless a single spatial map of the infrared world that superimposes on the visual map in the tectum? In studying this question Haseltine (Haseltine, 1978; Haseltine, Kass and Hartline, 1977), found evidence for a remarkable degree of evolutionary plasticity of neural maps. The large anterior supralabial pits of pythons have overlapping infrared fields of view, but the center of the

Figure 2. In a series of electrode penetrations along the anterior–posterior axis of a tectum of *C. viridis*, both visual and infrared receptive fields were mapped, using a multi-unit electrode in the appropriate tectal layer. The anterior–posterior location (mm from the most rostral penetration) is plotted as the ordinate against the horizontal center coordinate of the visual (filled circles) and infrared (open circles) receptive fields. If there were perfect correspondence between visual and infrared representations of space, the two sets of points would coincide.

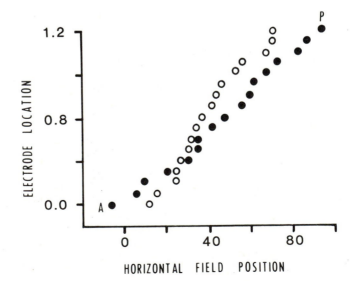

field of an anterior pit is more nasal than the center of a relatively posterior one. Each pit 'views' a field 100–120 degrees wide in the naso-temporal field, and all of them combined from one side cover from 50 degrees across the midline to 150 degrees behind the midline. Each pit, although not as obviously like a pinhole camera as the rattlesnake's pit, nonetheless has image-inverting properties. The anterior to posterior pit array, the overlapping fields of view, and the inverting optics of each pit all have corresponding features in the map of somatic connectivity from the pit to the tectum.

By isolating each pit (blocking the others with foil), while recording from an array of tectal loci, Haseltine delineated the tectal region that could be driven by each of the large pits. More anterior pits (which look at a more nasal portion of space) project to more rostral regions of the tectum. This qualitatively conforms to an expectation based on the conventional vertebrate somatotopic map.

By an elaboration of this technique Haseltine used a small intense infrared spot focused directly on the heat-sensitive membrane to map the area within each pit that could excite a given tectal locus (this technique was first used by Terashima and Goris, 1976, to delineate the 'receptive areas' of tectal neurons of pit vipers). The electrode was moved to a new rostro-caudal location, and the process was repeated.

Figure 3. Schematic cross-section of rattlesnake pit organ illustrating the pit's inverting optics. (From *The Infrared 'Vision' of Snakes*, by E. A. Newman and P. H. Hartline. Copyright (1982) by Scientific American, Inc. All rights reserved.)

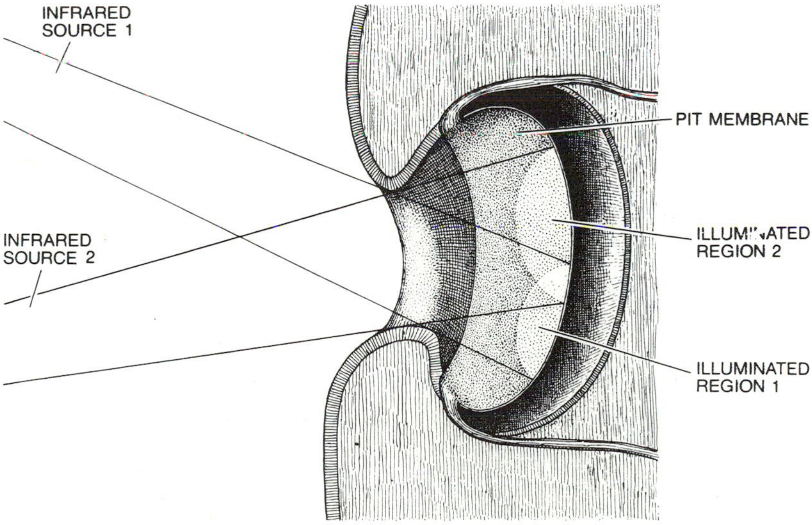

INFRARED SOURCE 1

INFRARED SOURCE 2

PIT MEMBRANE

ILLUMINATED REGION 2

ILLUMINATED REGION 1

The results are illustrated in Figure 4. Each pit is projected to a subset of the tectum termed its 'projection region'. More anterior pits have more rostral projection regions, which resembles the conventional vertebrate somatotopic map. However, as in rattlesnakes, the somatic map of each pit within its projection region is inverted compared to the conventional vertebrate map.

The inverted map from each pit to its projection region clearly helps to bring about similarity between visual and infrared spatiotopic maps. That more anterior pits project to more rostral tectum also clearly favors overall inter-modality spatial registration. However, the key to obtaining a single representation of space must be held in the overlap between projection regions of adjacent pits. Without the right overlap, each region of infrared space would have multiple representations in the

Figure 4. Somatotopic mapping in *Python reticularis*. Eight tectal penetration sites along an anterior–posterior transect of the tectum (bottom) and the receptive areas corresponding to each, delineated by the labeled outline of the heat-sensitive membrane at the bottom of the five largest superior labial pit organs. Within each pit, more anterior tectal sites were driven by more posterior (but often overlapping) regions of the pit membrane. More posterior pits are represented only at more posterior tectal locations. (Printed with permission of E. C. Haseltine.)

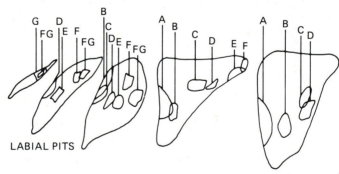

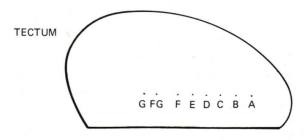

tectum. The extensive interpenetration of the projections from pits with overlapping fields of view is illustrated in Figure 4, where multiple occurrence of the letter A, for instance, indicates the regions of the front two pits that could drive neurons recorded by a multi-unit electrode in location A.

Infrared system considered as a somatic sense

There have been many examples in which there are non-uniformities of the magnification in sensory neural maps; the expanded receptotopic map of foveae (vision) and lips and fingers (tactile) are well-known examples. In Crotaline and Boid snakes, if one considers projections of the body's somatic receptors to the tectum, non-uniform magnification is particularly prominent. A very small part of the body surface (the pits) has a greatly expanded tectal representation, in fact filling most if not all of the tectal surface. (Note however that considering spatiotopic rather than receptotopic properties in the infrared system, magnification is relatively uniform.)

The rattlesnake gave the first example I have found of a naturally occurring receptotopic map rotation in a somatic system. The situation in the python is even more complex. The sensory surface has undergone fragmentation into fields (the pits) and each field independently exhibits a 180-degree rotation of its tectal receptotopic map similar to the rotation of the map of the rattlesnake's single pit. In addition, the projection of each field (pit) overlaps those of its neighbors extensively. Thus each tectal locus must receive input from many well separated areas of the total sensory epithelium. The final result of the complex somatic-tectal mapping found in Pythons is in fact a single infrared spatiotopic map that maintains approximate registration with the visual spatiotopic map (Haseltine, 1978; Haseltine et al., 1977).

Inter-modality map discrepancies

The degree to which the ancestral somato-tectal maps of these snakes has been rearranged to achieve sensible correspondence between visual and infrared neural representations of the world is quite impressive. At least in the rattlesnake, however, the spatial correspondence is not perfect. This can be seen in Figure 2. If spatial registration were perfect, the points representing infrared receptive field centers would fall on top of the points for visual field centers. But at the caudal part of the tectum, visual receptive fields are located much more temporally (posteriorly) than the corresponding infrared fields.

A possible reason for the failure of complete spatial correspondence of the two modalities lies in the differences in the total fields of view of the eye and pit organ. Each eye sees from a bit over the midline to almost directly behind the head. The infrared pit's total field of view has about two-thirds of this naso-temporal extent. Thus, if neurons representing the entire infrared field of view were spread in the infrared layer over the entire extent of the tectum, and if neurons representing the entire visual field of view were spread out over the entire tectum, one would expect the sort of mismatch between the two modalities that in fact occurs. This situation suggests that there is no mechanism for fine-tuning the connections of tectal afferents in the two modalities to achieve precise intermodality spatial correspondence. From studies of development of retinal connections to the optic tectum of amphibians (reviewed in Jacobson, 1970), it appears that retinal fibers spread out to occupy whatever tectal surface is available. The lack of precise intermodality spatial correspondence in snakes invites the speculation that during development, tectal or superior collicular afferents from each modality simply spread out to occupy all available sites within the appropriate tectal layer (Hartline et al., 1978), but that all modalities share the spatial axes intrinsic to the tectum. From these data it is not necessary to postulate the existence of a mechanism whereby one sensory map is able to influence the other, although from studies of owls (Knudsen, Knudsen and Esterly, 1982) there is evidence that plastic adjustment of intermodality correspondence can occur.

Receptive fields of multimodal neurons

Multimodal neurons have been reported in the superior colliculus in many mammalian species; they can be stimulated by vision and a second modality, particularly touch (Wickelgren, 1971; Gordon, 1973; Drager and Hubel, 1975, 1976; Stein et al., 1976). The locations of the visual fields of multimodal neurons have been found to correspond approximately to the locations of tactile fields in the same units. However, tactile fields are located at the animal's surface (i.e. the skin or close to it, as in the case of vibrissae). The spatial relationship between a particular patch of fur and the visual coordinate system is not obvious. Consequently, just what 'spatial correspondence' would mean for visual and tactile fields of a multimodal neuron is not easy to define. But, in snakes, both infrared and visual fields are projected into distant space, and spatial position has the same meaning for both modalities. Thus, snakes are nearly ideal for examining the spatial relationship between receptive fields in two modalities.

Several notable features of intermodality spatial correspondence are illustrated in Figure 5. First, the infrared-receptive fields of multimodal neurons that respond to stimulation by either modality alone (designated OR neurons) are quite a bit larger than the visual receptive fields. Over most of the tectum, the visual field is completely or largely contained within the infrared-receptive field. In this sense, the approximate spatial correspondence found in spatiotopic maps holds also for infrared-visual bimodal neurons. However, the fields are usually not concentric; in fact their non-concentricity varies systematically over the tectum, and follows the pattern set by the disparity between infrared and visual spatiotopic maps. Note that in Figure 5C, made at a penetration far caudal in the tectum, the visual field is located outside of and posterior to the infrared field. The trend is general, as Figure 6 illustrates. The experiment of Figure 2 is used to plot the infrared field center coordinate against the visual field center coordinate for a rostro-caudal series of electrode penetrations. On top of it is plotted one point for each OR neuron (pooled from three rattlesnakes). The relationship between infrared and visual spatiotopic maps satisfactorily

Figure 5. Visual receptive fields (hatched) and infrared-receptive fields (solid borders) of visual-infrared OR neurons of *C. viridis*. Visual fields were mapped with a thermoneutral black cardboard wand moved toward each field center. Infrared fields were mapped by moving a warm soldering iron toward each field center along horizontal, vertical, and the two 45-degree axes. A, B, and C are in anterior, mid-tectal, and far posterior tectal locations, respectively. The origin is a point directly in front of the snake.

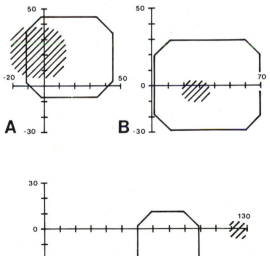

predicts the relationship between infrared and visual receptive field centers of the OR neurons' two modalities.

From this I conclude that the same sensible but imperfect spatial registration of the two modalities holds for OR neurons that holds for the tectal maps. Thus, there is no indication that OR neurons 'correct' the map disparities, as they might have by sending their dendrites to different tectal positions in the infrared and visual layers.

Multimodal integration

The optic tectum is thought of as having a prominent role in spatial shift of attention and in behaviors that are oriented with respect to a spatially localized stimulus (Schneider, 1969; Schaefer, 1970; Ingle, 1970; Schiller and Stryker, 1972; reviews: Sprague et al., 1973; Wurtz and Albano, 1980). Looking, or visual grasp, is an often cited example.

Figure 6. Spatial relationship between visual and infrared-receptive field centers of OR neurons of *C viridis*. Open circles are derived from Figure 2 and show the relationship between spatiotopic organization of visual and infrared neurons in their respective tectal layers. For each open circle the abscissa is the visual receptive field center coordinate and the ordinate is the infrared receptive field center coordinate and the ordinate is the infrared receptive field center coordinate at one tectal location. Each square is based on one unit's receptive fields, and shows visual field center (abscissa) *v*. infrared field center (ordinate). Data from OR neurons of three different snakes (1, 2, 3) are shown. The disparity between I.R. and visual maps (shown by deviation of the open circles from a line through the origin with unity slope) adequately predicts the disparity between infrared and visual field centers of OR neurons at different tectal locations.

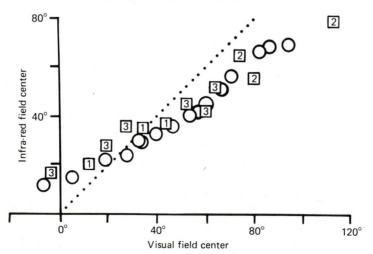

Not only vision, but many other modalities can provide information about the location of objects that are important for an animal's survival. Behavior oriented toward such objects would be efficiently coordinated if other localizing modalities had input to the command and output circuitry of the optic tectum (Gordon, 1973; Drager and Hubel, 1975; Stein et al., 1976; Hartline et al., 1978).

Perhaps multimodal neurons with spatially similar receptive fields, such as the OR neurons illustrated in Figure 5, occur as a necessary consequence of the convergence of two modalities on tectal output elements; they guarantee that an object at a particular spatial location will evoke orientation commands appropriate to the location of the object, regardless of the modality of the sense that localized it.

Newman and Hartline (1981, 1982) have investigated the question of whether the need for all modalities to share tectal output elements can account for all types of modality interactions in the tectum of rattle-snakes. We wished to identify neurons whose response properties depend on the relationship between infrared and visual stimulation resulting from an object that affects both senses. As a first step, our procedure has been to isolate a neuron, and roughly localize its receptive field center in whichever modalities are overtly excitatory. If either modality is not effective, we choose, for its stimulus location, one that was effective for other units in the same penetration. Then we present a sequence of stimuli: a visual stimulus (various sizes of light spots turned on, off, or moved), an infrared stimulus (a stationary spot turned on and off), and the same two stimuli simultaneously.

Figure 7A illustrates OR neurons, which for combined stimulation gives a greater response than either modality presented alone. It is indisputable that such neurons could be elements in the final common path for initiation of an orientation movement. However, if an object were marginally detectable in both infrared and visual modalities, such a neuron would respond more reliably than would unimodal neurons of either sense. Furthermore, in the few cases specifically tested, combining a near-threshold infrared stimulus with a near-threshold visual stimulus yields OR neuron responses greater than expected by linear summation. Both aspects of OR neuron response suggest some specialization for localizing dual modality objects.

We have also identified several more novel classes of modality interaction. Figure 7B illustrates the infrequently encountered class of AND neurons; they give no response or an unreliable one to either single modality stimulus. However, if the modalities are combined, they evoke a strong reliable response. While the OR neurons seem only slightly specialized for dual modality properties of an object, the AND neurons are extremely specialized. Such neurons might identify an object by its warmth and visibility, and by its similar spatial location and simultaneous appearance in both modalities. We imagine that they would be activated by the snake's warm-blooded prey.

Two classes of neurons display inhibitory or depressive cross-modality interactions. Figure 8A illustrates that a moderate response evoked by visual stimulation can be almost completely suppressed by the simultaneous onset of a suitable infrared stimulus. Figure 8B, in which the roles of the two modalities are reversed, shows an instance in which a modest decrement of the infrared response could be produced by visual stimulation. We have recorded examples of neurons where the cross-modality inhibition is so weak as to be inconsequential. But there remains the intriguing possibility that for neurons showing a weak interaction, there may be some particular stimuli in the inhibiting modality that exert a strong effect. What is equally significant is that some infrared-depressed visual neurons can be made to show enhance-

Figure 7. Raster displays showing the effects of separate and combined visual and infrared stimulation on bimodal neurons in *C. viridis*. Each vertical bar represents the time of occurrence of a nerve impulse. Each raster line represents a 15-s trial (the trials were contiguous, but each is plotted below the previous one). The infrared stimuli for Figures 7, 8, and 9 were one-second *on* flashes of a 3° infrared source. For the OR neuron, the visual stimulus was a stationary light spot that was turned off during the 0.5-s stimulus marker (*off* flash). The visual stimulus for the AND neuron was a one-second *on* flash. Note that the OR neuron's response to the combined stimulation is greater than the response to either modality presented alone. The AND neuron did not respond reliably to either stimulus alone, but gave a brief, high-frequency burst of about four spikes if both stimuli were presented simultaneously.

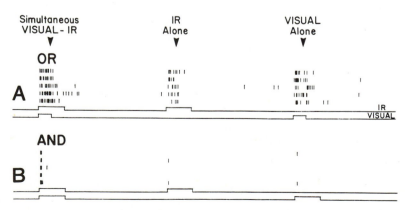

ment if the sign of the infrared stimulus is reversed. Such an IR-DEPRESSED VISUAL cell gives a moderate visual response, a weak response if onset of an infrared source coincides with the visual stimulus, and a strong response if offset of an infrared source coincides with the visual stimulus. Offset of an infrared source might occur in nature if an animal cooler than the surroundings enters the snake's infrared field of view.

A highly non-linear modality interaction is exhibited by two classes of ENHANCED neurons. For the neuron illustrated in Figure 9A, a visual stimulus, while effective if presented alone (thus designated 'primary'), could evoke a much stronger response if it was combined with the infrared stimulus (designated 'enhancing'). However, infrared stimulation alone was ineffective at even our highest stimulus level. In other neurons, the primary and enhancing modalities were reversed (Figure 9B). It should be mentioned that, for some OR neurons, reduction of one modality to below threshold while maintaining a low to moderate stimulus in the other modality can also show enhancement; the subthreshold modality becomes the enhancing one. It is possible that OR neurons and ENHANCED neurons are fundamentally similar types representing differing degrees of non-linear modality summation.

Enhancement and subthreshold summation may both be manifestations of a cross-modality attention mechanism. The enhancing modality,

Figure 8. Non-linear modality interaction in DEPRESSED neurons. Combining the ineffective modality stimulus with the effective one causes reduction in the response that would have been generated by the effective stimulus alone. In some IR-DEPRESSED VISUAL cells, offset of the infrared stimulus can cause enhancement. Raster and stimulus markers as in Figure 7. Visual stimulus: top, moving spot; bottom, *off* flash.

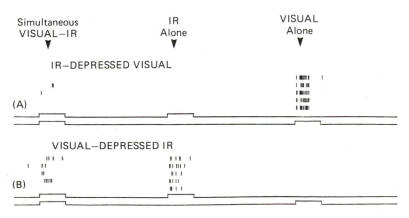

for instance infrared, may thus prime a region of the tectum correspond-ing to the spatial location of a source of warmth. IR-ENHANCED VISUAL neurons in this region would be particularly responsive to anything seen (visually) in the vicinity of the warmth. Given equal visual stimulation in an unprimed and a primed tectal region, the orientation output would be more likely for the one that was primed. In short, the animal would behave as if it were attending to visual occurrences in the region of space corresponding to the tectal region primed by the infrared sense.

Our study of cross-modality interactions is at an early stage; many of the most interesting questions remain to be asked. Do enhancement and depression have spatial distribution similar to the receptive fields of single modality infrared and visual neurons, or is there more complex spatial interaction? Can enhancement and depression occur in the same neuron, but have different spatial distributions? Can the relationship between infrared and retinal receptive field locations be modified during behavior (e.g. eye movements) or during development? To what extent are temporal simultaneity and spatial coincidence required in the two modalities for AND and ENHANCED neurons? Are the multimodal neurons tectal output cells, or if not, what relationship do they bear to the output?

Although the state of our knowledge is preliminary, it is already clear that there is more to multimodal integration than simple sharing of output circuity. The reports, from the past decade, of multimodal neurons in superior colliculus have all concerned OR neurons. As

Figure 9. Non-linear modality interaction in ENHANCED neurons. Note that in both cases, the enhancing modality alone produced no response, but caused the primary modality to evoke a greater response. Raster display and stimulus markers as in Figure 7. Visual stimuli: light spot that was moved during the indicated time but stationary otherwise.

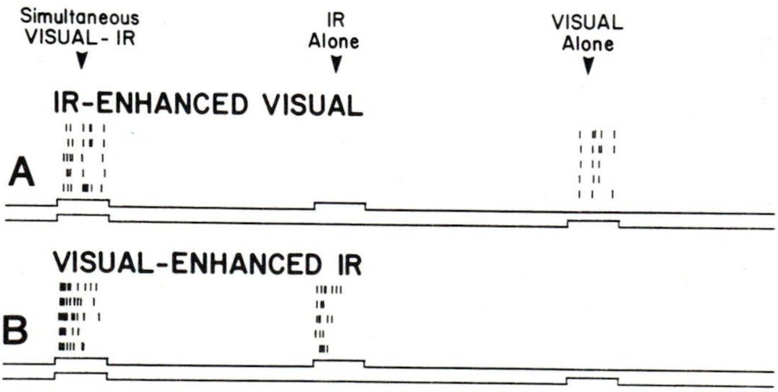

Newman and Hartline (1981) pointed out, this is due to the unimodal search stimuli and the use of only separate modality stimulation in those studies. The more interesting multimodal neurons found in rattlesnakes (the AND cells, DEPRESSED cells and ENHANCED cells) would have been labeled unresponsive or unimodal in those studies. Consequently, the mammalian superior colliculus remains fertile ground for comparative studies of modality integration.

References

Bastian, J. (1981). Visual and electrosensory responses in the optic tectum of a weakly electric fish. *Soc. Neurosci. Abstr. 7:* 845.

Bullock, T. H., and Cowles, R. B. (1952). Physiology of an infrared receptor – the facial pit of pit vipers. *Science 115:* 541–3.

Bullock, T. H., and Barrett, R. (1968). Radiant heat reception in snakes. *Comm. Behav. Biol. A 1:* 19–20.

Bullock, T. H., and Diecke, F. P. J. (1956). Properties of an infrared receptor. *J. Physiol., Lond. 134:* 47–87.

Drager, U. C., and Hubel, D. H. (1975). Responses to visual stimulation and relationship between visual, auditory, and somatosensory inputs in mouse superior colliculus. *J. Neurophysiol. 38:* 690–713.

Drager, U. C., and Hubel, D. H. (1976). Topography of visual and somatosensory projections to mouse superior colliculus. *J. Neurophysiol. 39:* 91–101.

Ewert, J. P. (1970). Neural mechanisms of prey-catching and avoidance behavior in the toad (*Bufo bufo* L.). *Brain Behav. Evol. 3:* 36–56.

Fish, S. E., and Voneida, T. J. (1979). Extra visual neurons in the optic tectum of a sighted and an unsighted fish. *Soc. Neurosci. Abstr. 5:* 784.

Gordon, B. G. (1973). Receptive fields in deep layers of cat superior colliculus. *J. Neurophysiol. 36:* 157–78.

Goris, R. C., and Terashima, S. (1973). Central response to infrared stimulation of the pit receptors in a crotaline snake, *Trimeresurus flavoviridis*. *J. Exp. Biol. 58:* 59–76.

Gruberg, E. R. (1969). Functional organization of the tectum of the tiger salamander (*Ambystoma tigrium*.). PhD thesis, University of Illinois, Urbana, Illinois.

Gruberg, E. R., Newman, E. A., and Hartline, P. H. (1982). 2-Deoxyglucose labeling of the infrared sensory system in the rattlesnake. *Soc. Neurosci. Abstr. 8:* 407.

Hartline, P. H. (1974). Thermoreception in snakes. In *Handbook of Sensory Physiology*, ed. A. Fessard, pp. 297–312. New York: Springer-Verlag.

Hartline, P. H., Kass, L., and Loop, M. S. (1978). Merging of modalities in the optic tectum: infrared and visual integration in rattlesnakes. *Science 199:* 1225–9.

Haseltine, E. (1978). Infrared and visual organization of the tectum of boid snakes. Doctoral Dissertation. Indiana University.

Haseltine, E., Kass, L., and Hartline, P. H. (1977). Infrared and visual organization of the tectum of boid snakes. *Soc. Neurosci. Abstr. 3:* 90.

Ingle, D. (1970). Visuomotor function of the frog optic tectum. *Brain Behav. Evol. 3:* 57–71.

Jacobson, M. (1970). *Developmental Neurobiology*. New York: Holt, Reinhart, and Winston. 465 pp.

Kass, L., Loop, M. S., and Hartline, P. H. (1978). Anatomical and physiological localization of visual and infrared cell layers in the tectum of pit vipers. *J. Comp. Neurol. 182:* 811–20.

Knudsen, E. I. (1982). Auditory and visual maps of space in the optic tectum of the owl. *J. Neurosci. 2:* 1177–94.

Knudsen, P. F., Knudsen, E. I., and Esterly, S. D. (1982). Early auditory experience modifies sound localization in barn owls. *Nature 295:* 238–40.

Newman, E. A., and Hartline, P. H. (1981). Integration of visual and infrared information in bimodal neurons of the rattlesnake optic tectum. *Science 213:* 789–91.

Newman, E. A., and Hartline, P. H. (1982). The infrared 'vision' of snakes. *Scient. Am. 246(3):* 116–27.

Otto, J. (1972). Das Grubenorgan, ein biologisches System zur Abbildung von Intrarotstrahlern. *Kybernetic 10:* 103–6.

Ramon, P. (1896). Estructura del encefalo del camaleon. *Rev. Trimest. Micrograf. 1:* 46–82.

Schaefer, K. P. (1970). Unit analysis and electrical stimulation in the optic tectum of rabbits and cats. *Brain Behav. Evol. 3:* 222–40.

Schiller, P. H., and Stryker, M. (1972). Simple unit recording and stimulation in superior colliculus of the alert rhesus monkey. *J. Neurophysiol. 35:* 915–24.

Schneider, G. E. (1969). Two visual systems. *Science 163:* 895–902.

Sprague, J. M., Berlucci, G., and Rizzolatti, G. (1973). The role of the superior colliculus and pretectum in visually guided behavior. In *Handbook of Sensory Physiology* VII/3, ed. R. Jung, pp. 27–101. Berlin: Springer-Verlag.

Stein, B. E., and Gaither, N. S. (1981). Sensory representation in reptilian optic tectum: some comparisons with mammals. *J. Comp. Neurol. 202:* 69–87.

Stein, B. E., Magalhaes-Castro, B., and Kruger, L. (1976). Relationship between visual and tactile representations in cat superior colliculus. *J. Neurophysiol. 39:* 401–19.

Terashima, S.-I., and Goris, R. C. (1975). Tectal organization of pit viper infrared reception. *Brain Res. 83:* 490–4.

Terashima, S.-I., and Goris, R. C. (1976). Receptive area of an infrared tectal unit. *Brain Res. 101:* 155–9.

Wickelgren, B. G. (1971). Superior colliculus: some receptive field properties of bimodally responsive cells. *Science 173:* 69–72.

Wurtz, R. H., and Albano, J. E. (1980). Visual-motor function of the primate superior colliculus. *A. Rev. Neurosci. 3:* 189–226.

3.5

Neuropeptides in retina: morphological and biochemical aspects

M. SCHORDERET and P. J. MAGISTRETTI

It is generally conceived that the retina of vertebrates subserves two major functions. One, performed by the photoreceptors, is to transduce part of the information contained in the optical image into neural (i.e. electrical) signals. The other, achieved by an intricate neuronal circuitry, is to extract some features of the visual world from photoreceptor signals and transfer this partially processed information to the brain via the optic nerve fibers (Rodieck, 1973). Therefore, many biophysical and biochemical aspects of energy transduction processes, local neuronal interactions and integration mechanisms can conveniently be studied in this relatively simple and accessible region of the central nervous system. From the structural point of view, neuroanatomical studies have shown that the retina, like the cerebral cortex, is a laminar structure of the central nervous system, in which a restricted range of synaptic interactions is engaged by each cell type with another one (Rodieck, 1973). Furthermore, the early work of Ramon y Cajal (1893) has shown that basic retinal cell types are limited in number and are morphologically well defined. Thus, tremendous progress has been achieved in the morphology and physiological function(s) of the vertebrate retina and they have been extensively reviewed (Dowling, 1970; Rodieck, 1973; Kaneko, 1979). However, less is known about the biochemistry and pharmacology of retinal neurotransmitters, although several candidates, similar to classical brain transmitters, have been identified and their role in retinal neurotransmission often proven in various conditions (Bonting, 1976). A very well-defined biochemical and pharmacological tool for the study of a catecholamine as a retinal transmitter was introduced ten years ago by Brown and Makman (1972), when they showed that dopamine receptors were linked to the

421

enzyme adenylate cyclase. From that time, the vertebrate retina *in vitro* was used extensively as a specific model for pharmacological and/or binding studies of dopamine receptors, in order to screen dopamine-related drugs and to develop new potential agents for the treatment of Parkinson's disease, schizophrenia or hyperprolactinemia (see Schorderet and Magistretti, 1983, for review).

More recently, several neuropeptides have been localized by im-muno-histochemical techniques, in mammalian and non-mammalian retina (Stell et al., 1980; Karten and Brecha, 1981). The possible physiological role(s) of neuropeptides in the visual organ are still a matter of speculation, although recent electrophysiological and biochemical data have suggested a transmitter-like function for substance P, neurotensin and enkephalins (Dick, Miller and Behbehani, 1980; Glickman, Adolph and Dowling, 1980; Djamgoz, Stell, Chin and Lam, 1981; Dick and Miller, 1981; Dubocovich, Stewart and Weiner, 1982). On the other hand, some of these peptides, such as VIP and glucagon, are known to stimulate nervous- and non-nervous adenylate cyclase (Said, 1980). Thus, it was demonstrated recently that both neuropeptides were also able to stimulate the activity of this enzyme in retinal preparations (Longshore and Makman, 1981; Schorderet, Sovilla and Magistretti, 1981). Furthermore, the biochemical signal in response to VIP or glucagon seemed to be species-specific (Schorderet et al., 1981), corroborating the immuno-histochemical experiments, by which specificity for the localization of VIP (in mammals and avians) or glucagon (in avians) was also shown (Stell et al., 1980). Therefore, a change in cyclic AMP (cAMP) levels may be considered as an indicator of a possible physiological role of a given substance. This experimental approach has been applied to many putative retinal neurotransmitters such as dopamine (see above), adenosine (Schorderet, 1982a,b), and various neuropeptides (Schorderet and Magistretti, 1983). This type of investigation also affords the opportunity to study possible interactions, at the intracellular level, of neuropeptides with aminergic neurotransmission. For example, neurotensin and substance P have been shown to interact with dopamine function in other areas of the central nervous system (Nemeroff, Luttinger and Prange, 1980; Hanson, Alphs, Pradham and Lovenberg, 1981; Hanson et al., 1981; Palacios and Kuhar, 1981).

In this article we shall focus on three aspects of the biochemistry and pharmacology of retinal neurotransmission: first we shall attempt to evaluate the actual status of neurotransmitters in vertebrate retina, second we shall summarize the immunohistochemical localization of retinal neuropeptides, and third we shall comment on a few further electrophysiological, biochemical and pharmacological approaches used for investigating putative role(s) of retinal peptides and their possible significance for visual physiology.

Neurotransmitters in vertebrate retina: the present status

It has been stressed that the study of central neurotransmitters should be more feasible in the retina, due to the accessibility of the tissue, its relative anatomical simplicity and its remarkable metabolic survival (Starr, 1977; Watling, 1981; Ames III and Nesbett, 1981). In addition, the responses to the natural stimulus (i.e. light) can be recorded, precisely from individual cells or more grossly from the ERG, optic nerve or higher centers in the brain (Starr, 1977). Despite these advantages over other areas of the CNS, and paramount progress achieved in this field during the last decade, most retinal neurotransmitters are still referred to as 'alleged', 'putative', 'probable' and 'possible' candidates (Rodieck, 1973; Starr, 1977; Bonting, 1976; Voaden, 1979). The reasons are that first, it is commonly agreed that numerous criteria, using histochemical, physiological, biochemical and pharmacological techniques, have to be fulfilled before attributing an unequivocal neurotransmitter role to a substance (Bonting, 1976; Dismukes, 1979; Bloom, 1980). Secondly, a candidate could be a physiological neurotransmitter in one only or possibly more of the different types of retinal neurons, its precise localization and function remaining thus difficult to establish. Thirdly, species specificity and concomitant differences related to localization and function are not infrequent (Watling, 1981; Starr, 1977). Despite these restrictions, one can attempt, as shown in Table 1, to review the present status of retinal neurotransmitters. It is generally admitted that acetylcholine and dopamine (but not noradrenaline or serotonin) are more than 'candidates'. Both agents have transmitter function elsewhere in the CNS and a variety of electrophysiological, biochemical and, more recently, pharmacological experiments have confirmed a similar role in the retina of most species (Table 1). The other 'candidates' are amino-acid neurotransmitters, which have been shown to have diverse and strong effects on neuronal excitability in the retina and mainly in other areas of the central nervous system (Davidson, 1976; Neal, 1976; DeFeudis and Mandel, 1981).

Neuropeptides in vertebrate retina: localization and putative function(s)

Immunochemistry

During the last three years, several neuro- as well as gut-peptides have been detected by RIA or localized by immuno-histo-

Table 1. *Neurotransmitters in vertebrate retina*[a]

Substance	Localization of neurotransmitter function	Type of action
Classical candidates		
Acetylcholine	photoreceptors[b] bipolar cells[b] amacrine cells[c]	excitatory
Dopamine	dopaminergic junctional or interplexiform cells[c]	inhibitory
Amino-acid candidates		
Aspartate	photoreceptors[b]	excitatory
GABA	horizontal cells[b] amacrine cells[b]	inhibitory
Glutamate	photoreceptors[b]	excitatory
Glycine	horizontal cells[b] amacrine cells[b]	inhibitory
Taurine	photoreceptors[b] horizontal cells[b] amacrine cells[b]	inhibitory

[a] Related references: Bonting, 1976; Neal, 1976; Starr, 1977; Voaden, 1979; Watling, 1981.
[b] possible function.
[c] proven function.

chemical techniques in the retina of various species, mostly vertebrates, mammals and non-mammals (Table 2). Peptides of strictly CNS origin are TRH (the only one for which binding sites have been looked for), somatostatin and GnRH, whereas VIP, glucagon and CCK were initially detected in the gut. The detection of the presence of a neural substance is one of the criteria which have to be met for a proof of its possible neurotransmitter function (see above). Furthermore, this approach has to be completed by the other biochemical and pharmacological criteria (Bonting, 1976; Dismukes, 1979; Bloom, 1980). Thus, it appears that most of the retinal neuropeptides are located within the amacrine cell region (Table 2), where a physiological function of proven or possible neurotransmitters (Table 1) has been fully or partially demonstrated, respectively. It is thus postulated that a relationship might exist between classical neurotransmitters and one or another newly detected retinal peptides (Table 2), in analogy with what seems also to be existing in the brain (Hökfelt et al., 1980). Further fine immunohistochemical analysis even led to the visualization of reactive cells, which in morphological aspect and intraneuronal connections are characteristic for almost every retinal peptide (Stell et al., 1980; Karten and Brecha, 1981). Based on these morphological considerations, it is not illogical to imagine some possible specific role(s) linked with visual or cellular metabolic events for each retinal peptide, in a way dependent or independent of other known transmitters.

Biochemistry

As previously mentioned at the beginning of this chapter, homogenized or intact retinae of rat and calf were used successfully by Brown and Makman (1972) to reveal a link between dopamine receptors and cAMP metabolism. This important finding was confirmed in subsequent similar studies performed with retinal preparations of *Octopus bimaculatus* (invertebrate) as well as with those of several mammalian and non-mammalian vertebrates (see Schorderet and Magistretti, 1983, for review). These studies have firmly established the existence of specific and selective D_1-type of dopamine receptors (linked with adenylate cyclase stimulation, Kebabian and Calne, 1979) in the visual organ of most species and were further substantiated by radioligand-binding studies (Magistretti and Schorderet, 1979; Makman, Dvorkin, Horowitz and Thal, 1980; Redburn, Clement-Cormier and Lam, 1980; Schaeffer, 1980; Watling and Iversen, 1981).

On the other hand, VIP and glucagon are also known to activate adenylate cyclase in gastro-intestinal organs (Makman and Sutherland, 1964; Laburthe et al., 1978; Dupont et al., 1980), and VIP also stimulates cAMP generation in various brain regions (Quik, Iversen and Bloom, 1978; Kerwin, Pay, Bhoola and Pycock, 1980) or in brain cells in culture (Van Calker, Müller and Hamprecht, 1980). As a result, the retina of various mammalian and non-mammalian vertebrates has been used recently to investigate possible similar biochemical effects of VIP and glucagon (including secretin which shares structural homologies with VIP and glucagon) as well as of several other retinal neuropeptides. Table 3 shows that VIP stimulates adenylate cyclase in all species tested, whether intact or homogenized tissues are used. However, the rabbit retina (intact preparation) seems to be particularly sensitive to the stimulating effects of VIP, since a concentration of 1 nM already induces significant cAMP increases, whereas a concentration of 1 μM is needed to stimulate cAMP formation in pigeon and carp retina (Table 3). In addition, VIP induces a 25-fold increase of cAMP over control tissues at the highest concentration tested (0.5 μM) (Schorderet et al., 1981). For comparison with another agent promoting cAMP formation (e.g. dopamine), threshold-stimulation was observed at

Table 2. *Neuropeptides in vertebrate retina*[a]

Neuropeptides	Detected by	Species	Concentrations and/or localization	Authors
Tripeptide TRH (thyrotropin-releasing hormone) (thyroliberin)	Binding studies RIA RIA	sheep rat *mammals:* rat, rabbit, guinea-pig, monkey, cow *avians:* chick *amphibians:* bullfrog *fish:* eel	 hardly detectable: 0.1–0.3 pg/mg, w/w id. 95 pg/mg, w/w inner retinal cells and/or ganglion cells 64 pg/mg, w/w	Burt (1979) Schaeffer, Brownstein and Axelrod (1977) Eskay, Long and Iuvone (1980)
Pentapeptide Methionine – and Leucine – enkephalin	Immunohisto-fluorescence	*avians:* chick, pigeon *reptiles:* turtle	subclass of amacrine cells	Brecha, Karten and Laverack (1979) Humbert, Pradelles, Gros and Dray (1979) Fukuda (1982)
Decapeptide Gn-RH (gonadotropin-releasing hormone)	RIA	variety of species (not specified) *avians:* chick	subclass of amacrine cells	Stell et al. (1980) Fukuda (1982)
Undecapeptide Substance P	RIA, Immunohisto-fluorescence	*mammals:* rat, rabbit, guinea-pig, monkey, cow *avians:* chick, pigeon *amphibians:* bullfrog, mud-	subclass of amacrine cells	Brecha et al. (1979) Eskay et al. (1980) Fukuda et al. (1981a) Karten and Brecha (1980) Stell et al. (1980), Fukuda (1982) Eskay, Furness and Long (1981)

fish: carp

	Method	Species	Localization/Concentration	References
Tridecapeptide Neurotensin	RIA, Immunohisto-fluorescence	*avians:* pigeon	subclass of amacrine cells 59 fmol/whole retina 15.4 fmol/mg protein	Stell et al. (1980) Brecha, Karten and Schenker (1981) Fukuda et al. (1981b) Fukuda (1982)
Tetradecapeptide Somatostatin (SRIF)	RIA, Immunohisto-fluorescence	*mammals:* rat, rabbit, guinea-pig, cow, monkey, man *avians:* chick, pigeon	subclass of amacrine cells 102 pg/mg, w/w 2209 fmol/whole retina	Rorstad, Brownstein and Martin (1979) Shapiro, Kronheim and Pimstone (1981) Rorstad, Senterman, Hoyte and Martin (1980) Stell et al (1980); Brecha et al. (1981) Buckerfield, Oliver, Chubb and Morgan (1981) Morgan, Oliver and Chubb (1981) Fukuda (1982)
		amphibians: bullfrog, frog *fishes:* goldfish	527 fmol/mg protein 46 pg/mg, w/w	Eskay et al. (1980) Yamada et al. (1980) Yamada et al. (1980)
Octacosapeptide VIP (Vasoactive intestinal peptide)	Immunohisto-fluorescence	*avians:* chick, pigeon *mammals:* rat	subclass of amacrine cells	Stell et al. (1980); Fukuda et al. (1981b) Fukuda (1982) Loren, Tornqvist and Alumets (1980)
Nonacosapeptide Glucagon	Immunohisto-fluorescence	Variety of non-mammalian species (avians, amphibians, reptiles)	subclass of amacrine cells	Stell et al. (1980) Fukuda (1982)
Triacontapeptide CCK, Cholecystokinin	Immuno-fluorescence	*mammals:* man, calf *amphibian:* frog	subclass of amacrine cells	Osborne, Nicholas, Cuello and Dockray (1981)

(a) Modified from Schorderet and Magistretti (1983).

$0.5 \mu M$ and maximal increase of cAMP (about 2.5-fold over controls) was obtained at one up to $100 \mu M$ (Schorderet and Magistretti, 1980). In contrast, glucagon was inactive in intact preparation but active in homogenates of rabbit retina, as found independently by two groups of investigators (Table 3). Glucagon was also able to stimulate cAMP production in intact pigeon retina (Table 3), thus corroborating histochemical data demonstrating the presence of glucagon immunoreactivity only in retinae of non-mammalian species (Table 2). Interestingly, secretin was to some extent able to mimic the effects of VIP and glucagon in rabbit and pigeon retina, respectively, although it was considerably less potent and less efficient in both species (Table 3 and Schorderet et al., unpublished). These results contrast with those obtained in brain cells in culture (Van Calker et al., 1980) where secretin was even more potent than VIP.

The VIP-induced accumulation of cAMP measured in intact rabbit retina was studied in the presence of various dopamine antagonists such as (+)-butaclamol, haloperidol and fluphenazine (Schorderet et al., 1981) since both VIPergic and dopaminergic neurons coexist in the inner nuclear layer in subclasses of amacrine cells (Tables 1 and 2). Thus, a mutual interaction between the two neuronal systems could be postulated. However, neuroleptics were unable to affect the VIP-stimulted adenylate cyclase in intact rabbit retina (Schorderet et al., 1981). Similar data were also shown recently in intact carp retina exposed to VIP ($10 \mu M$) in the presence of $100 \mu M$ haloperidol (Watling and Dowling, 1981). In addition, drugs related to other neuronal systems, such as phenoxybenzamine (α-blocking agent) or betanechol (cholinomimetic) were also devoid of antagonist activity against VIP-mediated stimulation of cAMP formation (Schorderet et al., 1981). These results suggested that the biochemical effects of VIP were not directly related to other cAMP-dependent catecholaminergic or cholinergic pathways (Brown and Rietow, 1981). Rather, VIP may directly stimulate specific receptors (coupled to an adenylate cyclase), as recently demonstrated in various regions of brain by radioligand-binding studies (Taylor and Pert, 1979). On the other hand, we and others have found recently that adenosine and adenosine analogs were also able to stimulate, in a dose-dependent manner, the activity of adenylate cyclase in rabbit and chick retina (Schorderet, 1982a,b; Paes de Carvalho and de Mello, 1982). However, at the lower range of concentrations ($1 \mu M$), adenosine and its analog, L-phenylisopropyl-adenosine (L-PIA) partially inhibited the stimulating effects of VIP (Schorderet, in preparation). It is worth noting that a similar pharmacological interaction between VIP and

Table 3. *Neuropeptide-sensitive adenylate cyclase in vertebrate retina*[a]

	Active neuropeptides[b]	Inactive neuropeptides	Type of preparation	Authors
Avians Pigeon	VIP (1–10 μM) glucagon (1–10 μM) secretin (10 μM)		intact	Schorderet et al. (1981)
Fishes Carp	VIP (1–10 μM)	substance P (1 mM) 2-D-ala,5-D-leu- enkephalin (0.1 mM) somatostatin (0.1–1 mM)	intact	Dowling and Watling (1981) Watling and Dowling (1981)
Mammals Rat	VIP (10 μM) glucagon (10 μM) secretin (10 μM)		homogenates[c]	Longshore and Makman (1981)
Rabbit	VIP (10 μM) secretin (10 μM) glucagon (10 μM)		homogenates[c]	Longshore and Makman (1981)
Rabbit	VIP (1 nM–0.5 μM) secretin (10 nM–0.5 μM) neurotensin (10–50 μM)	glucagon (100 nM–10 μM) α-MSH (10 μM) pentagastrin (10 μM) substance P (100 μM) somatostatin (1–10 μM)[d]	intact	Schorderet et al. (1981)
Calf	VIP (10 μM)		homogenates[c]	Longshore and Makman (1981)

(a) Modified from Schorderet and Magistretti (1983).

(b) The range of concentrations promoting minimal and maximal activity is given in parentheses. One number is given when only the corresponding concentration was tested. Active neuropeptides are listed for each species according to the rank of potency.

(c) Since Gpp(NH)$_p$ influences the activity of neuropeptide-stimulated adenylate cyclase (Longshore and Makman, 1981), results given here are for experiments performed in absence of the guanine nucleotide analog.

(d) Somatostatin was also tested as a possible antagonist of VIP-sensitive adenylate cyclase in the same range of concentrations indicated in parentheses. The test was negative.

adenosine has been also shown recently in nerve cells in culture (Van Calker et al., 1980). Adenosine has been shown to have bimodal effects on cAMP levels in nervous and other tissues: it inhibits the formation of cAMP by interacting with high-affinity receptors, called A_1, while it has stimulatory effects on the cAMP formation, via low affinity, A_2 receptors (Daly, Bruns and Snyder, 1981). It therefore appears that at least two populations of receptors, for dopamine and for VIP, coupled to cAMP-generating systems, exist in the retina. These receptors may be differentially modulated by adenosine's interactions with A_1 and A_2 receptors. A schematic operational model is presented in Figure 1. The

cAMP-dependent receptors in vertebrate retina

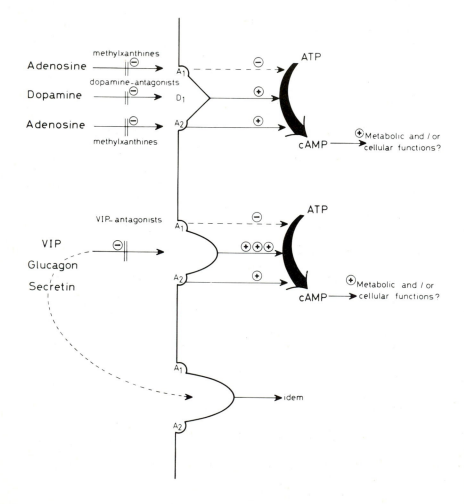

functional implications of increases in intracellular cAMP are diverse and have been reviewed recently (Greengard, 1981). It is, however, interesting to note that VIP has been recently shown to stimulate glycogenolysis in cerebral cortex in mice, possibly through a cAMP-dependent mechanism (Magistretti et al., 1981). It is therefore conceivable that in the retina also, VIP might play a similar role in the regulation of carbohydrate metabolism.

Finally, we have attempted to antagonize the VIP-induced formation of cAMP by somatostatin as found recently in some other nervous and non-nervous systems (Carter, Khalil, Zfass and Makhlouf, 1978; Van Calker et al., 1980). Somatostatin was inactive at concentrations as high as 10 μM when tested in intact rabbit retina exposed to VIP (Table 3). Several other peptides, such as substance P, neurotensin, α-MSH and pentagastrin have also been tested in intact rabbit retina for a possible activation effect on adenylate cyclase (Table 3). Only neurotensin (at 10–50 μM) was able slightly to stimulate the production of cAMP (Table 3). These concentrations are very high for an effect *in vitro* of a peptide.

Figure 1. Vertebrate retina appears to contain two populations of cAMP-dependent receptors: (1) The dopamine receptors (of D_1-type, also detected by binding studies, see text page 425), which generate cAMP ($\oplus$) in response to dopamine or dopamine agonists (such as apomorphine or substituted aminotetralins). cAMP in turn may be responsible for mediating metabolic and/or other cellular actions *in vivo*. Dopamine antagonists (such as classical neuroleptics) block D_1-receptors ($\ominus$) and inhibit the cAMP increase induced by the agonists. In addition, the activity of the enzyme generating cAMP from ATP (adenylate cyclase) is modulated by adenosine. Adenosine interacts with extracellular receptors of A_1-type (inhibitory, high-affinity, nM–μM range, $\ominus$) or of A_2-type (stimulatory, low-affinity, μM–mM range, $\oplus$). Thus, adenosine (or adenosine analogs), at low or high concentration, can inhibit or potentiate, respectively, the effects of dopamine on cAMP production. Finally, methylxanthines are antagonists of adenosine at both A_1 and A_2 sites. (2) The VIP-receptors, which generate cAMP ($\oplus\oplus\oplus$) in response to VIP or other peptides sharing structural homologies with VIP, such as glucagon or secretin. (It is not excluded that in some species, such as avians, specific receptors for glucagon exist; see Table 2). VIP antagonists, such as secretin 5–27 (Van Calker et al., 1980), not tested yet in retina, may block VIP receptors and the concomitant increase of cAMP. The three $\oplus\oplus\oplus$ indicate that in rabbit retina, VIP is much more efficacious than dopamine applied under similar experimental conditions. (Schorderet and Magistretti, 1980.) Finally, as shown for dopamine-D_1 receptors, adenosine may influence the VIP effects in both directions ($\ominus$ and $\oplus$, A_1 or A_2 sites), depending upon the concentrations of adenosine (see above).

However, a mutual interaction between neurotensin and dopaminergic neurons (both also located in subclasses of amacrine cells, Tables 1, 2) has been suggested to occur in brain by a variety of experimental data (Nemeroff et al., 1980; Ervin, Birkemo, Nemeroff and Prange, 1981). Possible interactions between neuropeptides and other classical neurotransmitters are also investigated now in the retina by various experimental approaches and will be discussed in the next paragraph.

Physiological and/or functional studies
     A few electrophysiological studies of substance P, neurotensin and opioids have been performed recently in isolated retinae of fish and amphibians (Glickman et al., 1980; Dick et al., 1980; Dick and Miller, 1981; Djamgoz et al., 1981). Light-evoked and/or spontaneous activity of ganglion cells was recorded with extracellular electrodes, following nebulization of substance P or its application by iontophoresis. In both cases, substance P and neurotensin were able to evoke spontaneous activity and to enhance light-dependent responses, suggesting that in both species (fish and amphibian) it may have a transmitter or neuromodulator function. Opposite results were found with opioids applied to amphibian retina under similar iontophoretic experimental conditions (Dick et al., 1980; Dick and Miller, 1981). In the latter case, enkephalinamide, morphine or even naloxone gave rise to a long-lasting inhibition of light-evoked responses and aspartate-activated spike activity in all ganglion cell types. Comparable (but not identical) results were also found recently by Djamgoz et al. (1981) in recording ganglion-cell unit activity from the isolated, inverted retina of goldfish using metal microelectrodes.
     Studies of presumed interactions of neuropeptides with known or putative retinal neurotransmitters were also performed. By loading isolated retinae with ^{3}H-dopamine or ^{3}H-GABA, it is possible to measure, under well defined conditions, their subsequent release, triggered by high potassium for labeled GABA (Djamgoz et al., 1981) or by electrical stimulation for labeled dopamine (Dubocovich et al., 1982), in absence and in presence of various opioids. Enkephalin (1 μM) and morphine (10 μM) were able to inhibit the K^{+}-stimulated release of ^{3}H-GABA from amacrine cells of goldfish retina, the inhibition being reversed by 10 μM naloxone (Djamgoz et al., 1981). It was thus concluded that in goldfish retina exogenous opiates affect both the release of GABA from GABA-ergic amacrine cells and the firing pattern of ganglion cells (see above). In physiological situations, it is postulated that opioid neuronal pathways inhibit, by releasing enkepha-

lins, GABA-ergic amacrine cells; thus by antagonizing the inhibitory actions of the amino acid, disinhibition of ON-centre ganglion cells occurs (Djamgoz et al., 1981).

Similarly, morphine (0.01–3 μM) and synthetic enkephalins (0.001–1 μM) were able to inhibit the electrically-evoked release of ^{3}H-dopamine from isolated rabbit retina, the inhibition being reversed by 1 μM (−)naloxone but not by (+)-naloxone (Dubocovich et al., 1982). Furthermore, S-Sulpiride, an antagonist of dopamine at presumed D_2-receptor subtype (autoreceptors involved in the modulation of release through a negative feedback mechanism, Dubocovich and Weiner, 1981) did not affect the opioid-induced inhibitory effects. It was thus concluded that in addition to the dopamine-inhibitory autoreceptors (D_2), rabbit retina is endowed with inhibitory opiate receptors (possibly located on dopamine-containing amacrine cells). When activated, those receptors inhibit the release of dopamine evoked by electrical stimulation (Dubocovich et al., 1982).

Another experimental approach used for unmasking a possible interaction of neuropeptides with the formation, storage and release of dopamine was recently exploited by Sovilla and Schorderet (1982) in isolated rabbit retina. It was known that the immediate precursor of dopamine, L-dopa, was able to induce significant increase in cAMP levels *in vitro* (Sovilla and Schorderet, 1982). Several lines of evidence indicated that the L-dopa effect was mediated by the formation *in situ* of new dopamine, which in turn stimulated the post-synaptic D_1-receptor subtype with concomitant increases in cAMP concentrations. Among several dopaminergic and GABA-ergic drugs, or neuropeptides tested simultaneously with L-dopa, substance P potentiated the generation of cAMP induced by the dopamine precursor, but not that mediated by dopamine itself. It appears likely that substance P, acting at presynaptic level, facilitates the release of newly-formed dopamine. However, the potentiation of L-dopa effect by substance P was observed at rather high concentrations (minimal effects at 1 μM, maximal effects at 100 μM). It is conceivable that in these experiments *in vitro*, substance P adhered to the internal glass surface of assay tubes (Franco, Costa and Furness, 1979) or was rapidly inactivated. Thus, high concentrations were required to achieve a detectable pharmacological effect. In any case, a relationship between substance P and dopaminergic activity has been demonstrated in brain (Hanson et al., 1981) and further studies *in vivo* and *in vitro* are now needed to establish more firmly similar functional interactions in retina.

Conclusions

It is now well established that the retina *in vitro* represents a useful preparation for studying various aspects of neurotransmission, such as neurotransmitter identification and localization, release and possibly, functions. Particularly during the last decade, this alternative to brain slices was used specifically to investigate dopaminergic transmission at the level of a relevant biochemical signal (cAMP generation) and has led to the pharmacological characterization of a population of dopamine-receptors of D_1-subtype, detected in binding studies, and similar to striatal-D_1-receptors.

Recently, the immunohistochemical localization of several neuropeptides was elegantly performed in the retina of various vertebrate and invertebrate species. These findings open a new fertile trend of research for studying neuropeptide transmission and function, at the morphological, biochemical, pharmacological and electrophysiological level. Interestingly, most retinal peptides have generally been localized in subclasses of amacrine cells, where proven and putative neurotransmitters seem to be functional. Furthermore, the immunohistochemical findings have been partially corroborated by electrophysiological studies. For example, exogenously applied peptides such as substance P and opioids have been shown to have direct effects on the neuronal circuitry of the inner nuclear layer. The same neuropeptides seem also to interact with other neurotransmitters contained in amacrine cells, such as GABA and dopamine, at the presynaptic level, by modulating their release from nerve terminals. Finally, at the biochemical level, VIP, glucagon, and to some extent neurotensin, increase retinal cAMP via an interaction, at least for VIP and glucagon, with specific receptors coupled to the cAMP-generating system. The biochemical response induced by VIP is even more pronounced than that induced by dopamine, at least in some mammalian species. At the functional level, the role of such an increase of cAMP remains speculative. However, it is interesting to note here that VIP has been demonstrated to influence energy metabolism in mouse cortex, through an increase in cAMP. In addition, VIP and glucagon can modulate dopaminergic transmission at the level of post-synaptic receptors for potentiating the biochemical signal (i.e. cAMP increases) which is also under the negative or positive control of adenosine through A_1- and A_2-receptors, respectively.

Thus, questions about the role and regulation of peptide-mediated neurotransmission can now be constructively addressed and in certain instances hopefully answered by use of retinal preparations.

Supported by the Swiss National Science Foundation, grant No. 3.345.0.81.

We would like to express our gratitude to Mrs G. Gilliéron, S. Bonnet and N. Collet for their excellent technical and secretarial assistance and to Mr F. Pillonel for elegant artwork.

References

Ames III, A., and Nesbett, F. B. (1981). *In vitro* retina as an experimental model of the central nervous system. *J. Neurochem.37:*867–77.

Bloom, F. E. (1980). Neurohumoral transmission and the central nervous system. In *The Pharmacological Basis of Therapeutics*, 6th edn, ed. A. Goodman Gilman, L. S. Goodman and A. Gilman, pp. 235–57. New York: MacMillan.

Bonting, S. L. (1976). *Transmitters in the Visual Process.* Oxford: Pergamon Press.

Brecha, N., Karten, H. J., and Laverack, C. (1979). Enkephalin-containing amacrine cells in the avian retina: immunohistochemical localization. *Proc. Narn. Acad. Sci. USA 76:* 3010–14.

Brecha, N., Karten, H. J., and Schenker, C. (1981). Neurotensin-like and somatostatin-like immunoreactivity within amacrine cells of the retina. *Neuroscience 6:* 1329–40.

Brown, J. H., and Makman, M. H. (1972). Stimulation by dopamine of adenylate cyclase in retinal homogenates and of adenosine 3'-5'-cyclic monophosphate formation in intact retina. *Proc. Natn. Acad. Sci. USA 69:* 539–43.

Brown, J. H., and Rietow, M. (1981). Muscarinic-dopaminergic synergism on retinal cyclic AMP formation. *Brain Res. 213:* 388–92.

Buckerfield, M., Oliver, J., Chubb, I. W., and Morgan, I. G. (1981). Somatostatin-like immunoreactivity in amacrine cells of the chicken retina. *Neuroscience 6:* 689–95.

Burt, D. R. (1979). Thyrotropin releasing hormone: apparent receptor binding in retina. *Expl Eye Res. 29:* 353–65.

Carter, R. F., Khalil, N. B., Zfass, A. M., and Makhlouf, G. M. (1978). Inhibition of VIP-stimulated intestinal secretion and cyclic AMP production by somatostatin in the rat. *Gastroenterology 74:* 726–30.

Daly, J. W., Bruns, R. F., and Snyder, S. H. (1981). Adenosine receptors in the central nervous system: relationship to the central actions of methylxanthines. *Life Sci. 28:* 2083–97.

Davidson, N. (1976). *Neurotransmitter Amino-acids.* New York: Academic Press.

DeFeudis, F. V., and Mandel, P. (1981). Amino acid neurotransmitters. In *Advances in Biochemical Psychopharmacology*, vol. *29*, ed. E. Costa and P. Greengard. New York: Raven Press.

Dick, E., Miller, R. F., and Behbehani, M. M. (1980). Opioids and substance P influence ganglion cells in amphibian retina. *Investigative Ophthalmology Visual Science ARVO Supplement 19:* 132.

Dick, E., and Miller, R. F. (1981). Peptides influence retinal ganglion cells. *Neurosci. Lett. 26:* 131–6.

Dismukes, R. K. (1979). New concept of molecular communication among neurons. *The Behavioral and Brain Sciences 2:* 409–48.

Djamgoz, M. B. A., Stell, W. K., Chin, C. A., and Lam, M. K. (1981). An opiate system in the goldfish retina. *Nature 292:* 620–3.

Dowling, J. E. (1970). Organization of vertebrate retinas. *Investigative Ophthalmology 9:* 655–80.

Dowling, J. E., and Watling, K. J. (1981). Dopaminergic mechanisms in the teleost retina. II. Factors affecting the accumulation of cyclic AMP in pieces of intact carp retina. *J. Neurochem. 36:* 569–79.

Dubocovich, M. L., Stewart, J., and Weiner, N. (1982). Enkephalins modulate dopamine release from the isolated rabbit retina. *Fed. Proc. 41:* 1532.

Dubocovich, M. L., and Weiner, N. (1981). Modulation of the stimulation-evoked release of ^{3}H-dopamine in the rabbit retina. *J. Pharmacol. Exp. Therapeutics 219:* 701–7.

Dupont, C., Laburthe, M., Broyart, J. P., Bataille, D., and Rosselin, G. (1980). Cyclic AMP production in isolated colonic epithelial crypts: a highly sensitive model for the evaluation of vasoactive intestinal peptide action in human intestine. *Eur. J. Clin. Invest. 10:* 67–76.

Ervin, G. N., Birkemo, L. S., Nemeroff, C. B., and Prange, A. J. (1981). Neurotensin blocks certain amphetamine-induced behaviors. *Nature 291:* 73–6.

Eskay, R. L., Furness, J. F., and Long, R. T. (1981). Substance P activity in the bullfrog retina: localization and identification in several vertebrate species. *Science 212:* 1049–51.

Eskay, R. L., Long, R. T., and Iuvone, P. M. (1980). Evidence that TRH, somatostatin and substance P are present in neurosecretory elements of the vertebrate retina. *Brain Res. 196:* 554–9.

Franco, R., Costa, M., and Furness, J. B. (1979). Evidence for the release of endogenous substance P from intestinal nerves. *Naunyn-Schmiedeberg's Arch. Exp. Path. Pharmak. 306:* 195–201.

Fukuda, M. (1982). Localization of neuropeptides in the avian retina: an immunohistochemical analysis. *Cell. Molec. Biol. 28:* 275–83.

Fukuda, M., Kuwayama, Y., Shiosaka, S., Ishimoto, I., Shimizu, Y., Takagi, H., Inagaki, S., Sakanaka, M., Senba, E., Takatsuki, K., and Tohyama, M. (1981a). Demonstration of a substance P-like immunoreactivity in retinal cells of the rat. *Neurosci. Lett. 23:* 239–42.

Fukuda, M., Kuwayama, Y., Shiosaka, S., Ishimoto, I., Shimizu, Y., Takagi, H., Sakanaka, M., Takatsuki, K., Senba, E., and Tohyama, M. (1981b). Localization of vasoactive intestinal polypeptide and neurotensin immunoreactivities in the avian retina. *Curr. Eye Res. 1:* 115–18.

Glickman, R. D., Adolph, A. R., and Dowling, J. E. (1980). Does substance P have a physiological role in the carp retina? *Investigative Ophthalmology Visual Science ARVO Supplement 19:* 281.

Greengard, P. (1981). Intracellular signals in the brain. *The Harvey Lectures*, series 75: 277–331.

Hanson, G., Alphs, L., Pradhan, S., and Lovenberg, W. (1981). Response of striatonigral substance P systems to a dopamine receptor agonist and antagonist. *Neuropharmacology 20:* 541–8.

Hanson, G. R., Alphs, L., Wolf, W., Levine, R., and Lovenberg, W. (1981). Haloperidol-induced reduction of nigral substance P-like immunoreactivity: a probe for the interactions between dopamine and substance P neuronal systems. *J. Pharmac. Exp. Ther. 218:* 568–74.

Hökfelt, T., Johansson, O., Ljungdahl, A., Lundberg, J. M., and Schultzberg, M. (1980). Peptidergic neurones. *Nature 284:* 515–21.

Humbert, J., Pradelles, P., Gros, C., and Dray, F. (1979). Enkephalin-like products in embryonic chicken retina. *Neurosci. Lett. 12:* 259–63.

Kaneko, A. (1979). Physiology of the retina. *A. Rev. Neurosci. 2:* 169–91.

Karten, H. J., and Brecha, N. (1980). Localisation of substance P immunoreactivity in amacrine cells of the retina. *Nature 283:* 87–8.

Karten, H. J., and Brecha, N. (1981). Biochemical and morphological specificity of retinal amacrine cells: immunohistochemical findings. In *Monoclonal Antibodies to Neural Antigens*, ed. R. McKay, M. C. Raff and L. F. Reichardt, pp. 203–7. Cold Spring Harbor: Cold Spring Harbor Laboratory.

Kebabian, J. W., and Calne, D. B. (1979). Multiple receptors for dopamine. *Nature 277:* 93–6.

Kerwin, R. W., Pay, S., Bhoola, K. D., and Pycock, C. J. (1980). Vasoactive intestinal polypeptide (VIP)-sensitive adenylate cyclase in rat brain: regional distribution and localization on hypothalamic neurons. *J. Pharm. Pharmac. 32:* 561–6.

Laburthe, M., Rousset, M., Boissard, C., Chevalier, G., Zweibaum, A., and Rosselin, G. (1978). Vasoactive intestinal peptide: a potent stimulator of adenosine $3':5'$-cyclic monophosphate accumulation in gut carcinoma cell lines in culture. *Proc. Natn. Acad. Sci. USA 75:* 2772–5.

Longshore, M. A., and Makman, M. H. (1981). Stimulation of retinal adenylate cyclase by vasoactive intestinal peptide (VIP). *Eur. J. Pharmac. 70:* 237–40.

Loren, I., Tornqvist, K., and Alumets, J. (1980). VIP (Vasoactive Intestinal Polypeptide)-immunoreactive neurons in the retina of the rat. *Cell Tiss. Res. 210:* 167–70.

Magistretti, P. J., and Schorderet, M. (1979). Dopamine receptors in bovine retina: characterization of the H-spiroperidol binding and its use for screening dopamine receptor affinity of drugs. *Life Sci. 25:* 1675–86.

Magistretti, P. J., Morrison, J. H., Shoemaker, W. J., Sapin, V., and Bloom, F. E. (1981). Vasoactive intestinal polypeptide induces glycogenolysis in mouse cortical slices: a possible regulatory mechanism for the local control of energy metabolism. *Proc. Natn. Acad. Sci. USA 78:* 6535–9.

Makman, M. H., Dvorkin, B., Horowitz, S. G., and Thal, L. J. (1980). Properties of dopamine and antagonist binding sites in mammalian retina. *Brain Res. 194:* 403–18.

Makman, M. H., and Sutherland, E. W. (1964). Use of liver adenyl cyclase for assay of glucagon in human gastrointestinal tract and pancreas. *Endocrinology 75:* 127–34.

Morgan, I. G., Oliver, J., and Chubb, I. W. (1981). Discrete distribution of putative cholinergic and somatostatinergic amacrine cell dendrites in chicken retina. *Neurosci. Lett. 27:* 55–60.

Neal, M. J. (1976). Amino acid transmitter substances in the vertebrate retina. *Gen. Pharmac. 7:* 321–32.

Nemeroff, C. B., Luttinger, D., and Prange, A. J. (1980). Neurotensin: central nervous system effects of a neuropeptide. *Trends Neurosci. 3:* 212–15.

Osborne, N. N., Nicholas, D. A., Cuello, A. C., and Dockray, G. J. (1981). Localization of cholecistokinin-immunoreactivity in amacrine cells of the retina. *Neurosci. Lett. 26:* 31–5.

Paes de Carbalho, R., and de Mello, F. G. (1982). Adenosine-elicited accumulation of adenosine 3′,5′-cyclic monophosphate in the chick embryo retina. *J. Neurochem. 38:* 493–500.

Palacios, J. M., and Kuhar, M. J. (1981). Neurotensin receptors are located on dopamine-containing neurons in rat midbrain. *Nature 294:* 587–9.

Quik, M., Iversen, L. L., and Bloom, S. R. (1978). Effect of vasoactive intestinal peptide (VIP) and other peptides on cAMP accumulation in rat brain. *Biochem. Pharmac. 27:* 2209–13.

Ramon y Cajal, S. (1893). La rétine des vertébrés. *Cellule 9:* 17–257.

Redburn, D. A., Clement-Cormier, Y., and Lam, D. M. K. (1980). Dopamine receptors in the goldfish retina: ^{3}H-spiroperidol and ^{3}H-domperidone binding; and dopamine-stimulated adenylate cyclase activity. *Life Sci. 27:* 23–31.

Rodieck, R. W. (1973). *The Vertebrate Retina, Principles of Structure and Function.* San Francisco: W. H. Freeman and Co.

Rorstad, O. P., Brownstein, M. J., and Martin, J. B. (1979). Immunoreactive and biologically active somatostatin-like material in rat retina. *Proc. Natn. Acad. Sci. USA 76:* 3019–23.

Rorstad, O. P., Senterman, M. K., Hoyte, K. M., and Martin, J. B. (1980). Immunoreactive and biologically active somatostatin-like material in the human retina. *Brain Res. 199:* 488–92.

Said, S. I. (1980). Peptides common to the nervous system and the gastrointestinal tract. In *Frontiers in Neuroendocrinology*, vol. 6, ed. L. Martini and W. F. Ganong, pp. 293–331. New York: Raven Press.

Schaeffer, J. M. (1980). Identification of dopamine receptors in the rat retina. *Expl Eye Res. 30:* 431–7.

Schaeffer, J. M., Brownstein, M. J., and Axelrod, J. (1977). Thyrotropin-releasing hormone-like material in the rat retina: changes due to environmental lighting. *Proc. Natn. Acad. Sci. USA 74:* 3579–81.

Schorderet, M. (1982a). Adenosine-A_2-receptors in isolated rabbit retina: a neurochemical study. *Neuroscience 7* (Suppl.), S187.

Schorderet, M. (1982b). Pharmacological characterization of adenosine-mediated increase of cyclic AMP in isolated rabbit retina. *Fedn Proc. 41:* 1707.

Schorderet, M., and Magistretti, P. J. (1980). The isolated retina of mammals: a useful preparation for enzymatic-(adenyl cyclase) and/or binding studies of dopamine receptors. *Neurochemistry 1:* 337–53.

Schorderet, M., and Magistretti, P. J. (1983). Comparative aspects of the adenylate cyclase system in retina. In *Progress in Nonmammalian Brain Research*, vol. II, ed. G. Nistico and L. Bolis, pp. 185–211. Boca Raton: CRC Press, Inc.

Schorderet, M., Sovilla, J. Y., and Magistretti, P. J. (1981). VIP- and glucagon-induced formation of cyclic AMP in intact retinae *in vitro. Eur. J. Pharmac. 71:* 131–3.

Shapiro, B., Kronheim, S., and Pimstone, B. (1981). The presence of immunoreactive somatostatin in rat retina. *Hormonal Metabolism Research 11:* 79–80.

Sovilla, J. Y., and Schorderet, M. (1982). L-dopa accumulation of cyclic AMP in isolated rabbit retinae *in vitro.* Effects of light and/or pharmacological factors. *Life Sci. 31:* 2081–92.

Starr, M. S. (1977). Prospective neurotransmitters in vertebrate retina. In *Essays in Neurochemistry and Neuropharmacology*, ed. M. B. H. Youdim, W. Lovenberg, D. F. Sharman and J. R. Lagnado, pp. 152–74. Chichester: John Wiley.

Stell, W., Marshak, D., Yamada, T., Brecha, N., and Karten, H. J. (1980). Peptides are in the eye of the beholder. *Trends Neurosci. 3:* 292–5.

Taylor, D. P., and Pert, C. B. (1979). Vasoactive intestinal polypeptide: specific binding to rat brain membranes. *Proc. Natn. Acad. Sci. USA 76:* 660–4.

Van Calker, D., Müller, M., and Hamprecht, B. (1980). Regulation by secretin, vasoactive intestinal peptide, and somatostatin of cyclic AMP accumulation in cultured brain cells. *Proc. Natn. Acad. Sci. USA 77:* 6907–11.

Voaden, M. J. (1979). Vision: the biochemistry of the retina. In *Companion to Biochemistry*, vol. *2*, ed. A. T. Bull, J. R. Lagnado, J. R. Thomas and K. F. Tipton, pp. 451–73. London: Longman.

Watling, K. J. (1981). Transmitter candidates in the retina. *Trends Pharmac. Sci. 2:* 244–7.

Watling, K. J., and Dowling, J. E. (1981). Vasoactive intestinal peptide stimulates cAMP accumulation in the carp retina. *Investigative Ophthalmology Visual Science ARVO Supplement 20:* 167.

Watling, K. J., and Iversen, L. L. (1981). Comparison of the binding of ^{3}H-spiperone and ^{3}H-domperidone in homogenates of mammalian retina and caudate nucleus. *J. Neurochem. 37:* 1130–43.

Yamada, T., Marshak, D., Basinger, S., Wals, J., Morley, J., and Stell, W. (1980). Somatostatin-like immunoreactivity in the retina. *Proc. Natn. Acad. Sci. USA 77:* 1691–5.

3.6

Lack of relations between dopaminergic and GABA-ergic mechanisms in chick retina

G. NISTICÒ, A. DE SARRO, G. URNA,
A. PUJIA AND R. IENTILE

On the basis of its morphology, embryology and function, the retina is considered part of the CNS and several transmitters have been identified. Amongst the other transmitters, attention has been focused in recent years on dopamine and GABA and it has been proposed that these substances play a functional inhibitory role in the intraretinal circuits of mammalian and non-mammalian species.

Dopaminergic cell bodies are found in the inner nuclear layer mostly among the amacrine cells and more rarely in interplexiform cells, ganglion cells and eremite cells of the inner plexiform layer (see Ehinger, 1977, and Magistretti, 1979). Since amacrine cells possess no axons but only dendrites or processes, they appear to be a model for local circuit neurons. Dopaminergic processes ramify within the inner plexiform layer with considerable species variation. In rabbits they form a set of interneurons solely connecting amacrine cells, whereas in goldfish and cebus monkey, dopamine processes extend from the inner plexiform to the outer plexiform layer, where synapses are formed on bipolars and cone horizontal cells (see Ehinger, 1977). Thus the processes of dopamine amacrine cells form complex synaptic interconnections since they have pre- and post-synaptic contacts with ganglion cells (Dowling, 1978).

In avian retina, dopamine seems to be the only monoamine (Ehinger, 1967; Stoeckel et al., 1976), since no indoleamine fluorescence was detectable in normal retinae of chick embryo, newborn and older chickens or pigeons (Florén, 1979).

The physiological role of dopamine in the retina is not completely known although it has been shown that stimulation by light is able to increase dopamine release and turnover (Kramer, 1971; Da Prada,

441

1977) and electrophysiological experiments with exogenously applied dopamine indicate that this amine may function as an inhibitory transmitter (Ames and Pollen, 1969). The physiological effects of dopamine in retina seem to be mediated by cAMP since a dopamine-sensitive adenylate cyclase linked to dopamine receptors has been shown to be present at the retinal level (Brown and Makman, 1972; Schorderet, 1977). Recently it has been reported that other dopaminergic agonists, i.e. LSD and apomorphine increase cAMP formation in rat retina and that in rats kept in the dark, dopamine and dopaminergic agonists produce a further increase of dopamine-sensitive adenylate cyclase activity, suggesting the development of supersensitivity of dopamine receptors (Spano et al., 1977). In view of the existence of multiple receptors for dopamine in the brain (see Seeman, 1980) it has been shown that in retina all dopamine receptors seem to be linked to adenylate cyclase (Watling, Dowling and Iversen, 1979; Magistretti, 1979). Neuroleptic drugs such as haloperidol, chlorpromazine and flufenazine selectively antagonize dopamine-sensitive adenylate cyclase in calf and carp retina (Brown and Makman, 1973; Watling and Dowling, 1981).

On the other hand, several studies have shown the existence of GABA and glutamate-decarboxylase activity, the rate-limiting step in GABA biosynthesis, in mammalian and non-mammalian retina; in particular, it appears that GABA is predominantly located in the amacrine and horizontal cells (see Neal, 1976; Dowling, 1970; Macaione, 1972; Nakamura, McGuire and Starling, 1980).

It is well established that in CNS strict functional relations exist between dopaminergic and GABA-ergic mechanisms (Fahn, 1976; Hornykiewcz, Lloyd and Davidson, 1976). We have previously reported that in chicks an oral subacute treatment with l-DOPA (Di Giorgio, Macaione, Lanotte and Nisticò, 1979) or an intraventricular treatment with apomorphine (Nisticò, Ientile, Lanotte and Di Giorgio, 1980) increases GAD activity and consequently GABA content in the avian paleostriatum augmentatum, homologous to the mammalian caudate nucleus. Recently we have found that in chicks only large doses of apomorphine, acting on dopamine post-synaptic receptors linked to the adenyl-cyclase activity, are able to increase GABA synthesis in avian paleostriatum augmentatum (Nisticò et al., 1982).

On the other hand the effects of l-DOPA on the GABA system in the retina are not unequivocal since in rat a single dose of l-DOPA *in vivo* produced a decrease of GABA content and GAD activity (Macaione, Di Giorgio and Ruggeri, 1973), whereas in chick retina l-DOPA increased GABA content as the consequence of an inhibition of GABA-transaminase, the enzymatic activity involved in GABA break-down (Di Giorgio et al., 1979).

In an attempt to demonstrate whether relations between dopamine and GABA neurons in the chick retina exist, we have studied the effects on GABA mechanisms of drug manipulations by using agonists and antagonists at dopamine multiple receptors having a different profile (see Seeman, 1980). Thus the effects of apomorphine and bromocriptine on GABA content, GAD and GABA-T activities both in conditions of a light cycle of 12 h/day and in conditions of light deprivation (exposure to darkness for 72 h) were studied. In addition, the effects of a treatment with haloperidol and l-sulpiride on GAD activity and GABA content in the retina were assessed.

Materials and methods

Rhode Island Red chicks, two weeks old, were used. After decapitation, retinae were quickly dissected out and rapidly homogenized in 0.1 M sodium phosphate buffer, pH 6.8.

GAD activity was assayed using the conditions of Beaven, Wilcox and Terpestra (1978), slightly modified. A 30-μl sample of the tissue homogenate (1:10) was mixed with 20 μl of reagent inside a 1.5-ml polypropylene Eppendorf vial. The vial was placed inside a 20-ml screw-cap liquid scintillation counting vial. A drop (20 μl) of 30% 2-phenylethylamine in methanol was adsorbed on a paper square (1 cm^2 of filter paper, Whatman 3MM), placed at the bottom of the counting vial away from the Eppendorf vial. The reagent consists of (a) L-[U-^{14}C]glutamic acid, 20 nCi; (b) unlabelled L-glutamic acid to bring the concentration of amino acid to 1.5×10^{-3}M; (c) 1×10^{-5}M PLP; and (d) 0.1 M sodium phosphate buffer, pH 6.8; (e) Triton X 100 (final concentration 0.5%). Reaction blanks were prepared by substituting buffer for the sample. The counting vials were capped tightly and incubated at 37°C for 30 min; for deproteinization the vials were then placed on ice and uncapped one at a time and 20 μl of 2 N perchloric acid were added to the Eppendorf vials. The counting vials were quickly recapped and reincubated for 30 min. At the end of the second incubation, the Eppendorf vials were removed from the counting vials and discarded. Ten millilitres of liquid scintillation mixture (2.5 g PPO and 150 mg POPOP/litre toluene) were added to each counting vial and radioactivity was measured by a Beckman LS 7500 liquid scintillator at room temperature. Preliminary experiments have shown that in our experimental conditions ^{14}CO$_2$ loss was approximately 2%. In addition, under our experimental conditions the rate of enzyme reaction was linear as a function of time (up to 30 min) as well as of protein (up to 0.150 mg).

GABA-aminotransferase (GABA-T) was assayed in reaction mixtures containing 250 nmol Tris-HCl buffer, pH 8.3; 1.3 nmol pyridoxal phosphate; 75 nmol [4-^{14}C]-γ-aminobutyric acid (0.58 μCi/μmol), and 39 nmol sodium α-ketoglutarate in a total volume of 10 μl. Final pH of the reaction mixture after addition of enzyme was 8.2. The tubes were placed in an ice bath and after addition of 10 μl of a retina homogenate (15 μg protein) the tubes were incubated at 37°C for 30 min.

After the enzyme incubation, the tubes were replaced in the ice bath and 5 μl of 15 mM 2,4-dinitrophenylhydrazine in 1M H$_2$SO$_4$ were added followed by 150 μl of ethyl acetate.

The contents of the tubes were mixed and centrifuged, and a 100-μl aliquot of the organic phase was removed and mixed with 50 μl 0.3M HCl to wash out trace amounts of labelled substrate. The mixture was again centrifuged and 50 μl of the organic phase were removed for counting in 10 ml of scintillation fluid containing 2.5 g PPO and 150 mg POPOP/litre toluene.

GABA content was determined by the enzymatic fluorimetric procedure of Graham and Aprison (1966), as modified by Balcom, Lenox and Meyerkoff (1975).

Thirty microlitres of deproteinized sample (diluted to the 10 mg tissue/ml range) was added to 30 μl of reaction mixture composed of: 5 vol. of 0.1% sodium pyrophosphate buffer pH 8.4, 1 vol. 1.1 mM NAD, 1 vol. 60 mM β-mercaptoethanol, 1 vol. 60 mM α-ketoglutaric acid pH 7 and 1 vol. of GABAse solution containing 2.5 U/ml.

Samples in duplicate were incubated at 38°C for 1 h. One hundred microlitres of 0.6 M sodium phosphate buffer pH 11.4 were added; the tubes were recapped, mixed, and incubated at 60°C for 15 min. One hundred microlitres of the sample solution were then transferred into another tube containing 0.2 ml of alkaline-peroxide solution, 0.2 ml of 3% H$_2$O$_2$ plus 19.8 ml of 10 N NaOH).

The contents of the tubes were mixed, covered and incubated at 60°C for 10 min; 1.5 ml of H$_2$O was added, the contents of the tubes were mixed and their relative fluorescence was determined with a Perkin-Elmer model 3000 spectrophotofluorometer (EXC. 365 Em. 470). At the same time standard solutions of GABA were examined.

Protein content was determined by the Lowry method with bovine serum albumin as standard.

Results

Effects of apomorphine and bromocriptine on GAD, GABA-T and GABA content

Apomorphine (0.025 and 2 mg kg^{-1} intraperitoneally) and bromocriptine (20 mg kg^{-1} intraperitoneally) did not produce any significant change in GAD activity, GABA content or GABA-transaminase in chick retina 15 (Figures 1, 2, 3), 30 and 60 min. after administration. Also, in chicks kept in the dark for 72 h, apomorphine (2 mg kg^{-1} intraperitoneally) was unable to change GAD activity or GABA content in the retina (Figures 4, 5).

Effects of neuroleptic drugs on GABA-ergic mechanisms in the chick retina

In order to determine whether dopamine exerts a tonic regulatory role on GAD activity we studied the effects of two neuroleptic agents, haloperidol which acts selectively on post-synaptic D$_1$ and D$_2$ receptors and l-sulpiride which is a weak antagonist at D$_1$ receptors

Figure 1. Effects of an *in vivo* treatment with apomorphine (APO, 2 mg kg^{-1} i.p.) and bromocriptine (BRO, 20 mg kg^{-1} i.p.) on retinal GAD activity 15 min later. In comparison to control animals (CON), no significant changes were detected in the two experimental groups. Each column is the mean ±S.E.M. of at least six experiments each in triplicate assay.

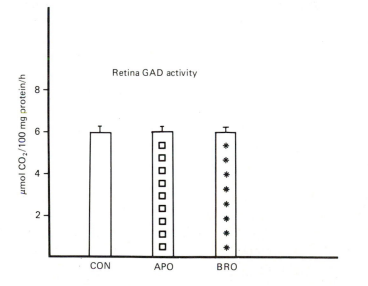

Figure 2. Effects of an *in vivo* treatment with apomorphine (APO, 2 mg kg⁻¹ i.p.) and bromocriptine (BRO, 20 mg kg⁻¹ i.p.) on retinal GABA content 15 min later. In comparison to control animals (CON), no significant changes were detected in the two experimental groups. Each column is the mean ± s.e.m. of at least six experiments each in triplicate assay.

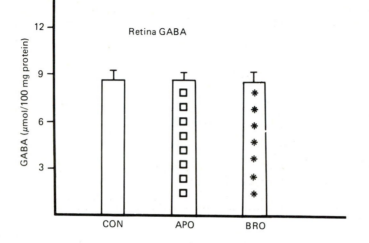

Figure 3. Effects of an *in vivo* treatment with apomorphine (APO, 2 mg kg⁻¹ i.p.) and bromocriptine (BRO, 20 mg kg⁻¹ i.p.) on retinal GABA-T activity 15 min later. In comparison to control animals (CON), no significant changes were detected in the two experimental groups. Each column is the mean ± s.e.m. of at least six experiments each in triplicate assay.

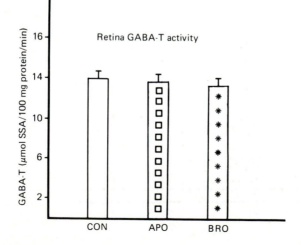

Figure 4. Effects of apomorphine (APO, $2\,mg\,kg^{-1}$ i.p.) on retina GAD activity in chicks kept in the dark for 72 h, 30 min after the administration. Each column represents mean values ± s.e.m. of at least six assays each in triplicate.

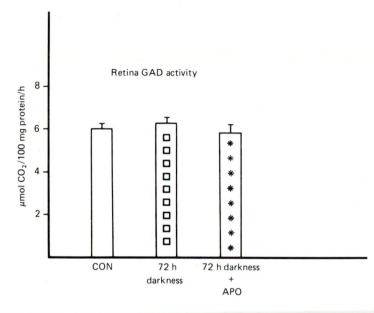

Figure 5. Effects of apomorphine (APO, $2\,mg\,kg^{-1}$ i.p.) on retinal GABA content in chicks kept in the dark for 72 h, 30 min after the administration. Each column represents mean values ± s.e.m. of at least six assays each in triplicate.

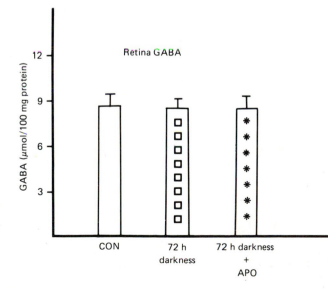

Figure 6. Effects of a systemic administration of l-sulpiride (SUL, 0.1 mg kg^{-1} i.p.) or haloperidol (HAL, 1 mg kg i.p.) on retinal GAD activity at 15 min after the administration; CON, control. Each column represents mean values ± s.e.m. of six to eight experiments, each in triplicate.

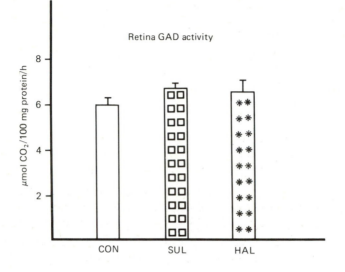

Figure 7. Effects of a systemic administration of l-sulpiride (SUL, 0.1 mg kg^{-1} i.p.) or haloperidol (HAL, 1 mg kg^{-1} i.p.) on retinal GABA content at 15 min after the administration. CON, control. Each column represents mean values ± s.e.m. of six to eight experiments, each in triplicate.

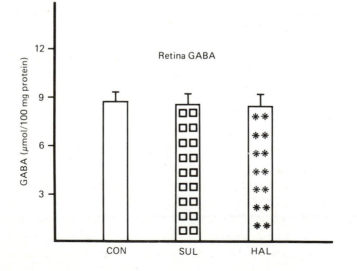

linked to adenylate cyclase (see Seeman, 1980). However neither drug was able to affect the GABA-ergic system in the chick retina (Figures 6, 7).

Conclusions

In previous studies it has been reported that a single dose of l-DOPA *in vivo* significantly decreases GABA content and GAD activity in rat retina (Macaione et al., 1973). However a longer treatment with l-DOPA affects the GABA-ergic system in the chick retina in a different way, i.e. GABA content increases as a consequence of GABA-T inhibition (Di Giorgio et al., 1979).

In the chick brain apomorphine given systemically or intraventricularly, at a dose level which produces behavioral and electrocortical arousal and stereotyped movements, is able to increase GABA synthesis by stimulating GAD activity in the paleostriatum augmentatum, an area homologous to the mammalian caudate nucleus (Nisticò et al., 1980, 1982). The increase in GAD activity is not due to an increase in GAD for PLP but to an increase in its V_{max} (Nisticò et al, 1982). The increase in GAD activity seems to be due to an increase in cAMP since GAD activity was also increased (Nisticò et al., 1980) after intraventricular administration of dibutyryl-cAMP.

The finding that apomorphine at various dose levels, acting presumably on dopamine pre- and post-synaptic receptors, was unable to affect GABA-ergic mechanisms in the chick retina demonstrates that although some anatomical connections may exist between the two types of neurons, no functional link between them is evident. Such a concept is also reinforced by the fact that after exposing the chicks to 72 h of darkness, i.e. in conditions in which presumably in chicks as in rats dopamine receptors linked to adenylate cyclase become supersensitive (Spano et al., 1977), administration of apomorphine did not lead to any change in retina GAD activity or GABA content.

The finding that neuroleptic drugs, acting as antagonists at post-synaptic D_1 and D_2 receptors, did not affect GABA-ergic mechanisms, excludes the possibility that, under physiological conditions, dopamine exerts a control on GAD activity. Also l-sulpiride, which is a poor antagonist at dopamine receptors linked to adenylate cyclase, was found ineffective in changing GAD activity or GABA content.

In conclusion, the present findings show that after different drug manipulations leading to a change in activity of dopamine receptors, GABA-ergic mechanisms in the chick retina were not affected and our results do not support the idea of a functional relation between dopaminergic and GABA-ergic neurons in chick retina.

Partial support from the Italian Council for Research (CNR) and Ministry of Public Education is gratefully acknowledged. Our thanks to Mrs Adriana Mastroeni for typing the manuscript.

References

Ames, A., and Pollen, D. A. (1969). Neurotransmission in central nervous tissue – a study of isolated rabbit retina. *J. Neurophysiol. 32:* 424–42.

Balcom, G. J., Lenox, R. N., and Meyerkoff, J. L. (1975). Regional γ-aminobutyric acid levels in rat brain determined after microwave fixation. *J. Neurochem. 24:* 609–13.

Beaven, M. A., Wilcox, G., and Terpestra, G. K. (1978). A microprocedure for the measurement of ^{14}C or release from ^{14}C carboxyl-labeled aminoacids. *Analyt. Biochem. 84:* 638–41.

Brown, J. H., and Makman, M. H. (1972). Stimulation by dopamine of adenylate cyclase in retinal homogenates and of adenosine-3′,5′-cyclic monophosphate formation in intact retina. *Proc. Natn. Acad. Sci. USA 69:* 539–43.

Brown, J. H., and Makman, M. H. (1973). Influence of neuroleptic drugs and apomorphine on dopamine-sensitive adenylate cyclase of retina. *J. Neurochem. 21:* 477–9.

Da Prada, M. (1977). Dopamine content and synthesis in retina and n. accumbens septi: pharmacological and light-induced modifications. *Adv. Bioch. Psychopharmac. 16:* 311–19.

Di Giorgio, R. M., Macaione, S., Lanotte, M., and Nisticò, G. (1979). Effects of l-DOPA on GABA metabolism in chick brain and retina. *Neuropharmacology 18:* 771–81.

Dowling, J. E. (1970). Organisation of vertebrate retinas. *Invest. Ophthalmol. 9:* 655–80.

Dowling, J. E. (1978). The interplexiform cell system. I. Synapses of the dopamine neurons of the goldfish retina. *Proc. Roy. Soc. B201:* 7–26.

Ehinger, B. (1967). Adrenergic nerves in the avian eye and ciliary ganglion. *Z. Zellforsch. mikrosk. Anat. 82:* 577–88.

Ehinger, B. (1977). Synaptic connections of the dopaminergic retinal neurons. *Adv. Biochem. Psychopharmac. 16:* 299–306.

Fahn, S. (1976). Regional distribution studies of GABA and other putative neurotransmitters and their enzymes. In *GABA in Nervous System Function*, ed. E. Roberts, T. N. Chase and D. B. Tower, pp. 169–86. New York: Raven Press.

Florén, I. (1979). Indoleamine accumulating neurons in the retina of chicken and pigeon. A comparison with the dopaminergic neurons. *Acta Ophthalmol. 57:* 198–210.

Graham, G. J., and Aprison, M. H. (1966). Fluorimetric determination of aspartate, glutamate and GABA in nerve tissue using enzymatic methods. *Analyt. Biochem. 15:* 487–97.

Hornykiewicz, O., Lloyd, K. G., and Davidson, L. (1976). The GABA system, function of the basal ganglia and Parkinson's disease. In *GABA in Nervous System Function*, ed. E. Roberts, T. N. Chase and D. B. Tower, pp. 479–85. New York: Raven Press.

Kramer, S. G. (1971). Dopamine: a retina neurotransmitter. I. Retinal uptake, storage and light-stimulated release of (^{3}H)-dopamine *in vivo. Invest. Ophthalmol. 10:* 438–52.

Lowry, O. H., Rosebrough, N. J., Farr, A. L., and Randall, R. J. (1951). Protein measurement with the Folin phenol reagent. *J. Biol. Chem. 193:* 265–75.

Macaione, S. (1972). Localization of GABA system in rat retina. *J. Neurochem. 19:* 1397–1400.

Macaione, S., Di Giorgio, R. M., and Ruggeri, P. (1973). Azione in vivo della l-DOPA sul contenuto in GABA e sull'attività glutammicodecarbossilasica (GAD) della retina di ratto. *Boll. Soc. Ital. Biol. Sper. 49:* 903–7.

Magistretti, P. (1979). Ph.D. Thesis n. 3765: Etude de la liaison spécifique du ^{3}H-spiropéridol dans la fraction membranaire de la rétine de mammifère: son intérêt pour l'évaluation de l'affinité dopaminergique des substances psychotropes. Genève.

Nakamura, Y., McGuire, B. A., and Starling, P. (1980). Interplexiform cell in cat retina: identification by uptake of γ-[H^3]-aminobutyric acid and serial reconstruction. *Proc. Natn. Acad. Sci. USA 77:* 658–61.

Neal, M. J. (1976). Amino acid transmitter substances in the vertebrate retina. *Gen. Pharmac. 7:* 321–32.

Nisticò, G., Ientile, R., Lanotte, M., and Di Giorgio, R. M. (1980). Evidence to suggest that dopamine-induced increase in GABA concentrations in chick brain is mediated through cyclic AMP. *J. Pharm. Pharmac. 32:* 663–4.

Nisticò, G., Rotiroti, D., Faraone, V., De Sarro, G. B., and Ientile, R. (1982). Effects of apomorphine on glutamate decarboxylase activity in chick paleostriatum augmentatum. *Neuropharmacology 21:* 847–50.

Schorderet, M. (1977). Pharmacological characterization of the dopamine mediated accumulation of cyclic AMP in intact retina of rabbit. *Life Sci. 20.:* 1741–8.

Seeman, P. (1980).Brain dopamine receptors. *Pharmac. Rev. 32:* 229–313.

Spano, P. F., Govoni, S., Hofmann, M., Kumakura, K., and Trabucchi, M. (1977). Physiological and pharmacological influences on dopaminergic receptors in the retina. In *Adv. Biochem. Psychopharmac. 16:* 307–10.

Stoeckel, M. E., Roussel, G., Zwiller, J., Medarasz, B., and Porte, A. (1976). Concentration of dopaminergic fibers in the marginal zone of the bird retina. A nonvisual photoreceptor system? *Cell Tiss. Res. 173:* 335–41.

Watling, K. J., Dowling, J. E., and Iversen, L. L. (1979). Dopamine receptors in the retina may all be linked to adenylate cyclase. *Nature 281:* 578–80.

Watling, K. J., and Dowling, J. E. (1981). Dopamine-sensitive adenylate cyclase in homogenates of carp retina; effects of agonists, antagonists and ergots. *J. Neurochem. 36:* 559–68.

4
Magnetic and electric fields

4.1

Neuroethological basis for electrocommunication

THOMAS SZABO and PETER MOLLER

Electric fish and electrocommunication

The African mormyriform fishes comprising the Mormyridae and the monospecific *Gymnarchus niloticus*, as well as the South American gymnotoid knifefish possess the ability to generate and perceive weak electric organ discharges (EODs). The EODs are produced by specialized electric organs whose embryonic origin is in most cases myogenic (Bennett, 1971a; Baillet-Derbin, 1978). The electroreceptors are related to the lateral line organs and are of two types, the ampullary and tuberous organs (Szabo, 1965; Bennett, 1971b).

A comprehensive understanding of electroperception necessitates a two-level approach, evaluating both the overt behavioral phenomena and the underlying anatomical and physiological substrates. At first, Lissmann's (1951, 1958) discovery of this new, electric sense, suggesting a role in object (electro) location and social (electro) communication, inspired a host of neurophysiological and neuroanatomical studies, all focusing in great detail on electroreceptors and the fate of electroreceptive input (see reviews by Fessard and Szabo, 1974; Bell, 1979; Bullock, 1982). In the early 1970s, a number of ethologists became fascinated with the electric sense and have been hooked ever since (see reviews by Scheich and Bullock, 1974; Hopkins, 1977, 1980; Moller, 1980a,b; Westby, 1981; and literature cited therein). While neurobiologists, neurophysiologists and ethologists worked independently for a while, we have seen in recent years a fruitful combination of the three disciplines in a neuroethology of perception, addressing questions about the underlying sensory processes and pathways, stimulus filtering, selection and integration, as well as adaptive function and evolutionary history (Hopkins, 1976, 1981; Hopkins and Bass, 1981; Heiligenberg, 1977; Moller and Szabo, 1981; Bullock, Northcutt and Bodznick, 1982).

Social communication requires some form of information transfer between sender and receiver organisms. The information may be extremely stable and long-lived, such as identity information about species membership, development stage and sex, or less stable and short-lived, such as motivational information about reproductive readiness, threat or submission.

Description and analytical studies on social communication in weak electric fish, carried out both in the field and laboratory, have clearly established that the EODs can or could transmit both types of information. The single EOD (in pulse type species, including all mormyrids and some gymnotoids) and the EOD frequency bands (in wave type species, mostly gymnotoids and *G. niloticus*) are species-typical (Hopkins, 1974, 1980; Moller, 1980a,b; Kramer, Tautz and Markl, 1981) and in some species show even age-class related differences and sexual dimorphism (Hopkins, 1974, 1980; Luecker and Kramer, 1981; Hopkins and Bass, 1981; Westby and Kirschbaum, 1982).

The undisturbed EOD activity (resting pattern) is individual-specific in *G. petersii* and *B. niger* (Malcolm in Moller, 1980a). Characteristic changes of this discharge activity are caused by a variety of energy forms, including light (reviewed in Moller, Serrier, Belbenoit and Push, 1979; Teyssèdre and Moller, 1982), sound (Kramer et al., 1981), chemical (Jager, 1974), thermal (Toerring and Serrier, 1978) and electromagnetic energy (see reviews by Scheich and Bullock, 1974; Kalmijn, 1974).

The student of animal communication is for obvious reasons most interested in the electric modality, and specifically in intra- and interspecific EOD interactions and their associations with overt behavioral displays. There exists now a comprehensive catalogue of these associations between electric and non-electric overt behaviors, and in many cases, the information content of the EODs has been extracted in carefully designed playback experiments. Most of the laboratory work has been focused on non-reproductive, competitive interactions (Black-Cleworth, 1970; Westby, 1974, 1975a,b; Bauer, 1972, 1974; Bauer and Kramer, 1973, 1974; Bell, Myers and Russell, 1974; Russell, Myers and Bell, 1974; Kramer, 1974, 1976a,b, 1979; Crockett, 1982) and some of the field studies have also investigated the role of EODs as courtship signals (Hopkins, 1974, 1980; Hopkins and Bass, 1981).

The biologically effective range of electrocommunication depends on species characteristics and the ionic content of the aquatic environment.

Under conditions of low conductivity, typical of the fishes' blackwater habitats, such range does extend to about one meter for *G. petersii* and *B. niger* (Moller and Szabo, 1981; Squire and Moller, 1982). While other sensory modalities may play supportive roles in the fishes' social behavior (Moller, Serrier, Squire and Boudinot, 1982) the electric modality remains the most efficient one.

The higher-order neural processing and integration of electroreceptive input has been studied in physiological, restrained preparations (Zipser and Bennett, 1976a,b; Russell and Bell, 1978; Bell, 1979; Szabo, Enger and Libouban, 1979). Recently, we have contributed to the neuroethology of electroperception by testing the EOD behavior in fish with their electrosensory pathways/relays selectively impaired (Moller and Szabo, 1981).

Electroreceptors and neural pathways

We distinguish two categories of electroreceptors: (i) the mormyromasts and ampullary receptors; and (ii) the tuberous Knollenorgans. The function of the receptors in these two categories is quite different. In the first, the receptors are essentially intensity coders and provide grade information about the variations of the fish's own electric field, caused by nearby objects or d.c. fields. In the second, the receptors are dubbed pulse-markers which give off a single afferent impulse for each exogenous electric pulse, for example in response to a conspecific EOD. The pulse marker also furnishes an afferent impulse for each of the fish's own EODs, but these afferent impulses are cancelled at the rhombencephalic input, so that the foreign signal remains undisturbed on its arrival at higher encephalic levels.

An important difference between the two categories of electroreceptors is their threshold. The pulse-marker threshold is about 100 times lower than that of the intensity coder (Figure 1), which means that an exogenous signal (of the same intensity and amplitude) can excite the pulse-marker receptors from a much greater distance than can the intensity coders. Tuberous pulse markers are therefore much more likely candidates for mediation of electrocommunication than are intensity coders.

The two receptor categories are connected to different central nervous pathways (Figure 2):

(1) The peripheral afferent fibers of the intensity coders, which represent the major part of the electroreceptive fibers, project to the cortex of the posterior lateral line lobe in the rhombencephalon. The output, represented by the ganglion cell axons of the latter, courses in

the lateral lemniscus and projects bilaterally to the mesencephalic lateral nucleus.

(2) The peripheral afferent fibers of pulse-marker receptors project to the nucleus of the posterior lateral line lobe; in return, this nucleus sends its axons via the lateral lemniscus, to the anterior mesencephalic extrolateral nucleus.

Although the coursing of the two systems is very much parallel up to this level, the information processing in them is quite different. The information channelled by the intensity-coding system is first integrated at the rhombencephalic, and then, a second time, at the mesencephalic level. The information in the pulse-marker system is only relayed at these two levels and the input signal is encountered at the extrolateral nucleus in a 1:1 relationship.

From the mesencephalon on, the two electrosensory pathways diverge. The intensity-coder system projects from the mesencephalic lateral nucleus directly to the cerebellum to the median leaf of the valvula (Figure 2). The pulse-marker system, on the contrary, is somewhat more complex: it is relayed several times before arriving at the cerebellum (Figure 3a, b). The anterior extrolateral nucleus develops two parallel pathways to the cerebellum via the posterior mesencephalic extrolateral nucleus (Haugedé-Carré, 1979): one of them projects via the medio-ventral mesencephalic nucleus, the other via the mesencephalic ganglion isthmi to the lateral leaf of the valvula (Figure 3b). We may consider the valvula as the terminal of the electrosensory pathway.

Figure 1. Threshold curves for the three types of electroreceptors in the mormyrid fish *Gnathonemus* sp.: tuberous knollenorgan (filled circle), ampullary organ (circle) and mormyromast (triangle). Note the marked threshold difference between the pulse-marker tuberous receptor and the intensity-coder mormyromast. Abscissa, relative stimulus intensity; ordinate, number of sensory impulses.

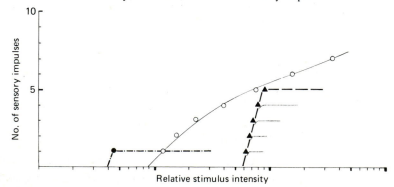

Figure 2. Schematic drawing of the pulse-marker (solid line) and the intensity-coder (dashed line) systems. The pulse-marker system originates from the knollenorgan receptors (Kn); relayed in the lateral line lobe nucleus (nLLL) it projects to the mesencephalic extro-lateral nucleus (n. extro-lat.). The intensity-coder system originates from the ampullary receptors (Amp) and the mormyromasts. The peripheral impulses are integrated in the posterior lateral line lobe (lat. line lobe) and conveyed in the lateral lemniscus path toward the mesencephalic lateral nucleus (n. lat.) from where the sensory information is conducted to the median leaflet of the valvula into two distinct regions (Amp, Mo). NLL, lateral line nerve; lat. lem. commissure, lateral lemniscal commissure. (Szabo et al., 1979.)

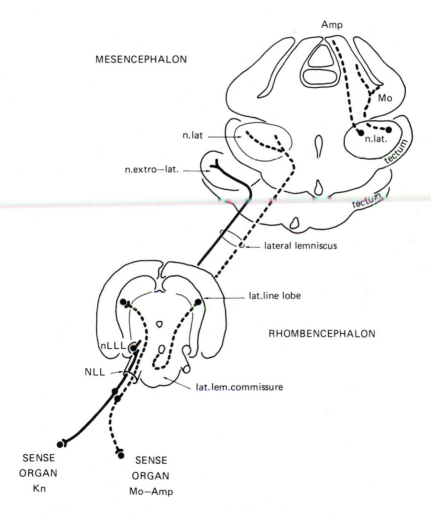

The most important neural elements of the valvula, the so-called basal cells, which, according to Nieuwenhuys, Pouwels and Smulders-Kersten (1974) receive the afferent input of a large number of Purkinje cells, project back again to the basal region of the posterior mesencephalic brainstem (Szabo, personal observation). However, this region is rather distant from the medullary brainstem region, where the medullary center which commands the fish's electric discharge (Szabo, Enger, unpublished observations) is located. On the other hand, recent investigations (Bell, Libouban and Szabo, 1982) have shown that the

Figure 3a. Schematic drawing of the efferent connections of the posterior mesencephalic extrolateral nucleus (gray area, nELp) in a mormyrid fish (*Brienomyrus niger*) represented in serial transverse sections. Solid black line indicates the nELp projections to the medioventral nucleus (nMV) and to the ganglion isthmi (GI). Both projections are ipsi and contralateral; the contralateral contingent of this pathway courses within the post chiasmatic commissure (co.p.ch.). Fine dashed line indicates the connection between anterior (nELa) and posterior (nELp) mesencephalic extrolateral nuclei. Cc, corpus cerebelli; ll, lemniscus lateralis; nELa, nucleus extrolateralis anterior; nL, nucleus lateralis mesencephali; nP, nucleus preeminentialis; nSP, nucleus sub-preeminentialis; nVP, nucleus ventralis posterior; tect., optic tectum; TM, tectum Marklager; v, ventricle; valv., valvula; A–P arrow indicates antero-posterior axis. (From Haugedé-Carré, 1979.)

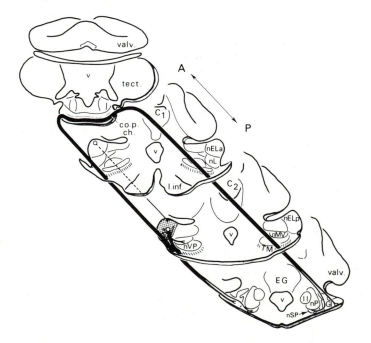

medullary command is connected to several specific brainstem structures, the activity of which is closely associated with that of the electric-organ discharge. This may suggest that the valvular projection influences the EOD command activity via one of these specific brainstem structures, though the link between the valvular projection area and the command system is not yet established.

Once these pathways are established we could determine the level of a lesion within the electrosensory system to test its role in mediating foreign EODs in electrocommunication.

Behavioral studies

In the following experiment we used pairs of mormyrid fish, *Gnathonemus petersii* (10–12 cm standard length).

The experimental cement tank measured 400×70 cm. The water level was maintained at 28 cm, water temperature at 26°C and water conductivity at 141 μS cm^{-1}. Between experiments the fish were kept individually in 30-l tanks under a light–dark regimen of 12:12 and fed once a week with tubifex worms.

Figure 3b. Schematic drawing of the mesencephalo-valvula projection of the pulse-marker system. Both projections appear to be at this level ipsilateral, GI, ganglion isthmi; nMV, medio ventral nucleus; nPe, nucleus preeminentialis; Kn, pulse-marker projection area in the lateral leaflet of the valvula.

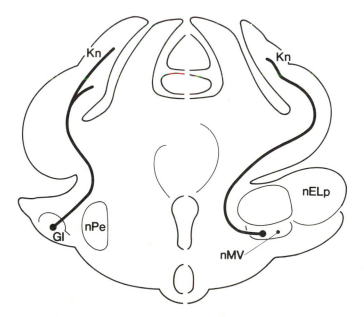

The experimental device consisted of a track running the length of the tank 25 cm above the water surface. Two porous ceramic tubes (15 × 5 cm) were suspended on the two ends of the track by means of a wheeled carriage. A motor-driven system allowed movement of one of the carriage/tube assemblies back and forth along the track at a speed of 2 cm s⁻¹, while the other tube remained stationary.

During the experiment one fish was confined to each tube, blind ended at one extremity, excluding visual and mechanical interactions. The EODs of both fish were monitored with a pair of carbon electrodes fixed to the ends of each tube, differentially amplified and recorded on tape.

After an equilibration period of five minutes, one fish, within its shelter tube, was moved towards the other fish until the tubes faced each other; then the fish which had been moved was returned to its original position. During such an approach, different kinds of EOD interactions can be observed. We will consider here only a temporary cessation in either fish's EOD activity. Figure 4 gives an example of EOD inter-action between two *G. petersii* as a function of interfish distance

Figure 4. Electric organ discharge activities of *Gnathonemus petersii* A (dashed line) and B (solid line) at a distance of 34 cm, final 45 s recording time (control); and at 24 cm, 45 s recording time (experiment). Graphs show number of fish impulses (EOD) per successive 400-ms time period (ordinate) illustrating both fish discharge rates at corresponding and comparable time intervals. Black horizontal triangle indicates time during which fish A was moved toward fish B (6 s). Note long duration discharge cessation of fish A (hollow arrow) concommittant with discharge rate increase (black arrow) of fish B. (From Moller and Bauer, 1973.)

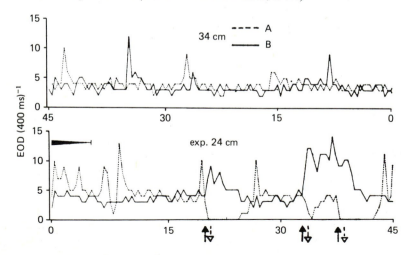

(Moller and Bauer, 1973). At an interfish distance of 34 cm, frequency increases in either fish show neither excitatory nor inhibitory effects upon the other's EOD rate. However, when the interfish distance was changed to 24 cm, the moved fish (A) ceased discharging.

In the present study, we monitored the interfish distance at which either fish ceased discharging for at least 500 ms and that at which it subsequently resumed its EOD activity. The periods of EOD cessation were determined from the differences between the cessation and the resumption distances and expressed in distances (cm) and time measures. EOD cessation began to occur at an interfish distance of about 70 cm and 9% of all cessations occurred within 50 cm.

The electric display 'discharge cessation' was studied in animals in which the tuberous, pulse-marker system was lesioned at the limit of the n. mes. ext. lat. anterior and posterior which is the projection area of the second-order neurons within the pulse-marker electrosensory system. Figure 5 shows a schematic representation of the histological control. The lesion does not appear very large but it interrupts the connection between the two nuclei. Figure 6 illustrates how the second-order neurons of this pathway which receives strictly ipsilateral input from the periphery project bilaterally to the mesencephalic nuclei.

Figure 5. Lesions in the mesencephalic extrolateral nucleus.
(A) Schematic drawing of serial histological transverse sections through the mesencephalic extrolateral nucleus (nELa and p) showing the depth of the lesion (hatched area). nELa and nELp, anterior and posterior mesencephalic extrolateral nucleus. (B) Dorsal view of the surface of the nELa and p indicating the antero-posterior extension of the lesion (hatched area). The lesions were restricted to the nELa and p and never extended to the other neighboring mesencephalic nuclei, nucleus lateralis and nucleus medio dorsalis. Scale bar, 0.5 cm. (From Moller and Szabo, 1981, modified.)

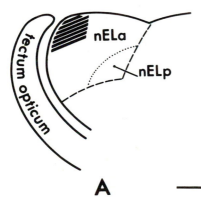
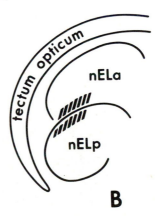

Therefore, the same lesion was carried out on both sides. Experiments were started four weeks after the second operation. The occurrence of EOD cessation was investigated in both moved and stationary fish. The following dyadic interactions were tested: (1) operated fish moved towards intact fish; (2) intact towards operated; (3) operated towards operated animals; and as controls (a) intact fish moved towards intact

Figure 6. Schematic drawing of the bilateral rhombo-mesencephalic projections within the pulse-marker system. The projection contains a majority of crossed fibers. nLLL, lateral line lobe nucleus; NLLa and p, anterior and posterior lateral line nerve; n. mes. ext. lat. ant., anterior mesencephalic extrolateral nucleus; torus sem., torus semicircularis; t. opt., optic tectum; lob. caud., lobus caudalis; lob. lat., posterior lateral line lobe.

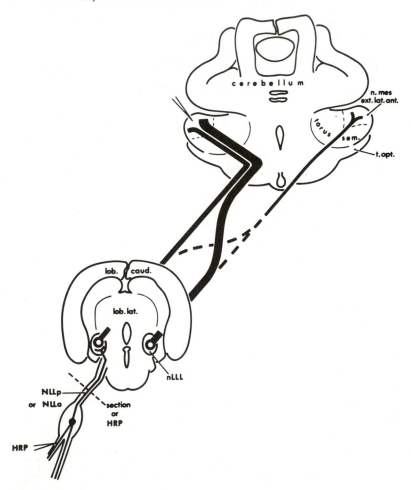

fish; (b) the empty tube towards intact fish or operated fish; and (c) vice versa, intact or operated animals towards the empty tube.

The 190 trials of this group of fish clearly established the effects of the lesion (Figure 7). Intact animals ceased discharging in 74%, while lesioned fish ceased in only 9% of the trials. When occurrence and duration of EOD stops were considered, the difference between intact and lesioned fish was even more pronounced: intact fish stopped in 93% of trials and were 'silent' for 97% of the total time, while lesioned fish, under the same conditions, stopped in only 7% of the trials and were 'silent' for 2.5% of the total time. The control trials, with an intact fish moved towards an intact conspecific, show that EOD cessations occurred in both the moved and stationary fish. The other controls indicate that EOD cessation was a social response and not due to tube movement. When the empty tube was moved toward an intact fish, EOD cessation occurred in only a few interactions.

Our results have established that EOD cessation in intraspecific dyadic interactions is almost exclusively found in the intact fish. This EOD response is abolished when the specific electrosensory pathway is bilaterally interrupted at the mesencephalic extro-lateral nucleus.

To trace the fate of EOD cessation to the next cerebellar relay, as neuroanatomical studies would suggest, we inflicted lesions at the surgically accessible higher level.

Russell and Bell (1978) showed that the pathway of pulse-marker receptors projects to a well defined, restricted area in the cerebellum, into the outer leaf of the valvula. This mesencephalic cerebellar projection involves a double – two neuronal – pathway. Figure 8 shows a schematic dorsal view of the mormyrid cerebellum. The valvula covers the brain dorsally. The projection areas of both electrosensory pathways are as follows: the pulse-marker system (Kn) is located somewhat laterally while the ampullary intensity-coder system (Amp) lies close to the midline. Lesions were made in either area by sucking away the valvular cortex. Animals lesioned in the intensity-coder area served as controls. Figure 8 also shows the extension of the actual bilateral lesions in both cases.

According to Russell and Bell (1978), both projection areas involve one distinct leaflet. The histological inspection revealed the extension of the lesion. Figure 9 shows that the corresponding valvular area was removed, the outer leaflet in one case and the top of the medium leaflet in the control animal.

Using the same experimental paradigm as described below, we investigated EOD cessation in fish with their cerebellar pulse-marker

Figure 7. Occurrence of electric organ discharge cessations in the mormyrid fish *Gnathonemus petersii*: with bilateral lesion in the mesencephalic extrolateral nucleus (above) and in the valvular cerebellum (below). In interaction trials (first four pairs of columns) an intact (I) or an operated (O) fish was moved toward (→) an intact or operated conspecific. In control trials (last four columns, above) an empty shelter tube (e) was moved toward an intact or operated fish, or vice versa, the fish was moved toward the empty shelter. In control trials (last two pairs of columns, below) fish which had been sham-operated (SHA) or lesioned in the ampullary region (OA) were used. Numbers on tops of columns indicate number of trials. Note the comparable effects in fish with lesion in the mesencephalic extrolateral nucleus and in the valvula cerebellum.

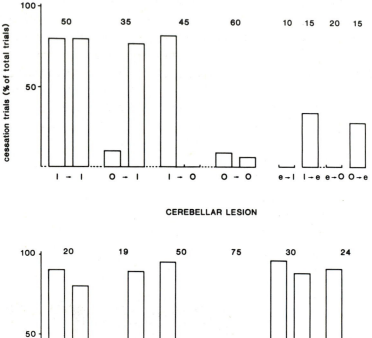

area removed. The following pairings were tested: (1) pulse-marker operated fish moved toward intact fish; (2) intact fish toward pulse-marker operated fish; and (3) pulse-marker operated fish toward each other. Control interactions included: (a) intact fish moved toward intact fish; (b) sham-operated toward sham-operated; and (c) 'intensity-coder' operated against each other. Again the lesioned fish showed a pronounced effect. In 208 trials, intact fish ceased discharging in 88% of the trials, while pulse-marker operated fish ceased discharging in only 18% (Figure 7). This lack of responsiveness to conspecific EODs was evident for operated fish, regardless of whether they were moved or stationary.

The control trials with intact fish moved toward intact fish, showed again that EOD cessation occurred in both (moved and stationary) fish. Results obtained with sham-operated fish being moved toward each other were not distinguishable from those obtained with intact fish. In the other controls, we found that fish operated in the ampullary region also ceased discharging with a somewhat smaller percentage recorded for the stationary animal. The results obtained in fish with mesencephalic lesions are comparable to those obtained in animals with pulse-marker cerebellar lesions (Figure 7). Our data indicate that both mesencephalic and cerebellar lesions effected similar deficits in the fish's exhibiting EOD cessation.

Figure 8. Left: Dorsal view of the mormyrid cerebellum showing schematically the valvular projection area of the pulse-marker system (Kn) and that of the ampullary contingent (Amp) of the intensity-coding system. (From Russell and Bell, 1978.) Photographs: Dorsal views of the brains of two experimental fish with bilateral lesion in the Kn (middle) and in the Amp (right) valvular cortex areas. × 3.5 approx.

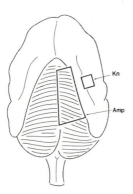
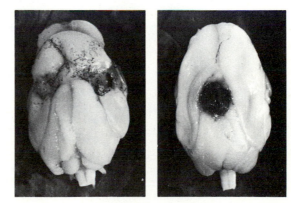

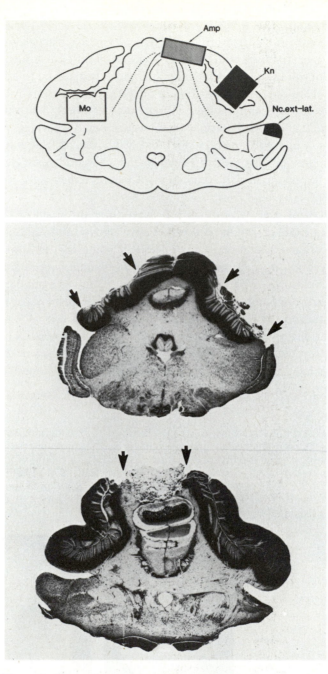

Figure 9. Above: Schematic representation of a frontal section through the midbrain of the mormyrid fish *Gnathonemus* sp. showing the valvular projection area of the three types of electroreceptors: Median leaflet for the ampullary organs (Amp) and mormyromasts (Mo) and

Discussion

We can assume that EOD cessation, as a form of social behavior, is mediated by the fish's tuberous electroreceptors, the low-threshold Knollenorgans and the associated electrosensory pathway which may serve in electrocommunication. Our lesions interrupted this pathway either in the mesencephalic extrolateral nucleus or at the valvular cortex of the cerebellum. In both instances the fish were electrically 'blind' and failed to respond appropriately to conspecific EODs.

An interesting observation emerges from these findings. Sensory information elicited by conspecific signal is relayed and integrated several times along the electrosensory pathway before it reaches the cerebellar cortical level, from which it effects a change in the pacemaker system in the form of EOD cessation, as in the present case. In other words, the sensory integration which occurs at different mesencephalic levels is not sufficient to elicit this response which evidently depends on the integrity of the specific cerebellar area which was investigated. It is important to realize that the neural mechanism which controls EOD cessation remains intact. The removal of the cerebellar cortical area does not abolish the fish's ability to stop discharging altogether; it abolishes responsiveness under conditions of social communication. Under different experimental conditions, the fish can still break his EOD activity (Moller, in preparation). Thus, it seems that the lesion in the specific mesencephalic or cerebellar areas only removed the input to an EOD-inhibitory center.

Fish with either type of lesion, at the ext. lat. as at the cerebellum, can still exhibit other EOD responses. The 'echo response' or 'preferred latency response' (Russell and Bell, 1978; Bauer and Kramer, 1974) which consists of short latency (10–12 ms) EODs to exogenous stimuli, can be obtained with a single artificial stimulus (Serrier, 1982) and in social encounters in response to conspecific EODs (Kramer, personal communication).

While each lesion impairs the fish's electrocommunication channel, its electrolocation capabilities are not affected: operated fish still respond

---

Caption for Fig. 9 (*cont.*)
lateral leaflet for the Knollenorgans (Kn). Lesions are indicated by gray and solid-black rectangles. Lesion (solid black) in the mesencephalic extrolateral nucleus (Nc.ext.-lat.) is also indicated. (Slightly modified after Russell and Bell, 1978.) Photographs: histological sections of the two brains shown in Figure 8; the lesion (between arrows) involves in one case the lateral valvula leaflet (upper) and the other, top of the median leaflet (below). × 8.

with an EOD rate change (novelty response) to impedance changes produced by means of a short circuit of two external electrodes. Also, fish lesioned in the mesencephalic extrolateral nucleus still exhibit stereotyped electrolocating motor behavior and associated EOD patterns in the presence of conductive and insulating objects (Toerring, 1979), and when restrained, produce the novelty response to moving objects (Moller et al., in preparation). This was to be expected since both operations left intact the second electrosensory channel through which the fish monitors changes in his own electric field.

EOD cessation in intraspecific encounters begins to occur well outside the fish's electrolocation range which extends to about 10 cm from the fish (Toerring and Belbenoit, 1979; Push and Moller, 1979) and is severely impaired by one of two central lesions, in the n. mes. extrolateralis or the valvula cerebelli: i.e., in areas that in neuroanatomical studies were clearly implicated to be part of the fish's fast-electrocommunication pathway. From this we concluded that EOD cessation, as a social response, is mediated through this electrocommunication channel.

The question arises as to how specific this response is. Do the interacting fish recognize each other as members of the same species or

Figure 10. Examples of interspecific EOD interactions between *Mormyrops deliciosus* and *Mormyrops zanclirostris*. Note 'long discharge cessation' of *M. deliciosus* (short duration EOD, thin spikes) occurring twice in response to high-frequency bursts (arrows) of *M. zanclirostris*. (From Szabo in Lissmann, 1961.)

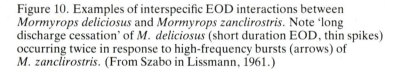

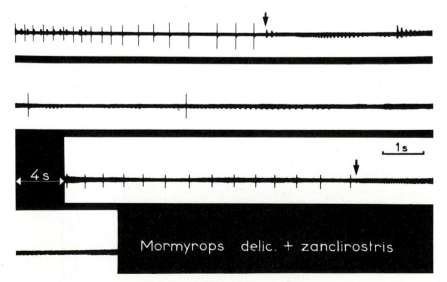

is EOD cessation a universal mormyrid-specific electric display? We have elucidated earlier the evidence for EODs serving in species recognition. Neuroethological studies (Hopkins and Bass, 1981) have shown that males of *Brienomyrus brachyistius* t.p. (an Ivindo River mormyrid) respond to phase-spectral cues of the female's EOD. The fact that sympatric species could not elicit the specific courtship 'rasp' in the *B. brachyistius* t.p. male points to a species recognition or discrimination mechanism possibly associated with the electrocommunication pathway (Hopkins and Bass, 1981).

EOD cessation is typical not only for electric interactions between two *G. petersii*, but has also been established in *Brienomyrus niger* (Squire and Moller, 1982) as well as in *Brienomyrus brachyistius* and *Marcusenius cyprinoides* (Moller, in preparation). We have also observed the cessation response in dyadic interactions between mixed species, including *G. petersii*, *M. cyprinoides* and *B. niger* (Moller, in preparation). One of the first recorded EOD interactions (between *Mormyrops zanclirostris* and *Mormyrops deliciosus*) clearly shows interspecific EOD cessation (Figure 10). Here, the phase-spectral cues of the interacting fish's EODs are quite different. Thus, we conclude that while electric displays associated with courtship necessitate unambiguous species recognition, EOD cessation, as a social 'hiding response', may serve a broader, interspecific, adaptive function. Future studies on EOD displays associated with other adapted behaviors will test the biologically effective specificity of mormyrid electric signals.

This investigation was supported by the Fondation pour la Recherche Médicale Française. The behavioral studies were supported in part by a CUNY Research Award: PSC-BHE-12225 and the Animal Behavior – Biopsychology Program (NIMH Training grant: MH 15341). We also express our thanks to the Department of Ichthyology, AMNH and Dr C. L. Smith for generous logistic support and D. Rouilly for the histological preparations.

References

Baillet-Derbin, C. (1978). Cytodifferentiation of the regenerating electrocyte in an electric fish. *Biol. Cell. 33:* 15–24.

Bauer, R. (1972). High electrical discharge frequency during aggressive behaviour in a mormyrid fish, *Gnathonemus petersii. Experientia 28:* 669.

Bauer, R. (1974). Electric organ discharge activity of resting and stimulated *Gnathonemus petersii* (Mormyridae). *Behaviour 50:* 306–23.

Bauer, R., and Kramer, B. (1973). Relation entre le comportement agressif du mormyridé *Gnathonemus petersii* et sa décharge électrique. *J. Physiol., Paris 67(2):* 240–1a.

Bauer, R., and Kramer, B. (1974). Agonistic behaviour in mormyrid fish: latency-relationship between the electric discharges of *Gnathonemus petersii* and *Mormyrus rume. Experientia 30:* 51–2.

Bell, C. C. (1979). Central nervous system physiology of electroreception, a review. *J. Physiol., Paris 75:* 361–79.

Bell, C. C., Libouban, S., and Szabo, T. (1982). Central pathways of the electric organ discharge command in mormyrid fish. *Abstr. Soc. Neurosci. 30:* 641–50.

Bell, C. C., Myers, J. P., and Russell, C. J. (1974). Electric organ discharge patterns during dominance related behavioral displays in *Gnathonemus petersii* (Mormyridae). *J. Comp. Physiol. 92:* 201–28.

Bennett, M. V. L. (1971a). Electric organs. In *Fish Physiology*, vol. V, ed. W. S. Hoar and D. J. Randall, pp. 347–491. New York and London: Academic Press.

Bennett, M. V. L. (1971b). Electroreception. In *Fish Physiology*, vol. V, ed. W. S. Hoar and D. J. Randall, pp. 493–574. New York: Academic Press.

Black-Cleworth, P. (1970). The role of electrical discharges in the non-reproductive social behavior of *Gymnotus carapo* (Gymnotidae, Pisces). *Animal Behav. Monogr. 3:* 3–77.

Bullock, T. H. (1982). Electroreception. *A. Rev. Neurosci. 5:* 121–70.

Bullock, T. H., Northcutt, R. G., and Bodznick, D. A. (1982). Evolution of electroreception. *Trends Neurosci.* 50–3.

Crockett, D. P. (1982). The role of the electric organ discharge in facilitating social interactions of mormyrid fish. Ph.D. Thesis, City University of New York.

Fessard, A., and Szabo, T. (1974). Physiology of electroreceptors. In *Handbook of Sensory Physiology*, vol. III/3, ed. A. Fessard, pp. 59–124. Berlin, Heidelberg, New York: Springer-Verlag.

Haugedé-Carré, F. (1979). The mesencephalic extrolateral posterior nucleus of the mormyrid fish *Brienomyrus niger*: efferent connections studied by the HRP method. *Brain Res. 178:* 179–84.

Heiligenberg, W. (1977). Principles of electrolocation and jamming avoidance in electric fish. A neuroethological approach. In *Studies of Brain Function*, vol. 1, ed. V. Braitenberg, pp. 1–85. Berlin, Heidelberg, New York: Springer-Verlag.

Hopkins, C. D. (1974). Electric communication in fish. *Am. Scient. 6:* 426–37.

Hopkins, C. D. (1976). Stimulus filtering and electroreception: tuberous electroreceptors in three species of gymnotoid fish. *J. Comp. Physiol., 111:* 171–207.

Hopkins, C. D. (1977). Electric communication. In *How Animals Communicate,* ed. T. A. Sebeok, pp. 263–89. Indiana University Press.

Hopkins, C. D. (1980). Evolution of electric communication channels of mormyrids. *Behav. Ecol. Sociobiol. 7:* 1–13.

Hopkins, C. D. (1981). The neuroethology of electric communication. *Trends Neurosci. 4:* 4–6.

Hopkins, C. D., and Bass, A. H. (1981). Temporal coding of species recognition signals in an electric fish. *Science 212:* 85–7.

Jäger, U. (1974). Geruchsrezeption und Entladungsaktivität bei dem schwachelektrischen Fisch *Gnathonemus petersii* (Gthr. 1862) (Mormyridae, Teleostei). Thesis, Saarbrücken.

Kalmijn, Ad. J. (1974). The detection of electric fields from inanimate and animate sources other than electric organs. In *Handbook of Sensory Physiology*, vol. III/3, ed. A. Fessard, pp. 147–200. Berlin, Heidelberg, New York: Springer-Verlag.

Kramer, B. (1974). Electric organ discharge interaction during interspecific agonistic behaviour in freely swimming mormyrid fish. A method to evaluate two (or more) simultaneous time series of events with a digital analyser. *J. Comp. Physiol. 93:* 203–35.

Kramer, B. (1976a). Electric signalling during aggressive behaviour in *Mormyrus rume* (Mormyridae, Teleostei). *Naturwissenschaften 63:* 48.

Kramer, B. (1976b). The attack frequency of *Gnathonemus petersii* towards electrically silent (denervated) and intact conspecifics, and towards another mormyrid (*Brienomyrus niger*). *Behav. Ecol. Sociobiol. 1:* 425–46.

Kramer, B. (1979). Electric and motor responses of the weakly electric fish *Gnathonemus petersii* (Mormyridae) to play-back of social signals. *Behav. Ecol. Sociobiol. 6:* 67–79.

Kramer, B., and Bauer, R. (1976). Agonistic behaviour and electric signalling in a mormyrid fish, *Gnathonemus petersii*. *Behav. Ecol. Sociobiol. 1:* 45–61.

Kramer, B., Tautz, J., and Markl, H. (1981). The EOD sound response in weakly electric fish. *J. Comp. Physiol. 143:* 435–41.

Lissmann, H. W. (1951). Continuous electrical signals from the tail of a fish, *Gymnarchus niloticus* Cuv. *Nature 167:* 201–2.

Lissmann, H. W. (1958). On the function and evolution of electric organs in fish. *J. Exp. Biol. 35:* 156–91.

Lissmann, H. W. (1961). Ecological studies on gymnotids. In *Bioelectrogenesis*, ed. C. Chagas and A. Paes de Carvalho, pp. 215–26. Amsterdam: Elsevier.

Luecker, H., and Kramer, B. (1981). Development of a sex difference in the preferred latency response in the weakly electric fish *Pollimyrus isidori*. *Behav. Ecol. Sociobiol. 9:* 103–9.

Moller, P. (1980a). Electroreception and the behaviour of mormyrid electric fish. *Trends Neurosci. 3:* 105–9.

Moller, P. (1980b). Electroperception. *Oceanus 23:* 44–54.

Moller, P., and Bauer, R. (1973). 'Communication' in weakly electric fish, *Gnathonemus petersii* (Mormyridae). II. Interaction of electric organ discharge activities of two fish. *Anim. Behav. 21:* 501–12.

Moller, P., Serrier, J., Belbenoit, P., and Push, S. (1979). Notes on ethology and ecology of the Swashi river mormyrids (Lake Kainji, Nigeria). *Behav. Ecol. Sociobiol. 4:* 357–68.

Moller, P., Serrier, J., Squire, A., and Boudinot, M. (1982). Social spacing in the mormyrid fish *Gnathonemus petersii* (Pisces): a multisensory approach. *Anim. Behav. 30:* 641–50.

Moller, P., and Szabo, T. (1981). Lesions in the nucleus mesencephali exterolateralis: effects on electrocommunication in the mormyrid fish *Gnathonemus petersii* (Mormyriformes). *J. Comp. Physiol. 144:* 327–33.

Nieuwenhuys, R., Pouwels, E., and Smulders-Kersten, E. (1974). The neuronal organization of cerebellar lobe C1 in the mormyrid fish *Gnathonemus petersii* (Teleostei). *Z. Anat. Entw. Gesch. 144:* 315–56.

Push, S., and Moller, P. (1979). Spatial aspects of electrolocation in the mormyrid fish, *Gnathonemus petersii*. *J. Physiol., Paris 75:* 355–7.

Russell, C. J., and Bell, C. C. (1978). Neuronal responses to electrosensory input in the mormyrid valvula cerebelli. *J. Neurophysiol. 41:* 1495–1510.

Russell, C. J., Myers, J. P., and Bell, C. C. (1974). The echo response in *Gnathonemus petersii* (Mormyridae). *J. Comp. Physiol. 92:* 181–200.

Scheich, H., and Bullock, T. H. (1974). The detection of electric fields from electric organ. In *Handbook of Sensory Physiology*, vol. III/3, ed. A. Fessard, pp. 300–75, Berlin, Heidelberg, New York: Springer-Verlag.

Serrier, J. (1982). Comportement électrique des Mormyridae (Pisces). Electrogénèse en réponse à un signal exogène. Thèse Dr ès Sciences, Université Paris XI, Orsay.

Squire, A., and Moller, P. (1982). Effects of water conductivity on electrocommunication in the weak-electric fish *Brienomyrus niger* (Mormyriformes). *Anim. Behav.* 30: 375–82.

Szabo, T., Ravaille, M., Libouban, S., and Enger, P. S. (1983). The Mormyrid rhombencephalon: I. Light and EM investigations on the structure and connections of the lateral line lobe nucleus with HRP labelling. *Brain Res. 266:* 1–19.

Szabo, T. (1965). Sense organs of the lateral line system in some electric fish of the Gymnotidae, Gymnarchidae and Mormyridae. *J. Morphol. 117:* 229–50.

Szabo, T., Enger, P. S., and Libouban, S. (1979). Electrosensory systems in the mormyrid fish *Gnathonemus petersii*: special emphasis on the fast conducting pathway. *J. Physiol., Paris 75:* 409–20.

Teyssèdre, C., and Moller, P. (1982). The optomotor response in weak electric mormyrid fish: can they see? *Z. Tierpsych. 60:* 306–12.

Toerring, M. J. (1979). Etude du comportement exploratoire moteur et électrique de Mormyridae. Thèse, Paris VI.

Toerring, M. J., and Serrier, J. (1978). Influence of water temperatures on the electric organ discharge (EOD) of the weakly electric fish *Marcusenius cyprinoides* (Mormyridae). *J. Exp. Biol. 74:* 133–50.

Toerring, M. J., and Belbenoit, P. (1979). Motor programmes and electroperception in mormyrid fish. *Behav. Ecol. Sociobiol. 4:* 369–79.

Westby, G. W. M. (1974). Assessment of the signal value of certain discharge patterns in electric fish, *Gymnotus carapo*, by means of playback. *J. Comp. Physiol. 92:* 327–41.

Westby, G. W. M. (1975a). Has the latency-depending response of *Gymnotus carapo* to discharge-triggered stimuli a bearing on electric fish communication? *J. Comp. Physiol. 96:* 307–41.

Westby, G. W. M. (1975b). Comparative studies of the aggressive behaviour of two gymnotid electric fish (*Gymnotus carapo* and *Hypopomus artedi*). *Anim. Behav. 23:* 192–213.

Westby, G. W. M. (1981) Communication and jamming avoidance in electric fish. *Trends Neurosci. 4:* 205–10.

Westby, G. W. M., and Kirschbaum, F. (1977). Emergence and development of the electric organ discharge in the mormyrid fish, *Pollimyrus isidori*. I. The larval discharge. *J. Comp. Physiol. 122:* 251–71.

Westby, G. W. M., and Kirschbaum, F. (1978). Emergence and development of the electric organ discharge in the mormyrid fish, *Pollimyrus isidori*. II. Replacement of the larval by the adult discharge. *J. Comp. Physiol. 127:* 45–59.

Westby, G. W. M., and Kirschbaum, F. (1982). Sex differences in the wave-form of the pulse-type electric fish, *Pollimyrus isidori* (Mormyridae) *J. Comp. Physiol. 145(3):* 399–404.

Zipser, B., and Bennett, M. V. L. (1976a). Responses of cells of posterior lateral line lobe to activation of electroreceptors in a mormyrid fish. *J. Neurophysiol. 39:* 693–712.

Zipser, B., and Bennett, M. V. L. (1976b). Interaction of electrosensory and electromotor signals in lateral line lobe of a mormyrid fish. *J. Neurophysiol. 39:* 713–21.

4.2
Neural mechanisms of electrolocation and jamming avoidance behavior in electric fish

WALTER HEILIGENBERG

Almost 25 years have passed since Lissmann and Machin (1958) first demonstrated that certain species of fish can exploit weak electric signals for the detection and localization of objects in their environment. A large volume of behavioral, neurophysiological and neuro-anatomical studies on this subject has accumulated since. Various reviews have focused on the physiology and anatomy of electroreceptors and electric organs (Bennett, 1971a,b; Szabo and Fessard, 1974; Bell, 1979) as well as on central nervous mechanisms and behavioral performances (Scheich and Bullock, 1974; Kalmijn, 1974; Heiligenberg, 1977, 1980a,b; Bullock, 1982). In a few instances, such as in the case of the Jamming Avoidance Response (JAR) of gymnotoid fish, investigators have been particularly successful in linking behavioral phenomena to functional and structural properties of the central nervous system.

The electric sense displays a number of basic design features, such as center-surround organization of receptive fields, topographically orga-nized neuronal maps, looped central nervous pathways, efferent control of afferent information flow, etc. Although such features are long known from the study of other sensory modalities, their functional significance in several instances is still obscure. This is obviously due to the fact that we have failed to identify behavioral responses and facets of their sensory control which are intricately linked to such designs. Only to the extent that we know the natural mode of operation of a given piece of neuronal hardware are we able to conceive experiments which will lead us to an understanding of its relevant features rather than trap us in a blind occupation with epiphenomena. For this very reason, the simplicity of the electric sense and the existence of robust behavioral responses which still function in neurophysiological preparations have rendered this sensory modality a most suitable model system for the study of central nervous mechanisms which govern the processing of sensory information.

The significance of electric organ discharges (EODs) for orientation and communication

By continually discharging an electric organ, electric fish generate a current field which emanates from their anterior body surface and converges upon the tip of their tail. This field is distorted by objects which differ electrically from the surrounding water, and local changes in transepidermal current flow which are caused by such field distortions yield cues about the appearance and motion of objects. The animal's ability to 'electrolocate' objects in this manner may be hampered if electric fields of neighbors interfere with its own field, and various forms of jamming avoidance responses (JARs) have evolved which minimize the detrimental effects of signal interference by changing the frequency or the timing of the animal's electric organ discharges (EODs, see review in Heiligenberg, 1977).

EODs are also employed in the context of social communication. Since their spectral and temporal features vary little within one species but commonly differ considerably between species, they offer reliable cues for species identification. In addition, sexual dimorphism in EOD waveforms and sex-specific modulations in the rate of discharging play an important role in reproductive behavior (Hopkins, 1972, 1974a,b; Hopkins and Bass, 1981).

Electric fish species can readily be classified into two groups, so-called 'wave' species, which fire EODs in a very regular manner, with a duty cycle near 50%, and 'pulse' species, which fire EODs in a less-predictable temporal sequence and with a duty cycle of not more than a few percent. The lack of species with intermediate types of EODs suggests that either extreme represents a particular adaptation and conveys specific advantages. This resembles the situation in echolocating bats which either use frequency-modulated (FM) signals or constant-frequency (CF) signals. But whereas at least some bat species are known to use both types of signals and to employ them with maximum benefit (Simmons et al., 1978), we know of no electric fish species which can modify its EODs in a similar manner.

Various advantages and disadvantages are linked to the use of wave- and pulse-type EODs. The former, with their narrow power spectra, carry all energy in narrow frequency bands and can thus achieve high signal to noise ratios even if signal amplitudes are weak. This should not only benefit the electrolocation of objects but also enhance the detection of species members and social communication between them. It would, however, also help a predator on electric fish in zeroing in on its victim. Pulse-type EODs, on the other hand, have broad power spectra, and higher signal amplitudes are needed for sufficient signal-to-noise ratios. Their broad power spectra may convey advantages for the assessment of capacitive features in the environment, since mormyrid species with very short EOD pulses (and thus substantial power in the high-frequency range) are particularly sensitive to small capacitive loads in the water (Meyer, 1982). Particularly the highly irregularly firing pulse species, such as the mormyrids, are much more difficult to detect electrically than wave species with their narrowly concentrated spectral power. Whereas this may protect them from predators which cue in on electrical signals it also may make social communication more difficult. The more regular repetition of EOD pulses in the context of courting, called 'rasping' (Hopkins and Bass, 1981), certainly makes a mormyrid sender more detectable to a potential mate.

Apart from their respective advantages for electrolocation and communication, wave- and pulse-type EODs also offer different strategies for jamming avoidance. Whereas wave-species minimize signal interference by shifting their fundamental EOD frequency away from those of near neighbors, pulse-species instead time their pulses in a manner that makes coincidences with pulses of neighbors least likely (for review see Heiligenberg, 1977, 1980a,b).

Like all temporal functions, EODs can equally well be described in terms of their Fourier transforms which consist of an amplitude spectrum and a phase function. In contrast to our own auditory system, which responds poorly to alterations of the phase function alone, electric fish have been shown to be extremely sensitive to this aspect of the signal, and they are able to distinguish waveforms with identical amplitude spectra but different phase functions (Heiligenberg and Altes, 1978; Hopkins and Bass, 1981). On the basis of this sensory capacity, electric fish are able to assess the orientation of the electric field of neighbors (Westby, 1974) and to distinguish EOD waveforms which appear identical to our auditory system. This phase sensitivity should make electric fish particularly susceptible to capacitive features in their environment.

Electrosensory structures and pathways in gymnotiform electric fish

Two aspects of the animal's EOD are modified by the appearance of objects as well as by the interference with EODs of neighbors. These are, for a given spectral frequency, local instantaneous amplitude and local instantaneous phase. In the case of wave-type EODs, instantaneous phase of the fundamental frequency is equivalent to the relative timing of the zero crossing of the signal. The importance of amplitude and phase modulations in electrosensory feedback is reflected in various neuronal specializations which allow for the detection and evaluation of these two variables.

(1) Receptors, primary afferents and posterior lateral line lobe (PLLL)

Various types of electroreceptors are found on the electric fish's body surface: ampullary receptors, which respond to low-frequency electric signals of biological and geophysical origin, and tuberous receptors, which respond to local modulations of the transepidermal current flow linked to the animal's own EODs. Whereas one type of tuberous receptor may be specialized to detect modulations in instantaneous phase of this signal, another type may be specialized to detect modulations in instantaneous amplitude. By monitoring local changes in the animal's transepidermal current flow, tuberous electroreceptors are instrumental in the detection of nearby objects and interfering electric fields of discharging neighbors. The pattern of local changes in transepidermal current flow which is caused by the presence of an object can indeed be considered the electric 'image' of the object, and electrolocation can thus be viewed as a way of 'seeing' with the body surface.

The input from electroreceptors is mapped in a somatotopic, or 'dermatotopic', manner onto various laminated structures in the central nervous system (CNS). The following description of this organization focuses on the case in the South American gymnotiform fish. A similar, but not identical, pattern is found in the non-related African electric fish, the mormyriformes (Haugedé-Carré, 1979; Bell, Finger and Russell, 1981; Finger, Bell and Russell, 1981).

A simplified neuronal flow diagram is given in Figure 1 which is based upon more recent neuroanatomical studies on the genera *Eigenmannia* and *Apteronotus* (Maler, Finger and Karten, 1974; Maler, Sas and Rogers, 1981; Maler, Sas, Carr and Matsubara, 1982; Maler, 1979; Scheich and Ebbesson, 1981; Carr, Maler, Heiligenberg and Sas, 1981; Carr, Maler and Sas, 1982; Heiligenberg and Dye, 1982). Primary afferents from ampullary receptors (A-input in Figure 1) project in a somatotopic manner upon the most medial part of the posterior lateral line lobe (PLLL), whereas primary afferents from tuberous receptors project to three different somatotopic maps in the more lateral portions of the PLLL. Most peculiarly, each tuberous afferent projects to all three maps so that the animal obtains three tuberous maps with identical sensory input.

The same anterior lateral line nerve ganglion through which electro-sensory afferents enter the brain also carries mechanosensory afferents

Figure 1. Flow diagram of electrosensory stations and pathways in the central nervous system of gymnotoid fish. Primary afferents from ampullary electroreceptors (A-input) project to the medial part of the posterior lateral line lobe (PLLL) which in turn projects predominantly to lamina 7 of the torus semicircularis, with collaterals entering the nucleus praeeminentialis. Primary afferents from tuberous electroreceptors which encode phase information (T-input) project to the layer of spherical cells (O) in the central and lateral portions of the PLLL, and spherical cells in turn project to lamina 6 of the torus semicircularis. Primary afferents from tuberous electroreceptors which encode amplitude modulations (P-input) project to more-dorsal layers of the central and lateral portions of the PLLL, and two types of higher-order cells, E- and I-units, which respond to a rise and fall respectively in stimulus amplitude, project predominantly to laminae 3, 5 and 7 of the torus semicircularis, with collaterals entering the nucleus praeeminentialis. Electroreceptor afferents project to the ipsilateral PLLL which in turn projects predominantly to the contralateral torus semicircularis. The lobus caudalis receives input from the nucl. praeem., and both structures project back to the PLLL. The lobus caudalis also projects to lamina 8 of the contralateral torus semicircularis. This flow diagram does not contain the medullary pacemaker or the prepacemaker nucleus of the midbrain.

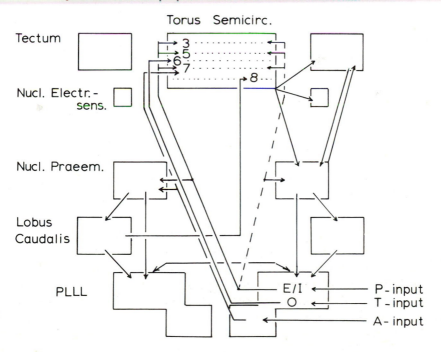

of the ordinary lateral line system. Mechanosensory afferents, however, project to different parts of the hindbrain, such as the anterior lateral line lobe (or medial nucleus), the eminentia granularis and part of the lobus caudalis. Different modalities are thus processed in different nuclei of the hindbrain, and even the two types of electrosensory afferents, ampullary and tuberous, project to separate portions of the PLLL. The somatotopic organization of these projections is shown in Figure 2.

Figure 2. Dorsal view of the posterior lateral line lobe (PLLL) showing four somatotopic maps of primary electrosensory afferent projections. Whereas the medial (med.) portion of the PLLL receives ampullary afferents, the three remaining portions, central–medial, central–lateral and lateral, receive identical tuberous input as each tuberous afferent sends one branch to each map. Maps were constructed on the basis of physiologically identified, intracellularly labelled primary afferents whose receptor pores were localized on the body surface. The hatched area, which is the dorsal portion of the head, was held above the water surface, and its receptor pores could not be studied for this reason. Although the pectoral fins do not carry electroreceptors, they were drawn into the maps as landmarks. Note the exaggerated representation of the head region, which also shows the highest density of receptors. The orientation of the animal's body axes is shown in the upper right. (From Heiligenberg and Dye, 1982.)

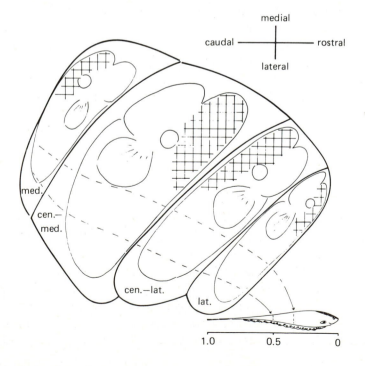

The neuroanatomy of those portions of the PLLL which receive afferents from tuberous electroreceptors has been studied in great detail by Maler and his associates (Maler, 1979; Maler et al., 1981), and it appears that part of the circuitry is devoted to the encoding of phase and amplitude modulations in local receptive fields on the body surface. In electric fish genera, such as *Eigenmannia*, which fire their electric organ in a continual, near-sinusoidal manner, two types of tuberous electro-receptors are distinguished: T-units which fire one spike per EOD cycle, phase-locked to the zero crossing of the signal, and P-units which fire intermittently and raise their rate of firing if the amplitude of the signal increases (Scheich, Bullock and Hamstra, 1973). The relative timing of T-unit firing thus reflects local phase, and the rate of P-unit firing thus reflects local amplitude of the stimulus. These two classes of receptors, however, do not encode phase and amplitude in a strictly orthogonal manner, as some T-units are still sensitive to modulations in amplitude as they advance the timing of their firing as amplitude rises (Bullock and Chichibu, 1965), and P-units statistically reflect phase by the average timing of their rather irregular firing (see Figures 3 and 4 in Bastian and Heiligenberg, 1980a).

Primary afferents, bipolar cells whose somata are located in the anterior lateral line nerve ganglion (ALLG in Figure 3), relay responses of tuberous receptors to various targets in the PLLL. According to Maler's analysis of neuroanatomical fine structure, primary afferents from T-type receptors are assumed to form electrical synapses on the spherical cells in the most ventral layer of the PLLL (see Figure 3). Possibly, T-type electroreceptors also form electrical synapses with their primary afferents (Szabo and Fessard, 1974) which would allow for quickest conduction of phase information from the periphery to the central nervous system. According to Maler's estimates, approximately four T-type afferents converge upon one spherical cell, but this number could be larger if one afferent contacted several spherical cells. The synaptic organization and spike-initiating mechanism of the spherical cell suggest that a spike will be transmitted only in response to near-synchronous arrival of spikes on several afferents. This may account for the fact that the phase of firing of a spherical cell shows even less jitter than the phase of firing of single T-type afferents, and whereas some T-type afferents may advance their phase of firing in response to a rise in stimulus amplitude, the spherical cells of the PLLL are immune to modulations in amplitude (Maler, personal communication). The axon of the spherical cell reaches lamina #6 of the torus semicircularis where further computation of phase information takes place (see below). T-type receptors, afferents and spherical cells (all filled in black in Figure 3) thus constitute a separate pathway (the 'rapid electrosensory pathway' of Szabo and Fessard, 1974) which only transmits phase information to the torus semicircularis of the midbrain.

According to Maler's analysis, primary afferents from P-type receptors synapse on granule, basilar pyramidal and polymorphic cells of the PLLL. Whereas the role of the latter cell type is still not clear, very plausible assumptions can be made about the function of the pyramidal cells (see schematic diagram in Figure 3). Basilar pyramidals are characterized by a long basilar dendrite which receives excitatory input from P-type afferents and inhibitory input from more distant granule cells which in turn receive excitatory input from P-type afferents. Under the assumption that the spatial order in the layers of the PLLL reflects the spatial order on the body surface, this organization of synaptic input would imply that a basilar pyramidal cell is excited by a rise in stimulus amplitude in the center of its receptive field and that it is inhibited by a rise in amplitude in the periphery of its receptive field. Maler estimates

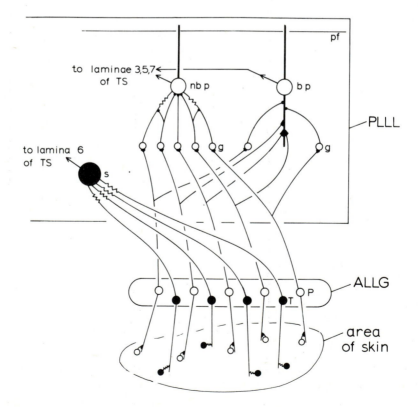

that approximately eight primary afferents converge upon one basilar pyramidal cell.

Whereas basilar pyramidal cells are excited by a rise in stimulus amplitude in the center of their receptive field, nonbasilar pyramidal cells should be inhibited: nonbasilar pyramidal cells, which lack the basilar dendrite typical for basilar pyramidals, receive inhibitory input from nearest granule cells and excitatory input, via electrical synapses, from more distant granule cells. Input from more distant granule cells, however, is inhibited by collaterals from more proximal granule cells. Since all granule cells receive excitatory input from P-type afferents, and if one again assumes that the spatial relations between granule cells reflect the spatial relations among their corresponding receptor inputs, then a basilar pyramidal cell should be inhibited by a rise in stimulus amplitude in the center of its receptive field and should be excited by a lowering in stimulus amplitude. Maler estimates that approximately eight primary afferents converge upon one nonbasilar pyramidal cell.

Axons of pyramidal cells terminate predominantly in laminae 3, 5 and 7 of the torus semicircularis (see below), and their firing reports local

Figure 3. The recipients of tuberous electroreceptor afferent projections in the PLLL, schematized after Figure 17 in Maler et al. (1981). ALLG is the anterior lateral line nerve ganglion, which contains the somata of all primary electrosensory afferents. T-type afferents (filled, T) are assumed to synapse electrotonically upon spherical cells (filled, s), in the most ventral layer of the PLLL. P-type afferents (open, P) are assumed to form excitatory synapses (triangles) on granule cells (g) and on the basilar dendrites of 'basilar pyramidal' cells (bp). The same basilar pryamidal cells also receive inhibitory (dots) input from more-distant granule cells, believed to represent the periphery of the cell's receptive field on the body surface. 'Nonbasilar pyramidal' cells (nbp) are inhibited by proximal granule cells and excited, via electrotonic synapses (resistor symbol), by more distant granule cells. This excitatory input, in turn, is inhibited by the more proximal granule cells, believed to represent the center of a receptive field on the body surface. The dorsal dendrites of both types of pyramidal cells are contacted by parallel fibers (pf) which originate from the lobus caudalis of the cerebellum. The spherical cells send axons to lamina 6 of the torus semicircularis, whereas the pyramidal cells send axons predominantly to laminae 3, 5 and 7. It is likely, but not certain, that basilar and nonbasilar pyramidal cells share the same primary afferents within a receptive field on the body surface. They could also share the same sets of granule cells, although separate sets were chosen in this figure for clarity. The ratio between granule cells and primary afferents is not known. Between 5 and 16 primary afferents are estimated to converge on one pyramidal cell, and at least four afferents are assumed to contact one spherical cell.

rises and falls in stimulus amplitude on the animal's body surface. Two types of cells have been recorded in the PLLL: E-type cells, which are excited by a rise in stimulus amplitude, and I-types, which are excited by a fall in stimulus amplitude (Bastian and Heiligenberg, 1980a; Bastian, 1981), and as one would have expected, intracellular labeling of these cells with HRP has shown that E-types are basilar pyramidal cells and I-types are nonbasilar pyramidal cells (Bastian, personal communication). By studying the receptive field size of E- and I-units as well as local receptor densities, Bastian (1981) estimated that 6 to 15 receptors converge upon one E- or I-cell in the PLLL, a number close to Maler's estimate of eight.

Since P-type afferents fire in a preferred phase range of the EOD cycle, they still convey some phase information. Very little of this information, however, is retained in the firing of E-type cells in the PLLL and none is seen in the firing of I-type cells, which are even further removed from the receptor input (see diagram in Figure 3). These two cell types thus encode amplitude information more exclusively than do their primary afferents. The fact that the animal has cells which are specialized to recognize rises and falls in stimulus amplitude respectively is in good agreement with the observation that these two features are of crucial importance in the control of the Jamming Avoidance Response (JAR) (Heiligenberg and Bastian, 1980b; Heiligenberg, 1980) as well as for the identification of the conductive properties of objects (Bastian, 1981).

The diagram in Figure 3 assumes a strict distinction between T- and P-type afferents. It seems, however, that these two types are better described as the ends of a continuous spectrum of tuberous afferents rather than as discrete classes (see Figure 2 in Heiligenberg and Bastian, 1980, and Viancour, 1979). Moreover, EM studies of synaptic contacts of physiologically identified primary afferents which were filled with intracellular injection of HRP (Maler and Heiligenberg, in preparation) have shown that one and the same primary afferent may contact spherical cells as well as granule cells, a seeming violation of the rules laid out in Figure 3. It appears now that, in accordance with the more statistical distinction of T- and P-type afferents, the pattern of connections of these cells in the PLLL also follows a more statistical and quantitative rather than a strictly qualitative rule. Such a rule could specify that a given primary afferent, the more it leans towards the T-type end of the spectrum, predominantly contacts spherical cells, whereas to the extent that it leans toward the P-type end of the spectrum, it predominantly contacts granule, basilar pyramidal and polymorphic cells. This strategy would still yield a clear separation of phase and amplitude information at the level of the PLLL.

The center-surround organization of the receptive fields of pyramidal cells in the PLLL obviously enhances the detection of local contrast in spatial patterns of amplitude modulations on the animal's body surface. The animal should thus be particularly sensitive to the edges of electric images and less so to broadly and evenly distributed amplitude modulations as they result if its own field interferes with that of a neighbor. As a consequence, the animal's ability to analyse electric images should be less vulnerable to jamming by conspecifics. The extreme of this evolution is seen in the genus *Sternopygus* which appears to be immune to jamming and also displays no Jamming Avoidance Response (Matsubara, 1981).

(2) Torus semicircularis, nucleus praeeminentialis and lobus caudalis of the cerebellum

The next higher stations in the processing of electrosensory information are the torus semicircularis (TS) and nucleus praeeminentialis (NP) (see Figure 1). The TS is a multilayered structure (Scheich, 1977; Scheich and Ebbesson, 1981; Carr et al., 1981) in which each horizontal layer apparently contains only one somatotopic map, and all maps are vertically in register. Most significantly, the single ampullary map and the three tuberous maps of the PLLL are superimposed in the TS (see Figure 4). Details of this organization still have to be worked out, but so far the following features have emerged:

(a) The spherical cells from all three tuberous sections of the PLLL project to lamina 6 of the TS and almost exclusively to its contralateral side. Massive horizontal connections within this lamina obviously form a substrate in which the animal can compare phase information from different parts of the body surface, a crucial operation for the control of the JAR. Horizontal fibers originate from large spherical cells in lamina 6 which receive direct input from axons of the spherical cells of the PLLL (Carr et al., 1981). Lamina 6 in the genera *Eigenmannia* and *Apteronotus* is obviously homologous to the nucleus magnocellularis mesencephali (NMM) described for gymnotiform fish with pulse-type (rather than wave-type) EODs, such as *Gymnotus* and *Hypopomus* (see Szabo and Fessard, 1974). The particular cell type which ultimately computes local differences in phase has not yet been identified anatomically, but extracellular recordings near and possibly below lamina 6 have

monitored cells which indeed encode differences in arrival time of
T-unit spikes from different parts of the body surface (Bastian and
Heiligenberg, 1980a,b).

(b) The basilar and nonbasilar pyramidal cells of the PLLL, which
respond to a rise and fall respectively in stimulus amplitude, project
predominantly to the contralateral side of the TS and most heavily to

Figure 4. The posterior lateral line lobe (bottom) projects most heavily
to the contralateral torus semicircularis (top), and its four somatotopic
maps merge into one. Letters indicate HRP injection sites in the torus
and their respective retrogradely-labelled sources in the PLLL.
Whereas the two central injections (e and j) yield substantial labelling
in both PLLLs, all other injections almost exclusively label the
contralateral PLLL. Note the even further exaggeration of the head
region at the level of the torus.

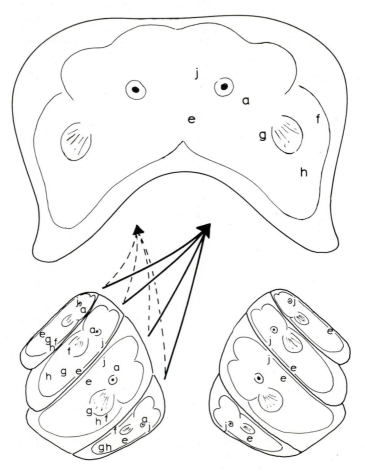

laminae 3, 5 and 7. Quite commonly, a collateral branch will travel through the ipsilateral lemniscus lateralis and thus land on the ipsilateral side of the TS. In contrast to axons of spherical cells, axons of pyramidal cells send collaterals to the nucleus praeeminentialis (NP, see Figure 1). The input of pyramidal cells can be recorded in the higher laminae of the TS. In deeper laminae of the TS, at the level between lamina 7 and lamina 9, cell types can be recorded which obviously receive higher-order input from these pyramidal cells which is gated by cells which evaluate differential phase (Partridge, Heiligenberg and Matsubara, 1981).

(c) Small injections of HRP in the most medial part of the PLLL, the target of ampullary afferents, have labelled terminals mostly in lamina #7 and some in lamina #5 of the TS. Since all laminae are in somatotopic register with one another, the animal could, in principle, compile an electric representation of its surrounding which contains information from both ampullary and tuberous receptors. The role of the separate representations at the level of the PLLL could be that they allow for separate, modality-specific preprocessing of this information, such as possible sharpening of contours in electric image representations, etc.

The role of the NP in electroreception is not yet clear. With the exception of the spherical cells, all cells in the PLLL which project to the TS also send collaterals to the NP, and each of the four somatotopic maps in the PLLL has a separate representation in the NP (Maler et al., 1982). The projection of the NP to the lobus caudalis (LC) seems to be the only electrosensory input to this structure (Figure 1). Bastian (1975) demonstrated a somatotopic organization of the LC and recorded higher-order cells with complex receptive fields on the body surface: a center-surround, excitatory–inhibitory organization was commonly found, and some units responded predominantly to movement of objects in one particular direction. Such elaborate features are not found at the level of the PLLL, although the receptive field organization of pyramidal cells clearly shows the beginning of a center-surround organization (see Figure 4). The LC strongly projects to lamina #8 of the contralateral TS. The function of this connection is still unknown.

Both LC and NP project back to the PLLL, thus closing a loop in electrosensory processing of still unknown significance. It is possible that the three tuberous maps of the PLLL receive different descending inputs and thus may be specialized for different tasks of feature extraction. These looped pathways could certainly serve as a substrate for iterative image analysis.

(3) The tectum opticum and the prepacemaker nucleus of the midbrain

The TS projects heavily and in a topographic manner to the tectum opticum, and it appears that the somatotopic map of the TS is in spatial register with the retinotopic map of the tectum so that a given column in the tectum receives electrical and visual input from a specific spatial angle in the animal's environment (Carr et al., 1981). Bastian (1982) indeed has recorded multimodal tectal units which respond to the motion of an object in a specific part of the fish's environment if either the object can be seen or if it can be perceived on the basis of its distortion of the animal's electric field. Some units respond better when both modalities are available, and the vulnerability of such units to electrical jamming is lessened if visual cues are simultaneously available.

Whereas the dorsal TS is strictly electrosensitive, the ventral TS contains acoustical and mechanosensory units (Matsubara, Finger, Maler and Carr, 1981). Dorsal and ventral TS both project topographically to the tectum, and it appears that the tectum thus receives a multimodal, spatially ordered image of the environment which serves as a basis for spatially oriented behavioral responses. A similar situation is found in higher vertebrates: Newman and Hartline (1981) found tectal units in snakes which respond to visual and thermal stimuli originating from specific spatial angles. Similarly, Knudsen (personal communication) reported tectal units in owls responding to acoustical and visual stimuli, and Dräger and Hubel (1976) reported superior collicular (a tectal homologue) units in mice responding to visual and somatosensory inputs.

The picture in Figure 1 is further complicated by a descending connection from TS to NP and reciprocal connections between tectum and NP. Nothing is known about the functional role of these pathways. The same holds for additional descending connections from TS to the pretectal nucleus electrosensorius, to the thalamus and to various regions of the reticular formation.

In the context of the Jamming Avoidance Response (JAR), the animal is able to modulate the frequency of its medullary pacemaker. The only known input to this pacemaker originates in a paired prepacemaker nucleus in the midbrain (Heiligenberg, Finger, Matsubara and Carr, 1981). Since crucial computations of sensory information which drives the JAR take place in the TS, one should expect at least an indirect pathway from TS to prepacemaker nucleus. This connection, however, has still not been traced.

General characteristics of electrosensory central nervous structures and pathways

The processing of electrosensory information follows principles widely known from the study of other senses which evaluate spatially structured information. These principles are:

(1) Parallel distribution of afferent information to various stations in the CNS which evaluate different aspects and features of images perceived at the periphery.

(2) Reciprocal connections and recurrent loops between different central stations.

(3) Eventual convergence of information flow from separate central stations and combination with information obtained from other sensory modalities with the ultimate purpose of controlling oriented responses.

(4) The use of laminated structures which receive spatially ordered images of the environment, with different layers specialized for the processing of particular aspects of these images.

(5) Center-surround organization of receptive fields. This feature, first discovered in vision (Kuffler, 1953), seems to be employed wherever images are evaluated in a two-dimensional stratum upon which spatially ordered aspects of the environment are mapped. Most remarkably, it is also found in the acoustical spatial map represented in the owl's inferior colliculus (Knudsen and Konishi, 1978a,b) and here too obviously serves the sharpening of spatial contrasts. The case of a central nervous acoustical map intrigues us for the following reason: in all other senses which handle spatially ordered information, a spatial map originates in a two-dimensional array of sensors upon which sections of the environmental 'shell' which surrounds the animal are projected, such as a 'retina' in vision and infrared reception, or the whole body surface in electroreception. As these receptors project to layers of higher-order units by maintaining their neighborhood relations – possibly an embryological necessity – a central nervous map of the environment is readily obtained. In the case of hearing, however, no spatial image exists at the receptor level, and the nervous system has to go through much computing of binaural information in order to reconstruct a spatial map. Apparently, a two-dimensional neuronal array which simulates the appearance and movement of images in a spatially ordered manner offers advantages; at least, it should be economical with respect to the total amount of 'wiring' needed for interconnecting neurons.

Extraordinary features of the electric sense and their potential as model systems for the study of sensory and motor organization

The electric sense, apart from being a rather exotic modality, excels in a number of evolutionary accomplishments which challenge our understanding of neuronal organization, function and development.

(1) A biological clock of unparalleled precision

Electric fish with wave-type EODs are capable of firing their medullary electric-organ pacemaker at a highly constant rate: over thousands of successive cycles, the coefficient of variation in the length of the discharge cycle can be as low as 10^{-4}. For a fish with a 1000-Hz EOD frequency, this amounts to a jitter in interval length of not more than $0.1\,\mu s$ (Bullock, Behrend and Heiligenberg, 1975). Although much has been learned about the synaptic organization of the pacemaker (Bennett, Pappas, Gimenez and Nakajima, 1967; Bennett, 1971a; Tokunaga, Akert, Sandri and Bennett, 1980), the source of this precision is still unknown.

(2) Accuracies in neuronal timing in efferent and afferent pathways

EOD pulses in some species of electric fish may be as short as $0.3\,ms$, and they thus belong to the shortest known electrical signals in neuronal systems. Since the electric organ consists of long stacks of electrocytes, a short EOD pulse requires highly synchronous discharging of all electrocytes in the stack. Bennett (1971a) demonstrated that synchronous arrival of the motor command at all sites of the electric organ is achieved by systematic variation in axon diameters and total lengths of efferent fibers, but how this system remains tuned while the animal grows is still unknown.

A similar problem exists on the afferent side: electroreceptors which mark particular electrical events, such as the moment of the positive zero crossing of the EOD signal, are located in widely separated regions of the animal's body surface. Differences in their distance from the central nervous system (CNS) would introduce differences in the arrival time of their messages if speed of nerve conduction were identical for all afferents, and a synchronous electrical event would thus be reported asynchronously in the CNS. In the genus *Eigenmannia*, where control of the Jamming Avoidance Response requires rather accurate coding in phase differences of the electric signal across distant parts of the body surface, delayed arrival of spikes from more distant electroreceptors is largely compensated for by higher nerve conduction speed (Heiligenberg and Dye, 1982).

(3) Electroreceptor tuning to sender's dominant frequency

Electric fish with wave-type EODs have individually different fundamental frequencies which lie within a band which is typical for a given species. Stimulus frequencies at which a given individual's electroreceptors respond with the lowest threshold, also referred to as 'best frequencies', cluster near the animal's fundamental EOD frequency so that each individual is most sensitive in the range of its own signal frequency. Moreover, as EOD frequency changes with temperature, the best frequency of the receptors follows (Hopkins, 1976). Since individuals undergo drastic changes in EOD frequency during their ontogeny, and since electroreceptors always appear to be most sensitive in the range of the current EOD frequency, effector and receptor characteristics must be continually adjusted to each other. Animals of the wave-type genus *Sternopygus* lower their frequency under the influence of androgens, which appears to account for the fact that, under reproductive conditions, males have lower EOD frequencies than females. As animals change their EOD frequency under the influence of steroid hormones, the tuning of their receptors follows (Meyer and Zakon, 1982). The mechanism of continual receptor retuning is still unknown.

(4) The efference copy in mormyrid electric fish

Electric fish with pulse-type EODs might benefit from being able to distinguish between feedback from their own EODs and sensations caused by EODs of neighbors. The most elegant solution to this problem was chosen by the mormyrids which send a corollary discharge of their pacemaker command to various stations of their brain involved in the analysis of electrosensory inputs (Bennett and Steinbach, 1969; Zipser and Bennett, 1976b; Bell, 1981). The timing of this corollary discharge matches the arrival of sensory input caused by the animal's own discharges and thus allows for selective gating of sensory feedback. Most recently, Bell (1981) identified cells in the posterior lateral line lobe which are driven by input from ampullary receptors and, over the course of minutes, become less sensitive to any input caused by the animal's own EODs. It appears that the mormyrid continually updates a template of expected electrosensory input linked to its own EOD activity, and that this template serves as a background against which true novelties can be detected. A similar mechanism obviously exists in gymnotoid pulse species (Heiligenberg, 1980b), but its neuronal basis is definitely different from the case in mormyrids.

Acknowledgement: This work is supported by grants from NIMH and NSF. I thank Catherine E. Carr for helpful comments on this manuscript.

References

Bastian, J. (1975). Receptive fields of cerebellar cells receiving electro-receptive input in a gymnotoid fish. *J. Neurophysiol. 38(2):* 285–300.

Bastian, J., and Heiligenberg, W. (1980a). Neural correlates of the Jamming Avoidance Response in *Eigenmannia. J. Comp. Physiol. 136:* 135–52.

Bastian, J., and Heiligenberg, W. (1980b). Phase-sensitive midbrain neurons in *Eigenmannia*: neural correlates of the Jamming Avoidance Response. *Science 209:* 828–31.

Bastian, J. (1981). Electrolocation I and II. *J. Comp. Physiol. 144:* 465–94.

Bastian, J. (1982). Vision and electroreception: integration of sensory information in the optic tectum of the weakly electric fish, *Apteronotus albifrons. J. Comp. Physiol. 147:* 287–98.

Bell, C. C. (1979). Central nervous system physiology of electroreception, a review. *J. Physiol., Paris 75:* 361–79.

Bell, C. C. (1981). An efference copy which is updated by reafferent input. *Science 214:* 450–2.

Bell, C. C., Finger, T. E., and Russell, C. J. (1981). Central connections of the posterior lateral line lobe in mormyrid fish. *Expl. Brain Res. 42:* 9–22.

Bennett, M. V. L., Pappas, G. D., Gimenez, M., and Nakajima, Y. (1967). Physiology and ultrastructure of electrotonic junctions. IV. Medullary electromotor nuclei in gymnotoid fish. *J. Neurophysiol. 30:* 236–300.

Bennett, M. V. L., and Steinbach, A. B. (1969). Influence of electric organ control system on electrosensory afferent pathways in mormyrids. In *Neurobiology of Cerebellar Evolution and Development*, ed. R. Llinas, pp. 207–14. Chicago: Am. Med. Assoc.

Bennett, M. V. L. (1971a). Electric organs. In *Fish Physiology*. vol. 5, ed. W. S. Hoar and D. J. Randall, pp. 347–491. New York: Academic Press.

Bennett, M. V. L. (1971b). Electroreception. In *Fish Physiology*, vol. 5, ed. W. S. Hoar and D. J. Randall, pp. 493–574. New York: Academic Press.

Bullock, T. H., and Chichibu, S. (1965). Further analysis of sensory coding in electroreceptors of electric fish. *Proc. Natn. Acad. Sci. USA 54(2):* 422–9.

Bullock, T. H., Hamstra, R. H., and Scheich, H. (1974). The jamming avoidance response of high frequency electric fish. *J. Comp. Physiol. 77:* 1–48.

Bullock, T. H., Behrend, K., and Heiligenberg, W. (1975). Comparison of the jamming avoidance response in gymnotoid and gymnarchid fish: a case of convergent evolution of behavior and its sensory basis. *J. Comp. Physiol. 103:* 97–121.

Bullock, T. H. (1982). Electroreception. *A. Rev. Neurosci. 5:* 121–70.

Carr, C. C., Maler, L., Heiligenberg, W., and Sas, E. (1981). Laminar organization of the afferent and efferent systems of the torus semicircularis of gymnotiform fish:

morphological substrates for parallel processing in the electrosensory system. *J. Comp. Neurol. 203:* 649–70.

Carr, C. E., Maler, L., and Sas, E. (1982). Peripheral organization and central projections of the electrosensory nerves in gymnotiform fish. *J. Comp. Neurol. 211:* 139–53.

Dräger, U. C., and Hubel, D. H. (1976). Topography of visual and somatosensory projections to mouse superior colliculus. *J. Neurophysiol. 39:* 91–102.

Finger, T. E., Bell, C. C., and Russell, C. J. (1981). Electrosensory pathways to the valvula cerebelli in mormyrid fish. *Expl. Brain Res. 42:* 23–33.

Haugedé-Carré, F. (1979). The mesencephalic exterolateral posterior nucleus of the mormyrid fish *Brienomyrus niger*: efferent connections studied by the HRP method. *Brain Res. 178:* 179–84.

Heiligenberg, W. (1977). Principles of electrolocation and jamming avoidance. In *Studies of Brain Function*, vol. 1, pp. 1–85. Berlin, Heidelberg, New York: Springer-Verlag.

Heiligenberg, W., and Altes, R. (1978). Phase sensitivity in electroreception. *Science 199:* 1001–4.

Heiligenberg, W. (1980a). The evaluation of electroreceptive feedback in a gymnotoid fish with pulse-type electric organ discharges. *J. Comp. Physiol. 138:* 173–85.

Heiligenberg, W. (1980b). The Jamming Avoidance Response in the weakly electric fish *Eigenmannia. Naturwissenschaften 67:* 499–507.

Heiligenberg, W., Baker, C., and Matsubara, J. (1978). The Jamming Avoidance Response in *Eigenmannia* revisited: The structure of a neuronal democracy. *J. Comp. Physiol. 127:* 267–86.

Heiligenberg, W., and Bastian, J. (1980). The control of *Eigenmannia*'s pacemaker by distributed evaluation of electroreceptive afferences. *J. Comp. Physiol. 136:* 113–33.

Heiligenberg, W., and Dye, J. (1982). Labelling of electroreceptive afferents in a gymnotoid fish by intracellular injection of HRP: the mystery of multiple maps. *J. Comp. Physiol. 148:* 287–96.

Heiligenberg, W., Finger, T., Matsubara, J., and Carr, C. C. (1981). Input to the medullary pacemaker nucleus in the weakly electric fish, *Eigenmannia. Brain Res. 211:* 418–23.

Heiligenberg, W., and Partridge, B. L. (1981). How electroreceptors encode JAR-eliciting stimulus regimes: reading trajectories in a phase-amplitude plane. *J. Comp. Physiol. 142:* 295–308.

Hopkins, C. D. (1972). Sex differences in electric signaling in an electric fish. *Science 176:* 1035–7.

Hopkins, C. D. (1974a). Electric communication: functions in the social behavior of *Eigenmannia virescens. Behaviour 50:* 3–4, 270–305.

Hopkins, C. D. (1974b). Electric communication in the reproductive behavior of *Sternopygus macrurus. Z. Tierspychol. 35:* 518–35.

Hopkins, C. D. (1976). Stimulus filtering and electroreception: tuberous electroreceptors in three species of gymnotoid fish. *J. Comp. Physiol. 111:* 171–208.

Hopkins, C. D., and Bass, A. H. (1981). Temporal coding of species recognition signals in an electric fish. *Science 212:* 85–7.

Kalmijn, A. J. (1974). The detection of electric fields from inanimate and animate sources other than electric organs. In *Handbook of Sensory Physiology*, vol. III/3, ed. A. Fessard, pp. 147–200. Berlin, Heidelberg, New York: Springer-Verlag.

Knudsen, E. I., and Konishi, M. (1978a). A neural map of auditory space in the owl. *Science 200:* 795–7.

Knudsen, E. I., and Konishi, M. (1978b). Center-surround organization of auditory receptive fields in the owl. *Science 202:* 778–80.

Kuffler, S. W. (1953). Discharge patterns and functional organization of the mammalian retina. *J. Neurophysiol. 16:* 37–68.

Lissmann, H. W., and Machin, K. E. (1958). The mechanism of object location in *Gymnarchus niloticus* and similar fish. *J. Exp. Biol. 35:* 451–86.

Maler, L. (1979). The posterior lateral line lobe of certain gymnotoid fish: quantitative light microscopy. *J. Comp. Neurol. 183(2):* 323–64.

Maler, L., Finger, T., and Karten, H. J. (1974). Differential projections of ordinary lateral line and electroreceptors in the gymnotoid fish, *Apteronotus albifrons. J. Comp. Neurol. 158:* 363–82.

Maler, L. Sas, E., and Rogers J. (1981). The cytology of the posterior lateral line lobe of high-frequency weakly electric fish (Gymnotoidei): dendritic differentiation and synaptic specificity in a simple cortex. *J. Comp. Neurol. 195:* 87–139.

Maler, L., Sas, E., Carr, C. E., and Matsubara, J. (1982). Efferent projections of the posterior lateral line lobe in gymnotiform fish. *J. Comp. Neurol. 211:* 154–64.

Matsubara, J. A. (1981). Neural correlates of a nonjammable electrolocation system. *Science 211:* 722–5.

Matsubara, J., Finger, T. E., Maler, L., and Carr, C. E. (1981). Electrosensory, auditory and lateral line nuclei in the midbrain of a gymnotiform weakly electric fish, *Sternopygus. Neurosci. Abstr.* 28.11, Los Angeles, 1981.

Meyer, J. H. (1982). Behavioral responses of weakly electric fish to complex impedances. *J. Comp. Physiol. 145:* 459–70.

Meyer, J. H., and Zakon, H. (1982). Androgens alter the tuning of electroreceptors. *Science 217:* 635–7.

Newman, E. A., and Hartline, P. (1981). Integration of visual and infrared information in bimodal neurons of the rattlesnake optic tectum. *Science 213:* 789–91.

Partridge, B. L., and Heiligenberg, W. (1980). Three's a crowd? Predicting *Eigenmannia*'s responses to multiple jamming. *J. Comp. Physiol. 136:* 153–64.

Partridge, B. L., Heiligenberg, W., and Matsubara, J. (1981). The neural basis of a behavioral filter: no grandmother cells in sight. *J. Comp. Physiol. 145:* 153–68.

Scheich, H. (1977). Neural basis of communication in the high frequency electric fish, *Eigenmannia virescens* (Jamming Avoidance Response). *J. Comp. Physiol. 113:* 181– 255.

Scheich, H., and Bullock, T. H. (1974). The role of electroreceptors in the animal's life, II. The detection of electric fields from electric organs. In *Handbook of Sensory Physiology*, vol. III/3, ed. A. Fessard, pp. 201–56. Berlin, Heidelberg, New York: Springer-Verlag.

Scheich, H., Bullock, T. H., and Hamstra, R. H. (1973). Coding properties of two classes of afferent nerve fibers: high frequency electroreceptors in the electric fish, *Eigenmannia. J. Neurophysiol. 36:* 39–60.

Scheich, H., and Ebbesson, S. O. E. (1981). Inputs to the torus semicircularis in the electric fish *Eigenmannia virescens. Cell Tiss. Res. 215:* 531–6.

Simmons, J. A., Lavender, W. A., Lavender, B. A., Childs, J. E., Hulebak, K., Rigden, M. R., Sherman, J., and Woolman, B. (1978). Echolocation by free-tailed bats (Tadarida). *J. Comp. Physiol. 125:* 291–9.

Szabo, T., and Fessard, A. (1974). Physiology of electroreceptors. In *Handbook of Sensory Physiology*, vol. III/3, ed. A. Fessard, pp. 39–124. Berlin, Heidelberg, New York: Springer-Verlag.

Tokunaga, A., Akert, K., Sandri, C., and Bennett, M. V. L. (1980). Cell types and synaptic organization of the medullary electromotor nucleus in a constant frequency weakly electric fish, *Sternarchus albifrons. J. Comp. Neurol. 192:* 407–26.

Viancour, T. A. (1979). Electroreceptors of a weakly electric fish I and II. *J. Comp. Physiol. 133:* 317–38.

Watanabe, A., and Takeda, K. (1963). The change of discharge frequency by AC stimulus in a weakly electric fish. *J. Exp. Biol. 40:* 57–66.

Westby, G. W. M. (1974). Assessment of the signal value of certain discharge patterns in the electric fish, *Gymnotus carapo*, by means of playback. *J. Comp. Physiol. 92:* 327–41.

Zipser, B., and Bennett, M. V. L. (1976a). Responses of cells of the posterior lateral line lobe to activation of electroreceptors in a mormyrid fish. *J. Neurophysiol. 39(4):* 693–712.

Zipser, B., and Bennett, M. V. L. (1976b). Interaction of electrosensory and electromotor signals in the lateral line lobe of a mormyrid fish. *J. Neurophysiol. 39(4):* 713–21.

4.3

Navigation by polarized skylight

RÜDIGER WEHNER

Due to the scattering of light within the earth's atmosphere, skylight is polarized. In 1809 this phenomenon was discovered accidentally by the French physicist Etienne Malus when he was looking out of his window through a mineral crystal, but it was not until 1871 that John William Strutt, better known as Lord Rayleigh, gave a full mathematical description. However, almost a thousand years ago, the Vikings had already taken advantage of the polarized light in the sky by using it as a celestial compass while sailing west from Iceland and Greenland to Newfoundland. As pointed out by the Danish archeologist Thorkild Ramskou (1969), the sunstones described in the old sagas were nothing other than birefringent and dichroic crystals that could serve as polarization analysers. In more recent times, an airplane was steered with fair precision from Norway to Sondre Storm Fjord airfield in Greenland with such a crystal as the only compass aid, and even commercial airplanes have been equipped with polarization compasses. The most useful application of such a Sky Light Compass (see Kollman Instrument Corporation in References) is in polar regions and during twilight periods, when the sun is low on the horizon, or even below the horizon. Then, as can be deduced from Figure 1a, skylight emanating from the zenith is strongly polarized. It is this zenith polarization that is exploited by technical skylight compasses.

Recently it has been surmised that there are also some non-human vertebrates such as *fish* (reviewed by Waterman, 1975, see also Quinn and Brannon, 1982) and *amphibians* (reviewed by Taylor and Auburn, 1978) which are able to steer compass courses by polarized skylight. In the latter case it seems to be the pineal complex rather than the pair of lateral eyes that mediates the response. Even *birds* are now believed to

(a)   (b)

(1)

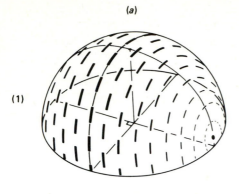
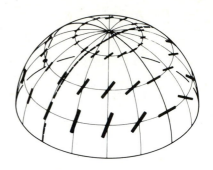

(2)

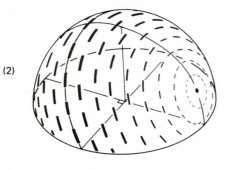
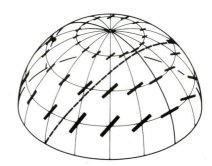

(3)

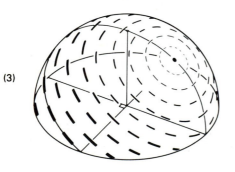
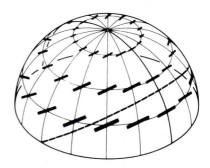

(4)

The caption to Figures 1–4 will be
found at the foot of page 500.

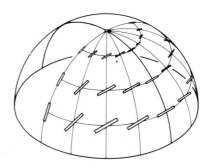

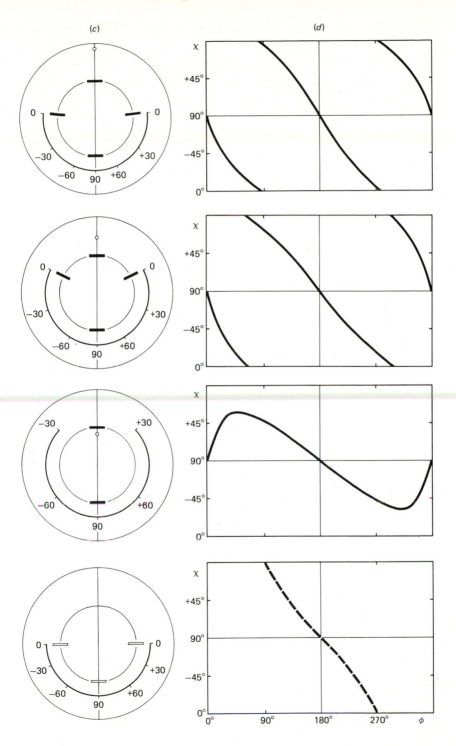

use skylight polarization for navigational means. In the laboratory, pigeons have been trained to discriminate between visual stimuli that differed in the state of polarization (Kreithen and Keeton, 1974; Delius, Perchard and Emmerton, 1976). As already reported much earlier by Kramer and St. Paul (1950), starlings can use skylight information as a compass even when the sun is not visible, but other investigators have

---

Figures 1–4. The patterns of polarized light in the sky (*1–3*) and the bee's celestial map (*4*). The skylight patterns are shown for three different elevations of the sun (*black disc*): 6° (*1*), 24° (*2*), and 53° (*3*). (*a*) Three-dimensional models of the patterns of polarized light in the sky. The directions and widths of the black bars mark the angles and degrees of polarization, respectively. Two great circles are shown, one including the solar and antisolar meridian, the other symbolizing the line of maximum polarization. Whereas direct light from the sun is unpolarized, light scattered by 90° is maximally polarized. In all figures (*a*) the solar meridian runs to the right. The pattern of polarized light is depicted in a celestial (sun-related) system of coordinates where the sun (and the antisun) form the poles of the sphere and the line of maximum polarization runs along the equator. Due to the laws of Rayleigh scattering, in such a system of coordinates the e-vectors are aligned with small circles running parallel to the equator. Apparently, the sun-related system of coordinates is the most convenient way of illustrating the geometry of the skylight patterns not only to the human observer but also to the navigating bee. What strikes the reader immediately about any of these patterns is its line of symmetry comprising the line of maximum polarization, and it is just this conspicuous feature of the pattern on which the bee's celestial map is based. In the horizon system of coordinates as shown in (*b*) another line of symmetry becomes apparent: the great circle consisting of the solar and antisolar meridian. The line of maximum polarization forms a symmetry line of the full sky only when the sun is at the horizon. (*b*) The same patterns of polarized light as shown in (*a*) but now presented in a horizon system of coordinates where the zenith (and the nadir) form the poles of the sphere and where the observer's horizon runs along the equator. Relative to (*a*) the celestial hemisphere is rotated by 180°, so that it is now the antisolar meridian that runs to the right. The *dashed line* marks the line of maximum polarization. As the sun moves up, this line tilts down. The distribution of e-vector directions is given for three parallels of altitude (22.5°, 45°, 67.5°). (*c*) The distribution of e-vectors for an elevation of 45° above the horizon. The azimuthal positions of horizontal (90°) and vertical (0°) e-vectors as well as the 30° and 60° e-vectors are indicated. (*d*) χ/φ functions relating e-vector direction (χ) with azimuthal distance from the sun (φ). The χ/φ functions are given for an elevation of 45° above horizon; compare (*c*) and the middle parallel of altitude in (*b*). The vertical and horizontal e-vectors are denoted by $\chi = 0°$ and 90°, respectively. $\varphi = 0°$, solar meridian; $\varphi = 180°$, antisolar meridian.

later stated that they had 'never obtained evidence that any other visual clue from the daylight sky, as for example the pattern of polarization, can guide the birds' (Hoffmann, 1960: p. 379). Recently, it has been suggested again that birds deduce some kind of navigational information from the polarization patterns in the sky (Able, 1982; Phillips and Waldvogel, 1982). After all, however, the animals in which navigation by polarized skylight has been demonstrated most convincingly and studied most extensively are the *insects* (for recent reviews see Waterman, 1981; Wehner, 1982a, and in press).

In this article, two questions will be raised dealing first with the polarization sensitivity of the eye and second with the compass strategy of the brain. Why is it that the visual systems of certain animals are sensitive to polarized light, and what are the strategies used by these animals to derive compass information from the pattern of polarized light in the sky? While the former question has attracted much attention from neuroanatomists and neurophysiologists, the latter has remained enigmatic.

(1) Polarization sensitivity

As is now well established, insects – and other arthropods as well – use the dichroism of their photoreceptor membranes as a means of analysing linearly polarized light. Rhabdomeric photoreceptors of many invertebrates are highly sensitive to polarized light because (1) the photoreceptor membranes are rolled into narrow tubes, the microvilli; (2) the molecular absorption vectors of the visual pigment are aligned, in the mean, parallel to the axes of the microvilli; and (3) the microvilli are aligned within the rhabdomere of the photoreceptor (for references see review articles in Snyder and Menzel, 1975; Goldsmith and Wehner, 1977; Wehner, in press).

In vertebrates, however, the photoreceptor membranes form flat discs. The disc membranes are fluid mosaics in which the rhodopsin molecules undergo rapid rotational diffusion (Brown, 1972; Cone, 1972), thus rendering on-axis dichroism impossible. How then do vertebrate eyes analyse polarized light? Three possibilities will be mentioned: (1) Light scattered within the retina could reach the outer segments of the photoreceptor cells in off-axis rather than on-axis directions (Snyder, 1973). Due to the disc array of their photoreceptor membranes, vertebrate photoreceptors are highly dichroic when stimulated perpendicularly to their optical axes, i.e. side-on (Liebman, 1962). (2) Some types of photoreceptor could be sensitive to polarized light owing either to structural specializations of the photoreceptors or to special geometrical arrangements of the photoreceptor cells within the retina. For example, in some groups of teleost fish the outer segments of particular cones are arranged in a way that betokens specialization. They are positioned side-on to the incident light (Fineran and Nicol, 1978). No one, however, has studied polarization vision in these teleosts. (3) Entoptic phenomena such as Haidinger's brushes (1844) or Boehm's brushes (1940) rather than the structure of the photoreceptors could be responsible for the polarization sensitivity of vertebrate eyes.

While Haidinger's brushes comprise a small foveal entopic image caused by the *dichroism of the yellow macular pigment* overlying the photoreceptors in the foveal region of the retina, Boehm's brushes are a parafoveal phenomenon due to *intraocular light scattering*. Either image can be described as a cross in which the two arms aligned at right angles to the direction of polarization are either dark (Haidinger's brushes) or light (Boehm's brushes). The latter effect is consistent with the observation that in a colloidal medium a light double cone occurs at right angles to the e-vector direction of a beam of light passing through the medium. The former effect arises from the circumferential alignment of the dichroic macular pigment, as already hypothesized by v. Helmholtz (1867: p. 422). Thus, looking through a polarizer at a brightly lit blue surface will reveal a dark brush oriented perpendicularly to the direction of polarization. The reason is that the dichroic pigment preferentially absorbs blue light (Wald, 1945). Yellow brushes appear instead of dark brushes when a white surface of polarized light is viewed. These are the 'flying phantoms of yellowish colour' described by Haidinger in 1844. Recently, it has been shown that the orientation of the brushes is further influenced by the birefringence of the collagen fibrils in the cornea (Shute, 1974).

The possibility that entoptic phenomena such as Haidinger's or Boehm's brushes could be exploited by vertebrates has lurked off and on in the wings ever since Waterman (1972) presented the first detailed account of polarization vision in vertebrates. It has even gained some support from electrophysiological studies on the optic tectum of the goldfish (Waterman and Aoki, 1974), but direct evidence for any such hypothesis is still missing. In humans at least, Haidinger's brushes are far too faint and unreliable to be able to serve for polarized-light navigation.

(2) Skylight compass

We would have little appreciation of the polarization sensitivity of any photoreceptor if we were unaware that the animal in question possessed the ability to use the pattern of polarized light in the sky as a compass. Of course, one can also conceive of other functions that are possibly mediated by polarization-sensitive photoreceptors (Wehner, in press), but until now most is known about the insect's polarization compass. Thus, this chapter deals exclusively with the perception of polarized skylight.

What strategy does the insect apply in deriving compass information from the pattern of polarized light in the sky? Attempts to answer this question were limited after von Frisch's (1949) early discovery until very recently when there was a remarkable recrudescence of interest in this subject. As nothing is known about the strategies applied by vertebrates, the following account will focus exclusively on insects.

The mere fact that bees and ants can navigate by using only a single small patch of polarized light in the sky is fascinating indeed. However, in trying to understand how the insect's celestial compass works this finding seems to have generated more speculative enthusiasm than experimental discipline. As tacitly assumed in most accounts, the insect should somehow be able to infer the position of the sun from analysing a single e-vector in the sky. In more specific hypotheses, the insect has been considered either to remember the skylight pattern last seen and later to match it with whatever pattern it experiences in the current sky (Stockhammer, 1959), or to perform three-dimensional geometry in the sky (Kirschfeld, Lindauer and Martin, 1975). No experimental results have been published to favour either hypothesis.

To understand the bee's strategy, one remarkable eccentricity must first be mentioned. As already surmised by von Frisch (1965: p. 409) and later shown by Rossel, Wehner and Lindauer (1978) and Brines and Gould (1979), bees do not use the degree of polarization as a compass cue, but rely exclusively on the direction of polarization. This is a sensible strategy, because the degree of polarization is affected severely by haze or clouds, but the direction of polarization is not (as recently confirmed by the comprehensive skylight measurements of Brines and Gould, 1982). However, disregarding the degree of polarization as a possible compass cue creates certain problems. As outlined in detail elsewhere (Wehner, in press), ambiguities arise whenever a compass direction must be inferred from a single point of polarized light in the sky and when the only information read off this point in the sky consists of the direction of polarization. Our curiosity was aroused when we found that even then the bees oriented unambiguously. How did they solve the problem of ambiguity?

The solution is charmingly simple. The bee does not perform

three-dimensional geometry in the sky, neither does it depend exclusively on the pattern last seen, nor does it rely on an astronomical almanac in which all possible skylight patterns are laid down. What it seems to have adopted instead is a simplified master-image of the sky, a highly generalized version of the celestial e-vector pattern. This master-image reflects the mean distribution of the maximally polarized e-vectors as they occur across the celestial canopy during the course of the day (Rossel and Wehner, 1982; Wehner, 1982b). Whereas the actual e-vector patterns in the sky vary with the elevation of the sun, the bee's celestial map does not. It only rotates about the zenith as the sun's azimuth changes during the day.

Using a simplified rather than correct map implies that navigational errors must occur. As the bee's celestial map (Figure 4b–d) is based exclusively on the maximally polarized e-vectors in the sky, it is confined to only one half of the celestial hemisphere, namely to the half lying opposite to the sun. In the real sky, this half is more highly polarized than the one around the sun. It had already been shown earlier by two independent research groups that whenever a single e-vector was presented to a dancing bee, the bee invariably interpreted this e-vector as lying in the highly- rather than the less-polarized part of the sky, even though this e-vector direction occurred in both halves of the sky (Rossel et al., 1978; Brines and Gould, 1979). The disagreement, however, was over whether the bee expected any particular e-vector exactly where it actually occurred in the sky (Brines and Gould, 1979) or whether the bee instead used a stereotyped celestial map and thus, under certain stimulus conditions, exhibited systematic navigational errors (Rossel et al., 1978). All recent experimental evidence at hand favours the latter hypothesis (Rossel and Wehner, 1982; Wehner, 1982a).

However intriguing the concept of the insect's generalized celestial map may be, there are at least three additional questions that spring to mind immediately. First, there is the question of *economics*: How can the insect afford to use a map that at any time of the day is an inaccurate map? No errors occur whenever the insect has access to the whole celestial hemisphere or to patches of skylight centred around the symmetry line of the highly polarized part of the sky, the antisolar meridian. The errors which occur under other circumstances are usually small. Consider, too, that in the less-polarized part of the sky the sun serves as an additional (unequivocal) compass cue. Thus, it is only when the bee has to rely exclusively on small patches of polarized light presented in the less-polarized part of the sky that navigational errors become really large. In all cases studied so far, however, the errors actually made by the dancing bee could be predicted exactly from the bee's celestial map as depicted in Figure 4b–d. In the foraging bee, any such error is certainly kept down by the additional use of some powerful backup systems such as piloting (Wehner, 1981).

Secondly, there is the question of *evolutionary and developmental biology*. How has the simplified map of the e-vector pattern in the sky been incorporated into the insect's visual system? Certainly, this map is not a figment of the insect's mind. As natural selection does not favour piecemeal tinkering, there must be a rule by which the insect has derived its celestial map from the actual skylight patterns. As outlined above, this rule is indeed rather simple. There is only one aspect of skylight polarization that contributes to the map: the distribution of the maximally-polarized e-vectors in the sky.

Thirdly, of course, there is the question of *neurobiology*. What does such a map mean in physiological terms? Is it laid down at a peripheral, even retinal, level? Or is there a more central map? The neuroanatomy and neurophysiology of the polarization analysers within the insect's retina have been studied in detail, and retinal maps of receptor arrays have been drawn recently for bees and ants (for review see Wehner, 1982a, and in press), but nothing at all is known about the routes along which the information about polarized skylight might travel beyond the level of the retina. No one has recorded yet from any insect interneuron that is sensitive to polarized light. However, the discovery of the bee's strategy to deal with skylight polarization may be a powerful spur to define the problems with which neurophysiologists must contend. The race is now on to unravel the insect's neural map of the sky.

References

Able, K. P. (1982). Skylight polarization patterns at dusk influence migratory orientation in birds. *Nature 299:* 550–1.

Bernard, G., and Wehner, R. (1977). Functional similarities between polarization vision and color vision. *Vision Res. 17:* 1019–28.

Boehm, G. (1940). Ueber ein neues entoptisches Phänomen im polarisierten Licht. 'Periphere' Polarisationsbüschel. *Acta Ophthalmol. 18:* 143–60.

Brines, M. L., and Gould, J. L. (1979). Bees have rules. *Science 206:* 571–3.

Brines, M. L., and Gould, J. L. (1982). Skylight polarization patterns and animal orientation. *J. Exp. Biol. 96:* 69–91.

Brown, P. K. (1972). Rhodopsin rotates in the visual receptor membrane. *Nature 236:* 35–8.

Cone, R. A. (1972). Rotational diffusion of rhodopsin in the visual receptor membrane. *Nature 236:* 39–43.

Delius, J. D., Perchard, R. J., and Emmerton, J. (1976). Polarized light discrimination by pigeons and an electroretinographic correlate. *J. Comp. Physiol. Psychol. 90:* 560–71.

Fineran, B. A., and Nicol, J. A. C. (1978). Studies on the photoreceptors of *Anchoa mitchilli* and *Anchoa hepsetus* (Engraulidae) with particular reference to the cones. *Phil. Trans. Roy. Soc. Lond. Biol. 283:* 25–60.

Frisch, K. v. (1949). Die Polarisation des Himmelslichts als orientierender Faktor bei den Tänzen der Bienen. *Experientia 5:* 142–8.

Frisch, K. v. (1965). *Tanzsprache und Orientierung der Bienen.* Berlin, Heidelberg, New York: Springer-Verlag.

Goldsmith, T. H., and Wehner, R. (1977). Restrictions of rotational and translational diffusion of pigment in the membranes of a rhabdomeric photoreceptor. *J. Gen. Physiol. 70:* 453–90.

Haidinger, W. (1844). Ueber das direkte Erkennen des polarisierten Lichts und der Lage der Polarisationsebene. *Ann. Phys. (Leipzig) 63:* 29–39.

Helmholtz, H. v. (1867). *Handbuch der physiologischen Optik.* Leipzig: L. Voss.

Hoffmann, K. (1960). Experimental manipulation of the orientation clock in birds. *Cold Spring Harb. Symp. quant. Biol. 25:* 379–87.

Kirschfeld, K., Lindauer, M., and Martin, H. (1975). Problems of menotactic orientation according to the polarized light of the sky. *Z. Naturf. 30c:* 88–90.

Kollman Instrument Corporation. *Installation, Operation and Service Instructions of the Polarized Sky Light Compass.* Elmhurst, NY, USA: Kollman Instrument Corp.

Kramer, G., and St. Paul, U. v. (1950). Stare (*Sturnus vulgaris*) lassen sich auf Himmelsrichtungen dressieren. *Naturwissenschaften 37:* 526–7.

Kreithen, M. L., and Keeton, W. T. (1974). Detection of polarized light by the homing pigeon, *Columbia livia. J. Comp. Physiol. 89:* 83–92.

Liebmann, P. A. (1962). In situ microspectrophotometric studies on the pigments of single retinal rods. *Biophys. J. 2:* 161–78.

Malus, E. (1809). Sur une propriété de la lumière réfléchie par les corps diaphanes. *Bull. Sci. Soc. Philom. (Paris) 1:* 266–9.

Phillips, J. B., and Waldvogel, J. A. (1982). Reflected light cues generate the short-term deflector-loft effect. In *Avian Navigation*, ed. F. Papi and H. G. Wallraff, pp. 190–202. Berlin, Heidelberg, New York: Springer-Verlag.

Quinn, T. P., and Brannon, E. L. (1982). The use of celestial and magnetic cues by orienting sockeye smolts. *J. Comp. Physiol. 147:* 547–52.

Ramskou, T. (1969). *Solstenen. Primitiv Navigation i Norden før Kompasset.* København: Rhodos.

Rossel, S., and Wehner, R. (1982). The bee's map of the e-vector pattern in the sky. *Proc. Natn. Acad. Sci. USA 79:* 4451–5.

Rossel, S., Wehner, R., and Lindauer, M. (1978). E-vector orientation in bees. *J. Comp. Physiol. 125:* 1–12.

Shute, C. C. D. (1974). Haidinger's brushes and predominant orientation of collagen in corneal stroma. *Nature 250:* 163–4.

Snyder, A. W. (1973). How fish detect polarized light. *Invest. Ophthalmol. 12:* 78–9.

Snyder, A. W., and Menzel, R., eds (1975). *Photoreceptor Optics.* Berlin, Heidelberg, New York: Springer-Verlag.

Stockhammer, K. (1959). Die Orientierung nach der Schwingungsrichtung linear polarisierten Lichtes und ihre sinnesphysiologischen Grundlagen. *Erg. Biol. 21:* 23–56.

Strutt, J. W. (1871). On the light from the sky, its polarization and colour. *Phil. Mag.* *41:* 107–20, 274–9.

Taylor, D. H., and Auburn, J. S. (1978). Orientation of amphibians by linearly polarized light. In *Animal Migration, Navigation, and Homing*, ed. K. Schmidt-Koenig and W. T. Keeton, pp. 334–46. Berlin, Heidelberg, New York: Springer-Verlag.

Wald, G. (1945). Human vision and the spectrum. *Science 101:* 653–8.

Waterman, T. H. (1972). Visual direction finding by fishes. In *Animal Orientation and Navigation*, ed. S. R. Galler, K. Schmidt-Koenig, G. J. Jacobs and R. E. Belleville, pp. 437–56. Washington, DC: National Aeronautics and Space Administration.

Waterman, T. H. (1975). Natural polarized light and e-vector discrimination by vertebrates. In *Light as an Ecological Factor*, vol. II, ed. G. C. Evans, R. Bainbridge and O. Rackham, pp. 305–35. Oxford: Blackwell.

Waterman, T. H. (1981). Polarization sensitivity. In *Handbook of Sensory Physiology*, vol. VII/6B, ed. H. Autrum, pp. 281–469. Berlin, Heidelberg, New York: Springer-Verlag.

Waterman, T. H., and Aoki, K. (1974). E-vector sensitivity patterns in the goldfish optic tectum. *J. Comp. Physiol. 95:* 13–27.

Wehner, R. (1981). Spatial vision in arthropods. In *Handbook of Sensory Physiology*, vol. VII/6C, ed. H. Autrum, pp. 287–616. Berlin, Heidelberg, New York: Springer-Verlag.

Wehner, R. (1982a). Himmelsnavigation bei Insekten. Neurophysiologie und Verhalten. *Neujahrsbl. Naturf. Ges. Zürich 184:* 1–132.

Wehner, R. (1982b). The bee's celestial map – a simplified model of the outside world. In *The Biology of Social Insects*, ed. M. D. Breed, C. D. Michener and H. E. Evans, pp. 375–9. Boulder (Colorado): Westview Press.

Wehner, R. The perception of polarized light. In *The Biology of Photoreceptors*, ed. D. Cosens and D. Vince-Prue. Cambridge: Cambridge University Press (in press).

4.4

Electroreceptor mechanisms in teleost and non-teleost fishes

S. OBARA and Y. SUGAWARA

Electroreceptors in fish are secondary sensory organs specialized to detect a weak electric field in the water. They are derivatives of the acousticolateralis system, and share many morphological and functional features in common with more familiar mechanosensitive hair cells. Morphological adaptations in their accessory structures and ciliary appendages have been reviewed (see Szabo, 1974). Response properties of various receptor types have been extensively studied. Detailed analysis of receptor mechanisms is also available in a few cases, which will be the main topics in this paper.

This presentation attempts to deduce certain general features in electroreceptor mechanisms despite apparent diversity among various receptor types. Trends of convergent evolution toward their high detection sensitivity may also provide some clues in understanding sensitive receptor mechanisms of other modalities.

Overview

Basic morphology and operation of electroreceptors are summarized in Figure 1 (see Bennett and Clusin, 1979). The sensory epithelium forms an ampulla which lies beneath epidermis. The ampullary lumen is connected to the outside through a duct of varying length. The receptor cells (RC) are joined to neighboring supporting cells (SC) by occluding or tight junctions (ZO) which prevent current leakage through intercellular clefts. The receptor cell membrane is thus divided into two parts: *apical* (lumenal, outer or ciliated) face and *basal* (serosal, inner or presynaptic) face. A lumen-positive (anodal) stimulus tends to hyperpolarize the apical face, and to depolarize the basal face. A lumen-negative (cathodal) stimulus has the reverse effect. Ensuing

509

differential polarization of the two opposing membranes may activate voltage-sensitive ionic channels in either or both faces (thick arrows). The receptor cell response under physiological conditions shows diverse variety in different receptors, ranging from almost linear response to graded oscillation, and even to an all-or-none receptor spike (Bennett, 1967). The net result is to produce presynaptic depolarization in the basal face which is then transmitted synaptically to the afferent nerves (N) to be encoded into various impulse patterns (see Bullock, 1973). In most cases the synaptic transmission is mediated chemically, but electrical transmission is also known to occur in certain species. In contrast to most mechanosensitive hair cells, efferent synapse is absent. Efferent control on afferent information flow occurs only within the CNS (see Hopkins, 1981).

Non-teleost receptors

Since the early study on elasmobranchs (Murray, 1965), search for likely electroreceptive species has been greatly extended. It now appears that nearly all non-teleosts are electroreceptive (see Bullock, Northcutt and Bodznick, 1982). Evidence is not yet complete, but judging by the few well-studied cases, all non-teleost receptors appear to be uniform (Figure 1); the receptor cell has a single kinocilium at the apical face, and the afferent nerve discharge is facilitated by a lumen-negative stimulus (and suppressed by a lumen-positive stimulus). This polarity effect comes from the presence of an electrically-excitable membrane at the apical face as will be discussed below. In addition, they are all *ampullary receptors* in structure, and sensitive to low-frequency signals (*low-frequency receptor*). There is usually 'resting' afferent discharge of fairly regular frequency, which is gradedly modulated by applied stimuli (*F coder*). 'Off' rebounds are usually observed to occur after the end of stimuli.

Ampullae of Lorenzini of skate, a marine elasmobranch, are extremely sensitive electroreceptors, capable of detecting changes of a few microvolts. The ampullae are buried deep beneath the body surface to which they are connected by long jelly-filled ampullary ducts. This is generally regarded as an adaptation to high-conductivity milieu (see Kalmijn, 1974). Because of this structure they can be removed easily from the fish for *in vitro* experiments.

An early microelectrode study recording from ampullary lumen and afferent nerve has proposed a somewhat complex receptor mechanism (Obara and Bennett, 1972). Briefly, a lumen-negative stimulus depolarizes and excites the apical face. Apical inward current thus evoked flows outward across and depolarizes the basal face, which then releases excitatory transmitter to the afferent (Figure 1). Also postulated is an ongoing activity of the apical face in the absence of stimuli. A lumen-positive stimulus hyperpolarizes the apical face and suppresses this ongoing activity, which results in decreased transmitter release, and finally in afferent suppression – or more appropriately called – disfacilitation (see Obara and Oomura, 1973). In other words, the apical face behaves as a receptive membrane, and the basal face as a presynaptic and secretory membrane.

In a later series of current- and voltage-clamp experiments, an individual ampulla was isolated electrically by exposing the long duct to the air. Thus isolated, the ampulla shows a lumen-positive d.c. potential (10–30 mV), and a large lumen-negative receptor spike (up to 100 mV and lasting *c.* 100 ms) on stimulation. In voltage-clamp analysis, the following four types of ionic currents were described in addition to leakage current: (a) at the apical face (Clusin and Bennett, 1977a,b); (1) V-sensitive Ca current and (2) Ca-induced late current (presumably K),

Figure 1. Diagram of electroreceptor cells of non-teleost (skate) and teleost (*Plotosus*). RC, receptor cell; SC, supporting cell; ZO, zonula occludens; N, afferent nerve. Receptor cell membrane is divided by ZO into apical and basal faces. Main inward current components, Ca current, are shown by thick arrows. Upper insets: *In situ* responses to facilitatory stimuli are shown schematically. I, stimulus; V, lumen potential, positivity shown up, N, single afferent response. Note different stimulus polarity for afferent facilitation. Lower insets: Epithelial current pattern. $I_{ep.}$, active current, inward in respective membrane site shown downward.

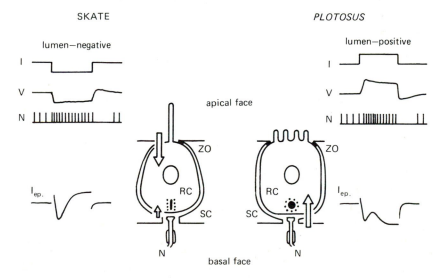

and (b) at the basal face (Clusin and Bennett, 1979b); (3) V-sensitive Ca current and (4) V-sensitive K current (also Ca-induced?). Of these, the apical components are dominant in generating the receptor spike. It may be worth noting that apical Ca current acts only as the charge carrier, while basal Ca current controls transmitter release. The basal components normally show only small conductance changes, but can modulate the ampullary response, as will be described below.

Combined operation of these currents under *in situ* conditions was nicely simulated by shunting the isolated ampulla with a salt bridge (Clusin and Bennett, 1979a). The ongoing epithelial current hypothe-sized previously was confirmed to flow inward across the apical face (Figure 2a). A lumen-negative stimulus enhances the epithelial current, and a lumen-positive stimulus suppresses it, also in support of the

Figure 2. Ampullary receptor of skate. The isolated ampulla is shunted by a salt bridge to simulate the *in situ* responses. (*a*) Presence of d.c. epithelial current and of spontaneous oscillation. (A1)– (A3), spontaneous voltage oscillations in the ampulla (lumen-negative up). (B), active d.c. current is flowing inward through the apical face (inward shown down). (*b*) Responses of the shunted ampulla to small stimuli. V, ampullary potential (lumen-negative up); N, PSP recorded external from the afferent nerve (spikes are abolished by TTX); I, epithelial current (inward shown down). (A) and (B), small lumen-negative and -positive stimuli can produce discernible de- and hyperpolarization in N. (C), slightly larger lumen-positive stimulus suppressed oscillations in V and I, and produced clear hyperpolarization in N. OFF oscillation was followed by similar PSP oscillation with a delay of about 20 ms. (D), spontaneous oscillation and associated PSP with similar delay. (Modified from Clusin and Bennett, 1979a.)

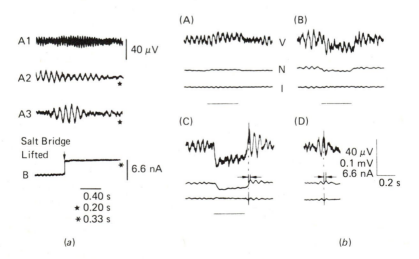

hypothesis. This epithelial current is superposed by small irregular oscillations of fixed frequency (*c.* 20 Hz) which are associated with similar PSP oscillation (Figure 2b). The oscillations appear to result from modulation of the predominant apical current through an inter-action with K and Ca conductances activated in the opposing basal face. Correlation of the ampullary responses with PSP outputs indicates that *in situ* the ampulla is operating in the negative impedance region of the apical face (Figure 3). It may deserve attention that PSP maxima occur with very small excursion ($\pm 400 \,\mu$V) in the negative impedance region which may span over 20–30 mV in an isolated ampulla (see Figure 3 in Clusin and Bennett, 1979b, for comparison).

Figure 3. Voltage-current relations with PSP in the shunted skate ampulla. (*a*) Sample records. Stimulus strength in mV is indicated to the left. Note that facilitatory stimuli (lumen-negative) are defined as positive. Epithelial current is shown inward down. Depolarizing PSP is shown up. Damped oscillations were produced in the epithelial current records. (*b*) Voltage-current relations with PSP amplitude. In (A), peak current is linearly related to voltage between -0.6 and 1.0 mV, with a negative slope. For larger suppressive stimuli, the V–I relation shows a positive slope. PSP changes steeply and saturates on ± 400-μV changes in V, indicating sensitive transduction process. In (B), epithelial current just before stimulus termination is plotted. Linearity of the relation and the negative slope features remain for moderate stimuli, but the slope is less steep. Maximum PSP deflections are smaller. (Modified from Clusin and Bennett, 1979a.)

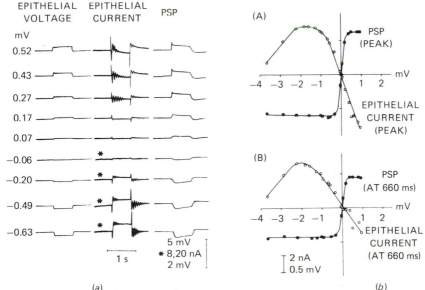

One interesting corollary of the receptor mechanism may be pointed out. Referring again to the diagram in Figure 1, the basal face of non-teleost receptors may be assumed to receive two opposing currents, *extrinsic* due to external voltage source and *intrinsic* due to the apical face activity. Normally, the intrinsic current is much larger, and dominates basal face polarization and hence transmitter release. Very strong stimuli, however, can override the intrinsic current and directly polarize the basal face. The stimulus polarity effect then will be reversed compared to that of weaker stimuli (Obara and Bennett, 1972). Thus, the skate might perceive very strong stimuli as being weak and of wrong polarity! This 'overstimulation phenomenon' was first described, but erroneously, by Murray (1965). An elegant demonstration was recently obtained in sturgeon (Teeter, Szamier and Bennett, 1980).

Teleost receptors

In contrast to non-teleosts, electroreception is found only in three orders of teleosts: Mormyriformes, Gymnotiformes and Siluriformes. There is a diverse variety of receptor types suggesting their independent evolution. All teleost receptors, however, share certain properties in common, and are distinctly different from those in non-teleosts (Figure 1). The receptor cell has no kinocilium, but bears microvilli at the apical face. The afferent discharge is facilitated by a lumen-positive stimulus since excitable membrane is in the basal face (see Bennett, 1971).

Ampullary receptors in teleost are found in both electric and non-electric fishes. Their response properties as *low-frequency receptor* and *F coder* are similar to non-teleost receptors, except with the 'inverted' polarity effect as noted above. Aside from the early example in weakly electric fish (Bennett, 1965), most data on receptor mechanisms were obtained from non-electric catfishes, one marine *Plotosus* (Obara, 1976) and another freshwater *Kryptopterus* (Bennett, 1971).

Plotosus ampullary receptors have long ducts, similar to those in skate (Friedrich-Freksa, 1930). This is a marked example of convergent evolution of common adaptive processes toward high-conductivity milieu, and also an excellent adaptation for neurophysiological use! The receptor mechanism proposed for *Plotosus* (Obara, 1976) is very similar to that of skate, except that the excitable membrane is now localized experimentally in the basal face (Akutsu and Obara, 1974). The apical face is inactive (Sugawara and Obara, 1979) and probably of low resistance as was suggested for gymnotid small receptors (Bennett, 1967), and confirmed by intracellular recording in transparent catfish *Kryptopterus* (Bennett, 1971). Much of the stimulus voltage, therefore, will develop across the basal face. The basal face of an ampulla *in situ* is spontaneously active as indicated by the 'resting' afferent discharge. Though opposite in polarity from skate receptor, the ongoing basal face activity is similarly modulated gradedly by incoming stimuli. The voltage sensitivity in terms of afferent frequency outputs is high, approaching that of the skate receptor.

The ongoing basal face activity in *Plotosus* receptor is induced by a shunt pathway external to the sensory epithelium (Obara, 1974). When the ampulla is electrically isolated (or current-clamped), the ampullary lumen changes negatively by 16–20 mV, and transmitter release virtually stops judging by near absence of the afferent activity. The ampulla shows large positive-going response with finite voltage threshold at near zero level (Figure 4, inset). The response is long-lasting and Ca-dependent, which is associated with transmitter release (Akutsu and

Figure 4. Ampullary receptor of *Plotosus*. (A) Comparison of I–V relations of the same ampulla under two conditions, *in situ* (filled circles) and electrically isolated (open circles). Note that the *in situ* ampulla is shunted by its own duct, and held biased near zero level. (B), Non-linear responses of the *in situ* ampulla around the resting level, recorded at higher gain. UNDERSHOOT: lumen potential with suppressed receptor cell activity following a strong activation. (C) Sample records. N, afferent impulses with PSP, external recording; I, stimulus current; V, ampullary lumen potential (lumen-positive up). Responses to lumen-negative (cath.) and lumen-positive (an.) stimuli are superimposed as marked in N traces. Symbols at the end of stimulus indicate the measurements plotted in (A) and (B). (Modified from Obara, 1974.)

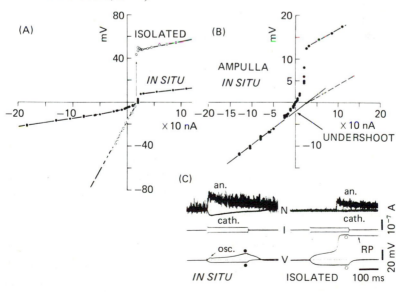

Obara, 1974). Prior to isolation, the ampulla *in situ* shows a much smaller d.c. potential near zero level, and also smaller voltage responses which may become oscillatory (osc. in inset) or gradedly regenerative upon stronger lumen-positive stimuli. There is a continual transmitter release leading to 'resting' afferent discharge. Comparison of their I-V relations (Figure 4A) clearly indicates that the *in situ* ampulla is shunted by the low-impedance of the duct, and held biased near zero level.

Closer inspection further suggests additional peculiarity of the biased sensory epithelium. When polarized beyond some $\pm 5\,mV$, the ampullary responses are quite linear, with a suggestion of fully activated state in the depolarized quadrant. In between and around the resting level, however, the responses are non-linear, showing slight upward concavity (Figure 4B). Evidently, the basal face is contributing voltage-dependent graded activity over a passive I-R drop. The amount of this contribution at the resting level may be inferred by extrapolation of the passive I-R drop line to ordinate (marked by arrow in Figure 4B). The ampulla becomes hyperpolarized to this level during undershoot immediately after strong activation, which indicates a d.c. bias current flowing outward to the basal face. Thus activated, the basal face is normally giving the receptor activity at 'rest' (Obara, 1974).

Voltage-clamp experiments on *Plotosus* receptor revealed a complex inward current pattern with two distinct peaks, fast and slow (Figure 1). As shown already in skate receptor, the transepithelial voltage-clamp suffers several inherent drawbacks because the two membranes are present in series in the current path. Some insight, however, can be gained by considering the differential polarization of the two opposing membranes (see Overview). A tentative summary may be given: (a) apical face (Sugawara and Obara, 1979); (1) slowly developing outward current (presumably K), which may prove essential for the low-resistance of the apical face, although demonstrated as yet only at very high level over $-150\,mV$; (b) basal face (Obara and Sugawara, 1979; Sugawara and Obara, 1979); (2) V-sensitive Ca current; and (3) small transient outward current (Ca-induced K current), which is partially abolished by 4-aminopyridine or by Ba replacement of Ca. In addition, (4) a larger maintained outward current (Ca-induced, and presumably non-specific) is strongly suggested in the basal face, but not yet identified.

Combined operation of these currents may best be demonstrated by responses of the *in situ* ampulla (Figure 5). The ampullary responses to moderate stimuli are symmetrical at a hyperpolarized level. The responses are larger and asymmetrical at the resting level, and show marked oscillations in depolarizing direction, associated with similar PSP oscillations (Figure 5B). The oscillations are abolished by 4-aminopyridine. Addition of Ca blocker, Co or Cd, further abolishes the resting Ca activation so that the responses at the resting level become smaller and symmetrical, approaching those at the hyperpolarized level. The synaptic transmission is also blocked. Thus, V-sensitive Ca current (2) and Ca-induced transient K current (3) play major roles in receptor operation. The Ca-induced maintained component (4) is probably involved in sensory adaptation (Obara and Higuchi, 1978).

Notice that the ampullary oscillations are apparent only when driven to supermaximal levels for the afferent output. The ampulla behaves quite linearly within the system's operating range which is less than one millivolt in terms of afferent frequency output. Overall input-output property of *Plotosus* receptor is shown together with normalized contributions of intermediate processes in Figure 6 (Obara, Higuchi and Nagai, 1981), in which only a small part of the receptor activity is engaged to produce PSP maxima. In recent experiments the ampulla was shunted by an electronic shunt circuit, similar in principle to the patch-clamp circuit (Neher, Sakmann and Steinbach, 1978). The PSP maxima proved to occur by small changes in epithelial current in its negative impedance property as shown in skate receptor (see Figure 3).

The high-gain synaptic transfer in secondary sensory organs was first suggested in small receptors of electric fish (Bennett, 1965). The high-gain transfer characteristics shown in Figure 6 have been discussed elsewhere. Briefly, the synaptic transfer in terms of PSP output is

Figure 5. Non-linear responses of *Plotosus in situ* ampulla and ionic channels in the basal face. Abbreviations for the traces are the same as in Figure 4. Afferent impulses are abolished by TTX. (A) Control responses at resting and hyperpolarized levels, showing the voltage-dependent non-linearity in the *in situ* ampulla. (B) 4-aminopyridine (4-AP, 2 mM) in the bath abolishes oscillation in V, but the V-dependent non-linearity persists. (C) Addition of Cd (0.1 mM) blocks the non-linear responses in V and also synaptic transmission.

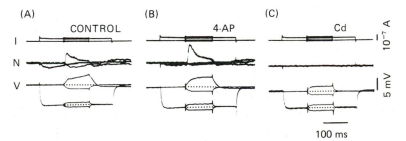

a steep sigmoid against the ampullary potential input, and shifted to the left along the input axis to the extent to produce 'resting' outputs. The shift of the transfer property is the direct consequence of the biased sensory epithelium.

Tuberous receptors are another class of teleost receptors which have evolved only in weakly electric fish, Mormyriformes and Gymnotiformes. Since they are apparently specialized to detect the electric field produced by electric-organ discharges (EOD), they are best discussed in connection with electrolocation or electrocommunication. Only relevant properties with respect to receptor mechanism will be reviewed (see Bennett, 1967, 1971; Bennett and Clusin, 1979).

In tuberous receptors, mechanical shielding is almost complete because the ampullary lumen is loosely packed with a small cell cluster (hence the tuberous appearance). Their afferent nerve shows little or no 'resting' discharge, and responds only to higher-frequency signals (*high-frequency receptor*). Normally, they are driven by the fish's own EOD, and fire afferent impulses with specific patterns (various *encoding types*). Receptor cell activity can be recorded as positive-going response

Figure 6. Input–output property of *Plotosus in situ* ampulla. Contributions of intermediate processes are shown normalized to each respective output maximum. Ordinate: outputs of each of the processes, normalized to respective output maxima. Abscissa: ampullary potential. Maximum values for each process are: PSP, c. 50 mV p–p, recorded internally from the afferent nerve; frequency, c. 400 s^{-1} at the peak and 200–250 s^{-1} at 200 ms; and receptor activity, c. 12 mV. The receptor activity is estimated as the active increments in ampullary potential as shown in Figure 4B. Insets to the right, composite sample records. I, V and N, as in Figures 4 and 5. P, externally recorded PSP, with afferent impulses attenuated by low-pass filtering; F, instantaneous frequency display of the single unit discharges shown in N trace. (From Obara, Higuchi and Nagai, 1981.)

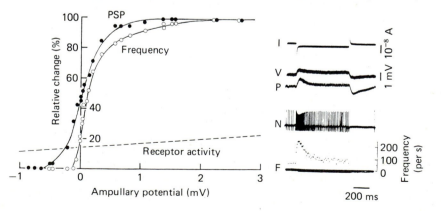

at the receptor opening. Graded oscillations or sharp receptor spikes are evoked by lumen-positive stimuli of a few tenths of a millivolt to a few millivolts. The responses become larger and, in some cases, begin to fire spontaneously, when the receptor opening is exposed over the water. Evidently, the receptors are normally shunted and loaded down by the water.

These response properties suggest that, first, the apical face is inactive and acts in a blocking capacity (d.c. insensitivity), and second, the basal face is excitable and is held biased close to the threshold level. Little is known of the ionic mechanisms involved in these processes. The receptor responses are insensitive to TTX, which suggests Ca conductance in the basal face (Zipser and Bennett, 1976). Receptor oscillations and spikes may also involve Ca-induced outward currents, similar to those in ampullary receptors.

The most conspicuous property of these receptors is that they are tuned to the fish's own EOD (see Viancour, 1979). Some receptor afferents are known to be as sharply tuned as cochlear afferents. This property resides mainly in receptor cells, because receptor oscillations and spikes are critically tuned to the EOD frequency spectrum. In other words, tuberous receptors behave as an active filter. Curiously, although the afferent impulses are evoked with specific patterns, individual impulses are only poorly correlated in phase with the receptor response. Their synaptic transfer properties need further clarification.

Strategies for high detection sensitivity

It is generally presumed that electroreceptors have evolved from mechanoreceptors of an ancestral lateral line system through a combination of adaptive processes; a reduction in mechanical sensitivity through loss of sensory hairs at the apical face and changes in accessory structures as for mechanical shielding, and an increase in electrical sensitivity which is potentially present due primarily to their strategic location. Electrical sensitivity is well known in receptors over the body surface, such as lateral-line organs and taste buds.

Aside from the morphological adaptations, electroreceptors are characterized by an increased density of voltage-sensitive Ca channels in the receptive membrane. This membrane process clearly serves for signal amplification over a simple I-V drop which would be induced in a passive membrane. Voltage amplification could not be made too excessive to become fully regenerative, if stimulus increments are to be encoded. Fully regenerative response, a receptor spike, does occur in some cases for detection of other fishes' EOD in electrocommunication.

The receptor spike can be shown, under certain conditions, even in ampullary receptors which normally behave quite linearly. The high sensitivity, either incremental or absolute, thus apparently was achieved by a common membrane process. In contrast, hair cell receptors have receptive membrane at the apical face which involves conductance changes to K (Corey and Hudspeth, 1979; Crawford and Fettiplace, 1981). The basal face presumably has some Ca channels for synaptic transmission, but their voltage contribution is rarely observed (Hudspeth and Corey, 1977). Fairly linear response of the basal face, however, proved to serve for high-gain synaptic transfer in teleost electroreceptors (Bennett, 1967; Obara, 1976; Obara et al., 1981), and may also play a similar role in hair cell synapses.

Despite the vast variety in receptor responses and different membrane loci, certain prevalent strategies for the high detection sensitivity may be deduced. First, their sensory epithelium is *held biased* for their optimum operation. In ampullary receptors this biased condition is achieved by a low-impedance shunt pathway external to the epithelium. It is worth noting that the essentially non-linear property of V-sensitive Ca channels is tamed to serve as a gradedly linear signal transfer with certain amplification. In tuberous receptors the d.c. bias is probably supplied by a built-in process within the basal membrane. The external shunt, however, does provide low resistance loading, by which optimum damping is obtained for a potentially oscillating reactive basal face.

Second, it may be amusing to note that we have arrived only recently at a technique of *modulation of carrier signals* to improve S/N ratio for effective signal transmission. A simple FM system is apparently in use in ampullary receptors, their carrier signal being a regular 'resting' discharge. In tuberous receptors the carrier signal is more complex, and consists of an EOD-driven afferent impulse pattern of various encoding modes. Complex but stereotyped carrier signals, specific to each receptor type, allow information extraction of more complex nature. The receptors driven by EOD can also be relatively immune to external electrical noise. The tuberous receptors are often called 'phasic', because in EOD-silenced preparations they give only transient response to d.c. stimulation. This term, however, may be misleading in view of the modulation mechanism outlined above. Normally they are driven by EOD, and known to signal the presence of an external object 'tonically'.

Finally, *electrical tuning* of passive and active nature has been shown further to improve S/N ratio. Ampullary receptors have accessory structures which provide passive low-pass filter property (see Waltman, 1966). Sensory adaptation further provides very-low-frequency cutoff, thus presumably ensuring a stable operation of the high-sensitivity systems. In contrast, tuberous receptors have blocking capacity at the apical face as a part of passive high-pass filter (Bennett, 1967). In most receptors, afferent discharges are critically tuned to the fish's own EOD (see Hopkins, 1976); oscillatory responses of the basal face may provide active filtering. Ionic mechanisms involved in tuned oscillation are unknown, but Ca-induced K conductance has been implied (Bennett and Clusin, 1979).

Notice that these strategies in fact are not unique to electroreception, but can also be found in other sensory modalities. The biased sensory epithelium has long been proposed in auditory transduction hypothesis (Davis, 1965), although the postulated bias current was experimentally confirmed only in ampullary receptors. In combination with similarly biased receptor cells, the modulation mechanism of various kinds of carrier signal is almost ubiquitous among sensitive receptors, e.g. vertebrate retina or vestibular apparatus. The electrical tuning through specific membrane properties was recently demonstrated in hair cell receptors (Crawford and Fettiplace, 1981).

Summary

Electroreceptors of non-teleost and teleost fishes were compared with particular reference to their common evolutional target, the high sensitivity to weak electric field. Voltage-sensitive Ca channels in the receptive membrane, though occurring in different membrane sites, proved to provide a basis of high-gain transduction process. Stable operation of such a high-gain system might further involve Ca-induced ionic channels, as demonstrated in certain species. Despite apparent diversity in various receptor types, several prevalent strategies for the high detection sensitivity can be recognised. A number of these mechanisms, such as the biased sensory epithelium, may be relevant to operation of mechanosensitive hair cells in the related acousticolateralis system, and also of higher-order receptors of other sensory modalities.

This work was supported in part by the grant from the Ministry of Education, Science and Culture, 00548101.

References

Akutsu, Y., and Obara, S. (1974). Calcium dependent receptor potential of the electroreceptor of marine catfish. *Proc. Japan Acad. 50:* 247–51.

Bennett, M. V. L. (1965). Electroreceptors in Mormyrids. *Cold Spring Harbor Symp. Quant. Biol. 30:* 245–62.

Bennett, M. V. L. (1967). Mechanisms of electroreception. In *Lateral Line Detectors*, ed. P. Cahn, vol. *20:* 313–93. Indiana University Press, Bollmington.

Bennett, M. V. L. (1971). Electroreception. In *Fish Physiology*, ed. W. S. Hoar and D. S. Randall, vol. V, 493–574. New York: Academic Press.

Bennett, M. V. L., and Clusin, W. T. (1979). Transduction at electroreceptors: origins of sensitivity. In *Membrane Transduction Mechanisms*, ed. R. A. Cone and J. E. Dowling, pp. 91–116, New York: Raven Press.

Bullock, T. H. (1973). Seeing the world through a new sense: electroreception in fish. *Am. Scient. 61:* 316–25.

Bullock, T. H., Northcutt, R. G., and Bodznick, D. A. (1982). Evolution of electroreception. *Trends Neurosci. 5:* 50–3.

Clusin, W. T., and Bennett, M. V. L. (1977a). Calcium-activated conductance in skate electroreceptors. Current clamp experiments. *J. Gen. Physiol. 69:* 121–43.

Clusin, W. T., and Bennett, M. V. L. (1977b). Calcium-activated conductance in skate electroreceptors. Voltage clamp experiments. *J. Gen. Physiol. 69:* 145–82.

Clusin, W. T., and Bennett, M. V. L. (1979a). The oscillatory responses of skate electroreceptors to small voltage stimuli. *J. Gen. Physiol. 73:* 685–702.

Clusin, W. T., and Bennett, M. V. L. (1979b). The ionic basis of oscillatory responses of skate electroreceptors. *J. Gen. Physiol. 73:* 703–23.

Corey, D. P., and Hudspeth, A. J. (1979). Ionic basis of the receptor potential in a vertebrate hair cell. *Nature 281:* 675–7.

Crawford, A. D., and Fettiplace, R. (1981). An electrical tuning mechanism in turtle cochlear hair cells. *J. Physiol., Lond. 312:* 377–422.

Davis, H. (1965). A model for transducer action in the cochlea. *Cold Spring Harb. Symp. Quant. Biol. 30:* 181–90.

Friedrich-Freksa, H. (1930). Lorenzinische Ampullen bei dem Siluroiden, *Plotosus anguillaris* Bloch. *Zool. Anz. 87:* 49–66.

Hopkins, C. D. (1976). Stimulus filtering and electroreception: tuberous electroreceptors in three species of Gymnotoid fish. *J. Comp. Physiol. 111:* 171–207.

Hopkins, C. D. (1981). The neuroethology of electric communication. *Trends Neurosci. 4:* 4–6.

Hudspeth, A. J., and Corey, D. P. (1977). Sensitivity, polarity and conductance change in the response of vertebrate hair cells to controlled mechanical stimuli. *Proc. Natn. Acad. Sci. USA 74:* 2407–11.

Kalmijn, A. J. (1974). The detection of electric fields from inanimate and animate sources other than electric organs. In *Handbook of Sensory Physiology*, vol. III/3, ed. A. Fessard, pp. 147–200. New York: Springer-Verlag.

Murray, R. W. (1965). Electroreceptor mechanisms: the relation of impulse frequency to stimulus strength and responses to pulsed stimuli in the ampullae of Lorenzini of elasmobranchs. *J. Physiol., Lond. 180:* 592–606.

Neher, E., Sakmann, B., and Steinbach, J. H. (1978). The extracellular patch clamp: a method for resolving currents through individual open channels in biological membranes. *Pflügers Arch. ges. Physiol. 375:* 219–28.

Obara, S. (1974). Receptor cell activity at 'rest' with respect to the tonic operation of a specialized lateralis receptor. *Proc. Japan Acad. 50:* 386–91.

Obara, S. (1976). Mechanism of electroreception in ampullae of Lorenzini of the marine catfish *Plotosus*. In *Electrobiology of Nerve, Synapse, and Muscle*, ed. J. P. Reuben, D. P. Purpura, M. V. L. Bennett and E. R. Kandel, pp. 129–47. New York: Raven Press.

Obara, S., and Bennett, M. V. L. (1972). Mode of operation of ampullae of Lorenzini of the skate, *Raja. J. Gen. Physiol. 60:* 534–57.

Obara, S., and Higuchi, T. (1978). Sensory transduction in the electroreceptor: high sensitivity and adaptation. *VI Int. Biophys. Congr. VII-21-(C1)*, 295 (Abstract).

Obara, S., Higuchi, T., and Nagai, T. (1981). High sensitivity processes in the sensory transduction of the *Plotosus* electroreceptors. *Adv. Physiol. Sci.*, vol. *31, Sensory Physiology of Aquatic Lower Vertebrates*, ed. T. Szabo and G. Czéh, pp. 41–56.

Obara, S., and Oomura, Y. (1973). Disfacilitation as the basis for the sensory suppression in a specialized lateralis receptor of the marine catfish. *Proc. Japan Acad. 49:* 213–17.

Obara, S., and Sugawara, Y. (1979). Contribution of Ca to the electroreceptor mechanism in *Plotosus* ampullae. *J. Physiol., Paris 75:* 335–40.

Sugawara, Y., and Obara, S. (1979). Voltage-clamp analysis of the Ca-dependent receptor potential in *Plotosus* electroreceptor. *Neurosci. Lett.*, Suppl. *2:* 83 (Abstract).

Szabo, T. (1974). Anatomy of the specialized lateral line organs of electroreception. In *Handbook of Sensory Physiology*, vol. III/3, ed. A. Fessard, pp. 13–58. New York: Springer-Verlag.

Teeter, J. H., Szamier, R. B., and Bennett, M. V. L. (1980). Ampullary electroreceptors in the sturgeon *Scaphirhynchus platorynchus* (Rafinesque). *J. Comp. Physiol. 138:* 213–23.

Viancour, T. A. (1979). Peripheral electrosense physiology: a review of recent findings. *J. Physiol., Paris 75:* 321–33.

Waltman, B. (1966). Electrical properties and fine structure of the ampullary canals of Lorenzini. *Acta Physiol. Scand.*, Suppl. *264:* 1–60.

Zipser, B., and Bennett, M. V. L. (1973). Tetrodotoxin resistant electrically excitable responses of receptor cells. *Brain Res. 62:* 253–9.

4.5

Theory of electromagnetic orientation: a further analysis

A. J. KALMIJN

Faraday's 1832 experimental researches in electricity suggest two modes of electromagnetic orientation applicable to marine sharks, skates, and rays: (1) a *passive mode* in which the animal estimates its drift with the flow of water from the electric fields that tidal and wind-driven ocean currents produce by interaction with the vertical component of the earth's magnetic field, and (2) an *active mode* in which the animal, when swimming relative to the water, derives its magnetic compass heading from the electric field it generates by interaction with the horizontal component of the earth's magnetic field (Kalmijn, 1974). In the active mode, marine elasmobranchs may detect the electrical signals resulting from their *forward* motion, whereas freshwater, terrestrial, and airborne animals would have to rely on the signals they induce by *turning* or by the relative motion of body parts. The present article extends the author's theory of electromagnetic orientation to include the latter animals, and offers a critical review of the evidence available at the time.

Physical principles

The study of electromagnetic orientation requires a thorough knowledge of the electric fields that the drift of the medium and the motions of the animals induce. Starting with Faraday's and Ohm's laws, the following discussion will develop the physical insights needed to conceive the motional-electric fields in the observer's frame of reference, to transform the fields to the animals' frames of reference, and to establish the information that these fields convey to the animals. Future research will demand a more formal, mathematical approach.

Fields due to the drift of ocean currents

According to Faraday's law, tidal and wind-driven ocean currents induce, by interaction with the *vertical* component of the earth's magnetic field, *horizontal* electric fields perpendicular to the flow of water (Figure 1a,b). In the northern hemisphere, the *induced electric fields* point to the left; in the southern hemisphere, they point to the right when viewed by an observer facing downstream. The strength and direction of the induced electric fields are given by the vector product $v \times B_v$, where v is the velocity of the flowing water and B_v the vertical component of the earth's magnetic field. The horizontal magnetic component B_h is of lesser importance for the detection of drift, as will be detailed below. The induced $v \times B_v$ has the dimensions of an electromotive force per unit length and, driven by the flow of water, provides the energy for the oceans' motional-electric fields. As a result of the induced electromotive force, an electric current tends to flow across the stream and back through the stationary environment with respect to which the motion takes place (Figure 1c).

According to Ohm's law, the electric current develops along its path an *ohmic electric field* $-\rho J$, where ρ is the resistivity of the water and J the current density (Figure 1a,c). The minus sign indicates that the $-\rho J$

Figure 1. Motionally-induced field of a steady, wind-driven ocean current flowing over deeper, stationary water layers, measured with a moored and with a drifting voltmeter. (a) Vector diagram, (b) $v \times B_v$ field, (c) J field, and (d) equivalent circuits. At a water velocity v, the flow of water interacts with the vertical component of the earth's magnetic field B_v, inducing an electric field $v \times B_v$. The induced field gives rise to an electric current of density J, which develops an ohmic field $-\rho J$. Because of the low resistance of the return path, the $-\rho J$ of the shallow stream effectively opposes the $v \times B_v$, and the total voltage gradient $v \times B_v - \rho J$, integrated across the stream, approaches zero. Thus, a moored voltmeter (V) hardly responds to the motional-electric field of the heavily loaded ocean current. When drifting with the stream, however, the measuring system induces fields along its connecting cables of the same strength and direction as the $v \times B_v$ in the water. As the two $v \times B_v$ contributions offset each other exactly and the voltmeter, ideally, does not draw any current, only the $-\rho J$, integrated over the distance between the electrodes, is measured. Yet, because of the heavy loading, the $-\rho J$ nearly equals the negative of $v \times B_v$, and thus offers the animal an excellent measure of its drift. In the equivalent circuits, the electromotive forces are indicated by batteries. V_{st} and V_{dr} are the readings of the high-ohmic, stationary and drifting voltmeters. The resistive elements represent the ohmic properties of the internal path (R_i) through the stream and the external path (R_e) through deeper water layers. The integral expressions for the induced electromotive forces and the ohmic voltage differences form the mathematical basis for the diagrams.

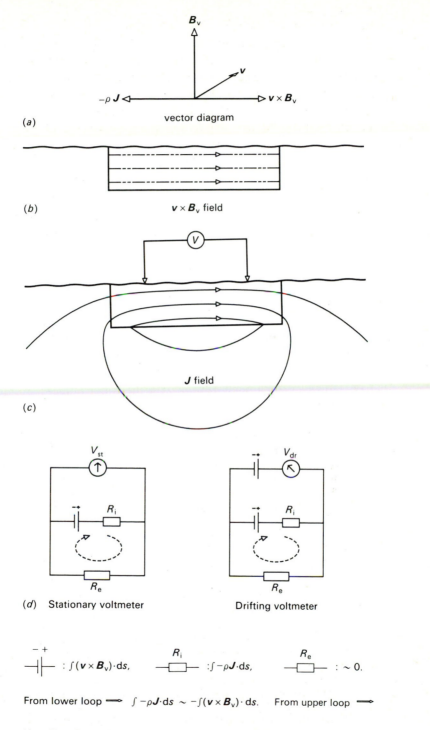

(a) vector diagram

(b) $\mathbf{v} \times \mathbf{B}_\mathrm{v}$ field

(c) $\mathbf{J}$ field

(d) Stationary voltmeter   Drifting voltmeter

$\dfrac{- \;\; +}{\dashv\vdash}$: $\int(\mathbf{v} \times \mathbf{B}_\mathrm{v})\cdot \mathrm{d}\mathbf{s}$, $\quad \overline{\underline{\square}}^{R_\mathrm{i}}$: $\int -\rho\mathbf{J}\cdot \mathrm{d}\mathbf{s}$, $\quad \overline{\underline{\square}}^{R_\mathrm{e}}$: ~ 0.

From lower loop $\longrightarrow$ $\int -\rho\mathbf{J}\cdot \mathrm{d}\mathbf{s} \sim -\int(\mathbf{v} \times \mathbf{B}_\mathrm{v})\cdot \mathrm{d}\mathbf{s}$.   From upper loop $\longrightarrow$

$V_\mathrm{st} = \int(\mathbf{v} \times \mathbf{B}_\mathrm{v} -\rho\mathbf{J})\cdot \mathrm{d}\mathbf{s} \sim 0,$ $\qquad V_\mathrm{dr} = \int(\mathbf{v} \times \mathbf{B}_\mathrm{v} -\rho\mathbf{J})\cdot \mathrm{d}\mathbf{s} - \int(\mathbf{v} \times \mathbf{B}_\mathrm{v})\cdot \mathrm{d}\mathbf{s} = \int -\rho\mathbf{J}\cdot \mathrm{d}\mathbf{s}$

field opposes the $v \times B_v$ field, thereby allowing the motional-electric energy to dissipate again. To balance the net energy gains and losses, the current field adjusts itself so that the resulting ohmic voltage *drop*, $\int \rho J \cdot ds$ equals the electromotive force of induction $\int (v \times B_v) \cdot ds$ around any closed loop through the stream and the stationary environment, where $\int \rho J \cdot ds$ and $\int (v \times B_v) \cdot ds$ are the line integrals of ρJ and $v \times B_v$ along the path *s*, and *v* and *B* are assumed to be independent of time. (Note that the ohmic voltage drop is the negative of $\int -\rho J \cdot ds$.) The current density *J* generated across a given stream depends on the resistance of the return path. A uniform flow cutting through a highly resistive bedrock, as in a fjord, may hardly generate any current. However, flowing over loose bottom sediments and deeper, slower-moving water layers, the same flow would induce currents of appreciable strengths. In short, Faraday's law predicts the induced electromotive force, but Ohm's law, applied to the complete circuit, determines whether and how much electric current will flow.

The induced electric fields of wind-driven ocean currents are usually loaded heavily by deeper water layers, so that most of the voltage drop takes place in the shallow flow of water (Figure 1a,d). The ohmic field, $-\rho J$, largely offsets the induced field, $v \times B_v$, leaving only a vanishingly small *total voltage gradient* $v \times B_v - \rho J$ for a *stationary* observer to detect. However, an animal *drifting* with the water induces an internal $v \times B_v$, exactly equal to that of the stream. In any conceivable measuring circuit through the animal and the water, the internally induced field cancels the $v \times B_v$ of the stream, reducing the total voltage gradient, $v \times B_v - \rho J$, to just the $-\rho J$ term. Thus, *drifting* with the flow of water is electromagnetically identical to being exposed to a virtually uniform $-\rho J$ field. Yet, as a consequence of the heavy loading, the $-\rho J$ that the animal detects nearly equals the negative of the $v \times B_v$ observed in the *stationary* frame of reference, and hence offers the animal a good estimate of the speed and direction of its drift *v* (except near the equator). B_v may be determined by operating the same sensory system in the active mode (cf. next section, page 534). (The relativistic differences of B_v and $-\rho J$ in the animal's and the observer's frames of reference are negligible, so that the Lorentz transformations of the electric and magnetic fields reduce to Faraday's law.)

However, without reference to the outside world, the animal cannot sense its drift solely from the local $-\rho J$ field, for that would violate Galileo's principle of relativity, elaborated by Einstein to cover not only mechanical, but electromagnetic phenomena as well. Nor can the animal be said to move relative to the ambient magnetic field *B*. The induced $v \times B$ is the result of the velocity v with respect to a reference frame in which there is a magnetic field B. Without a frame of reference, neither v nor B have meaning. Nevertheless, the animal may *infer* the presence of a reference frame in which it induces a $v \times B_v$ that fully accounts for the $-\rho J$ it detects. But to do so, the animal must know the relation between $-\rho J$ and $v \times B_v$ in the desired frame of reference. Although $-\rho J$ often approaches the negative of $v \times B_v$ closely, as was assumed in the above discussion, it normally will be less due to the finite resistance of deeper water layers and bottom sediments. In the open ocean $-\rho J$ averages ~90%, in the English Channel ~75%, and in some better-insulated channels as little as 16% of the $v \times B_v$ (cf. Kalmijn, 1974). To acquire the information needed to interpret $-\rho J$ correctly, the animals might occasionally dive to the bottom, or at least to well below the wind-driven surface flows, which can be several hundred meters in depth. In shallow water and near the bottom, the $-\rho J$ fields may serve a totally different orientational function, as will be explained on page 543.

How do the fields that the flow of water induces by interaction with the horizontal component of the earth's magnetic field relate to the detection of drift? It is important to note that electric, magnetic, and velocity fields are of vectorial nature and that any situation may be analysed in all its complexity or, more conveniently, component by component. Biologically, it seems reasonable to suppose that the recipient animals follow either one of these procedures, depending on the information desired. Ocean currents with velocity components along the east–west axis induce, by interaction with the *horizontal* magnetic component B_h, *vertically* directed $v \times B_h$ fields. Because the wind-driven flows are usually much shallower than wide (by a ratio of typically 1:1000) and the electrical return paths are largely obstructed by the air–water interface, the vertically induced fields are only lightly loaded and contribute relatively little to the $-\rho J$ fields that drifting animals detect. The vertically induced fields gain in importance when the flow of water narrows or widens laterally, especially near the equator where the horizontally induced fields are weak.

Considerable complications arise on the fringes of ocean currents. Just inside the stream, the ohmic field is no longer antiparallel to the induced field. On the outside, the field falls off only gradually, even though there is little, if any, flow of water (Figure 1c). The effects from interaction with the horizontal magnetic component are also more noticeable in these regions. Ocean currents often show large fluctuations and even gyrations, that make their ohmic fields even more complex. Moreover, surface waves, internal waves, upwellings, and geomagnetic variations add to the oceans' electric fields. In tidal flows and water movements of shorter period, the processes of self- and mutual-induction can be important as well, although they are not discussed in this paper. Temporal variations in the water velocity v and, consequently, in the current density J cause slight variations in the magnetic induction B, which induce secondary fields that feed back onto the primary fields (self-induction) and generate electric currents in adjacent waters and in the earth, of which the magnetic variations affect the original fields again (mutual-induction) (Cox, Filloux and Larsen, 1970). Interpretation of the various fields would require great expertise on the part of the animals.

The motional-electric fields of tidal and open-ocean flows were predicted by Faraday (1832), described mathematically by Longuet-Higgins, Stern and Stommel (1954), and treated more rigorously by Larsen (1968), Cox et al. (1970), Sanford (1971), and Chave (1983). Von Arx (1962) recorded fields of $50–500\,\mathrm{nV\,cm^{-1}}$ with electrodes towed near the surface of the Atlantic Ocean. Sanford (1975) and Sanford, Drever and Dunlap (1978) used a free-fall instrument equipped with two sets of sensors resembling the electroreceptors of elasmobranch fishes. In the SI system of units, the $v \times B$ fields are calculated as the product of [the velocity v in $\mathrm{m\,s^{-1}}$ ($=100\,\mathrm{cm\,s^{-1}}$)] × [the magnetic induction B in tesla or weber $\mathrm{m^{-2}}$ ($=10^4$ gauss)] × [the sine of the angle between v and B], giving $v \times B$ in $\mathrm{Vm^{-1}}$ ($= 10^7\,\mathrm{nV\,cm^{-1}}$). Its direction may be memorized as that of a right-hand screw turned from v into B. The numerical values of the velocity v, the magnetic induction B, and the strengths of $v \times B$ and $-\rho J$ will be given in the historically most common units of $\mathrm{cm\,s^{-1}}$ ($=10^{-2}\,\mathrm{m\,s^{-1}}$), gauss ($=10^{-4}$ tesla), and $\mathrm{nV\,cm^{-1}}$ ($=10^{-7}\,\mathrm{V\,m^{-1}}$). Thus, ocean currents flowing at velocities of $10–100\,\mathrm{cm\,s^{-1}}$ through a vertical magnetic field of 0.55 gauss induce $v \times B_v$ fields of $55–550\,\mathrm{nV\,cm^{-1}}$. If the streams are heavily loaded, the oppositely directed $-\rho J$ fields would measure only a few percent less. For time-independent v and B, the total field, $v \times B -\rho J$, may be expressed as the gradient of a potential function. However, the individual terms, $v \times B$ and $-\rho J$, are gradients of potential functions only if v and B are spatially uniform as well. In the static case, the electric field E is the negative of the total voltage gradient, $v \times B -\rho J$.

Fields due to the animals' forward motion

When a fish moves *relative to the water*, it also induces an electric field by *actively* interacting with the earth's magnetic field.

Crossing the horizontal magnetic component, B_h, the animal induces a *ventrodorsal* field when heading *east*, and a *dorsoventral* field when heading *west* (Figure 2a). Crossing the vertical magnetic component, B_v, the animal induces a right–left field when it is in the northern hemisphere and a left–right field when it is in the southern hemisphere. The resultant *induced electric field*, $v \times B$, causes an electric current to flow across the moving animal and back through the seawater environment with respect to which the motion takes place. This gives rise to an *ohmic electric field*, $-\rho J$, where J is the current density and ρ the resistivity of the medium. The current distributes itself again so that the ohmic voltage drop, $\int \rho J \cdot ds$, equals the induced electromotive force, $\int (v \times B) \cdot ds$, for any closed path s through the animal and the seawater environment. (Even though the velocity, v, varies greatly, the effects of self- and mutual-induction remain negligible because of the small size and the high resistivity of the animal.)

The field that a shark induces by interaction with the horizontal magnetic component will be described first (Figure 2a,b). Because the seawater return path has larger dimensions and appreciably lower resistivity ($\sim 20\,\Omega\,cm$) than the animal's skin and body tissues ($\sim 2000\,\Omega\,cm$), it virtually short-circuits the fish electrically. A near-maximal $-\rho J$ field develops within the animal, where it effectively counteracts the internally induced $v \times B_h$. (Only the dorso-ventrally-averaged resistivity is relevant here.) Consequently, for an observer *at rest* with the water, the *total voltage gradient*, $v \times B_h - \rho J$, averaged across the body, tends to zero. However, in the receptor system of the *swimming* fish a similar $v \times B_h$ is induced, precisely offsetting that of the skin and body tissues, leaving for the animal only the $-\rho J$ term to detect. Thus, moving with respect to the water is electrically identical to being exposed to an ohmic $-\rho J$ field acting across the body. Yet, given the heavy loading by the seawater, the animal may *interpret* the $-\rho J$ that it detects in terms of the $v \times B_h$ of its motion relative to the water. (This does not violate the principle of relativity, for the correctness of the fish's interpretation depends on a knowledge of the relations between $-\rho J$ and $v \times B_h$ in the frame of reference with respect to which the motion takes place.) Thus, swimming at a velocity v, a shark may infer the direction of B_h and hence its magnetic compass heading. The flow of water around the moving animal might enhance or diminish the $-\rho J$ depending on the hydrodynamic shape of the fish.

The dorsoventral voltage difference, $\int -\rho J \cdot ds$, integrated across the body, offers the shark complete information about its magnetic compass heading. Dorsal-minus/ventral-plus (V_-) denotes an easterly, dorsal-plus/ventral-minus (V_+) a westerly course of swimming. The magnitude of the dorsoventral voltage difference, relative to the maximum reached when the animal swims straight east or west, signals the angle between the actual compass direction and the east–west axis. The changes in dorsoventral voltage difference, δ^+ and δ^-, caused by the animal's swerving mode of swimming resolve the ambiguity of a northerly or southerly angle of deviation from the east–west axis. A change towards dorsal-more-negative/ventral-more-positive when the animal veers to the right means a northerly angle, and a similar change when it veers to the left, a southerly angle of deviation. The strengths of δ^+ and δ^- could also provide the magnitude of the angle of deviation. In short, the magnetic compass heading (relative to the east–west axis) may be derived from the $-\rho J$ field (cosine function) and its angular variations (sine function). Note that δ^+ and δ^- are the changes in the field resulting from the animal's forward motion. The fields that the swerving movements themselves induce remain virtually undetected (p. 538).

Figure 2. Rectilinearly-induced field of a swimming shark, as detected by a voltmeter at rest with the water and by the sensory system of the moving fish. (a) Vector diagram and J field, (b) equivalent circuits, and (c) electrical cues for various compass headings. The two sense organs indicated represent all those having ventrodorsal components. The contents of the ampullary canals have low resistivity, whereas the walls and sensory epithelia are high-ohmic. Moving with a velocity v through a magnetic field of horizontal induction B_h, the animal induces an electric field $v \times B_h$. The induced field gives rise to a current of density J, which produces an ohmic field $-\rho J$. Because of the low resistivity of the seawater, the ventrodorsally averaged ohmic $-\rho J$ practically cancels the induced $v \times B_h$, leaving little to detect for a voltmeter at rest with the water. However, the sensory system of the moving fish generates induced fields along the ampullary canals of the same strength and direction as the $v \times B_h$ in the skin and body tissues. As the two $v \times B_h$ contributions exactly null each other and the ampullary system draws hardly any current, the two sense organs are stimulated by the ohmic field, $-\rho J$, integrated over the height of the fish. Since the animal is heavily loaded by the water, the ohmic $-\rho J$ nearly equals the negative of the induced $v \times B_h$, and indirectly gives the shark its magnetic compass heading. In the equivalent circuits, V_{st} and V_{mv} are the signals received by the voltmeter at rest with the medium and by the moving fish. R_i is the internal resistance of the animal, R_e the resistance of the external medium. In the compass diagram, V_+ and V_- are the ohmic voltage differences between the dorsal and ventral surfaces of the fish, δ^+ and δ^- the changes thereof (Figure 3 in Kalmijn, 1981, gives the electromotive forces, which are of opposite sign).

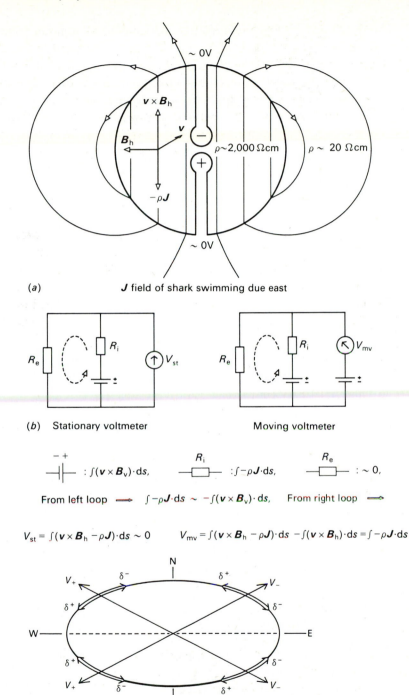

(a)　　　　　　　**J** field of shark swimming due east

(b)　Stationary voltmeter　　　　　　　　Moving voltmeter

$$-\vert\vert\!\!\!+ \; : \int (\boldsymbol{v}\times\boldsymbol{B}_v)\cdot d\boldsymbol{s}, \qquad R_i \;\; : \int -\rho\boldsymbol{J}\cdot d\boldsymbol{s}, \qquad R_e \;\; : \sim 0,$$

From left loop $\implies \int -\rho\boldsymbol{J}\cdot d\boldsymbol{s} \sim -\int(\boldsymbol{v}\times\boldsymbol{B}_v)\cdot d\boldsymbol{s}$, From right loop $\implies$

$$V_{st} = \int(\boldsymbol{v}\times\boldsymbol{B}_h - \rho\boldsymbol{J})\cdot d\boldsymbol{s} \sim 0 \qquad V_{mv} = \int(\boldsymbol{v}\times\boldsymbol{B}_h - \rho\boldsymbol{J})\cdot d\boldsymbol{s} - \int(\boldsymbol{v}\times\boldsymbol{B}_h)\cdot d\boldsymbol{s} = \int -\rho\boldsymbol{J}\cdot d\boldsymbol{s}$$

(c)　　　　　　　Sensory cues of compass headings

By interacting with the vertical component of the earth's magnetic field, the animal induces an electric field similar to that described above, except that it acts along the transverse, rather than the vertical axis. The ratio of the left–right $-\rho J$ and the maximal ventrodorsal $-\rho J$ gives the animal the inclination or dip of the earth's magnetic field and thereby the magnetic latitude of its position on the globe, both in magnitude (angular distance from the equator) and polarity (southern or northern hemisphere). So far, the animal has been assumed to swim horizontally, although the sensory system could conceivably function in other positions as well. In any event, to separate the effects of the horizontal and vertical magnetic components, detection of the vertical (gravity) is required. The animal need not know its swimming speed to orient electromagnetically, but must be able to reproduce it accurately. It may, of course, monitor its speed by other sensory systems, or even derive it from the horizontal $-\rho J$ (except near the equator). Conversely, the animal may estimate B_v from the $-\rho J$ produced by a given swimming effort.

The strength of the induced $v \times B$ that the animal may infer from the ohmic $-\rho J$, is calculated as the product of [the swimming velocity v in $m\,s^{-1}$ ($=100\,cm\,s^{-1}$)] × [the magnetic induction B in tesla or weber m^{-2} ($=10^4$ gauss)] × [the sine of the angle between v and B]. This gives $v \times B$ in $V\,m^{-1}$ ($= 10^7\,nV\,cm^{-1}$). Thus, a fish cruising due east along the magnetic equator at a speed of $100\,cm\,s^{-1}$, induces, at a horizontal intensity of 0.4 gauss, a ventrodorsally directed $v \times B_h$ of $400\,nV\,cm^{-1}$ (maximally). These values decrease to about 0.1 gauss and $100\,nV\,cm^{-1}$ (minimally) towards the northern and southern boundaries of the combined tropical and temperate regions in which most fish species occur. The same fish induces, by interaction with the vertical magnetic component, right–left and left–right $v \times B_v$ fields ranging from zero at the magnetic equator to over $600\,nV\,cm^{-1}$ near the northern and southern boundaries respectively. The dorsoventral electromotive forces across a fish 10 cm in height and width would range from 1000 to 4000 nV, the right–left and left–right electromotive forces from zero to 6000 nV. The ohmic voltage differences that the animal detects are of nearly the same strengths as the electromotive forces, but of opposite polarity.

The efficiency of the rectilinear mechanism of orientation, defined by the ratio $R_i/(R_i + R_e)$, with R_i the resistance of the internal and R_e the resistance of the external part of the circuit, depends critically on the resistivity of the external medium (Figure 2b). The electromagnetic mechanism is most plausible for marine animals, in which the efficiency can be as high as 98–99%. In freshwater fishes, which have average internal resistivities similar to those of the marine species, the ohmic field strength may range from ~75% of the induced field strength in near-brackish water, to less than 3% in almost pure rainwater. In land and airborne animals, the efficiency is orders of magnitude lower again. Besides reducing the efficiency, an increase in external resistance also gives rise to higher physical noise levels, rendering the mechanism even more problematic for freshwater, land, and airborne animals. The fields induced by an animal's turning movements or by the relative motion of body parts do not depend on the electrical properties of the medium, as will be explained below.

When swimming in an ocean current, an animal receives both the $-\rho J$ field of its drift *with* the water and the $-\rho J$ field of its motion *relative to* the water. The two fields add vectorially and would be difficult to resolve for a single instant in time. However, the actively and passively induced fields are entirely different functions of the animal's swerving movements. Moreover, the field along the vertical body axis is mainly compass-related, whereas the field along the horizontal body axis generally comprises both drift and swimming components. The principle of combining the two fields vectorially may also help the observer analyse more complicated situations. For instance, a fish swimming upstream with the same speed as the flow of water receives a ρJ that is the vector sum of the field due to its drift and the field of its swimming against the stream. When the animal settles on a rock bottom or buries under loose sand while the water is rushing by, it receives a similar field, although now additionally shaped by the presence of the insulating rock or by the loading of the seawater-soaked sand. Motionally-induced fields not due to the local flow of water or to the animal's movements will be discussed on page 543.

Fields due to the animals' turning movements

The electric fields resulting from angular, or turning, motion may be introduced as a logical extension of the fields due to rectilinear, or forward, motion. A fish heading east induces, by interaction with the horizontal component of the earth's magnetic field, equal ventrodorsal fields in the right and left halves of the body. Because of this basic symmetry, the net $v \times B_h$ around any closed path entirely within the body is zero, and all electric current takes the external route (Figure 2a). However, when the fish veers to the right, the left half of the body gains greater tangential speed and induces a stronger ventrodorsal field than the right half of the body (Figure 3a). Consequently, a net,

Figure 3. Rotationally-induced field of an animal veering to the right while heading east. (a) Vector diagram and *J* field, (b) wire circuits for rotational and rectilinear motion, (c) equivalent circuit, and (d) sensory cues of compass headings. Because the tangential velocity is greater in the left than in the right half of the body, a clockwise $v \times B_h$ is induced. A current of density *J* circulates within the animal and develops along its path an anticlockwise ohmic $-\rho J$, which depends only on the resistivity of the tissues, not on that of the outside medium. In the diagram, the forward velocity common to both halves of the body has been omitted to show the consequences of the differential velocity more clearly. The two wire circuits illustrate how the changes of magnetic flux, $d\Phi/dt$, arise in a rotating-coil and in a rectilinear magnetohydrodynamic generator. A high-ohmic voltmeter, inserted in an otherwise low-resistance loop $(R_e \ll R_i)$, indicates almost the full ohmic voltage increase, $\int -\rho J \cdot ds$, around the circuit, where R_i is the resistance shunting the meter and R_e the resistance of the remainder of the loop. Since $\int -\rho J \cdot ds$ equals the negative of $\int (v \times B_h) \cdot ds$, the meter reading, V_{rt}, also offers an excellent measure of the induced electromotive force. (The voltmeter indicates the full motionally-induced signal only if it is completely short-circuited around the loop.) The compass diagram illustrates the rotationally-induced signals as a function of the animals' magnetic compass headings. V_+ denotes a clockwise and V_- an anticlockwise ohmic voltage increase, while δ^+ and δ^- denote respectively the increments and decrements in V. All known electroreceptors connect to the outside and would be highly inefficient in detecting the rotationally-induced fields (cf. Figure 2a). Suitable internal measuring circuits have not yet been described. The semicircular canals show little promise because of their expected inefficiency $(R_i \ll R_e)$.

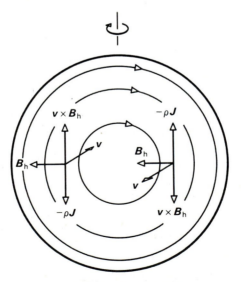

(*a*)   Animal turning to right

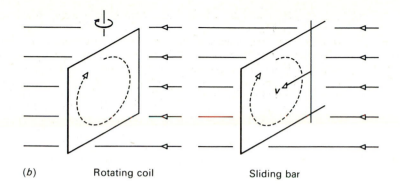

(*b*) Rotating coil Sliding bar

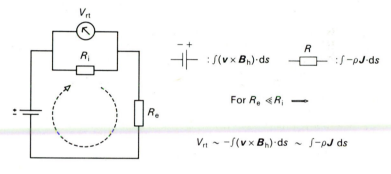

(*c*) Turning animal

$$-\!\!\!|\!\!\vdash \;\; : \int (\mathbf{v} \times \mathbf{B}_h) \cdot d\mathbf{s} \qquad -\!\!\boxed{}\!\!^{R}\!\!- \;\; : \int -\rho \mathbf{J} \cdot d\mathbf{s}$$

For $R_e \ll R_i \implies$

$$V_{rt} \sim -\int (\mathbf{v} \times \mathbf{B}_h) \cdot d\mathbf{s} \;\sim\; \int -\rho \mathbf{J}\, d\mathbf{s}$$

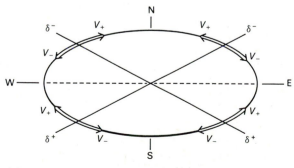

(d) Sensory cues of compass headings

clockwise $v \times B_h$ appears around all internal loops of non-zero vertical extent. This net induced field gives rise to a clockwise circulation of electric current that develops an anticlockwise ohmic field, $-\rho J$. (The induced field is anticlockwise and develops a clockwise $-\rho J$, when the animal veers left.) The current adjusts itself so that the ohmic voltage drop, $\int \rho J \cdot ds$, balances the induced electromotive force, $\int (v \times B_h) \cdot ds$, around all closed paths s within the body (the effects of self- and mutual-induction are negligible again). In short, when a fish turns right or left, a completely internal, closed-loop $-\rho J$ is superimposed on the dorso-ventral $-\rho J$ of the animal's forward motion. Note that the electro-receptors of sharks, skates, and rays detect the dorsoventral rather than the circular fields (cf. Figures 2a and 3a).

At this point, it is readily seen that the electromotive force induced by differential motion of the right and left sides of the body may also be described in terms of a decrease in magnetic flux Φ (or total number of field lines) enclosed by the circuit: $V = -d\Phi/dt$ (Figure 3b). This reveals the close analogy between the turning fish and the a.c. dynamo or rotating-coil generator. In terms of changing fluxes, the induced electromotive force is calculated as [the decrease of magnetic induction B along the axis of the loop, in tesla or weber m^{-2} ($= 10^4$ gauss) s^{-1}] $\times$ [the surface area enclosed by the loop, in m^2 ($= 10^4$ cm^2)], giving the answer in volts ($= 10^9$ nV), where a positive sign denotes that it increases in the clockwise direction. Thus, when a fish of 100 cm^2 cross-sectional area, while heading east along the magnetic equator, turns to the right at a rate of 1 radian s^{-1} (a full U-turn in π seconds), it induces, by interaction with the horizontal magnetic field, a 400-nV clockwise electromotive force and an equally strong anticlockwise ohmic voltage increase around an imaginary transverse loop just beneath the skin. A simultaneous forward speed of 100 cm s^{-1} would add a dorsoventral electromotive force of 4000 nV and a ventrodorsal ohmic voltage difference of nearly the same strength across a 10-cm-high fish.

In an attempt to apply the flux approach to the instance of rectilinear motion through a uniform magnetic field, one comes to the disturbing conclusion that there is no change of flux through any imaginary loop within the moving body. On careful inspection, however, there *is* a change of magnetic flux in the circuit formed by the animal and the surrounding water. This change of flux does not result from the translation of a rigid loop, but from a change in loop area due to the motion of one part of the circuit, that formed by the fish, relative to the rest of the circuit, that formed by the environment (Figure 3b). Therefore, electromagnetic induction by rectilinear motion relative to a low-resistive medium is more akin to the principle of a magnetohydro-dynamic generator (in which an ionized plasma is driven through a uniform magnetic field) than to the principle of the rotating-coil generator. Although flux considerations lead to exactly the same results, the analysis based on $v \times B$ and $-\rho J$ is often more enlightening for rectilinear motion. In fact, the 'hidden' change of flux of rectilinear motion has troubled biologists for years (page 553).

To evaluate the detectability of the rotationally-induced fields, consider a high-ohmic voltmeter inserted in an insulated, but otherwise low-ohmic, closed loop within the animal's body. When in the earth's frame of reference the animal veers either right or left, it induces an electromotive force equal to $\int (v \times B_h) \cdot ds$ integrated around the loop or, equivalently, to $-d\Phi/dt$ evaluated over the surface area enclosed by the loop. The induced electromotive force causes a loop current of density J that develops an ohmic field $-\rho J$. Because the electrical resistance is largely concentrated in the voltmeter, the meter reading indicates almost the full ohmic voltage increase, $\int -\rho J \cdot ds$, around the loop (Figure 3c). Since the ohmic voltage increase, $\int -\rho J \cdot ds$, equals the negative of the electromotive force, $\int (v \times B_h) \cdot ds$, around the loop, the voltmeter reading also offers an excellent measure of $\int (v \times B_h) \cdot ds$ or $-d\Phi/dt$. In the animal's frame of reference, where v is identically zero, $v \times B_h$ vanishes. The voltmeter reading still equals nearly $-d\Phi/dt$, but this time the change of flux is attributed to an apparent rotation of the ambient magnetic field.

From the foregoing, it may be concluded that the animal could sense its rotation relative to the earth's magnetic field without reference to the outside world, which is actually correct and does not contradict the principle of relativity. Although the interpretation of the rectilinearly-driven $-\rho J$ (due to a steady velocity) required a detailed knowledge of the environment relative to which the motion took place, the interpretation of the rotationally-driven $-\rho J$ (due to a change of velocity) depends only on the electrical properties of the internal measuring loop. The animal, which itself initiates the turning movements and is likely to monitor them mechanically, is fully justified to interpret the $-\rho J$ that it receives either as due to the rotation of the ambient magnetic field relative to its own reference frame, or as due to its own rotation relative to the reference frame in which the magnetic field is time-independent. Because the $-\rho J$ of the turning movements depends on the orientation of the animal with respect to the earth's magnetic field, it could serve as the physical basis of an alternative, rotational compass sense.

How the animal might interpret the voltage differences that develop around a transverse loop during turning can be seen as follows (Figure 3d). When the fish is heading in an easterly direction, it receives a clockwise ohmic voltage V_+ on veering left and an anticlockwise V_- on veering right. When the fish is heading in a westerly direction, it receives a V_+ on veering right and a V_- on veering left. The strongest signals are received when the animal goes through the magnetic east or west; the signal tends to zero when it goes through the magnetic north or south. Turning through intermediate compass points yields voltages proportional to the cosine of the angle of deviation from the east–west axis. Whether the animal deviates from this axis in a northerly or southerly direction is given by the changes δ^+ and δ^- in V, that are proportional to the sine of the angle of deviation. When the animal deviates from the east–west axis in a northerly direction, the V_+ decreases and the V_- becomes more negative (δ^-) during the turn. When it deviates in a southerly direction, the V_+ increases and the V_- becomes less negative (δ^+). Consideration of other than transverse loops leads to similar conclusions.

Since the rotational mechanism does not depend on the resistivity of the external medium (as the current paths close internally), it applies equally well to marine, as to freshwater, land, and airborne animals. In the ideal case discussed above, the ohmic voltage increase took place almost exclusively within the voltmeter, and the efficiency was nearly 100%. If, however, an appreciable flow of current is allowed to bypass the voltmeter, the efficiency reduces to $R_i/(R_i + R_e)$, where R_i is the resistance of the shunt around the meter and R_e the resistance of the remaining part of the circuit (Figure 3c). As a model for the electromagnetic mechanism, the semicircular canals of the inner ear have often been mentioned (cf. Jungerman and Rosenblum, 1980). The efficiency of these sensory structures depends, however, on the resistance of the gelatinous cupula (R_i) shunting the sensory crest relative to that of the remainder of the circuit (R_e). To block the current effectively, the cupular material would have to be at least two orders of magnitude more resistive than that of the endolymph in the canal, for which there is no evidence. Therefore, the electromagnetic efficiency of the semicircular canals is expected to be a few percent at most.

The strength of the electromagnetic stimulus depends not only on the efficiency, but also on the dimensions of the measuring circuit and on the angular rate of turning. Since both the strength of $v \times B$ and the length of the path of integration are proportional to the linear dimensions of the loop, the induced electromotive force is proportional to the surface area of the loop, as is the enclosed magnetic flux. Because $v \times B$

is also proportional to the angular rate of turning, small animals might, at least partially, compensate for their size disadvantage by turning faster (they have less inertia, but are limited by viscous drag). Circuits for the detection of rotationally-induced fields, taking full advantage of the size of the animal, have not been described in the literature, nor are smaller circuits of proven efficiency known to exist. This need not indicate their absence, for it is questionable whether anybody has seriously looked for the right structures. The biological feasibility of the rotational principle and of other, medium-independent induction mechanisms will be discussed on pages 554–6.

Biological evidence

Even the most comprehensive theory of electromagnetic orientation remains biologically irrelevant if not supported by hard experimental evidence. Conversely, even the most serious efforts to prove or disprove the biological reality of electromagnetic orientation are destined to fail if not founded on sound physical reasoning. In this section, the literature on electromagnetic orientation will be reviewed and carefully scrutinized 'in the high and pure philosophic desire to remove error as well as discover truth' (Faraday, 1832).

Orientation to the electric fields of ocean currents

Behavioral data. The notion that fishes might orient to the motional-electric fields of ocean currents was first mentioned in connection with the long-distance migrations of eel and salmon (Deelder, 1952; Royce, Smith and Hartt, 1968). Meanwhile, a sensitivity to extremely weak electric fields was observed in elasmobranch fishes. When tested with uniform square-wave fields of 5 Hz, the dogfish *Scyliorhinus canicula* and the skate *Raja clavata* exhibited behavioral reflexes at voltage gradients as low as $100\,\mathrm{nV\,cm^{-1}}$ (Dijkgraaf and Kalmijn, 1962). The skate showed unconditioned cardiac decelerations at even weaker fields, and based on the heartbeat response a formal threshold sensitivity of $10\,\mathrm{nV\,cm^{-1}}$ was established (Kalmijn, 1966). The sense organs mediating the observed reflexes were identified as the ampullae of Lorenzini (Murray, 1962; Dijkgraaf and Kalmijn, 1963, 1966). The biological relevance of these findings became evident from the animals' responses to the bioelectric fields of their prey (Kalmijn, 1966, 1971). Following a theoretical evaluation of the motional-electric fields and a review of the circumstantial evidence (Kalmijn, 1974), the elasmobranchs' ability to orient to the practically-uniform oceanic fields was ascertained in conditioning experiments (Kalmijn, 1978b, 1982; Kalmijn and Kalmijn, 1981).

The stingray *Urolophus halleri* was conditioned to enter an enclosure on the left, and to avoid a similar enclosure on the right relative to the direction of a uniform electric field (Figure 4a). After a correct choice the animals received a small piece of food; after an incorrect choice they were lightly prodded. Alternative cues were eliminated by applying the fields randomly either parallel or antiparallel to the local magnetic

Figure 4. Orientation of the stingray *Urolophus halleri* to a uniform electric field of $5\,\mathrm{nV\,cm^{-1}}$. (a) The stingrays are trained to enter an enclosure on the left with respect to the field in order to receive food. The electrodes are located in two separate seawater compartments (+ and −) that connect to the experimental tank by two current dividers of 18 salt bridges each. During the individual trials, the field is applied in a random sequence to point either north or south so as to eliminate the use of alternative cues. (b) Results of training experiments for two stingrays (1 and 2), tested under three different magnetic conditions: (A) in a magnetic null field, (B) in the presence of only the vertical component of the earth's magnetic field, and (C) in the normal earth's magnetic field as measured in the San Diego, California, area from where the animals were collected. The results were evaluated by the sequential probability ratio test (cf. Kalmijn, 1982, for details and references). The α and β errors associated with acceptance of orientation (0.75 or three out of four, upper critical line) and rejection of orientation (0.50 or random, lower critical line) were both set at 0.001.

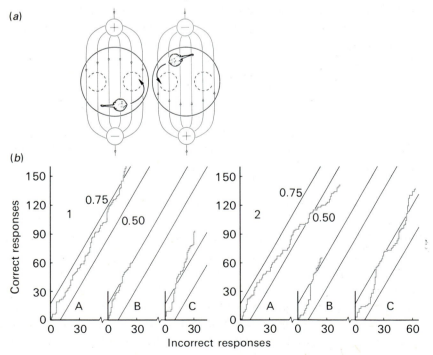

meridian. After an initial training at $160\,\mathrm{nV\,cm^{-1}}$ (d.c.), the strength of the field was successively lowered by factors of two. The results showed significant orientation, even at voltage gradients of only $5\,\mathrm{nV\,cm^{-1}}$ ($P \leqslant 0.001$ as determined by the sequential probability ratio test, Figure 4b), whereas the oceanic fields usually measure between 5 and $500\,\mathrm{nV\,cm^{-1}}$. The stingrays performed equally well in the presence as in the absence of the earth's magnetic field. The applied electric fields were very similar to those of ocean currents. Yet, that sharks, skates, and rays actually rely on the naturally occurring fields remains to be verified in experiments at sea. It may be noted that the freshwater catfish *Ictalurus nebulosus* learned to seek shelter in one out of twelve hiding tubes equally spaced along the periphery of their circular habitat (Kalmijn, Kolba and Kalmijn, 1976b), although freshwater fields tend to be stronger and are of electrochemical rather than electromagnetic origin (Kalmijn, 1974).

The theory of electromagnetic orientation shows its greatest potential when applied to fishes of the open sea. Nevertheless, the fields of ocean currents may play an important role in more protected areas as well. For example, the shallow waters of North and South Bimini (in the Bahamas) and the funnel-shaped bay that the islands enclose feature a steadily eastward $-\rho J$ field of 30–$60\,\mathrm{nV\,cm^{-1}}$ when measured with stationary electrodes (in collaboration with Dr Samuel H. Gruber). This regional field, which may be explained as due to the electrical return current of the adjacent Gulf Stream, could serve as a directional cue for the local sharks, skates, and rays as they move about the islands and in and out of the bay. The animals would have to take the fields of their drift into account in order to detect the regional field, but could do so because of their easy access to the bottom (cf. page 529). Further shallow-water data have been reported by Pals and Schoenhage (1979) and by Pals, Peters and Schoenhage (1982), who recorded motional-electric fields of 50–$350\,\mathrm{nV\,cm^{-1}}$ over sandy bottoms and much stronger electrochemical fields over clay and mud bottoms. The latter fields varied greatly on a scale of only $1\,\mathrm{m}$, averaging $6300\,\mathrm{nV\,cm^{-1}}$ at the bottom and $350\,\mathrm{nV\,cm^{-1}}$ at $30\,\mathrm{cm}$ above. The problem of evaluating these fields in terms relevant to electrosensitive fishes was not addressed by the authors (cf. Kalmijn, 1974). For further data on oceanic fields, including those induced by variations in the earth's magnetic field, see also Filloux (1974, 1980).

From experiments designed to study the responses of *Scyliorhinus canicula* to the fields over clay and mud bottoms, Pals, Valentijn and Verwey (1982) arrived at the disconcerting conclusion that it was 'impossible to train a dogfish to get its food at a certain place in an electric field'. However, if we may assume that the reported field strength of $500\,\mathrm{nV\,cm^{-1}}$ referred to the central, most uniform part of the field, then the strength a few centimeters over the electrodes must have been on the order of $10\,000\,\mathrm{nV\,cm^{-1}}$, which may have been too high for the animals. Nevertheless, in the light/dark experiments described by the same authors, the dogfishes seemed to accept these exceptionally potent fields as orientational cues. The 'electric wall' experiments from which the authors concluded that 'dogfish actually rely upon electric cues' simply showed a succession of avoidance reactions occurring each time the animals approached the individual electrodes and encountered field strengths of $1000-10\,000\,\mathrm{nV\,cm^{-1}}$ (cf. Kalmijn, 1971). The term 'electric fence' would have been more appropriate. Thus, the results were inconclusive as to whether *Scyliorhinus* might ignore, avoid, or orient to the local fields over clay and mud bottoms. Pals, Peters and Schoenhage (1982) considered the dogfish sufficiently sensitive to detect the local bottom fields, but doubted whether they would orient to the motionally induced fields, while skates would be able to use both. This curious remark was based on the fact that the highly sensitive cardiac deceleration technique was applied to determine the threshold sensitivity of *Raja* (Kalmijn, 1966), but not of *Scyliorhinus*. The dogfish *Mustelus canis* showed feeding responses at voltage gradients of only $5\,\mathrm{nV\,cm^{-1}}$ in experiments at sea (Kalmijn, 1982).

Although orientation to strictly uniform fields simulating those produced by the flow of water has been demonstrated only in the stingray *Urolophus halleri*, it should be noted that electrically-evoked feeding responses have been observed in a large variety of sharks, skates, and rays, and that the ampullae of Lorenzini are present in all species studied, including the plankton-feeding elasmobranchs: the whale shark *Rhiniodon typus* (Dr Compagno, personal communication), the basking shark *Cetorhinus maximus* (Matthews and Parker, 1950), the megamouth shark *Megachasma pelagios* (Dr Compagno, personal communication), and the devil fish *Manta birostris* (Chu and Wen, 1979). The presence of ampullae of Lorenzini in the plankton-feeding elasmobranchs could be construed as indirect evidence for the detection of orientational cues, except that the animals might use their electric sense to locate food-rich patches electrochemically as well (Kalmijn, 1974). Other electrosensitive fishes living or occurring in the ocean are the ratfish *Hydrolagus colliei* (Holocephali), the sturgeon *Acipenser sturio* (Chondrostei), and the marine catfish *Plotosus anguillaris* (Siluridae), which have not yet been tested on their orientational abilities (Fields and Lange, 1980; Jørgensen, Flock and Wersäll, 1972; Obara and Oomura, 1972; Kalmijn, 1974).

Attempts to demonstrate that eel and salmon detect the motional-electric fields of ocean currents have been unsuccessful, although it was for these migratory fishes that the electromagnetic principle was proposed (Deelder, 1952). By conditioning the cardiac reflex, Rommel and McCleave (1972, 1973) at first found that *Anguilla rostrata* and *Salmo salar* react to fields of only $60\,nV\,cm^{-1}$ in $40-\Omega\,cm$ water. However, all efforts to reproduce or confirm the original results have failed: McCleave, Albert and Richardson, 1974; Enger, Kristensen and Sand, 1976; Berge, 1979 (heartbeat); Bullock, 1982 (brain potentials). Kalmijn (1978a) also observed eels search for food, but remain totally indifferent to the electrically-simulated prey that the dogfish *Mustelus canis* attacked from distances of 25 cm and over. A partial explanation of the earlier, disputed data may be found in the use of stainless-steel electrodes and a low-voltage/low-ohmic stimulus circuit (a 1.5-V battery, attenuated by a *voltage* divider). On closing such a circuit, the electrodes produce transients that can be many times higher than the d.c. level of the stimulus, even if a (fast) 'click-free' switch is used. In later studies, the turning tendency of elvers was reported to depend on the strength of an applied field (Zimmerman and McCleave, 1975; McCleave and Power, 1978). However, the experiments did not corroborate the alleged sensitivity, despite the authors' favorable interpretation of the data (cf. Berge, 1979). No trace of electroreceptors or electroreceptive brain centers has been found in the eel (Leonard and Summers, 1976; Bullock, Bodznick and Northcutt, 1983). In summary, even though eels may be moderately sensitive to electric fields, they do not reliably rank even near those fishes with an established electric sense.

Biophysics of receptor system. The structural design of the elasmobranchs' ampullary system lends further support to the detection of the fields induced by ocean currents. The ampullary organs have well-insulating walls and low-resistance cores that allow only negligible ohmic voltage drop to develop within the often long, jelly-filled canals (Figure 5). Thus, nearly the full stimulus appears across the sensory epithelia forming the walls of the ampullae proper (Waltman, 1966). For the organs to detect the virtually uniform oceanic fields most effectively, sets of widely-separated skin pores should connect to ampullae having their sensory epithelia close together so as to avoid undue losses in the intervening tissues. Since the ampullae are usually arranged in clusters which are embedded in gelatinous stromata and surrounded by distinct capsules, this requirement seems adequately met. Viewed in this way, the distribution of the pores is the crucial characteristic for a spatial analysis of the imposed fields, whereas the lengths and directions of the canals 'merely' serve to bring the ampullae of far-separated pore populations into close apposition (Kalmijn, 1974, *vs* Murray, 1967, 1974). Although the ampullae themselves are single-ended input devices, their arrangement in clusters would allow the animals to measure the fields *differentially* by comparing the signals received from individual ampullae and suppressing their *common-mode* contents. Rejection of the common-mode signals would also make the animals less susceptible to interference from their own bioelectric fields, as those are expected to act predominantly on the capsular ends of the

Figure 5. Diagram illustrating the differential operation of the elasmobranchs' electroreceptor system. The individual ampullae detect the voltages at their skin pores relative to those of the capsular stromata to which they are connected. The ampulla on the left detects the voltage at pore A, the ampulla on the right detects the voltage at pore B, both with respect to capsular stroma C. By subtracting the responses of the two ampullae, the animal would measure the voltage difference between pores A and B, which contains the signal of interest, and reject the voltages that the two ampullae have in common, which are largely due to fluctuations in the fish's own bioelectric fields and offer little, if any, information (Kalmijn, 1974). The two ampullae depicted represent all those belonging to a single cluster. Most sharks, skates, and rays have three to four paired clusters, each with a few to well over a hundred ampullary organs. The resistive properties relevant to the operation of the ampullary system are labeled h = high-, i = intermediate-, and l = low-ohmic.

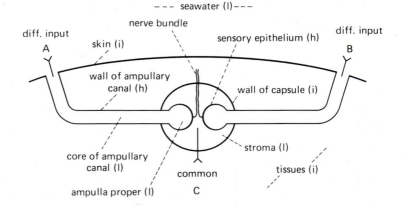

Differential pair of ampullary receptors

ampullary canals. Moreover, the high average resistivity of the skin and body tissues, as compared to that of the seawater medium, drastically affects the shape of the stimulus field, enhancing the available signal (Kalmijn, 1974), despite common belief that elasmobranch fishes would be electrically nearly transparent (Murray, 1967; Bennett and Clusin, 1978). Thus, the design of the peripheral system with the ampullae arranged in clusters and the skin pores covering the heads of sharks, and additionally spreading over the wing-like pectoral fins in skates and rays, would excellently suit the detection and spatial resolution of the oceans' electric fields.

The most sensitive nerve fibers of 2-cm-long ampullary canals showed clear neurophysiological responses to fields of $1000\,\mathrm{nV\,cm^{-1}}$ (Murray, 1962, 1974), which might suffice to explain the behavioral threshold of $5\,\mathrm{nV\,cm^{-1}}$ (Kalmijn, 1982), if the number of fibers per ampulla ($\sim$6), the total number of ampullae (several hundreds), and the distances between the skin pores of ampullae belonging to the same cluster (one-tenth to a third of the body length) are taken into account. When a step function was applied, the action potential rate changed rapidly to a new level (integrating time constant 20–30 ms) to adapt slowly to its former level (differentiating time constant $\sim$3 s), from which an approximate frequency range of 0.05 to at most 8 Hz (-3 db) may be derived. The behavioral responses to prey-simulating dipole fields also diminished sharply at $\sim$8 Hz (Kalmijn, 1974). For the longest ampullary canals, the higher frequencies are additionally attenuated by capacitive leakage through the canal walls (Waltman, 1966). Thus, the ampullae of Lorenzini, although responding to extremely low frequencies, are not true d.c. receptors. This is not surprising, for d.c. receptors would greatly suffer from offset voltages and thermal drift at the microvolt level. Nor does it contradict the animals' high responsiveness to the d.c. fields of prey and ocean currents, as the swimming movements modulate the stimulus fields, bringing them within the frequency range of the receptors (Kalmijn, 1971). For the transduction process at the membrane level, see Bennett and Clusin (1978).

The performance of the receptor system may also be judged from the signal-to-noise (S/N) power ratio of the circuits formed by differential pairs of ampullae and the outside medium (Figure 5). The thermal noise generated by a passive circuit element is given by the root-mean-square voltage $V_n = (4\,\mathrm{k}TBR)^{\frac{1}{2}}$ of an equivalent noise source in series with the impedance of the element, where k is the Boltzmann constant (1.38×10^{-23} Joule/degree Kelvin), T the absolute temperature ($\sim$300 °K), B the noise band-width under consideration

($\pi/2 \times \sim 8\,\text{Hz}$), and R the ohmic resistance of the element. Since the internal resistance, R_i, of the two sensory epithelia is high compared to the external resistance, R_e, of the two canals, the capsular stroma, and the outside medium, the noise voltage of each ampullary pair may be approximated by $V_n = (4\,\text{k}TBR_e)^{\frac{1}{2}}$. (The high noise voltages of the receptor epithelia are effectively shorted out by the external resistance R_e; the much lower noise voltages of the external parts of the circuit, including the ampullary canals, appear across the sensory epithelia practically unattenuated.) Furthermore, the core resistance of the ampullary canals is usually much higher than that of the outside medium and the capsular stroma, so that R_e is mainly determined by the canal dimensions and the resistivity of the core material ($\sim 25\,\Omega\,\text{cm}$, nearly that of seawater). For an ampullary pair with canals 10 cm in length and 0.12 cm in diameter, $R_e = \sim 44\,\text{k}\Omega$ and $V_n = \sim 100\,\text{nV}$. In comparison, a uniform field of 5-nV cm^{-1} threshold strength gives a signal V_s across the two sensory epithelia combined of $\sim 100\,\text{nV}$ also. Thus, regarding the thermal agitation of the charge carriers, the signal-to-noise (S/N) power ratio, $(V_s/V_n)^2$, is about unity for the selected pair of ampullae, if calculated over the neurophysiological bandwidth of $\sim 8\,\text{Hz}$. For the resistance values, see Murray and Potts (1961), Waltman (1966), and Bennett and Clusin (1978).

Since there are, say, 50 ampullae with 10-cm-long canals and a great many with shorter canals, the whole system would operate at an S/N power ratio of ~ 50 at most, depending on the distribution of the skin pores and the direction of the stimulus field (the noise is coherent for the $\sim 10\,000$ receptor cells of the same ampulla, but largely incoherent for the ~ 1000 individual ampullae). Any other sources of extrinsic (environmental) or intrinsic (physiological) noise will lower the S/N ratio. On the other hand, the animal may integrate single events over the duration of the response (thus limiting the bandwidth to the lower frequencies) or make the signal repetitive by exploratory movements and average the response (thus narrowing the bandwidth about the frequencies of interest). This sets the lower limit of the physical noise that the animals have to cope with, independent of how many receptor cells and nerve fibers they have, or how they process the data neurophysiologically. According to Bennett and Clusin (1978), the $8\text{-}\mu\text{m}^2$ electrosensitive luminal membrane of the individual receptor cell would have ~ 30 times higher resistance than the $500\text{-}\mu\text{m}^2$ inactive basal membrane. Nevertheless, the basal membranes of all receptor cells of a single ampulla combined would have a resistance five times higher than that of the jelly-filled canals, which, if correct, would mean a six-fold deterioration of the S/N power ratio. In other words, the thermal noise of the basal membranes of the individual receptor cells would, even when averaged over all 10 000 cells of the single ampulla, still increase the S/N ratio by a factor of six. Other noise calculations by Jungerman and Rosenblum (1980) have suffered from a poor choice of threshold value, canal length, and literature references.

Orientation to the earth's magnetic field: aquatic animals

Behavioral data. After discovering the neurophysiological responses of the ampullae of Lorenzini to weak electric fields, Murray (1962) remarked that elasmobranch fishes, if sensitive enough, could use the electric fields they induce by moving through the earth's magnetic field to decide whether they are heading in an easterly or westerly direction. Discouraged by a one-order of magnitude lack of sensitivity and the complications arising from the phasic nature of the nervous response, Murray wondered, however, whether such a mechanism would be feasible. Shortly thereafter, the notion of an electromagnetic compass sense received renewed attention, when it was learned that sharks and skates were behaviorally up to two hundred times more sensitive to electric fields than expected from the neurophysiological recordings (Dijkgraaf and Kalmijn, 1962; Kalmijn, 1966, 1982). Furthermore, a study of the physics involved revealed that the design of the ampullary system would allow the detection of the stimuli that the animals themselves induce as well as those of ocean currents and prey (Kalmijn, 1974).

Despite the electrical sensitivity of the animals and the biophysical adequacy of their electroreceptor system, it remained to be determined whether the fishes *are* capable of orienting to the earth's magnetic field, and if so, that they make use of the proposed electromagnetic mechanism. To address the first, most crucial question, the stingray *Urolophus halleri* was conditioned to procure food, this time, from an enclosure in the *magnetic east*, and not to visit a similar enclosure in the *magnetic west* of its seawater habitat (Kalmijn, 1978b, 1981, Figure 6a). Despite the random sequence of normal and reversed field conditions, instituted to prevent the use of alternative cues, the stingrays readily learned to base their choices on the direction of the ambient magnetic field ($P \leqslant 0.001$, Figure 6b). The strength and inclination of the magnetic test fields were those of the San Diego area from where the animals were collected (0.49 gauss and 58 degrees respectively). In recent tests (Figure 6b, unpublished data), the stingrays also showed significant orientation in strictly horizontal fields of equatorial strength (0.40 gauss), proving the vectorial nature of the response (detection of both the direction and the polarity of the field).

The second question, whether the animals detect the earth's magnetic field by the electric fields they themselves induce, may be addressed by first training the stingrays to orient to a *horizontal magnetic* field, and subsequently testing them in a magnetic null field on their responses to *vertical electric* fields simulating those they would have received if the magnetic field were still present. At the moment, the strongest argument in favor of the electromagnetic principle is the fact that the animals receive the appropriate signals even when swimming at speeds of only a few centimeters per second and that the signals suffice to explain the vectorial nature of the animals' magnetic compass sense (see above). Furthermore, the stingrays' ability to orient to imposed electric fields of $5\,\mathrm{nV\,cm^{-1}}$ while swimming through the earth's magnetic field would seem to require a thorough familiarity with the 10–$100\,\mathrm{nV\,cm^{-1}}$ fields they induce by their forward motion (p. 534). A good knowledge of the detection mechanism will also aid the design of magnetic orientation experiments at sea.

The remote possibility of an electromagnetic compass sense in the eel remains shrouded in controversy for lack of decisive data. Branover, Vasil'yev, Gleyzer and Tsinober (1971) reported non-random distributions of eels in the ambient magnetic field, but based their electromagnetic calculations on erroneous formulae, whereas McCleave and Power (1978) could not reproduce Branover et al.'s results. Tesch (1974) observed a north–south preference in eel, but argued against the use of the motional-electrical fields of either ocean currents or the animals themselves. For freshwater electrosensitive fishes, the electromagnetic principle is less plausible than for the marine species. Not that the *induced* electric fields are weaker, but the animals are expected to be much less effective in detecting the resulting *ohmic* fields (p. 535). The lowest voltage gradient at which the freshwater catfish *Ictalurus nebulosus* and the weakly electric fish *Hypopomus* sp. oriented to uniform electric fields was $1000\,\mathrm{nV\,cm^{-1}}$ (Kalmijn, Kolba and Kalmijn, 1976a), as compared with $5\,\mathrm{nV\,cm^{-1}}$ for the marine stingray *Urolophus halleri*. This difference is not merely due to the resistivity of the medium, for the threshold sensitivity of the catfish was not noticeably affected by dilution of the aquarium water from 2 to $40\,\mathrm{k\Omega\,cm}$ (unpublished data).

A few remarks on the definitions of *passive* and *active* electroreception may be helpful to avoid needless confusion. In keeping with engineering convention, a sensory system is called passive if the energy it receives originates from the environment, and is called active if the

Figure 6. Orientation of the stingray *Urolophus halleri* to the earth's magnetic field. (a) The stingrays are trained to obtain food from an enclosure in the magnetic east and to avoid a similar enclosure in the magnetic west. The magnetic field is controlled by two sets of Helmholtz coils having their axes along the local meridian and the vertical respectively. The horizontal direction of the field is either normal or reversed according to a random sequence. (b) Results of training experiments for six stingrays (two times 1–3) under two different magnetic conditions: (A) the field has a total strength of 0.49 gauss and an inclination of 58 degrees as in the San Diego area from where the animals were collected, (B) the field has a total strength of 0.40 gauss and an inclination of zero degrees as at certain locations along the magnetic equator. The latter experiments demonstrate that the animals derive both the direction and polarity from the ambient magnetic field. The results are evaluated by the sequential probability ratio test, mentioned in the legends of Figure 4. For the magnetic experiments, orientation is defined by a seven-out-of-ten (0.70) rather than a three-out-of-four (0.75) correct score.

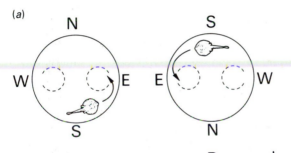

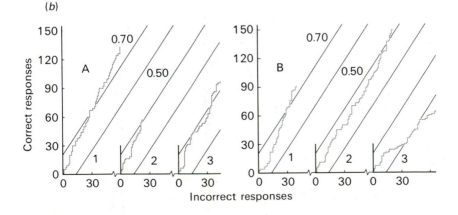

energy it receives is generated by the animal itself (Machin, 1962). Electrosensory systems may operate in either a passive or active *mode* (Kalmijn, 1974). Thus, weakly electric fishes can detect the electrical discharges of conspecifics (passive mode) or probe the environment with their own electric-organ discharges (active mode). Similarly, elasmobranch fishes can detect the fields of ocean currents (passive mode) or use the fields they induce themselves to detect their magnetic compass headings (active mode). Therefore, the use of the term active for the sensory systems of fishes with electric organs and the term passive for those of fishes without is improper. The terms active and passive electrosensitive fishes are amusing at best.

Biophysics of receptor system. Is it reasonable to assume that elasmobranch fishes detect both the uniform fields of ocean currents and the fields induced by their own swimming movements with the same receptor system, and is it really possible to simulate the fields induced by free-swimming animals? Although it may not be intuitively obvious, the answer is that the physical requirements for the two modes of operation are very similar, if not identical, and that the one type of field can mimic the effects of the other if we may approximate the fishes to highly-resistive bodies of ellipsoid shape (theorem of equivalence). Because the animals' dorsoventrally-averaged resistivities are about one hundred times higher than that of seawater, and their body shapes resemble, with some imagination, rostrocaudally elongated ellipsoids (for sharks) or ventrodorsally flattened ellipsoids (for skates and rays), this approximation is not unreasonable. Thus, according to physical theory, the ohmic voltage differences that the fish receive when exposed to uniform electric fields (pp. 526–30) are essentially the same as those they receive when actively moving through the earth's magnetic field, except for the probably minor, but as yet undetermined, effects of the flow of water around the swimming animal (p. 531). Normally, the two types of field are readily distinguished, as they act along different axes and are different functions of the animals' movements.

The neurophysiological responses of the ampullae of Lorenzini can be studied either by simulating the motional-electric fields, or by having the fish actually move with respect to water. Direct electrical stimulation requires imposed fields of uniform configuration applied perpendicularly to the imaginary swimming velocity, v, and to the earth's magnetic field, B, in conformity with the theorem of equivalence (except for the effect of the water flowing around the fish). This implies that Murray's

1962 experiments may have been more relevant to the active mode of orientation than he realized at the time. On the other hand, if the fish is stimulated by having it move or by towing it through the water, the motion should take place with respect to a mass of water sufficiently large to short-circuit the animal's body as a source of motional electricity. If the fish is kept stationary while the water rushes by, a long channel lined by walls of insulating material should be used to suppress the ohmic field of the flowing water. Moving both the fish and the aquarium through the earth's magnetic field (Rommel, 1973) does not offer a meaningful test situation due to the lack of a suitable return path.

A first attempt to test the ampullae of Lorenzini on their responses to induced electric fields was made by Andrianov, Brown and Ilyinsky (1974). The skate *Trygon pastinaca* was placed over one pole of an electromagnet, through the windings of which a linearly increasing current was passed, thus producing a steady change in ventrodorsal magnetic flux. However, Andrianov et al. were mistaken in equating the applied stimulus with that of rectilinear motion. Such a stimulus would only occur in nature when a skate passively somersaults or rolls over, carried by a mass of water trapped in a small, rocky pool. In the rectilinear case, the stimulus current flows across the animal; in their case it circulated in and around the animal (Figures 2a and 3a). The observed responses only confirmed that (1) electric fields can be obtained from changes in magnetic flux (Faraday, 1832), and (2) the ampullae of Lorenzini can be excited by electric fields (Murray, 1962), even by those rarely encountered in the natural habitat. This misconception of the physics involved was perpetuated by Akoev, Ilyinsky and Zadan (1976). Brown and Ilyinsky (1978) repeated the experiments once more and, without commenting on the fallacy of earlier statements, inferred that the skates may sense the natural variations in the earth's magnetic field. However, low-frequency magnetic variations of the reported threshold strength (0.8 gauss s^{-1}) are unheard of, and the electric fields induced by more natural magnetic variations tend to be uniform rather than concentric when measured over the volume occupied by the animal. At last, Brown and Ilyinsky (1978) conducted tests in which the fish were towed through the water or the water was rushed over a stationary fish. These experiments were interpreted in keeping with the theory and terminology introduced by Kalmijn (1974) and showed ampullary responses to genuine motional-electric fields, although not to the dorsoventral fields that the animals would use to orient to the earth's magnetic field.

Orientation to the earth's magnetic field: land and airborne animals

Behavioral data. With regard to rectilinear motion, even the fastest-flying birds would have great difficulty detecting the electric fields they induce, as the animals tend to short-circuit the highly resistive medium rather than being short-circuited by it (pp. 530–535). Nevertheless, there is some room for speculation (Yeagley, 1947; Neurath, 1964; Barnothy, 1964). In the absence of an external current path, opposing body surfaces collect electric charges of opposite polarity until the electrostatic field they produce offsets the internally induced field. Rapid changes in speed or direction of flight cause transient polarization currents flowing across the body to readjust the charge separations. However, the resulting ohmic fields that the animals would have to detect are on the order of only picovolts per centimeter. Birds also modulate the rectilinearly-induced fields by the flapping of their wings, but the resulting signals are as weak as those of the changes in speed or direction of flight. Thus, the high sensitivity required, together with the high level of atmospheric and frictional noise (Davis, 1948; Slepian, 1948; Varian, 1948), render the rectilinear mechanism highly implausible for airborne animals. It is unfortunate that Yeagley (1947) did not realize the need of an external current path for the detection of the motionally induced field, that Varian (1948) overlooked the theoretical feasibility of separating the signals induced by the bird and by its drift with the air, that Neurath (1964) confused the effects of rectilinear and angular motion, and that Barnothy (1964) incorrectly derived Faraday's law from the special theory of relativity as 'a physical phenomenon not yet considered'.

An anecdotal example of the need for a careful analysis is offered by the experiments in which pigeons were examined on their use of the earth's magnetic field during shipment to the release site (Papi et al., 1978). One group of pigeons was transported in an iron container that effectively excluded the earth's magnetic field from its interior, whereas the control birds were placed in a similar container made of aluminum. At the Tübingen (1977) conference where the paper was presented, it was suggested that the iron container deprived the birds of the electromagnetic information that the control birds might have received from their rectilinear motion through the earth's magnetic field. However, the aluminum container did not allow the control birds to receive such information either. Although in the reference frame of the aluminum container the magnetic field was quite normal, no motion took place and, consequently, no fields were induced. Certainly, by moving with respect to the earth's frame of reference, the container was exposed to a uniform electric field. However, the birds could not detect this field, for they were electrically shielded from it by the aluminum shell. An outside observer would explain the situation by saying that both the container and the birds induced electric fields, but that electric charges on the outside and inside of the shell, accumulating to expel the field from the highly conductive metal, produced an electrostatic field within the cavity exactly opposing the induced field, thus again leaving nothing for the poor pigeons to detect (cf. Smythe, 1968). Of course, the aluminum container did not prohibit the animals from monitoring the direction of the earth's magnetic field, whereas the iron container made even that impossible. The results of Papi et al.'s (1978) experiments actually showed large differences in the vanishing bearings of birds transported in iron and aluminum containers,

Biophysics of receptor system. If for land and airborne animals the detection of rectilinearly-induced fields offers so little promise, why then have the rotationally-induced fields, that do not depend on the resistivity of the medium, received so little attention? When an animal turns right or left, it is subject to a change of horizontal magnetic flux through any internal loop of vertical extent. When body parts move relative to one another, as in flying birds, deformations of the loops embracing those parts cause additional changes of magnetic flux. Thus, besides modulating the rectilinearly-induced fields, the turning movements of animals and the movements of body parts also induce electromotive forces of themselves (pp. 535–541). The signals could reach as much as 400 nV for an animal having a transverse loop enclosing a 100-cm^2 surface area and turning at a rate of 1 radian s^{-1} (a full U-turn in π seconds) or for an animal having a transverse loop of 10 cm^2, turning at a rate of 10 radians s^{-1} (a full U-turn in $\pi/10$ seconds), both of which would be quite natural. The signals induced by relative motion of body parts, if leading to sinusoidal changes of 10% in surface area, could reach 400 nV for loops of 100 cm^2 at a frequency of 1.6 Hz, and for loops of 10 cm^2 at a frequency of 16 Hz. The discouraging fact is that we do not know of any suitable sensory structures for the detection of these rotationally-induced fields. The semicircular canals form a three-dimensional set of fluid loops, but do not seem to qualify for lack of efficiency (p. 540).

Nevertheless, Jungerman and Rosenblum (1980) developed a mathematical model for the hypothetical loop detector and came to the conclusion that a ring canal of large outer diameter and very small inner diameter would be most desirable in order to attain an acceptable signal-to-noise level. A high-ohmic receptor membrane, inserted into the circular path of the canal, would supposedly collect the motionally-induced signal. However, they thereby stretched their model beyond repair and arrived at the physically inadvantageous situation in which the inner part of the single winding, instead of contributing to the signal, would tend to short the outer part for which the induced electromotive force was calculated. On the other hand, imagine a structure consisting of two ampullae of Lorenzini having their canals connected in series so as to form a closed, subcutaneous loop around the animal. The noise voltage of such a loop would only be slightly higher than the noise of two similar ampullae of Lorenzini connecting the dorsal and ventral surfaces of the animal, whereas the signals for the two configurations would be of the same strength for a fish of 100-cm^2 cross-sectional area and $10\,cm$ in height, turning at a rate of 1 radian s^{-1} at a forward speed of $10\,cm\,s^{-1}$. In short, the rotational principle cannot be rejected off-hand, although at the present time there is no evidence for its implementation.

Conclusions

Electric fields induced by tidal flows and ocean currents offer sharks, skates, and rays information about their drift at sea, and provide them with local orientational cues in shallow, protected waters. The electrochemical fields prevailing in the freshwater milieu could play a role in the ocean as well.

Sharks, skates and rays induce electric fields by their forward motion from which the animals may derive their magnetic compass headings. Animals in higher resistive media would have to rely on the electric fields they induce by turning or by the relative motion of body parts.

Marine stingrays are able to orient to uniform electric fields of oceanic strength as well as to magnetic fields of both equatorial and mid-latitude inclinations. For the orientation to electric fields, voltage gradients of $5\,nV\,cm^{-1}$ suffice. To detect their magnetic compass headings, the animals would have to swim at speeds of only a few centimeters per second.

The structural design of the elasmobranchs' electroreceptor system allows the animals to detect both the fields related to their drift and the fields signaling their magnetic compass headings. The same sensory system would also play a role in the detection of prey.

Freshwater, land, and airborne animals could conceivably determine their magnetic compass headings from the entirely internal motional-electric fields which are independent of the external medium. However, the lack of information on adequate sensory structures is not encouraging.

Drs George E. Backus, Theodore H. Bullock, Alan D. Chave, Charles S. Cox, James T. Enright, Jean H. Filloux, and Walter H. Munk have generously shared their time and wisdom with the author. Also his wife Vera and his son Jelger have offered invaluable help. The responsibility of any remaining errors rests solely with the author. This research was conducted under the auspices of the Office of Naval Research, Environmental Sciences, Drs Eric O. Hartwig and Bernhard J. Zahuranec, Program Directors.

References

Akoev, G. N., Ilyinsky, O. B., and Zadan, P. M. (1976). Responses of electroreceptors (ampullae of Lorenzini) of skates to electric and magnetic fields. *J. Comp. Physiol.* *106:* 127–36.

Andrianov, G. N., Brown, H. R., and Ilyinski, O. B. (1974). Responses of central neurons to electrical and magnetic stimuli of the ampullae of Lorenzini in the Black Sea skate. *J. Comp. Physiol. 93:* 287–99.

Barnothy, J. M. (1964). Proposed mechanisms for the navigation of migrating birds. In *Biological Effects of Magnetic Fields,* ed. M. F. Barnothy, pp. 287–93. New York: Plenum Press.

Bennett, M. V. L., and Clusin, W. T. (1978). Physiology of the ampulla of Lorenzini, the electroreceptor of elasmobranchs. In *Sensory Biology of Sharks, Skates, and Rays,* ed. E. S. Hodgson and R. W. Mathewson, pp. 483–505. Washington, DC: Government Printing Office.

Berge, J. A. (1979). The perception of weak electric a.c. currents by the European eel, *Anguilla anguilla. Comp. Biochem. Physiol. 62A:* 915–19.

Branover, G. G., Vasil'yev, A. S., Gleyzer, S. I., and Tsinober, A. B. (1971). A study of the behavior of the eel in natural and artificial and magnetic fields and an analysis of its reception mechanism. *J. Ichthyol. 11:* 608–14.

Brown, H. R., and Ilyinsky, O. B. (1978). The ampullae of Lorenzini in the magnetic field. *J. Comp. Physiol. 126:* 333–41.

Bullock, T. H. (1982). Electroreception. *A. Rev. Neurosci. 5:* 121–70.

Bullock, T. H., Bodznick, D. A., and Northcutt, R. G. (1983). The phylogenetic distribution of electroreception: evidence for convergent evolution of a primitive vertebrate sense modality. *Brain Res. Rev. 6:* 25–46.

Chave, A. D. (1983). On the theory of electromagnetic induction in the earth by ocean currents. *J. Geophys. Res. 88:* 3531–42.

Chu, Y. T., and Wen, M. C. (1979). A study of the lateral-line canals system and that of Lorenzini ampullae and tubules of Chondrichthyes fishes of China. *Monograph of Fishes of China,* No. 2. Shanghai: Science and Technology Press.

Cox, C. S., Filloux, J. H., and Larsen, J. C. (1970). Electromagnetic studies of ocean currents and electrical conductivity below the ocean-floor. In *The Sea*, ed. A. E. Maxwell, pp. 637–93. London, Sydney, Toronto: Wiley.

Davis, Jr. L. (1948). Remarks on: 'The physical basis of bird navigation'. *J. Appl. Phys. 19:* 307–8.

Deelder, C. L. (1952). On the migration of the elver (*Anguilla vulgaris* Turt.) at sea. *J. Cons. Int. Explor. Mer 18:* 187–218.

Dijkgraaf, S., and Kalmijn, A. J. (1962). Verhaltensversuche zur Funktion der Lorenzinischen Ampullen. *Naturwissenschaften 49:* 400.

Dijkgraaf, S., and Kalmijn, A. J. (1963). Untersuchungen über die Funktion der Lorenzinischen Ampullen an Haifischen. *Z. vergl. Physiol. 47:* 438–56.

Dijkgraaf, S., and Kalmijn, A. J. (1966). Versuche zur biologischen Bedeutung der Lorenzinischen Ampullen bei den Elasmobranchiern. *Z. vergl. Physiol. 53:* 187–94.

Enger, P. S., Kristensen, L., and Sand, O. (1976). The perception of weak electric d.c. currents by the European eel (*Anguilla anguilla*). *Comp. Biochem. Physiol. 54A:* 101–3.

Faraday, M. (1832). Experimental researches in electricity. *Phil. Trans. Roy. Soc. Lond. 122(1):* 125–94.

Fields, R. D., and Lange, G. D. (1980). Electroreception in the ratfish (*Hydrolagus colliei*). *Science 207:* 547–8.

Filloux, J. H. (1974). Electric field recording on the sea floor with short span instruments. *J. Geomag. Geoelectric. 26:* 269–79.

Filloux, J. H. (1980). Observation of very low frequency electromagnetic signals in the ocean. *J. Geomag. Geoelectric. 32:* Suppl. 1, SI 1–SI 12.

Jørgensen, J. M., Flock, A., and Wersäll, J. (1972). The Lorenzinian ampullae of *Polyodon spathula*. *Z. Zellforsch. 130:* 362–77.

Jungerman, R. L., and Rosenblum, B. (1980). Magnetic induction for the sensing of magnetic fields by animals – an analysis. *J. Theor. Biol. 87:* 25–32.

Kalmijn, A. J. (1966). Electro-perception in sharks and rays. *Nature 212:* 1232–3.

Kalmijn, A. J. (1971). The electric sense of sharks and rays. *J. Exp. Biol. 55:* 371–83.

Kalmijn, A. J. (1974). The detection of electric fields from inanimate and animate sources other than electric organs. In *Handbook of Sensory Physiology*, vol. III/3, ed. A. Fessard, pp. 147–200. Berlin, Heidelberg, New York: Springer-Verlag.

Kalmijn, A. J. (1978a). Experimental evidence of geomagnetic orientation in elasmobranch fishes. In *Animal Migration, Navigation, and Homing*, ed. K. Schmidt-Koenig and W. T. Keeton, pp. 347–53. Berlin, Heidelberg, New York: Springer-Verlag.

Kalmijn, A. J. (1978b). Electric and magnetic sensory world of sharks, skates, and rays. In *Sensory Biology of Sharks, Skates, and Rays*, ed. E. S. Hodgson and R. F. Mathewson, pp. 507–28. Washington, DC: Government Printing Office.

Kalmijn, A. J. (1981). Biophysics of geomagnetic field detection. *IEEE Trans. Magnetics 17:* 1113–24.

Kalmijn, A. J. (1982). Electric and magnetic field detection in elasmobranch fishes. *Science 218:* 916–18.

Kalmijn, A. J., and Kalmijn, V. (1981). Orientation to uniform electric fields in the stingray *Urolophus halleri*: sensitivity of response. *Biol. Bull. 161:* 347.

Kalmijn, A. J., Kolba, C. A., and Kalmijn, V. (1976a). Orientation of catfish (*Ictalurus nebulosus*) in strictly uniform electric fields: I. Sensitivity of response. *Biol. Bull. 151:* 415.

Kalmijn, V., Kolba, C. A., and Kalmijn, A. J. (1976b). Orientation of catfish (*Ictalurus nebulosus*) in strictly uniform electric fields: II. Spatial discrimination. *Biol. Bull. 151:* 415–16.

Larsen, J. C. (1968). Electric and magnetic fields induced by deep sea tides. *Geophys. J. Roy. Astr. Soc. Lond. 16:* 47–70.

Leonard, J. B., and Summers, R. G. (1976). The ultrastructure of the integument of the American eel, *Anguilla rostrata. Cell Tiss. Res. 171:* 1–30.

Longuet-Higgins, M. S., Stern, M. E., and Stommel, H. (1954). The electrical field induced by ocean currents and waves, with applications to the method of towed electrodes. *Papers Phys. Oceanog. Meteorol. 13:* 1–37.

Machin, K. E. (1962). Electric receptors. *Symp. Soc. Exp. Biol. 16:* 227–44.

Matthews, L. H., and Parker, H. W. (1950). Notes on the anatomy and biology of the basking shark (*Cetorhinus maximus* (Gunner)). *Proc. Zool. Soc. Lond. 120:* 535–76.

McCleave, J. D., Albert, E. H., and Richardson, N. E. (1974). Perception and effects on locomotor activity in American eels and Atlantic salmon of extremely low frequency electric and magnetic fields. *Final Rep. Office of Naval Res.* Contract No. N00014-72-C-0130, pp. 1–44.

McCleave, J. D., and Power, J. H. (1978). Influence of weak electric and magnetic fields on turning behavior in elvers of the American eel *Anguilla rostrata. Mar. Biol. 46:* 29–34.

Murray, R. W. (1962). The response of the ampullae of Lorenzini of elasmobranchs to electrical stimulation. *J. Exp. Biol. 39:* 119–28.

Murray, R. W. (1967). The function of the ampullae of Lorenzini of elasmobranchs. In *Lateral Line Detectors*, ed. P. Cahn, pp. 277–93. Bloomington: Indiana University Press.

Murray, R. W. (1974). The ampullae of Lorenzini. In *Handbook of Sensory Physiology*, vol. III/3, ed. A. Fessard, pp. 125–46. Berlin, Heidelberg, New York: Springer-Verlag.

Murray, R. W., and Potts, W. T. W. (1961). The composition of the endolymph, perilymph and other body fluids of elasmobranchs. *Comp. Biochem. Physiol. 2:* 65–75.

Neurath, P. W. (1964). Simple theoretical models for magnetic interactions with biological units. In *Biological Effects of Magnetic Fields*, ed. M. F. Barnothy, pp. 25–32. New York: Plenum Press.

Obara, S., and Oomura, Y. (1972). Receptor mechanism of a specialized lateralline organ in the sea catfish, *Plotosus anguillaris. J. Physiol. Soc. Japan 34:* 599.

Pals, N., and Schoenhage, A. A. C. (1979). Marine electric fields and fish orientation. *J. Physiol., Paris 75:* 349–53.

Pals, N., Peters, R. C., and Schoenhage, A. A. C. (1982). Local geo-electric fields at the bottom of the sea and their relevance for electrosensitive fish. *Netherlands J. Zool. 32:* 479–94.

Pals, N., Valentijn, P., and Verwey, D. (1982). Orientation reactions of the dogfish, *Scyliorhinus canicula*, to local electric fields. *Netherlands J. Zool. 32:* 495–512.

Papi, F., Ioalé, P., Fiaschi, V., Benvenuti, S., and Baldaccini, N. E. (1978). Pigeon homing: cues detected during the outward journey influence initial orientation. In *Animal Migration, Navigation, and Homing*, ed. K. Schmidt-Koenig and W. T. Keeton, pp. 65–77. Berlin, Heidelberg, New York: Springer-Verlag.

Rommel, S. A. (1973). Apparatus for simulating motion of animals through the geomagnetic field. *J. Fish. Res. Bd Can. 30:* 1581–2.

Rommel, S. A., and McCleave, J. D. (1972). Oceanic electric fields: perception by American eels? *Science 176:* 1233–5.

Rommel, S. A., and McCleave, J. D. (1973). Sensitivity of American eels (*Anguilla rostrata*) and Atlantic salmon (*Salmo salar*) to weak electric and magnetic fields. *J. Fish. Res. Bd Can. 30:* 657–63.

Royce, W. F., Smith, L. S., and Hartt, A. C. (1968). Models of oceanic migrations of Pacific salmon and comments on guidance mechanisms. *Fish. Bull. Fish Wildlife Serv. US 66:* 441–62.

Sanford, T. B. (1971). Motionally induced electric and magnetic fields in the sea. *J. Geophys. Res. 76:* 3476–92.

Sanford, T. B. (1975). Observations of the vertical structure of internal waves. *J. Geophys. Res. 80:* 3861–71.

Sanford, T. B., Drever, R. G., and Dunlap, J. H. (1978). A velocity profiler based on the principles of geomagnetic induction. *Deep-Sea Res. 25:* 183–210.

Slepian, J. (1948). Physical basis of bird navigation. *J. Appl. Phys. 19:* 306.

Smythe, W. R. (1968). *Static and Dynamic Electricity.* New York: McGraw-Hill.

Tesch, F. W. (1974). Influence of geomagnetism and salinity on the directional choice of eels. *Helgoländer wiss. Meeresuntersuch. 26:* 382–95.

Varian, R. H. (1948). Remarks on: 'A preliminary study of a physical basis of bird navigation'. *J. Appl. Phys. 19:* 306–7.

Von Arx, W. S. (1962). *An Introduction to Physical Oceanography.* Reading, London: Addison-Wesley.

Waltman, B. (1966). Electrical properties and fine structure of the ampullary canals of Lorenzini. *Acta Physiol. Scand. 66:* Suppl. 264, 1–60.

Yeagley, H. L. (1947). A preliminary study of a physical basis of bird navigation. *J. Appl. Phys. 18:* 1035–63.

Zimmerman, M. A., and McCleave, J. D. (1975). Orientation of elvers of American eels (*Anguilla rostrata*) in weak magnetic and electric fields. *Helgoländer wiss. Meeresuntersuch. 27:* 175–89.

5
Posture and muscle control

5.1

Cellular bases for gravistatic reception by invertebrates and vertebrates

CHRISTOPHER PLATT

Perspectives

Literature

Gravireceptive organs detect changes in orientation relative to the constant vertical pull of gravity, providing a signal for control of posture and locomotion. Nearly all classes of metazoans have gravireceptor cells, often in paired complex organs, where large numbers of sensory cells and neurons are organized into particular spatial arrays. Along with the peripheral organs, several levels of central neurons can be considered to form a gravistatic system in the central nervous system (CNS), producing behavioral responses to gravitational stimuli.

Several reviews in the last decade cover gravitational sensing systems, including whole volumes (Gordon and Cohen, 1971; Kornhuber, 1974; Schöne, 1975a; Mill, 1976) and major reviews (Markl, 1974; Goldberg and Fernández, 1975; Schöne, 1975b; Wilson and Peterson, 1978; Precht, 1979). Some cover particular animal groups such as molluscs (Vinnikov et al., 1968; Wolff, 1975; Budelmann, 1976), crustaceans (Schöne, 1971), insects (Horn, 1975a) and fishes (Lowenstein, 1971; Platt, 1983). Other extensive data appear in comparative works (Retzius, 1881; Hyman, 1940; Bullock and Horridge, 1965).

In this review, I will focus on recent studies on gravireceptive sensory cells, rather than provide a taxonomic or historical survey, or compare the central integration of gravistatic compensatory behaviors. Recently, some remarkable morphological similarities have been shown between the cephalopod and the vertebrate gravistatic receptors, and intracellular recordings have helped clarify the physiological transduction process in both arthropod and vertebrate gravistatic receptors.

563

Gravitational stimuli

Gravitational force has both magnitude and direction, so it is a vectorial quantity. The use of gravity as a distinct reference may depend on the constancy of gravitational input compared to the brief and variable linear accelerations produced by other forces (Mayne, 1974; see Lewis, this volume, for a discussion of acceleration and velocity detection).

A mass accelerated toward the earth by gravity exerts a force on a restraint that we call weight, $W = mg$, where m is the mass and g is the gravitational acceleration that is nearly constant over all the earth's surface. This force vector is directed toward the earth's center, defining a 'vertical' direction. If a mass is in a fluid, its effective weight is decreased by the buoyant force that depends on the density differential from the supporting fluid.

Conceptually, two different signals could be used for behavioral output (Figure 1). (1) The pressure component is maximal when the detecting surface is in the horizontal position. As the detector is tilted in any direction, the pressure magnitude decreases, going to zero when the vertical position is reached. Tilting past the vertical, the force then becomes a tension ('negative pressure') as the weight pulls instead of pushes on the surface, reaching a maximum when the detector is upside-down. (2) In contrast, the shearing component from gravity is zero when the detecting surface is horizontal, and will increase as the tilt

---

Figure 1. Pressure and shearing components of gravitational force. The relative magnitudes of separate components of the gravitational force vector depend on the orientation of the surface. The diagrammed line indicates a sensory surface, the arrow indicates the force applied to the surface from the gravity vector component. (A) A surface horizontal in the normal position (0°) is subject to maximum pressure that decreases with any tilt away from the normal. The pressure does not change direction when the surface is tilted in any direction from normal, but does go to zero (0) and changes sign from a push (+) to a pull (−) on tilting across the vertical. Stimulus magnitude follows a cosinusoidal relation around the tilting origin, as shown in the polar plot, with maxima at 0° and 180°, whatever the tilt direction. (B) A surface horizontal in the normal position (0°) is subject to no gravitational shear (0), which increases with any tilt away from the normal. Unlike pressure, the shear is a directional vector, aligned orthogonal to the axis of tilt; shear changes direction by 180° when crossing the horizontal, but not when crossing the vertical. Stimulus magnitude follows a sinusoidal relation around the tilting axis, with maxima at 90° and 270°; these maxima decrease in amplitude as a cosine function of the angle between the direction of the tilt and the directional sensitivity axis of the detector.

increases; furthermore, the component of shear in a given direction across the surface will depend on the direction of tilt. As the vertical position is reached and crossed, the shear vector becomes maximal, then declines in magnitude, but without changing its direction. So pressure (which is not a vectorial quantity) follows a cosine function of tilting angle, with uniform gain for tilts in any direction, and pressure changes sign when tilting to either side of the vertical. But the shearing force vector follows a sine function of tilting angle, with a gain that is a cosine function of the tilt direction relative to the axis of shearing sensitivity, and shear changes direction when tilting to either side of the horizontal.

A simple input–output control for gravistatic homeostasis thus would be by a shear detector that is horizontal when the animal is in its normal posture. This orientation would produce compensatory responses that increase in magnitude on increased tilt away from normal, and produce the directional reciprocity required for negative feedback stabilization.

Evolution

Gravistatic organs usually are such shear detectors having elements that can be bent when an attached mass is displaced by gravity (Figure 2). If this mass is stony, it is known as a statolith (Figure 2A), or an otolith (Figure 2B) if it is in the vertebrate ear. An organ that fully encapsulates the statolith is a statocyst, but some statolith organs are pendulous (Figure 2C) instead of enclosed (see Markl, 1974). The receptor cells often have cilia as mechanical elements (see Markl, 1974).

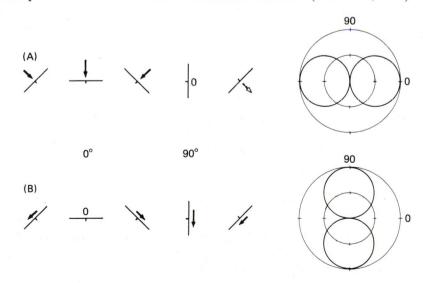

Phylogenetically, gravistatic organs have a venerable lineage. Indeed, the statocyst of coelenterates may have been the first true sensory organ (Hyman, 1940; Bullock and Horridge, 1965). Gravireceptors have not been found in sponges (Porifera) nor in many of the phyla of worms, especially among parasites, but at the other extreme, particularly complex gravistatic organs have evolved in two invertebrate classes, the crustaceans and the cephalopods, and similar complexity occurs in the vertebrates.

Gross structure

Statocysts and otolith organs are both structured to act as shear detectors. There are especially striking similarities between the octopus statocyst system and the vertebrate vestibular system (Young, 1977). Insect statocysts have not been discovered, and many insects utilize proprioceptors in or near joints to detect loading forces on different body parts (Mill, 1976); but recently, some insects have been found to use particular pendulous hairs on the cuticle (Figure 2D) as gravireceptors.

Statocysts

Statocysts are the gravireceptive organs in many invertebrates. In general, a statocyst is a spheroidal chamber filled with fluid, containing crystalline grains that adhere together to form a statolith (Figure 2A). The chamber lining may contain as few as only three hairs in an isopod crustacean (Rose and Stokes, 1981), to thousands of receptor cells in many molluscs (see Markl, 1974; Wolff, 1975), and these cells may be localized to form a patch called a sensory macula or cushion. The sensory cells in arthropods have dendrites linked to a cuticular hair, while many molluscs have ciliated hair cells. The paired statocysts of crustaceans may lie in the head as in amphipods and decapods, or instead near the tail as in isopods and mysid shrimps; the highly differentiated, paired statocysts in the head of both gastropods and cephalopods send projections to central ganglia (see Markl, 1974).

Otolith organs

The otolith organs of the paired inner ears in the head of a vertebrate are the peripheral gravireceptors of the vestibular system (see Lowenstein, 1974). Each otolith organ is a membraneous pouch containing a fluid endolymph and a mass of calcified crystals called the otolith or otoconia (Figure 2B). On one surface of the chamber wall is a macula of mechanosensory hair cells, each carrying a protruding ciliary bundle. There may be more than two hundred thousand hair cells in a single macula (Corwin, 1981). A gelatinous coating around the crystals called the otolithic membrane is believed to couple the mass to the cilia mechanically (Lim, 1979).

In gnathostome vertebrates, from elasmobranchs through mammals, each ear always contains at least two otolith organs. The utricle is the more dorsal organ, and has its sensory macula on the floor of the pouch, with the otolith lying upon it. The saccule is more ventral, and its sensory macula on the medial wall has the otolith hanging roughly vertically. A third otolith organ, the lagena, is present in most non-mammalian vertebrates as an outpouching posterior to the saccule, also with its macula on the medial wall. Behavioral responses after surgical removal of different otolith organs have verified that the utricle is the major gravistatic otolith organ in most vertebrates (Lowenstein, 1974). The saccule and lagena may be more involved in acoustic or vibrational reception than in gravireception, depending on the species (see Lowenstein, 1974; Hillman, 1976; Precht, 1976; Caston, Precht and Blanks, 1977; Platt and Popper, 1981).

Figure 2. Gravireceptor organs. Schematic sections show receptors (stippled) in relation to dense mass (shaded). (A) Statocyst. Statoliths if free to fall can stimulate sensory cells on the lowest side of the sphere. (B) Otolith organ. Statolith displacements are limited, and coupled to sensory macula by a gelatinous membrane (dashed outline). (C) Pendant statolith organ. Deflection of pendant mass stimulates receptors that surround it, or its own receptors. (D) Tricholith organ. Deflection of pendant mass bends a stalk that then stimulates an internal receptor.

(A)

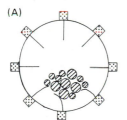

(B)

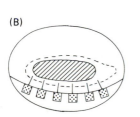

(C)

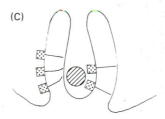

(D)

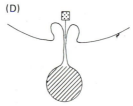

Other gravistatic organs

It is surprising that insects, as an immense and diverse group, generally lack statocysts. They do have hairlike cuticular organs and internal joint proprioceptors for detection of relative position of body parts (Mill, 1976). In several cases, especially in the stick insect *Carausius* and bees, there is evidence for specific gravireceptive use of these proprioceptors, and some aquatic insects utilize similar receptors with a buoyant bubble, instead of a dense mass or appendage, for gravireception (Jander, Horn and Hoffmann, 1970; Markl, 1974; Horn, 1975a,b; Wendler, 1975).

Another form of specific gravireceptor has been discovered recently in some insects that have small paired appendages, the cerci, extending caudally from the last abdominal segment. In certain crickets and roaches the ventral surface of each cercus has rows of small blunt sensillae, the clavate hairs or club hairs (trichobothria) (Figure 2D), that apparently control gravistatic orienting behavior (Bischof, 1975; Walthall and Hartman, 1981). As the body rolls or pitches, the massive tip is pulled by gravity and bends the slender innervated stalk. Bilaterally, the cerci are spread in a 'V' diverging away from the body, so that the rows of several tricholiths on one cercus are almost orthogonal to those on the other cercus.

Associated structures

Four features often are associated with gravireceptive organs; several may occur in a single organ. These features are the supporting cells, lymph, dense mass and gelatinous membrane.

Supporting cells are the cells in the sensory epithelium that are themselves not sensory; they usually are believed to provide structural and metabolic support (Lindeman, 1969; Markl, 1974; Wersäll and Bägger-Sjöbäck, 1974). Tight junctions may occur between the apical regions of the epithelial cells, and gap junctions in basal regions; such contacts may affect the flow of fluid, ions, and electrical currents from within the pouch to extracellular space (Hama and Saito, 1977).

The internal fluid that the apical sensory surfaces face often is a specialized lymph. In the vertebrates, this endolymph has a higher potassium and lower sodium ionic concentration than most cytoplasm (Peterson et al., 1978), and a density of $1.02–1.04 \, \mathrm{g \, cm^{-3}}$ (Trincker, 1962). At least in mammals, the utricle appears to secrete its own endolymph (Sellick, Johnstone and Johnstone, 1972), very unlike some of crustacean statocysts that apparently are open to the water (Markl, 1974).

The dense masses used for gravireceptors may be formed intracellularly, such as particles in the nemertean worm's 'statocyst chamber cell' (Brüggemann and Ehlers, 1981); or secreted extracellular structures such as the clavate hairs of crickets (Bischof, 1975) and calcified otoconia of vertebrates (Lim, 1979); or exogenous substances that are taken into the pouch, such as the statocyst sand grains taken up by crustaceans after molting (Markl, 1974). Statolith or otolith composition varies. Calcium is often the main mineral component, although it may appear in several different compounds (Vinnikov et al., 1981). Calcium carbonate in the crystalline form of aragonite forms the cephalopod statolith (Vinnikov et al., 1981) and the solid otoliths of teleost fishes (Trincker, 1962), but in mammals the small statoconia are formed of calcite; the density of aragonite (2.93) is slightly greater than that of calcite (2.71) (Trincker, 1962).

Often an organic matrix encases the dense extracellular crystalline mass. In molluscs, a mucus layer couples the statolith to the epithelium (Budelmann, 1976). In the vertebrates, the otolithic membrane may even have the ciliary bundles imbedded in pores on its macular side (Lewis, 1976; Lim, 1979). It is not yet clear how compliance of this gelatinous structure differs between the 'loaded' and 'unloaded' portions, when the membrane extends far beyond the otolith margin (Lowenstein and Roberts, 1949; see Platt and Popper, 1981).

Cellular morphology

Cuticular receptors

The statocyst hair of crustaceans is a modified cuticular sensory hair. Hundreds of these hairs may extend into the pouch from the sensory cushion of the statocyst, and they are innervated by neurons acting as stretch receptors (Figure 3A). In crayfish the basal part of a hair is the cask, thickened on one side to form a tooth with a hinge point, and having a thin flexible membrane on the opposite side. An internal strand, the chorda, attaches inside to a structure called the lingula, and connects the hair to the terminal dendrites of three sensory neurons (Schöne and Steinbrecht, 1968). Each dendrite contains a short, narrow ciliated segment, and these structures are stretched by the chorda when the hair bends. The structural orientation determines the axis around which the hair can bend, and hence the axis of maximum sensitivity for stretching the chorda (Stein, 1975).

Ciliated receptors

The hair cells that are found in many invertebrates and vertebrates have cilia as organelles formed from the surface membrane of the sensory cells. A true cilium, with the '9 + 2' arrangement of internal tubules and a basal body or foot inside the cell, is termed a kinocilium in these tissues.

In invertebrates, these ciliated hair cells usually are neurons, termed primary sensory cells, having an afferent axon projecting to the CNS (see Markl, 1974; Budelmann, 1976). There may be more than 500 cilia on a single hair cell in a gastropod, comprising almost half the total membrane area of the apical end of the cell (McKee and Wiederhold, 1974). Some invertebrate gravireceptor cells have been found to be secondary, without axons, in comb jellyfish (Ctenophora) (Krisch, 1973) and in cephalopods (Budelmann and Thies, 1977; Colmers, 1977, 1981). Such cells in *Octopus* have a variety of synaptic contacts with macular neurons (Colmers, 1981).

In cephalopods, each hair cell surface may contain up to 200 kinocilia, roughly six micrometers long, and usually arrayed in three to four rows of 20–30 cilia in a slight curve across the apical surface of the cell. The macula statica of an octopus may contain more than 5000 such cells (Budelmann, 1976). Because the basal feet of all cilia in a single cell point in the same direction, each cell has a structural orientation (Budelmann, 1979). It is believed that deflection of a cilium in the same

Figure 3. Receptor elements. In these schematic sections, the hollow arrow indicates the gravitational stimulus, the small arrow indicates direction of excitatory mechanical deflection in this tilted condition; the presumed transducing sites are stippled. (A) Crustacean (decapod) statocyst hair, with neuron dendrite (stippled) acting as a stretch receptor, and axon projecting to the CNS. (After Schöne and Steinbrecht, 1968.) (B) Molluscan (gastropod) statocyst ciliated cell, a primary sensory cell with several cilia having basal bodies (stippled) oriented in many directions, and an axon projecting to the CNS. (After Wolff, 1975.) (C) Vertebrate (Type II) hair cell, a secondary sensory cell with one kinocilium as a lever for deflecting a stereociliary bundle (stippled), and synapses to primary afferent axons to the CNS. (After Wersäll and Bagger-Sjöbäck, 1974.)

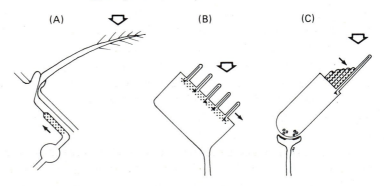

(A)   (B)   (C)

direction as its basal foot points is excitatory, giving directional sensitivity to the cell (Figure 3B) (Wolff, 1975).

In the vertebrate otolith organs, the hair cells are secondary sensory cells, without neurites, often considered not to be neurons. They make synaptic contacts with axons that form the eighth cranial nerve.

Vertebrate hair cells have an apical ciliary bundle that is unlike that of invertebrates (Flock, 1971; Lowenstein, 1974; Wersäll and Bagger-Sjöbäck, 1974). The bundle contains a single kinocilium at one end of an ordered array of roughly 50 stereocilia, which resemble elongated microvilli. The kinocilium may be up to 15 μm long in the utricular macula, and its intracellular basal foot is oriented pointing away from the bundle. The stereocilia form rows of graded lengths behind the kinocilium; the tallest stereocilia are next to, and never longer than, the kinocilium, and their heights decrease toward the far side of the bundle. Each cell has an orientation axis given by the kinocilium location, alignment of the basal foot and gradation of heights in the bundle. The stimulus causing maximal excitation is a bend of the bundle along this axis toward the side containing the kinocilium (Flock, 1971; Hudspeth and Corey, 1977).

Innervation

The statocyst hairs of decapod crustaceans are each innervated by three bipolar neurons; from each neuron, a single dendrite with its short ciliated segment extends toward the chorda (Schöne and Steinbrecht, 1968). Two of the neuron cell bodies are close to the cuticular surface, and from each of these two cells a thin axon of 1–2 μm in diameter is the afferent fiber to the brain. The third cell body lies somewhat deeper, and has an axon with a diameter of 3–4 μm.

In *Octopus*, three different kinds of synaptic contacts occur in the macula (Colmers, 1977, 1981). Perimacular neuron cell bodies form a ring around the macula, and these axons course radially inward, synapsing with overlying hair cells before forming the afferent macular nerve. Within this ring there are fewer intramacular neurons, which may have direct synapses from more than one hair cell onto each soma. A third innervation is the efferent system from the CNS, which synapses extensively on both hair cells and afferent axons. There are roughly 9000 axons in the nerve of a macula with about 5000 hair cells, and many may be efferent axons; axon diameters range from 0.2 to 18 μm (Budelmann, 1976).

The sensory maculae of the vertebrate otolith organs are innervated by a number of axons; a macula with 3000 hair cells may have roughly

1000 axons in its nerve branch (Goldberg and Fernández, 1975; Lewis and Li, 1975; Dunn, 1978). While some axons synapse on only two or three hair cells, others have terminal fields of more than a half dozen hair cells (Lewis, Baird, Leverenz and Koyama, 1982). Fiber sizes range from unmyelinated axons of less than one micrometer diameter to myelinated axons of more than 15 μm (Dunn, 1978).

Each cuticular hair in an insect sensillum is innervated by a single neuron; the soma is peripheral, the dendrite extends to the hair base, and the axon projects to a central ganglion (Thurm, 1964; Markl, 1974).

Diversity

Statocyst hairs of crustaceans are structurally and functionally diverse. Thick 'hook' hairs may contact the statolith or be free; the free ones, along with free 'thread' hairs, are believed to respond to rotational rather than gravitational accelerations (Sandeman and Okajima, 1972; Janse, 1980). Despite the variety in shapes and sizes of hairs in a statocyst of a crayfish, all the hairs seem to drive the 'sensory unit' of three characteristic neurons (Stein, 1975).

In ciliated statocysts of many invertebrates, the ultrastructure of the hair cells seems to be fairly uniform within a given species, even in complex statocysts. In cephalopods, even though synaptic contacts are variable, the ciliary array and the internal features of all the sensory cells are similar. There is some gradation in cell size, with larger cells spaced farther apart near the center of the macula, compared to the periphery (Budelmann, Barber and West, 1973; Colmers, 1977). Gastropods have hair cells different from cephalopods, but also show relatively homogeneous cellular structure within a species (Wolff, 1975). A famous exception to this uniformity of the hair cells of a mollusc is in some clams (Pelycepoda) with pronounced bilateral asymmetry. The upper statocyst of the scallop *Pecten* contains hair cells of two types, different in both length and orientations of the cilia, while the lower, smaller statocyst has cells with only one of these types (Barber and Dilly, 1969).

In the vertebrates there are several parameters of morphological diversity among the vestibular hair cells, even within a single otolith organ. Vestibular hair cells are distinguishable by transmission electron microscopy (TEM) into Type I hair cells that are flask-shaped, enclosed in a large synaptic cup of an afferent neuron, and are found only in mammals and birds; and Type II hair cells that are cylindrical, receive both afferent and efferent synaptic contacts from vestibular neurons, and occur in all vertebrates (Wersäall and Bagger-Sjöbäck, 1974). Often otolith organ maculae contain a zone called the striola (Lindeman, 1969; Rosenhall, 1970; Wersäll and Bagger-Sjöbäck, 1974; Lewis and Li, 1975; Dale, 1976; Lim, 1976; Platt, 1983), which is a broad band where the hair cells are larger than peripherally. The striola of mammals and birds is composed largely of Type I hair cells, with the Type II cells surrounding it (Lindeman, 1969; Jørgensen and Andersen, 1973).

Scanning electron microscopy (SEM) recently has revealed an extraordinary diversity in the forms of ciliary bundles on all the otolith organ maculae. In the utricle alone, at least three forms of bundle have been distinguished by the relative lengths of kinocilium and their tallest stereocilia. These different forms have particular distributions on the macula, and are similar in many fishes (Dale, 1976; Platt, 1977, 1983), amphibians (Lewis and Li, 1975; Hillman, 1976) and mammals (Lim, 1976; Kessel and Kardon, 1979). The striolar region of the utricle contains ciliary bundles with kinocilia ranging from four to eight micrometers long, and the tallest stereocilia in a given bundle usually are either about the same length or about half the length of the kinocilium in the same bundle. Most of the rest of the macular floor has bundles with kinocilia much shorter, 2–4 μm, and tallest stereocilia half the kinocilium length. A narrow zone around the striola contains bundles of a third form, with a kinocilium 10–15 μm long, but longest stereocilia of only 3–4 μm. Two additional forms sometimes are considered, depending on how the striolar population is subdivided (Platt and Popper, 1981; Platt, 1983).

An entirely new level of diversity is shown by these differences in bundle ultrastructure, because they are found even within maculae that have only Type II hair cells by TEM criteria. Recent identification of terminal fields for physiologically characterized afferents suggests that the tall striolar bundles are innervated by neurons with higher sensitivity and more phasic responses than those innervating the smaller marginal bundles (Lewis et al., 1982). The additional diversity in axon diameters leads to a range of conduction velocities, and is suspected to relate to background discharge rates and to sensitivity as well (Goldberg and Fernández, 1977).

Thus there are different degrees of diversity in cellular structure of gravireceptors. In a given crustacean, there is a variety of forms of the extracellular sensory hair, but there are common features in structure of the sensory units, each consisting of one hair and three identifiable neurons. In a given mollusc, cellular and ciliary morphology apparently are fairly homogeneous, although there can be variety in synaptic contacts. In the vertebrates, even a single otolith organ has ultrastructural diversity among its hair cells in cellular structure, ciliary form, and synaptic structures. In all cases where this diversity of elements occurs, it is spatially organized, forming a pattern in each macula that can be considered a receptor mosaic.

Physiology
Reception

The cellular basis of gravireception has been studied in three kinds of statolithic organs. In crustaceans, molluscs and vertebrates, hairlike processes are bent when the overlying dense mass is displaced by gravity, generating neural responses that often show a sensitivity to direction of tilt and its rate of change in addition to the tilt magnitude.

Transduction. The process of mechanosensory transduction is the conversion of mechanical energy into an electrochemical change in the receptor (Flock, 1971). Receptor potentials are produced intracellularly by changes in transmembrane ionic currents that occur when ionic conductances in the membrane change.

In the crustacean statocyst, the site of transduction for each neuron may be the ciliated segment of the dendrite that attaches to the chorda (Schöne and Steinbrecht, 1968). The shape of action potentials recorded in the soma, and their sensitivity to intracellular currents injected in the soma, suggest that the spike initiating zone is in the long dendrite itself, not the soma or afferent axon (Takahata, 1981).

In hair cells of vertebrates, the apical ciliary bundle apparently is the site of the early stages of transduction, since receptor currents can be localized to the stereociliary cluster (Hudspeth, 1982). Micromanipulation of individual bundles has shown that the stereocilia alone are necessary and sufficient for cellular responses (Hudspeth and Jacobs, 1979). The kinocilium may serve as a simple lever; in living preparations it is quite stiff, and adheres to the stereociliary bundle (Flock, Flock and Murray, 1977). Since the calcium ion is associated with many sensory transduction mechanisms, it is interesting that calcium-binding sites can be localized on stereocilia in both amphibian and mammalian hair cells, although in goldfish calcium binds instead to the ciliary necklace region of the kinocilium base (Moran, Rowley and Asher, 1981).

Despite the identification of transduction sites, the biophysical linkages between mechanical deformations and changing conductances remain unclear.

Receptor potentials. Intracellular receptor potentials in response to mechanical stimuli can depolarize hair cells by up to 20 mV in molluscan statocysts (Wiederhold, 1974, 1976; Detweiler and Fuortes, 1975) and vertebrate otolith organs (Hudspeth and Corey, 1977). Hair cells of the isolated bullfrog saccule (Hudspeth and Corey, 1977) have a reversal potential for the response that is near zero, and since the current channels show a low specificity for cations, even rather large ones, the ionic channel diameter has been estimated as more than 0.5 nm (Corey and Hudspeth, 1979). As these authors point out, these features are all similar to those of the acetylcholine-activated channels for synaptic transmission at the vertebrate neuromuscular junction.

The receptor potential may have a variety of relationships to the bending stimulus in these gravistatic systems (see Flock, 1971). The response to bending amplitude has both linear and non-linear regions in the bullfrog saccule, and the directionally dependent amount of de-polarization can be much greater than the amount of hyperpolarization from the resting potential (Figure 4) (Hudspeth and Corey, 1977). A sustained response to a maintained intracellular current injection occurs in some crayfish statocyst neurons, while some neurons in both crayfish and gastropods show only a transient change, indicating that the tonic and phasic properties of these receptors to hair bending can depend on neuronal and not just mechanical factors (Wiederhold, 1974; Takahata, 1981).

Receptor potentials can act as generator potentials to summate at the spike-initiating zone of the axon (Detweiler and Fuortes, 1975;

Figure 4. Transduction. Graph indicates the de- or hyperpolarization of the sensory cell during deflection of the ciliary bundle, showing saturation and asymmetry of the response voltage from the resting potential (zero here). (After Hudspeth and Corey, 1977.) The great sensitivity is shown by the sketches, drawn to scale. The cell on the left shows the deflection of 1 μm at the tip of a 10-μm bundle that, in the frog saccule, causes saturating hyperpolarization; the cell on the right shows a 1-μm deflection in the depolarizing direction.

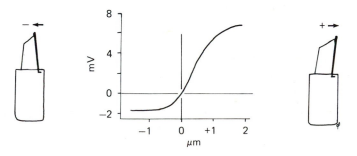

Takahata, 1981), or can modulate neurotransmitter release at synapses to afferent neurons (see Goldberg and Fernández, 1975). Depolarizing potentials in most gravireceptors are believed to produce excitatory responses, while hyperpolarizing potentials inhibit responses in the afferent axons.

Directional sensitivity. Directionally-dependent potential changes correlate with morphological orientation of mechanical elements. In most crayfish statocyst hairs, deflection toward the side of the tooth hinge stretches the chorda and excites the receptors, although some are excited by stimuli in any direction (Takahata and Hisada, 1979). In ciliated receptors, deflection of the cilium in the direction of its basal foot causes depolarization (Flock, 1971). In some snail statocyst hair cells with ciliary basal feet oriented in many directions, depolarizing stimuli are expected from any direction; but in other cells with all the

Figure 5. Macular directional arrays. Arrows indicate directions of structural orientation associated with excitation in these roughly horizontal maculae. (A) Crustacean (crayfish) statocyst cushion. (After Takahata and Hisada, 1979.) (B) Cephalopod (squid) macula neglecta posterior. (After Budelmann, 1979.) (C) Vertebrate (goldfish) utricle. (After Platt, 1977.) (D) Vertebrate (bullfrog) utricle. (After Lewis and Li, 1975.) (E) Vertebrate (cormorant) utricle. (After Jørgensen and Andersen, 1970.) A, anterior direction; L, lateral; not to scale.

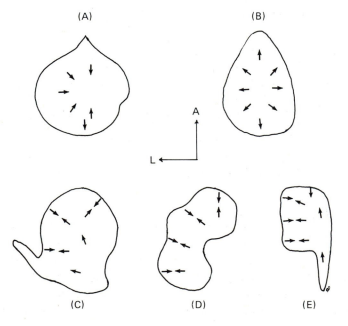

cilia oriented in the same direction, the response can be directionally sensitive (Wolff, 1975). In some cephalopods, all the kinocilia in a cell have the basal feet pointing the same way, so the ciliary bundle is believed to give each cell a directional polarization related to structural orientation (Budelmann, 1979). In vertebrate hair cells with their single kinocilium, the response also is directional, following a cosine function of stimulus direction, with the maximum depolarization when the bundle is bent in the direction toward the kinocilium (Flock, 1971; Hudspeth and Corey, 1977).

Structural orientation of receptors in a macula thus has functional significance. As noted by Schöne (1975c), gravistatic organs often have a 'fan' pattern of cellular orientations. Two-dimensional maps do not reveal the full extent of curvature of many sensory surfaces, but such maps of several statocyst and otolith organ maculae (Figure 5) show that cells are oriented with their polarization axes aligned in a radial fashion over the surface, facing either outward or inward (Schöne, 1975c; Jørgensen and Andersen, 1973; Lewis and Li, 1975; Budelmann, 1979; Takahata and Hisada, 1979; Janse, 1980; Platt and Popper, 1981). In many cases there is a boundary between inward- and outward-facing cells as a curving arc, around the anterior and lateral part of the sensory surface. Even among fishes with unusual postural swimming behavior, such as flatfishes that lie on their sides, rotated 90°, and upside-down catfish rotated 180°, this conservative pattern is retained (Platt and Popper, 1981; Platt, 1983).

Neural responses

Since cephalopods and vertebrates have secondary sensory cells presynaptic to the afferent axons, there can be spatial summation leading to their neuronal responses, unlike most invertebrates. Recent data from the crayfish statocyst (Ozeki, Takahata and Hisada, 1978; Takahata and Hisada, 1979; Takahata, 1981) are interesting to compare with those from molluscs (Wiederhold, 1974; Wolff, 1975) and vertebrates (Goldberg and Fernández, 1975; Precht, 1979), with regard to properties of sensitivity, adaptation, and channels of information.

Sensitivity. One measure of sensitivity in a receptor is the threshold for signal detection. Many gravireceptors show 'spontaneous activity', which may be operationally defined as activity when in the normal posture, without implying whether or not the cell is stimulated or has an endogenous pacemaker activity. In crayfish, such spontaneous firing is not seen in the normal position (Takahata, 1981). But in gastropod molluscs, neural activity in the normal position probably depends on the firing of the few cells that are contacted by the statolith (Wiederhold, 1974; Wolff, 1975). In the vertebrates, activity in the absence of tilt is common, with discharge rates ranging from a few to more than 50 spikes per second (Precht, 1979). Continual release of neurotransmitter from the hair cells to afferent terminals could produce this continual activity by tonically depolarizing the postsynaptic membrane back toward firing threshold shortly after each action potential (Highstein and Politoff, 1978). An ongoing signal in the normal position allows increased directional sensitivity, because the rate can be decreased by inhibition as well as increased by excitation, and because changes in rate can be infinitesimally small (Goldberg and Fernández, 1975). Such a 'push-pull' system also could convey great sensitivity if differential comparison of several receptor inputs is available.

Spiking rates of gravireceptive afferents often are very regular (Wolff, 1975; Precht, 1979; Takahata, 1981). In terms of information, a highly-regular discharge can be a sensitive indicator of change, because just a few intervals are needed to specify a new average rate.

Adaptation. Sensory adaptation in gravireceptors recently has been found as an extremely common property, despite the earlier assumption of great dependence on tonic responses (Precht, 1979). In crayfish, strongly phasic responses often occur to maintained bending stimuli, with rates declining to near zero in less than one second in over half the units sampled (Takahata, 1981). In pulmonate and opisthobranch gastropods, single-unit responses to tilt decline, often within several seconds, to a much lower steady rate that is relatively independent of tilt angle (Figure 6A) (Wolff, 1975). In the vertebrates, work particularly on frogs, cats and monkeys has shown many units with a purely phasic response to a maintained tilt, often with no resting activity, and even a large proportion of the tonic units have an initial phasic component (Figure 6B) (see Goldberg and Fernández, 1975; Blanks and Precht, 1976; Precht, 1979). It is also surprising that some units seem capable of changing their properties of regularity and adaptation. In an elasmobranch, the guitarfish, utricular unit activity may be modified from irregular to regular, and phasic to tonic, by introducing just a tiny positional 'jitter' as a background (Macadar, Wolfe, O'Leary and Segundo, 1975).

The overall impression is developing that, at least in the crayfish and gastropod statocyst and the vertebrate utricle, phasic properties of afferent activity during changes in position are very important for gravireception. While some adaptation mechanisms are present in some membranes to modulate the receptor potential, we do not yet know the contribution of micromechanics to adaptation.

Input channels. Tonic and phasic responses to tilt can provide static and dynamic positional information that may be carried by separate neurons. Tonic responses seem characteristic of regularly firing, small-diameter axons that have wide terminal branching and slow conduction velocities, while more phasic activity is associated with irregular large fibers innervating only a few cells, and having fast conduction (Goldberg and Fernández, 1977). However, many afferents combine a phasic initial activity with a different maintained tonic activity at a new tilt angle (Precht, 1979).

A consequence of the large dynamic component in many gravitational organs is the blurring of the distinction between positional sensors and velocity or acceleration sensors. Phasic units that respond briefly to any change of tilt away from a fixed position, in which they have been silent, occur in elasmobranch fishes and in frogs, and so can act also as 'out of position' detectors (Lowenstein and Roberts, 1949; Lowenstein and Saunders, 1975). The macular cells may act as arrays of filters for different frequencies of displacement oscillations (Lowenstein and Saunders, 1975), providing acoustic as well as gravistatic reception. In

Figure 6. Tonic and phasic afference. Polar plots show the activity, in spikes per second, of single afferent neurons from (A) a molluscan statocyst (snail, data from Wolff, 1975), and (B) a vertebrate otolith organ (elasmobranch ray, data from Lowenstein and Roberts, 1949). The solid lines connect the activity seen during a slow but continuous lateral roll, and show a peak response that appears to depend on position. But the dashed lines show the activity for the same neurons after each position was held for many seconds; the low positional discrimination of this tonic response alone is evident.

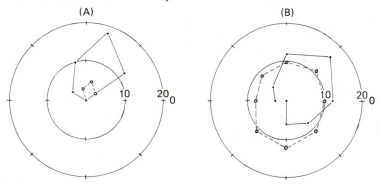

many fishes, some otolith organs are sensitive to vibrational or acoustic frequencies up to more than 1 kHz, far above the usual head movements producing dominant frequencies in the range 0.1–10 Hz (see Platt and Popper, 1981). The semicircular canal organs of the vertebrate inner ear, long considered exclusively angular acceleration detectors, under certain conditions may be sensitive to linear accelerations including gravity (Lowenstein and Compton 1978).

The vectorial quality of shearing force gives both a magnitude and direction to a stimulus across a gravireceptive surface (Flock, 1964). In gastropod molluscs, these properties may not be utilized; positional attitude may be indicated by the particular population of cells responding to statolith contact at a given tilt, with range fractionation so that each cell responds for only a part of the full sphere of tilt angles (Wolff, 1975). Among cephalopods, some utilize the directional information but not the shear magnitude to drive compensatory eye movements during tilt, while others may utilize both direction and magnitude (Budelmann, 1975, 1976). In the vertebrates, behavioral experiments on teleost fish by von Holst (1950) still remain an excellent demonstration of the central use of both shear direction and magnitude for positional information. Functional polarization vectors of single neurons have been described by many workers on vertebrates (see Goldberg and Fernández, 1975; Precht, 1979); these data support a gravistatic role for the mammalian saccule in addition to that for the utricle (Fernández, Goldberg and Abend, 1972; Fernández and Goldberg, 1976a,b).

The range and complexity of response parameters have made the early simple models of static responses less tenable. The role of differential densities and compliances in the accessory structures, the interaction of static and dynamic factors such as friction and viscosity, and even the transduction mechanism itself all remain in need of further clarification.

Integration

It is beyond the scope of this paper to cover the central integrative mechanisms by which gravistatic reception elicits postural behavior and visual stabilization. It should simply be mentioned that many animals show central properties of parallel processing, bilateral interactions, central efferent modulation of peripheral input, tactile and visual modulation, and central plasticity allowing recovery after partial functional losses (see reviews by Kornhuber, 1974; Goldberg and Fernández, 1975; Schöne, 1975a; Wilson and Peterson, 1978; Henn, Cohen and Young, 1981).

Future directions

There are four major areas in which current research seems likely to lead to exciting discoveries in gravireception. (1) Transduction. New microtechniques involving both biochemistry and biophysics allow labeling of subcellular compounds and structures having demonstrable cellular functions. The function of cilia is an obvious target. (2) Development. While it has been neglected in this paper, there already is work on the development of the inner ear in the vertebrates, and the invertebrate preparations may offer some unique advantages in studies of cell lineages, as they have in other aspects of neurobiology. The receptors in a macula develop into an organized array by mechanisms not yet understood. (3) Central organization. New anatomical and physiological techniques already have been used to clarify central auditory and visual systems in the brains of both vertebrates and invertebrates, and are just beginning to be used on the central projections of gravistatic systems. Gravistatic input might turn out to involve maps that are 'goniotopic', representing angles by spatial arrays of central neurons much as tonotopic projections occur in the auditory system. (4) System analysis. Most challenging because of its complexity is the analysis of the entire system from gravistatic input to postural behavior. A substantial amount of system modeling already has been done, and many aspects tested by behavioral work. Further work in this area will be useful in study of the plastic properties of the system during growth, compensation from injury or other deficits, or the sorting out of the particular gravistatic referent from all the other accelerations that may be present.

References

Barber, V. C., and Dilly, P. N. (1969). Some aspects of the fine structure of the statocysts of the molluscs *Pecten* and *Pterotrachea*. *Z. Zellforsch. mikrosk. Anat.* 94: 462–78.

Bischof, H.-J. (1975). Die keulenförmigen Sensillen auf den Cerci der Grille *Gryllus bimaculatus* als Schwererezeptoren. *J. Comp. Physiol. A* 98: 277–98.

Blanks, R. H. I., and Precht, W. (1976). Functional characterization of primary vestibular afferents in the frog. *Expl Brain Res.* 25: 369–90.

Brüggemann, J., and Ehlers, U. (1981). Ultrastruktur der Statocyste von *Ototyphlonemertes pallida* (Keferstein, 1882) (Nemertini). *Zoomorphologie* 97: 75–87.

Budelmann, B. U. (1975). Gravity receptor function in cephalopods with particular reference to *Sepia officinalis*. *Fortschr. Zool.* 23: 84–95.

Budelmann, B. U. (1976). Equilibrium receptor systems in molluscs. In *Structure and Function of Proprioceptors in the Invertebrates*, ed. P. J. Mill, pp. 529–66. London: Chapman & Hall.

Budelmann, B. U. (1979). Hair cell polarization in the gravity receptor systems of the statocysts of the cephalopods *Sepia officinalis* and *Loligo vulgaris*. *Brain Res. 160:* 261–70.

Budelmann, B. U., Barber, V. C., and West, S. (1973). Scanning electron microscopical studies of the arrangements and numbers of hair cells in the statocysts of *Octopus vulgaris, Sepia officinalis* and *Loligo vulgaris*. *Brain Res. 56:* 25–42.

Budelmann, B. U., and Thies, G. (1977). Secondary sensory cells in the gravity receptor system of the statocyst of *Octopus vulgaris*. *Cell Tiss. Res. 182:* 93–8.

Bullock, T. H., and Horridge, G. A. (1965). *Structure and Function in the Nervous Systems of Invertebrates*. 2 vols. San Francisco: W. Freeman.

Caston, J., Precht, W., and Blanks, R. H. I. (1977). Response characteristics of frogs lagenar afferents to natural stimulation. *J. Comp. Physiol. A 118:* 273–89.

Colmers, W. F. (1977). Neuronal and synaptic organization in the gravity receptor system of the statocyst of *Octopus vulgaris*. *Cell Tiss. Res. 185:* 491–504.

Colmers, W. F. (1981). Afferent synaptic connections between hair cells and the somata of intramacular neurons in the gravity receptor system of the statocyst of *Octopus vulgaris*. *J. Comp. Neurol. 197:* 385–94.

Corey, D. P., and Hudspeth, A. J. (1979). Ionic basis of the receptor potential in a vertebrate hair cell. *Nature 281:* 675–7.

Corwin, J. T. (1981). Audition in elasmobranchs. In *Hearing and Sound Communication in Fishes*, ed. W. N. Tavolga, A. N. Popper and R. R. Fay, pp. 3–38. New York: Springer-Verlag.

Dale, T. (1976). The labyrinthine mechanoreceptor organs of the cod *Gadus morhua* L. (Teleostei: Gadidae). *Norwegian J. Zool. 24:* 85–128.

Detweiler, P. B., and Fuortes, M. G. F. (1975). Responses of hair cells in the statocyst of *Hermissenda*. *J. Physiol., Lond. 251:* 107–29.

Dunn, R. F. (1978). Nerve fibers of the eighth nerve and their distribution to the sensory nerves of the inner ear in the bullfrog. *J. Comp. Neurol. 182:* 621–36.

Fernández, C., and Goldberg, J. (1976a). Physiology of peripheral neurons innervating otolith organs of the squirrel monkey. I. Response to static tilts and to long-duration centrifugal force. *J. Neurophysiol. 39:* 970–84.

Fernández, C., and Goldberg, J. (1976b). Physiology of peripheral neurons innervating otolith organs of the squirrel monkey. II. Directional selectivity and force-response relations. *J. Neurophysiol. 39:* 985–95.

Fernández, C., Goldberg, J., and Abend, W. K. (1972). Response to static tilts of peripheral neurons innervating otolith organs of the squirrel monkey. *J. Neurophysiol. 35:* 978–97.

Flock, Å. (1964). Structure of the macula utriculi with special reference to directional interplay of sensory responses as revealed by morphological polarization. *J. Cell Biol. 22:* 413–31.

Flock, Å. (1971). Sensory transduction in hair cells. In *Handbook of Sensory Physiology*, vol. 1, *Principles of Receptor Physiology*, ed. W. Loewenstein, pp. 396–441. Berlin: Springer-Verlag.

Flock, Å., Flock, B., and Murray, E. (1977). Studies on the sensory hairs of receptor cells in the inner ear. *Acta Otolaryngol. 83:* 85–91.

Goldberg, J. M., and Fernández, C. (1975). Vestibular mechanisms. *A. Rev. Physiol. 37:* 12–62.

Goldberg, J. M., and Fernández, C. (1977). Conduction times and background discharge of vestibular afferents. *Brain Res. 122:* 545–50.

Gordon, S. A., and Cohen, M. J., eds (1971). *Gravity and the Organism*. Chicago: University of Chicago Press.

Hama, K., and Saito, K. (1977). Gap junctions between the supporting cells in some acoustico-vestibular receptors. *J. Neurocytol. 6:* 1–12.

Henn, V., Cohen, B., and Young, L. R., eds (1980). Visual-vestibular interaction in motion perception and the generation of nystagmus. *Neurosci..Res. Prog. Bull.18:* 459–651.

Highstein, S. M., and Politoff, A. L. (1978). Relation of interspike baseline activity to the spontaneous discharges of primary afferents from the labyrinth of the toadfish, *Opsanus tau. Brain Res. 150:* 182–7.

Hillman, D. E. (1976). Morphology of peripheral and central vestibular systems. In *Frog Neurobiology*, ed. R. Llinás and W. Precht, pp. 452–80. Berlin: Springer-Verlag.

Horn, E. (1975a). The contributions of different receptors to gravity orientation in insects. *Fortschr. Zool. 23:* 1–17.

Horn, E. (1975b). Mechanisms of gravity processing by leg and abdominal gravity receptors in bees. *J. Insect Physiol. 21:* 673–80.

Hudspeth, A. J. (1982). Extracellular current flow and the site of transduction by vertebrate hair cells. *J. Neurosci. 2:* 1–10.

Hudspeth, A. J., and Corey, D. P. (1977). Sensitivity, polarity, and conductance change in the response of vertebrate hair cells to controlled mechanical stimuli. *Proc. Natn. Acad. Sci. USA 74:* 2407–11.

Hudspeth, A. J., and Jacobs, R. (1979). Stereocilia mediate transduction in vertebrate hair cells. *Proc. Natn. Acad. Sci. USA 76:* 1506–9.

Hyman, L. H. (1940). *The Invertebrates*, 6 vols. New York: McGraw-Hill.

Jander, R., Horn, E., and Hoffmann, M. (1970). Die Bedeutung von Gelenkrezeptoren in den Beinen für die Geotaxis der höheren Insekten (Pterygota). *Z. vergl. Physiol. 66:* 326–42.

Janse, C. (1980). The function of statolith-hair and free-hook-hair receptors in the statocyst of the crab, *Scylla serrata. J. Comp. Physiol. A 137:* 51–62.

Jørgensen, J. M., and Andersen, T. (1973). On the structure of the avian maculae. *Acta Zool., Stockh. 54:* 121–30.

Kessel, R. G., and Kardon, R. H. (1979). The shape, polarization and innervation of sensory hair cells in the guinea-pig crista ampullaris and macula utriculi. *Scanning Electron Microsc.* 1979/III, 967–73.

Kornhuber, H., ed. (1974). *Handbook of Sensory Physiology*, vol. VI, *Vestibular System*, parts 1 and 2. Berlin: Springer-Verlag.

Krisch, B. (1973). Über das Apikalorgan (Statocyste) der Ctenophore *Pleurobrachia pileus. Z. Zellforsch. mikrosk. Anat. 142:* 241–62.

Lewis, E. R. (1976). Surface morphology of the bullfrog amphibian papilla. *Brain, Behav. Evolut. 13:* 196–215.

Lewis, E. R., Baird, R. A., Leverenz, E. L., and Koyama, H. (1982). Inner ear: dye injection reveals peripheral origins of specific sensitivities. *Science 215:* 1641–3.

Lewis, E. R., and Li, C. W. (1975). Hair cell types and distributions in the otolithic and auditory organs of the bullfrog. *Brain Res. 83:* 35–50.

Lim, D. J. (1976). Morphological and physiological correlates in cochlear and vestibular sensory epithelia. *Scanning Electron Microsc.* 1976/II, 270–5.

Lim, D. J. (1979). Fine morphology of the otoconial membrane and its relationship to the sensory epithelium. *Scanning Electron Microsc.* 1979/III, 929–38.

Lindeman, H. H. (1969). Studies on the morphology of the sensory regions of the vestibular apparatus. *Ergebn. Anat. EntwGesch. 4:* 1–113.

Lowenstein, O. (1971). The labyrinth. In *Fish Physiology*, vol. V, *Sensory Systems and Electric Organs*, ed. W. S. Hoar and D. J. Randall, pp. 207–40. New York: Academic Press.

Lowenstein, O. (1974). Comparative morphology and physiology. In *Handbook of Sensory Physiology*, vol. VI, *Vestibular System*, part 1, Basic Mechanisms, ed. H. H. Kornhuber, pp. 75–120. Berlin: Springer-Verlag.

Lowenstein, O., and Compton, G. J. (1978). A comparative study of the responses of isolated first-order semicircular canal afferents to angular and linear acceleration, analysed in the time and frequency domains. *Proc. Roy. Soc. Lond. B202:* 313–38.

Lowenstein, O., and Roberts, T. D. M. (1949). The equilibrium function of the otolith organs of the thornback ray (*Raja clavata*). *J. Physiol., Lond. 110:* 392–415.

Lowenstein, O., and Saunders, R. D. (1975). Otolith-controlled responses from the first-order neurons of the labyrinth of the bullfrog (*Rana catesbeiana*) to changes in linear acceleration. *Proc. Roy. Soc., Lond. B191:* 475–505.

Macadar, O., Wolfe, G. E., O'Leary, D. P., and Segundo, J. P. (1975). Response of the elasmobranch utricle to maintained spatial orientation, transitions and jitter. *Expl Brain Res. 22:* 1–12.

Markl, H. (1974). The perception of gravity and of angular acceleration in invertebrates. In *Handbook of Sensory Physiology*, vol. VI, *Vestibular System*, part 1, Basic mechanisms, ed. H. H. Kornhuber, pp. 17–74. Berlin: Springer-Verlag.

Mayne, R. (1974). A systems concept of the vestibular organs. In *Handbook of Sensory Physiology*, vol. VI, *Vestibular System*, part 2, Psychophysics, applied aspects, and general interpretations, ed. H. H. Kornhuber, pp. 475–520. Berlin: Springer-Verlag.

McKee, A. E., and Wiederhold, M. L. (1974). *Aplysia* statocyst receptor cells: fine structure. *Brain Res. 81:* 310–13.

Mill, P. J., ed. (1976). *Structure and Function of Proprioceptors in the Invertebrates*. London: Chapman & Hall.

Moran, D. T., Rowley, J. C., and Asher, D. L. (1981). Calcium binding sites on sensory processes in vertebrate hair cells. *Proc. Natn. Acad. Sci. USA – Biol. 78:* 3954–8.

Ozeki, M., Takahata, M., and Hisada, M. (1978). Afferent response patterns of the crayfish statocyst with ferrite grain statolith to magnetic field stimulation. *J. Comp. Physiol. A 123:* 1–10.

Peterson, S. K., Frishkopf, L. S., Lechene, C., Oman, C. M., and Weiss, T. F. (1978). Element composition of inner ear lymphs in cats, lizards and skates determined by electron probe microanalysis of liquid samples. *J. Comp. Physiol. A 126:* 1–14.

Platt, C. (1977). Hair cell distribution and orientation in goldfish otolith organs. *J. Comp. Neurol. 172:* 283–98.

Platt, C. (1983). The peripheral vestibular system of fishes. In *Fish Neurobiology*, ed. R. G. Northcutt and R. E. Davis, pp. 89–123. Ann Arbor: University of Michigan Press.

Platt, C., and Popper, A. N. (1981). Fine structure and function of the ear. In *Hearing and Sound Communication in Fishes*, ed. W. N. Tavolga, A. N. Popper and R. R. Fay, pp. 3–38. New York: Springer-Verlag.

Precht, W. (1976). Physiology of the peripheral and central vestibular systems. In *Frog Neurobiology*, ed. R. Llinás and W. Precht, pp. 481–512. Berlin: Springer-Verlag.

Precht, W. (1979). Vestibular mechanisms. *A. Rev. Neurosci. 2:* 265–89.

Retzius, G. (1881). *Das Gehörorgan der Wirbelthiere: morphologisch-histologische Studien*, 2 vols. Stockholm: Centraldruckerei.

Rose, R. D., and Stokes, D. R. (1981). A crustacean statocyst with only three hairs: light and scanning electron microscopy. *J. Morphol. 169:* 21–8.

Rosenhall, U. (1970). Some morphological principles of the vestibular maculae in birds. *Arch. klin. exp. Ohren- Nasen- und Kehlkopfheilkunde 197:* 154–82.

Sandeman, D. C., and Okajima, A. (1972). Statocyst-induced eye movements in the crab *Scylla serrata*. I. The sensory input from the statocyst. *J. Exp. Biol. 57:* 187–204.

Schöne, H. (1971). Gravity receptors and gravity orientation in crustacea. In *Gravity and the Organism*, ed. S. A. Gordon and M. J. Cohen, pp. 223–35. Chicago: University of Chicago Press.

Schöne, H., ed. (1975a). Mechanisms of spatial perception and orientation as related to gravity. *Fortschr. Zool. 23:* 1–296.

Schöne, H. (1975b). Orientation in space: animals. In *Marine Ecology*. II. *Physiological Mechanisms*, ed. O. Kinne, pp. 499–553. London: Wiley.

Schöne, H. (1975c). On the transformation of the gravity input into reactions by statolith organs of the 'fan' type. *Fortschr. Zool. 23:* 120–7.

Schöne, H., and Steinbrecht, R. A. (1968). Fine structure of statocyst receptor of *Astacus fluviatilis*. *Nature 220:* 184–6.

Sellick, P. M., Johnstone, J. R., and Johnstone, B. M. (1972). The electrophysiology of the utricle. *Pflügers Arch., Eur. J. Physiol. 336:* 21–7.

Stein, A. (1975). Attainment of positional information in the crayfish statocyst. *Fortschr. Zool. 23:* 109–18.

Takahata, M. (1981). Functional differentiation of crayfish statocyst receptors in sensory adaptation. *Comp. Biochem. Physiol. 68A:* 17–23.

Takahata, M., and Hisada, M. (1979). Functional polarization of statocyst receptors in the crayfish *Procambarus clarkii* Girard. *J. Comp. Physiol. A 130:* 201–7.

Thurm, U. (1964). Mechanoreceptors in the cuticle of the honeybee: fine structure and stimulus mechanism. *Science 145:* 1063–5.

Trincker, D. (1962). The transformation of mechanical stimulus into nervous excitation by the labyrinthine receptors. In *Biological Receptor Mechanisms*, ed. J. W. L. Beament, pp. 289–316. New York: Academic Press.

Vinnikov, Y. A., Aronova, M. Z., Kharkeevich, T. A., Tsirulis, T. P., Lavrova, E. A., and Natochin, Y. V. (1981). Structural and chemical features of the invertebrate otoliths. *Z. mikrosk.-anat. Forsch. 95:* 127–40.

Vinnikov, Y. A., Gasenko, O. G., Bronstein, A. A., Tsirulis, T. P., Ivanov, V. P., and Pyatkina, G. A. (1968). Structure, cytochemical and functional organization of statocysts of Cephalopoda. In *Neurobiology of Invertebrates*, ed. J. Salánki, pp. 29–48. New York: Plenum Press.

von Holst, E. (1950). Die Arbeitsweise der Statolithenapparate bei Fischen. *Z. vergl. Physiol. 32:* 60–120.

Walthall, W. W., and Hartman, H. B. (1981). Receptors and giant interneurons signalling gravity orientation information in the cockroach *Arenivaga*. *J. Comp. Physiol. A 142:* 359–69.

Wendler, G. (1975). Physiology and systems analysis of gravity orientation in two insect species (*Carausius morosus, Calandra granaria*). *Fortschr. Zool. 23:* 33–45.

Wersäll, J., and Bägger-Sjöbäck, D. (1974). Morphology of the vestibular sense organ. In *Handbook of Sensory Physiology*, vol. VI, *Vestibular System*, part 1, Basic mechanisms, ed. H. H. Kornhuber, pp. 123–70. Berlin: Springer-Verlag.

Wiederhold, M. L. (1974). *Aplysia* statocyst receptor cells: intracellular responses to physiological stimuli. *Brain Res. 78:* 490–4.

Wiederhold, M. L. (1976). Mechanosensory transduction in 'sensory' and 'motile' cilia. *A. Rev. Biophys. Bioengng 5:* 39–62.

Wilson, V. J., and Peterson, B. W. (1978). Peripheral and central substrates of vestibulospinal reflexes. *Physiol. Rev. 58:* 80–105.

Wolff, H. G. (1975). Statocysts and geotactic behavior in gastropod molluscs. *Fortschr. Zool. 23:* 63–83.

Young, J. Z. (1977). Brain, behaviour and evolution of cephalopods. In *The Biology of Cephalopods*, ed. M. Nixon and J. B. Messenger, pp. 377–434. New York: Academic Press.

5.2

Inertial motion sensors

EDWIN R. LEWIS

Any clue at all to body movement is a clue to body velocity and acceleration. Drag forces in a viscous medium, motion of the visual field, sound-intensity changes, ambient-pressure changes, changes in electric or magnetic fields, intensity changes of chemical stimuli, all could provide velocity and acceleration information. However, I shall limit my discussion here to *inertial sensors*, which directly *detect and measure* body acceleration, *a*, by means of the reaction force, *f*, it imposes on a *sensing mass*, *m*,

$$f = -ma \tag{1}$$

or detect and measure body velocity by mechanical integration of *f* over time. Since the action of gravity on a mass at the earth's surface is equivalent to upward acceleration at approx. $980 \, \text{cm} \, \text{s}^{-2}$, dc inertial sensors also are gravity sensors. The previous chapter treated *body orientation* measurement by gravity sensors. This chapter treats *body velocity* and *acceleration* measurement by those same sensors and others. For extensive general discussions of the subject, I recommend Bullock and Horridge (1965), Cohen (1981), Keidel (1968), Mill (1976), Schöne (1975a), Schwartzkopff (1974, 1977), Talbot and Gessner (1973), Autrum (1977) and Wilson and Melvill Jones (1979).

Predation, a powerful evolutionary driving force, probably has been a prime mover in the evolution of sensitivity to substrate-borne vibrations (*seismic stimuli*). Ability to sense remote footfalls or other vibration-generating activities of potential predator or prey could provide a tremendous advantage to the animal that possessed it (e.g., Brownell and Farley, 1979; Vollrath, 1979). The most acute seismic sensitivities reported so far both among vertebrates and among invertebrates are associated with inertial sensors (Lewis and Narins, 1981; Autrum and Schneider, 1948). *Stability* of posture and orientation and *agility* of motor action during attempted prey capture or escape, mating, or other critical activities also provide tremendous advantage. Inertial sensors used either for direct control or feedback control in neuromuscular systems can enhance stability and help to defeat those two enemies of agility, *sluggishness* and *overshoot* (see Talbot and Gessner, 1973; Thaler and Brown, 1953). Thus, inertial sensors in animals play two roles, exteroceptive and proprioceptive.

Dynamic properties of inertial sensors

We shall consider sensors operating according to the following causal chain: acceleration of an inertial element (a simple mass such as a statolith, or perhaps a gyroscopic element such as a dipteran haltere) leads to a reaction force, which in turn acts against an elastic element to produce displacement, which in turn is sensed by a strain gauge or its equivalent. The requirement that the inertial element displace the elastic element limits the response dynamics of an inertial sensor. Consider the lumped, passive mechanical model depicted in Figure 1. It is represented as being in a cavity in a rigid body, L, and is designed to sense the motion of that body along the x axis. A rigid shaft bears the sensing mass, m, and pivots about the point x_o fixed to the body. Strain gauges, G, measure displacement of the shaft in response to body

Figure 1. Idealized model of an inertial motion sensor.

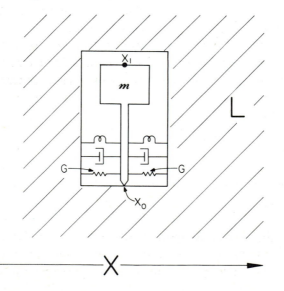

motion; elastic elements restore the mass to its original position ($x_1 = x_0$) in the cavity once motion of the body has ceased; and the inevitable frictional elements react to the velocity of the sensing mass within the cavity. For small values of displacement, ϕ,

$$\phi = x_1 - x_0 \tag{2}$$

the sensing system should behave linearly, in which case its dynamic behavior is described by

$$k\phi + b(d\phi/dt) + m(d^2x_1/dt^2) = 0 \tag{3}$$

where k, b and m are the equivalent elastance, viscous resistance, and sensing mass. The strain gauges measure displacement, ϕ, the dynamic equation for which is found by subtracting m times the x-axis acceleration (a) of the body from both sides of equation (3).

$$k\phi + b(d\phi/dt) + m(d^2\phi/dt^2) = -ma \tag{4}$$

This is the classic harmonic oscillator equation. It describes the dynamics of the strain gauge displacement in response to the driving force, ma. With inevitably finite viscous resistance, the equation represents two broad response regimes, *underdamped* and *overdamped*, separated by an infinitely narrow border representing *critical-damped response*. A system lying close to the critical-damp border (on either side of it) settles down to its steady-state relationship between displacement and acceleration more quickly than those remote from it. The border itself corresponds to parameter values for which

$$b^2 = 4km \tag{5}$$

The overdamp region corresponds to b^2 greater then $4km$, the underdamp region to the reverse. The *zero-state* relationship between ϕ and a (i.e., given that $t > 0$ and ϕ, $d\phi/dt$, and $d^2\phi/dt^2$ all equal *zero* when $t = 0$) conventionally is described by the transfer function T(s) in the Laplace transform domain:

$$T(s) = -\phi(s)/a(s) = 1/[s^2 + (b/m)s + (k/m)] \tag{6}$$

where s is the complex variable of the Laplace transform. For transient overdamped response, T(s) is most convenient in the form

$$T(s) = (m/k)/[(s\tau_1 + 1)(s\tau_2 + 1)] \tag{7}$$

which indicates that the response to an abrupt change in acceleration will include two decaying exponential terms, with time constants τ_1 and τ_2; or, equivalently, that the system will require approximately four times the longer of the time constants to complete its response to an abrupt change in acceleration. For steady-state response to a sinusoid with constant peak acceleration, A.

$$a(t) = A \cos[\omega t] \tag{8}$$

$T(s)$ is more convenient in its frequency-domain form,

$$T(i\omega) = 1/[(i\omega + \omega_1)(i\omega + \omega_2)] \tag{9a}$$

$$\omega_1 < \omega_2 \tag{9b}$$

$$\omega = 2\pi f \tag{9c}$$

where f is frequency in Hz; ω is frequency in rad s^{-1}. ω_1 and ω_2 are the lower and upper *corner frequencies*, respectively. For frequencies well below ω_1, the amplitude of $T(i\omega)$ is independent of frequency, and the phase shift imposed by $T(i\omega)$ is zero. For frequencies between ω_1 and ω_2, and far from either of them, the amplitude of $T(i\omega)$ is proportional to $1/\omega$, and the phase shift imposed by $T(i\omega)$ is $-\pi/2$ rad ($-90°$). For frequencies well above ω_2, the amplitude of $T(i\omega)$ is proportional to $1/\omega^2$, and the phase shift imposed by $T(i\omega)$ is $-\pi$ rad ($-180°$). Noting that

$$v(t) = \int a(t)dt = (1/\omega)A \cos[\omega t - \pi/2] \tag{10}$$

where $v(t)$ is the velocity of the body in Figure 1, and that

$$x_0(t) = \int v(t)dt = (1/\omega^2)A \cos[\omega t - \pi] \tag{11}$$

we see that for frequencies between ω_1 and ω_2, the response of the sensor is proportional to the *velocity* of the body, and for frequencies greater than ω_2, the response is proportional to the *displacement* of the body. Only for frequencies below ω_1 is the sensor a true accelerometer, with response proportional to the *acceleration* of the body. In every case acceleration is the ultimate stimulus. Thus, in the displacement- or velocity-sensing modes, the inertial motion sensor produces a response proportional to the displacement or velocity *of an accelerating body*.

For underdamped response, $T(s)$ is more convenient in the following forms:

$$T(s) = 1/[s^2 + 2\alpha s + \omega_0^2 + \alpha^2] \tag{12}$$

$$T(i\omega) = 1/[(\omega_c^2 - \omega^2) + i2\alpha\omega] \tag{13}$$

$$\alpha = b/2m \quad \omega_c^2 = k/m \quad \omega_0^2 = \omega_c^2 - \alpha^2 \quad \omega_r^2 = \omega_c^2 - 2\alpha^2 \tag{14}$$

Equation 12 indicates that the response to an abrupt change in acceleration will be a damped sinusoid, with frequency ω_0 and exponential-damping coefficient α. Equation 13 indicates that for frequencies well above the corner frequency, ω_c, the steady-state response to a sinusoid with constant peak acceleration [equation (8)] is proportional to $1/\omega^2$, with a phase shift of $-\pi$ rad with respect to the stimulus; the response is maximum at the frequency ω_r, and for frequencies well below ω_r, the response amplitude is independent of frequency and exhibits zero phase shift. Thus, for frequencies well above ω_c the response of the sensor is proportional to *displacement* of the body; and for frequencies well below ω_r the response is proportional to *acceleration* of the body. In the immediate vicinity of ω_c the response is proportional to the *velocity* of the body.

To use acceleration or velocity information effectively, a control system must have *measurements* of the acceleration or velocity amplitude and direction. For such purposes, an inertial sensor is useless in the frequency range over which its response is proportional to displacement rather than acceleration or velocity. Thus the upper corner frequency, ω_2 or ω_c of the inertial sensor of Figure 1 reflects its inherent sluggishness; it is inoperative at higher frequencies.

The lumped, passive, linear model depicted in the previous paragraphs very likely is a reasonably good one for the mechanics associated with biological inertial sensors employing exquisitely sensitive strain-gauge elements such as vertebrate hair cells or arthropod scolopale sense cells. The minute displacements sensed by such elements would be accompanied by comparably low velocities and therefore would tend to keep both elastic and viscous-resistance elements operating in their linear ranges. However, the principal message of this section does not depend upon linearity, passivity, or lumping. With or without those ingredients, the dynamics of any strain-gauge-based inertial sensor are limited by the inevitable sluggishness of the mechanical network that translates velocity or acceleration into displacement.

The seismic sense

In the evolutionary context that presumably gave rise to seismic sensitivity, sensitivity *per se* would be at a premium. Indeed, in seismic sensors we find biological mechanoreception honed to what presently seems to be its greatest sensitivity, comparable to that in the most sensitive auditory sensors (Autrum and Schneider, 1948; Walcott and van der Kloot, 1959; Hartline, 1971). The enemy of sensitivity is *noise*. Seismic sensors must contend with microseismic noise in the environment, mechanical noise generated within the body, and thermal noise generated in the mechanical and strain-gauge elements of the sensor itself and in the elements of the nervous system connected to the sensor. Conventional remedies for noise are bandwidth manipulation, signal amplification close to the input, temporal summation of signals, and spatial summation of signals. At the earth's surface, for frequencies above 2 to 3 Hz, microseismic noise spectra exhibit nearly constant mean acceleration amplitudes (typically between 0.00001 and 0.001 cm s^{-2}, depending on locale, over one-third-octave bandwidths); acceleration amplitudes increase drastically below 2 to 3 Hz (Brune and Oliver, 1959; Frantti, Willis and Wilson, 1962). Thus 3 Hz appears to be the lower edge of the environmental window for seismic signals. Even within that window there is an evolutionary design trade-off between the versatility of broad-band sensitivity and the noise rejection inherent in narrow-band sensitivity (in the face of inevitable noise-content increase with increasing bandwidth). One finds both extremes. For example, the tibial sense organs of many insects exhibit nearly uniform acceleration sensitivity over three or four octaves, but that of Autrum and Schneider's cockroach, *Periplaneta americana*, is tuned to a very narrow band (Autrum and Schneider, 1948; Schneider, 1950). Narrow-band tuning is observed in the exquisite seismic sensitivity of the snake inner-ear as well (Hartline, 1971). The spider has the advantage of both extremes in its tarsal lyriform organ, which, like the mammalian cochlea, covers a broad frequency band with many channels, each narrowly tuned to a different region (Walcott and van der Kloot, 1959).

Narrow-band tuning and temporal summation can be accomplished simultaneously in the sensor of Figure 1 by shifting far from the critical-damp border on the underdamp side, $b^2 \ll 4km$, leading to a peak of sensitivity in the immediate vicinity of frequency ω_r (see Figure 2). The conventional parameter Q provides measures of the peak's height and bandwidth:

$$Q \simeq (\text{peak sensitivity})/(\text{low-frequency sensitivity}) \simeq k/b\omega_r \quad (15)$$

$$\text{Bandwidth (at 0.707 of peak sensitivity)} \simeq \omega_r/Q \quad (16)$$

The amplitude of the system's response to a sinusoidal stimulus with frequency close to ω_r is an exponentially-weighted sum of the cycle-by-cycle stimulus amplitude; approximately Q cycles are required for the system to become fully excited by a constant amplitude sinusoid of frequency ω_r. Thus, as Q increases, the system becomes increasingly sluggish. It also becomes increasingly sensitive over an increasingly narrow band of frequencies.

The ultimate sensitivity of a strain-gauge-based accelerometer is established by the minimum peak-to-peak displacement of the strain-gauge element that can be discerned over the noise inherent in the element and its associated sensing-mass system (i.e., by the strain-gauge *displacement noise floor*). When operated at frequencies well below ω_1 or ω_r, the sensor of Figure 1 has peak-to-peak strain-gauge displacement, ϕ_{p-p}, that is directly proportional to peak body acceleration, A,

$$\phi_{p-p} = -2A/\omega_c^2 \quad \text{or} \quad \phi_{p-p} = -2A/\omega_1\omega_2 \tag{17}$$

When operated at frequency ω_r, the center of a sharp sensitivity peak, the sensor exhibits a summed strain-gauge displacement,

$$\phi_{p-p} \simeq -2QA/\omega_r^2 \tag{18}$$

Thus, the displacement noise floor of the strain-gauge element can be estimated from observations of the sensor's noise floor with respect to body acceleration and estimates of the sensor's corner frequencies (ω_1 and ω_2, or ω_c) or resonance frequency (ω_r). The most sensitive man-made inertial accelerometers have strain-gauge displacement noise floors in the neighborhood of 1 pm. Designed with corner frequencies in the

Figure 2. Sensitivity as a function of frequency, depicted in terms of asymptotes, for the idealized sensor of Figure 1. The overdamped system exhibits two corner frequencies, ω_1 and ω_2, with asymptotic slopes -1.0 between them and -2.0 beyond ω_2. The critically-damped system exhibits one corner frequency, ω_c, with asymptotic slope -2.0 beyond it. The underdamped system exhibits the same asymptotic slopes as the critically-damped system, but also has a resonance peak at frequency ω_r.

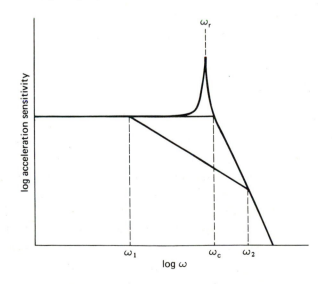

neighborhood of 1 kHz, such devices have input acceleration noise floors between 0.001 and 0.01 cm s^{-2}. By passing the accelerometer output through a spectrum analyser with effective bandwidths of less than 1 Hz (i.e., the analog of a super-cochlea or super-lyriform organ), one can reduce the acceleration noise floor of a vibration-monitoring system to the neighborhood of 0.0001 cm s^{-2}.

In searching the literature for comparable acceleration sensitivities among biological sensors, one must be careful to distinguish experiments in which the sensing mass is allowed to move freely from experiments in which the sensing mass is restrained or replaced by an effectively infinite mass. The former may provide direct measure of the sensor's acceleration noise floor and frequency response properties (which can be combined to yield estimates of strain-gauge displacement noise floors). The latter may provide direct measure of strain-gauge displacement noise floor, but cannot provide sufficient information for estimation of the sensor's acceleration noise floor. In crustacean and molluscan statocysts and vertebrate otolithic or otoconial organs, examples of each of which are known to have seismic sensitivity (Cohen, 1955; Maturana and Sperling, 1963; Budelmann, 1976; Lowenstein and Roberts, 1951; Ashcroft and Hallpike, 1934), the sensing masses apparently are confined to small volumes in the immediate vicinity of the sensors and normally are unrestrained during experiments. The same thing may be true for the spider lyriform organ and insect tibial organs, which also exhibit seismic sensitivity (Walcott and van der Kloot, 1959; Bullock and Horridge, 1965, p. 1058; Barth and Pickelmann, 1975; Autrum and Schneider, 1948). Other identified or potential sources of seismic sensitivity (Keidel, 1968; Burgess, 1974), including Pacinian corpuscles in mammals (Gray and Matthews, 1951; Keidel, 1956; Verrillo, 1966), Herbst corpuscles in birds (Dorward and McIntyre, 1971), various other tactile receptors in vertebrates or invertebrates (Keidel, 1968; Burgess, 1974; Tautz, 1977; Barth, 1980), and joint or muscle receptors in vertebrates or invertebrates (Roberts and Murray-Smith, 1970; Olivio, 1970), presumably employ either the entire body or a large part thereof (e.g., a limb, the visceral mass) as the sensing mass. Among the latter group, experiments with unrestrained sensing masses apparently are uncommon. When the situation is in doubt, the frequency–response properties of the sensor may provide a clue: sensors exhibiting tuning curves similar to those of Figure 2, with broad regions of frequency–independent acceleration sensitivity, probably have unrestrained sensing masses; those that exhibit frequency-independent displacement sensitivity extending to d.c. or to frequencies so low that adaptation becomes significant either are not acceleration sensors at all or are acceleration sensors with restrained sensing masses.

The most acute seismic sensitivity reported so far among invertebrates arises in the insect tibia, and in most cases is attributed to the subgenual organ, a special scolopophorous organ (Autrum, 1941; Autrum and Schneider, 1948; Schwartzkopff, 1974; Bullock and Horridge, 1965). Although the mechanics underlying the sensitivity of this organ were debated (see Schwartzkopff, 1974), its reported frequency–response properties usually conform well to those of the near-critical-damp case in Figure 2, with nearly frequency-independent acceleration sensitivity from 100 Hz or less up to a corner frequency ranging approximately from 600 to 2000 Hz, depending on the species, and, immediately above the corner frequency, nearly frequency-independent displacement sensitivity (see Autrum and Schneider, 1948, Figures 2, 3; Schneider, 1950, Figure 1). The outstanding exception to this pattern is the subgenual organ of Autrum and Schneider's cockroach (*Periplaneta americana*), which exhibited nearly frequency-independent acceleration sensitivity (with acceleration noise floors in the vicinity of $0.3 \, \text{cm s}^{-2}$) over three octaves, from 100 to 800 Hz, followed by a sharp sensitivity peak ($Q \simeq 15$, minimum acceleration noise floor approximately $0.02 \, \text{cm s}^{-2}$, $\omega_r/2\pi \simeq 1500 \, \text{Hz}$), followed in turn by acceleration-sensitivity decline as $1/\omega^1$ rather than $1/\omega^3$. Thus, contrary to the expectations from the model of Figure 1, the *Periplaneta* sensor exhibits no region of frequency-independent displacement sensitivity. Otherwise, it conforms well to the underdamped form of the model. Estimated on the basis of the model, the peak-to-peak strain-gauge displacement noise floor of the *Periplaneta* subgenual organ is in the range 40 to 70 pm. Among the most sensitive tibial seismic sensors in other insect species, the acceleration noise floors typically are greater than $0.1 \, \text{cm s}^{-2}$, and the estimated strain-gauge displacement noise floors are 100 pm or greater (Autrum and Schneider, 1948; Schneider, 1950). Seismic sensitivity over the same range of frequencies with $0.1 \, \text{cm s}^{-2}$ acceleration noise floor and 100 pm estimated strain-gauge displacement noise floor is found in the leg nerves of the beetle *Melolantha melolantha*, which lacks tibial subgenual organs (Schneider, 1950; Bullock and Horridge, 1965). Subgenual-organ responses exhibit adaptation to constant-amplitude sinusoids (Howse, 1962), and at least in one species, *Gryllus campestris*, the steady-state relationship between stimulus, S, and response, R, shows the classic logarithmic form (Dambach, 1970):

$$R = C \log S \tag{19}$$

This sort of adaptation cannot be explained in terms of the linear mechanisms (e.g., viscous coupling between sensing mass and strain gauge) often invoked to explain adaptation-like phenomena in the vertebrate ear.

In vertebrates, the most exquisitely sensitive seismic sensors reported so far reside in the ear rather than the leg (Hartline, 1971; Lewis and Narins, 1981). At the level of the midbrain, snakes exhibit seismic and auditory sensitivity with sharply-peaked tuning curves that match almost perfectly (Hartline, 1971). At the sensitivity peak ($f \simeq 250\,Hz$), the acceleration noise floor of the sensor is approximately $0.02\,cm\,s^{-2}$, the same level observed in *Periplaneta*. The corresponding externally-applied peak-to-peak displacement was approximately 100 pm; but owing to the complexity of the tuning curve this value is difficult to translate to strain-gauge noise floor. In a separate, somatic seismic sensor, snakes exhibit displacement sensitivity that is nearly frequency-independent from close to d.c. to at least 1000 Hz, with noise floors from 4 to 400 nm (Hartline, 1971).

Crude seismic sensitivity has been reported for the auditory endorgans of frogs and salamanders (Frishkopf and Goldstein, 1963; Smith, 1968), where coupling between the substrate and the oval window apparently is provided by the opercular plate and opercularis muscle (Lombard and Straughan, 1974). In frogs, however, the truly exquisite seismic sensitivity resides in non-auditory inner-ear endorgans, the sacculus and the lagena (Ashcroft and Hallpike, 1934; Caston, Precht and Blanks, 1977). Dye-injection studies revealed that seismic sensitivity resides over the entire saccular macula, but only at the very center of the lagenar macula (Lewis, Baird, Leverenz and Koyama, 1982). The more sensitive seismic afferent axons from the sacculus or lagena of the American bullfrog, *Rana catesbeiana*, exhibit acceleration noise floors in the neighborhood of $0.01\,cm\,s^{-2}$, with a few as low as $0.005\,cm\,s^{-2}$. The tuning bandwidths range from approximately 10 Hz to approximately 150 Hz, covering the frequency range approximately from 10 to 200 Hz (Koyama, Lewis, Baird and Leverenz, 1982; Lewis and Baird, 1981). The white-lipped frog, *Leptodactylus albilabris*, exhibits even greater sensitivity in single VIIIth-nerve seismic axons, with acceleration noise floors in the vicinity of $0.001\,cm\,s^{-2}$, covering approximately the same frequency range as those of the bullfrog (Lewis and Narins , 1981). The seismic sensitivity of this frog is so acute that the spike-rate responses of its more sensitive axons are thoroughly saturated at acceleration amplitude ($0.02\,cm\,s^{-2}$) corresponding to the noise floor of the snake ear or the *Periplaneta* tibia, and further increases in intensity apparently are coded by increasingly tight phase locking between stimulus and response (Narins and Lewis, in preparation). Spatial summation may play a special role in this exquisite sensitivity, inasmuch as individual afferent axons to the bullfrog sacculus terminate on more hair cells (typically 15 to 30, sometimes more than 200) than do the axons to any other inner-ear endorgan of that animal (Lewis et al., 1982).

Inertial sensors for increased agility and stability

The potential roles of inertial velocity and acceleration sensors in agility enhancement perhaps are most obvious in the context of the basic *servomechanism*, in which an *active motor element* attempts to drive a *mechanical load* in a particular manner, using position, velocity, acceleration, and possibly other clues measured by *sensing elements* and translated by *signal-processing elements* into appropriate motor commands. The agile servomechanism operates not only on the basis of the answers to 'where am I now and where do I want to be?', but also on the basis of answers to 'how fast do I want to get there?', 'is my destination moving; if so, how fast, what direction?', 'how fast and in what direction am I going now?', 'how fast and in what direction will I be going next?'. The answers to the last two questions can be provided by inertial accelerometers and velocity sensors. To understand the advantages of such sensors in a more formal respect, consider the case of a servomechanism whose load comprises the inevitable inertia, M, and viscous resistance, B, and whose motor element operates solely on the basis of the difference between the load's present position, y, and its desired position, $y_1(t)$, by generating force F given by

$$F = K(y_1 - y) \tag{20}$$

The dynamic equation for the system is

$$K(y_1 - y) = B(dy/dt) + M(d^2y/dt^2) \tag{21}$$

which leads to the following transfer function relating y to y_1:

$$y(s)/y_1(s) = 1/[(M/K)s^2 + (B/K)s + 1] \tag{22}$$

Once again we have the classic harmonic oscillator. If B^2 is much greater than $4KM$, y will approach the target (y_1) sluggishly, with error ($\varepsilon = y_1 - y$) that decreases exponentially in time for a target that is fixed. If B^2 is much less than $4KM$, y will overshoot a fixed target; and the error will take the form of a damped oscillation. Only if the system is in the vicinity of the critical-damp border, $B^2 = 4KM$, will it muster its maximum agility (minimum sluggishness, tolerable overshoot). Among near-critically-damped systems, those with higher values of ω_c or $\omega_1\omega_2$ (see equations 9–14) respond more quickly than those with lower values:

$$\omega_1\omega_2 = \omega_c^2 = K/M \simeq B^2/4M^2 \tag{23}$$

Thus, if K always is adjusted to place the system close to the critical-damp border, the system's agility will increase as the load's inertia decreases or its resistance increases.

The effective inertia and resistance of the load can be altered by appropriate velocity and acceleration control of the motor,

$$F = K_0(y_1 - y) + K_1(dy/dt) + K_2(d^2y/dt^2) \tag{24}$$

leading to

$$K_0(y_1 - y) = [B - K_1](dy/dt) + [M - K_2](d^2y/dt^2) \tag{25}$$

Thus, the active motor element is controlled so that it appears, in part, to be a positive or negative mass in parallel with *M* and a positive or negative frictional resistance in parallel with *B*, depending on the signs of K_1 and K_2. In order to achieve this effect, the servomechanism must have means of measuring the amplitudes of velocity and acceleration *and* means of sensing their directions. With adequate signal-processing elements, the algorithms for employing velocity and acceleration information could be improved over those of this relatively unsophisticated, linear servomechanism. For example, the use of velocity or acceleration information could be tempered directly by positional-error information to yield greater agility. No matter how sophisticated the nervous system's algorithms might be, the agility of a servomechanism ultimately is limited by the force it can devote to overcoming inertia and friction, by its sensitivity to motion, and by the speed with which it can conduct and process signals. Given the shared limitations of signal-conduction and processing delays, it can be no accident that our most agile appendages, our fingers, not only are driven by muscles far too large to be carried on the appendages themselves, but also are endowed with joint receptors 15 to 20 dB more sensitive to position and *velocity* than those of any of our other appendages except our toes (Provins, 1958). The same design factors that favor agility of action in a servomechanism also favor stability of the system when it faces external disturbances, such as load changes or positional shifts (Talbot and Gessner, 1973; Thaler and Brown, 1953).

In any animal with multiple moving parts, one expects at least two levels of control – coordinated control of all the parts for integrated motor action, and local control of each individual part to maintain its designated role in that action. Stability and agility are valuable at both levels and so, therefore, are velocity and acceleration sensors. Of course another critical role that can be played by velocity and acceleration sensors during coordinated action is maintenance of the animal's spatial orientation, accomplished solely by the motion sense itself or by other senses (e.g., vision) stabilized in space by means of the motion sense. Thus one might expect the senses of velocity and acceleration to be diffuse, with separate signal channels for each moving part and perhaps additional channels helping to provide global motion sense for overall coordination and orientation. This expectation is fulfilled at least in the more derived animals – arthropods, molluscs, vertebrates. Almost any mechanoreceptive sensor in those animals could be suspected of playing an important motion-sensing role, and many of those sensors could be inertial. In primates, for example, the cutaneous mechanoreceptors of the glabrous skin of hand and foot (Burgess, 1974), in association with the entire body serving as a sensing mass, presumably provide exquisite sensitivities to vertical and horizontal accelerations. The extraordinarily sensitive joint receptors of toes (Browne, Lee and Ring, 1954) presumably serve in the same way. With various appendages or portions of the trunk serving as sensing masses, the other, less-sensitive joint receptors also presumably provide acceleration sensitivity, i.e., the general kinesthetic sense (Gardner, 1950; Boyd and Roberts, 1953). The visceral mass coupled to the Pacinian corpuscles in the mesentery tissue presumably serves the same function (Loewenstein and Mendelson, 1965; Talbot, Darian-Smith, Kornhuber and Mountcastle, 1968). Many examples of analogous systems, with the entire body or major parts of it serving as the sensing mass and joint or cutaneous mechanoreceptors serving as strain-gauge elements, have been identified among the arthropods (Horn, 1975; Sandeman, 1976); and presumably such systems abound in the molluscs as well (e.g., see Janse, 1982; McClary, 1966).

In invertebrates and vertebrates, one also finds organs containing their own, specialized sensing masses and apparently dedicated to inertial sensing of orientation or motion. These are the otoconial or otolithic organs and canal organs of the vertebrate inner ear, the statocysts of invertebrates in general, and the halteres of the dipterans. According to equation (4), as long as the corner frequencies of an inertial motion sensor remain well above the range of expected stimulus frequencies, the sensitivity of the device will increase with increasing sensing mass. Thus, for example, by far the largest sensing mass in the frog inner ear is associated with the sacculus, the organ with acute seismic sensitivity. High sensitivity to motion in selected directions can be achieved with a modest sensing mass effectively amplified by being in motion at high velocity. The operating principles of such a sensor are based on

$$f = -\mathrm{d}p/\mathrm{d}t \qquad (26)$$

rather than on equation (1), where p is the momentum of the sensing mass. Very small motions in specific directions can constitute very large changes in the *direction* of the vector p, leading to very large reaction force, f. This is the basis of operation of the gyroscope, and it also appears to be the basis of operation of the haltere, a club-shaped, hind-wing derivative that vibrates at very high frequencies. With the bulk of its mass carried at its free-swinging distal end (*see* Figure 3), the vibrating haltere must exhibit high momentum, allowing it to serve as a gyroscopic inertial element (Pringle, 1948). An impressive array of sensory cells reside in its base, apparently measuring roll- or yaw-induced changes in the direction of the momentum vector (Bullock and Horridge, 1965, p. 1150; Tracy, 1975; Pringle, 1948).

The statocysts of crustaceans (Figure 4), the statocysts of cephalopods (Figures 5, 6), and the non-auditory endorgans of the vertebrate inner ear

Figure 3. s.e.m. A dipteran haltere (microgr. width $\approx 800\,\mu$m).

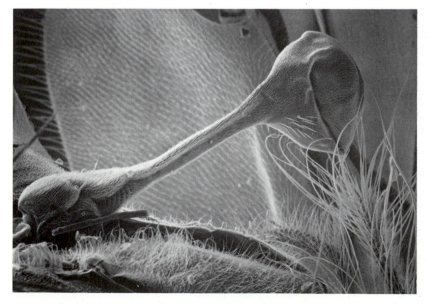

show remarkable convergence of structure and function (Cohen, 1955; Young, 1959; Retzius, 1881). All three sensors exhibit both linear inertial elements (statoliths, otoliths, or otoconia) and rotational inertial elements (fluid constrained to move in a circular path) (Janse and Sandeman, 1979a; Budelmann, 1977; Wilson and Melvill Jones, 1979). In all three sensors, the strain-gauge structures are morphologically and functionally polarized, each responding maximally to displacement in a specific direction (Cohen, 1955; Sandeman and Okajima, 1972; Takahata and Hisada, 1979; Budelmann, 1976, 1979; Lowenstein and Wersäll, 1959). In all three sensors, the arrays of receptor cells associated with linear inertial elements are separate from those associated with the rotational inertial elements. In each case the array associated with the linear inertial element is studded with receptors whose polarization axes fan out to cover virtually all directions in a given plane (Schöne, 1975b; Stein, 1975; Budelmann, 1979; Wersäll, Flock and Lundquist, 1965). All three sensors are linked directly to compensatory eye movement systems (Janse and Sandeman, 1979b; Dijkgraaf, 1959; Henn, Cohen and Young, 1980).

In all three sensors, the strain-gauge element (sensory cell) has or is associated with one or more hair-like projections into the statocyst or inner-ear cavity. In crustaceans, the projection is a cuticular hair; and the effective stimulus generally is presumed to be stretch or compression

Figure 4. s.e.m. Cuticular hairs of a lobster statocyst (microgr. width ≈ 0.33 cm).

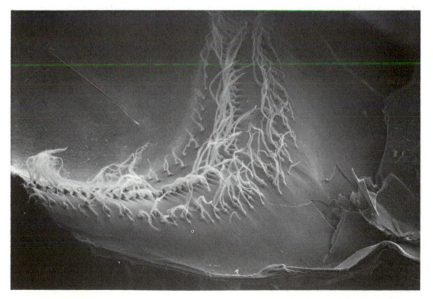

Figures 5, 6. s.e.m. An *Octopus* statocyst macula, and close-up of the hair cells, respectively (microgr. widths ≈ 0.1 cm, 60 μm).

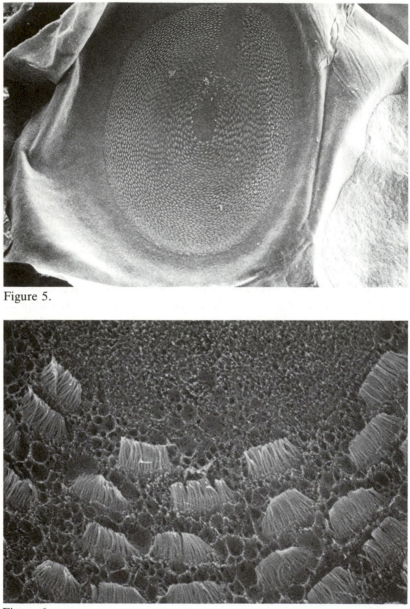

Figure 5.

Figure 6.

of the sensing-cell dendrite at the base of the hair (Mill, 1976). In cephalopods, the projections are the several cilia of the sensory cell (hair cell) itself. The micromechanical details of the effective stimulus are not known; but in similar hair cells in gastropods, transduction is mediated by a membrane conductance change, apparently induced indirectly by a relatively slow process initiated by cilia strain (Detweiler and Fuortes, 1975; Wiederhold, 1977). In vertebrates, the projections are the single true cilium (kinocilium) and the many microvilli-like stereocilia of the sensory cell (hair cell). The tips of the stereocilia evidently are endowed with displacement-sensitive, non-specific, ion conduction channels, which open very quickly in response to strain (Hudspeth and Corey, 1977; Hudspeth, 1982).

Although they appear in many ways to be similar, the rotational inertia systems of invertebrates and vertebrates have interesting structural differences. Assuming that its elastic cupula completely occludes d.c. flow of fluid (McLaren and Hillman, 1979) and that its walls are rigid, one can treat the vertebrate semicircular canal as a series combination of three lumped fluid-mechanical elements, an inertance i representing the mass of the fluid in the canal, a resistance r representing the viscosity of the fluid, and a compliance c representing the elastic properties of the cupula (Wilson and Melvill Jones, 1979). The sensory-cell strain apparently is, at least in part, coupled through the cupula directly to *fluid displacement* (Fernandez and Goldberg, 1971; McLaren and Hillman, 1979). Assuming that cupular displacements are sufficiently small to allow linear treatment, one is led to the following relationships between sensory-cell strain, ϕ, and rotational acceleration, $\ddot{\theta}$, in the plane of the canal:

$$T(s) = \phi(s)/\ddot{\theta}(s) = \beta_0/(s\tau_1 + 1)(s\tau_2 + 1) \tag{27a}$$

$$T(i\omega) = \beta_1/(i\omega + \omega_1)(i\omega + \omega_2) \tag{27b}$$

$$\omega_1^2 = 1/\tau_1^2 \simeq 1/ic; \quad \omega_2 = 1/\tau_2 \simeq r/i \tag{27c}$$

β_0 and β_1 being constants that depend on canal geometry. The sensory hairs of the crustacean semicircular canal do not occlude flow (Janse and Sandeman, 1979a). Through viscous drag on the hairs, sensory-cell strain apparently is coupled to *fluid velocity* (Sandeman, 1976). Assuming that individual hairs have elastic restoring forces, viscous-drag forces that totally overwhelm any inertial reaction forces, and that movement of the hair has negligible effect on the fluid, one is led to the same equations (27a and 27b) for the crustacean canal, with

$$\omega_1 = 1/\tau_1 = k/b; \quad \omega_2 = 1/\tau_2 = r/i \tag{28}$$

b and *k* being the local resistance and elastance of the individual hair, *i* and *r* being the inertance and resistance of the fluid in the canal.

In vertebrates, ω_1 and τ_1 have been estimated from psychophysical experiments and from direct observations on cupular deformation; ω_2 and τ_2 are estimated from canal geometry (i.e., assuming laminar flow of a Newtonian fluid in a rigid-walled cylindrical tube, bent with large radius of curvature):

$$\omega_2 = 32\eta/\rho d^2 \tag{29}$$

η and ρ being the viscosity and density of the fluid, *d* being the inside diameter of the canal. ω_2 for the human canal is in the neighborhood of $800\,\mathrm{rad\,s^{-1}}$ (130 Hz); estimates for ω_1 place it in the neighborhood of $0.1\,\mathrm{rad\,s^{-1}}$ (0.016 Hz) (Wilson and Melvill Jones, 1979). Between those two frequencies, the response of the canal is expected to be proportional to *rotational velocity*. In the squirrel monkey, *Saimiri sciureus*, that expectation is only partially fulfilled (Fernandez and Goldberg, 1971). The upper frequency limit is obscured by another dynamic component, leading to observed transfer functions of the form

$$T(i\omega) = T_0(i\omega + \omega_3)/[(i\omega + \omega_1)(i\omega + \omega_2)] \tag{30}$$

for single afferent axons, where ω_3 varies from one afferent to another, ranging from approximately $11\,\mathrm{rad\,s^{-1}}$ to approximately $80\,\mathrm{rad\,s^{-1}}$. The frequency range of velocity sensitivity is from ω_1 to ω_3 rather than to ω_2, which is estimated to be approximately $300\,\mathrm{rad\,s^{-1}}$ (50 Hz) for the squirrel-monkey canal. In some axons, the fluid dynamics of the system are further obscured by slow adaptation processes, with time constants ranging upward from 30 s.

The semicircular canal system of the crab *Scylla serrata* exhibits frequency-independent velocity sensitivity in the 0.3–2 Hz range, indicating that ω_1 and ω_2 are on opposite sides of that range (Fraser, 1977). In the same frequency range, the canal system of the crab *Carcinus maenas* apparently is shifting from acceleration to velocity sensitivity, indicating that ω_1 and ω_2 are within or above that range (Fraser, 1977). The diameters of crab canals are approximately five times those of vertebrate canals (Janse and Sandeman, 1979b), which according to equation (29) should shift ω_2 downward by a factor of approximately 25 (i.e., to the 2–6 Hz range).

The tonic responses of the linear-inertia systems of the invertebrate statocysts and the vertebrate inner ear were treated in the previous chapter; here I shall consider the phasic responses. In the context of gravity sensitivity the latter signal *changes* in orientation with respect to the gravity vector. In the context of dynamic acceleration sensitivity, they signal *changes* in acceleration rather than acceleration *per se.* Experiments usually have been carried out in the gravity context, stimuli being defined in terms of the declination, ψ, of the dorsoventral axis of the animal from its normal upright position, and the azimuth, θ (with respect to the anterior-posterior axis) along which the tilt occurred. For a directionally-sensitive sensory cell, it is convenient to define a *sensitivity vector* and to measure the stimulus strength as the projection of applied acceleration or its rate of change on that vector. If θ_0 and ψ_0 are the azimuth and declination of the sensitivity vector with respect to the anterior-posterior and dorsoventral axes of the animal, respectively, then the strength of the gravity stimulus is

$$S(\theta, \psi) = gD \cos (\psi - \xi) \tag{31a}$$

$$D = [\cos^2 \psi_0 + \sin^2 \psi_0 \cos^2 (\hat{\theta} - \theta_0)] \tag{31b}$$

$$\xi = \arctan [\cos (\hat{\theta} - \theta_0) \tan \psi_0] \tag{31c}$$

$$\hat{\theta} = \pi - \theta \text{ rad} \tag{31d}$$

g being the acceleration of gravity at the surface of the earth. The available evidence indicates that this measure of stimulus strength indeed is appropriate for tonic gravity sensitivity of the vertebrate inner ear (Fernandez and Goldberg, 1976a; Lowenstein and Saunders, 1975), and possibly for that of crustacean and cephalopod statocysts as well (Cohen, 1955; Budelmann, 1976). In the lobster *Homarus americanus*, the monkey *Saimiri scirueus*, and the frog *Rana catesbeiana*, where it has been examined carefully, the effective stimulus for phasic gravity sensitivity apparently is dS/dt, which, for constant-angular-velocity change of declination along a given azimuth ($\psi = \omega t$) is

$$dS/dt = gD \sin (\omega t - \xi) \tag{32}$$

Furthermore, in each case, the phasic response depends strongly on both the amplitude and the *sign* of dS/dt, typically reflected by a large increase in afferent-axon spike rate for large-amplitude dS/dt of one sign, and either spike-rate decrease (from a resting rate) or no change at all for large-amplitude dS/dt of the opposite sign (Cohen, 1955; Fernandez and Goldberg, 1976b; Baird, 1982; Lowenstein and Saunders, 1975). For a particular sensitivity vector, there are two orientations in which the amplitude of dS/dt is maximum: $\theta = \theta_0$, $\psi = \psi_0 - \pi/2$; and $\theta = \hat{\theta}_0$, $\psi = 3\pi/2 - \psi_0$. In both orientations, declination velocities in the same direction (both up or both down) will yield dS/dt of the same

606   *E. R. Lewis*

sign. However, since the azimuth is reversed, the effective stimulus will be clockwise in one case, anticlockwise in the other, to an observer at a fixed vantage point; the two orientations are antipodal. This prediction of the model has been tested only in the inner-ear afferent gravity axons of *Rana catesbeiana*, where it was verified (Lowenstein and Saunders, 1975).

Attempts to fit the sinusoidal steady-state responses of afferent axons from vertebrate otoconial organs to the simple inertial-sensor models of equations (9) and (13) so far have not succeeded. Phasic gravity axons from the inner ear of *Rana catesbeiana*, for example, exhibited amplitude-*v.*-frequency curves conforming reasonably well to those predicted by a model identical in form to equation (30); but the phase-shift of the responses did not conform at all well to those of that model (Lowenstein and Saunders, 1975). In *Saimiri sciureus*, good fits to amplitude and phase data were obtained with the following model:

$$T(s) = K(sk_a\tau_a + 1)[(s\tau_v)^{k_v} + 1]/(s\tau_a + 1)(s\tau_m + 1) \tag{33}$$

where τ_a and τ_v apparently are associated with adaptation processes (Fernandez and Goldberg, 1976c). Thus, the parameter τ_m, which was found to range from nearly 0 to approximately 50 ms, may be the only reflection of the sensing-mass system in the response dynamics, adaptation having obscured the rest.

I thank the University of California Committee on Research for providing a travel grant for this conference. My research is supported by the National Institutes of Health: Grant NS12359 from the National Institute of Neurological and Communicative Disorders and Stroke, and by the National Science Foundation: Grant BNS-8005834.

References

Ashcroft, D. W., and Hallpike, C. S. (1934). Action potentials in the saccular nerve of the frog. *J. Physiol., Lond. 81:* 23P.

Autrum, H. (1941). Übër Gehör und Erschütterungssinn bei Locustiden. *Z. vergl. Physiol. 28:* 580–637.

Autrum, H. (1977). Concept and method in sensory physiology. *J. Comp. Physiol. 120:* 87–100.

Autrum, H., and Schneider, W. (1948). Vergleichende Untersuchungen über den Erschütterungssinn der Insekten. *Z. vergl. Physiol. 31:* 77–88.

Baird, R. A. (1982). *Correspondence between Structure and Function in the Bullfrog Otoconial Organs* (doctoral dissertation). Berkeley: University of California.

Barth, F. G. (1980). Campaniform sensilla: another vibration receptor in the crab leg. *Naturwissenschaften 67:* 201–2.

Barth, F. G., and Pickelmann, P. (1975). Lyriform slit organs: modeling an arthropod mechanoreceptor. *J. Comp. Physiol. 103:* 39–54.

Boyd, I. A., and Roberts, T. D. M. (1953). Proprioceptive discharges from stretch-receptors in the knee joint of the cat. *J. Physiol., Lond. 122:* 38–59.

Browne, K., Lee, J., and Ring, P. A. (1954). The sensation of passive movement at the metatarso-phalangeal joint of the great toe in man. *J. Physiol., Lond. 126:* 448–58.

Brownell, P., and Farley, R. D. (1979). Detection of vibrations in sand by tarsal sense organs of the nocturnal scorpion, *Paruroctonus mesaenis. J. Comp. Physiol. 131:* 23–30.

Brune, J. N., and Oliver, J. (1959). The seismic noise of the earth's surface. *Bull. Seismol. Soc. Am. 49:* 349–53.

Budelmann, B.-U. (1976). Equilibrium receptor systems in molluscs. In *Structure and Function of Proprioceptors in the Invertebrates*, ed. P. J. Mill, pp. 529–66. London: Chapman & Hall.

Budelmann, B.-U. (1977). Structure and function of the angular acceleration receptor systems in the statocysts of cephalopods. *Symp. Zool. Soc., Lond. 38:* 309–24.

Budelmann, B.-U. (1979). Hair cell polarization in the gravity receptor systems of the statocysts of the cephalopods *Sepia officinalis* and *Loligo vulgaris. Brain Res. 160:* 261–70.

Bullock, T. H., and Horridge, G. A. (1965). *Structure and Function in the Nervous Systems of Invertebrates*, vols 1 and 2. San Francisco: Freeman.

Burgess, P. R. (1974). Cutaneous mechanoreceptors. In *Handbook of Perception*, vol. 3, ed. E. C. Carterette and M. P. Friedman, pp. 219–49.

Caston, J., Precht, W., and Blanks, R. H. I. (1977). Responses of lagena afferents to natural stimuli. *J. Comp. Physiol. 118:* 273–89.

Cohen, B., ed. (1981). *Vestibular and Oculomotor Physiology: International Meeting of the Barany Society (Ann. N.Y. Acad. Sci. vol. 374).* New York: New York Academy of Sciences.

Cohen, M. J. (1955). The function of receptors in the statocyst of the lobster *Homarus americanus. J. Physiol., Lond. 130:* 9–34.

Cohen, M. J. (1960). The response patterns of single receptors in the crustacean statocyst. *Proc. Roy. Soc. Lond. B152:* 30–49.

Dambach, M. (1970). Ein auf Substratvibration reagierendes Interneuron im Bauchmark der Grille. *Z. vergl. Physiol. 70:* 57–61.

Detweiler, P. B., and Fuortes, M. G. F. (1975). Response of hair cells in the statocyst of *Hermissenda. J. Physiol., Lond. 251:* 107–29.

Dijkgraaf, S. (1959). Kompensatorische Kopfbewegung bei Aktivdrehung eines Tintenfisches. *Naturwissenschaften 46:* 611.

Dorward, P. K., and McIntyre, A. K. (1971). Responses of vibration-sensitive receptors in the interosseus region of the duck's hind limb. *J. Physiol., Lond. 219:* 77–87.

Fernandez, C., and Goldberg, J. M. (1971). Physiology of peripheral neurons innervating semicircular canals of the squirrel monkey. II. Response to sinusoidal stimulation and dynamics of peripheral vestibular system. *J. Neurophysiol. 34:* 661–75.

Fernandez, C., and Goldberg, J. M. (1976a). Physiology of peripheral neurons innervating otolith organs of the squirrel monkey. I. Response to static tilts and to long-duration centrifugal force. *J. Neurophysiol. 39:* 970–84.

Fernandez, C., and Goldberg, J. M. (1976b). Physiology of peripheral neurons innervating otolith organs of the squirrel monkey. II. Directional selectivity and force-response relations. *J. Neurophysiol. 39:* 985–95.

Fernandez, C., and Goldberg, J. M. (1976c). Physiology of peripheral neurons innervating otolith organs of the squirrel monkey. III. Response dynamics. *J. Neurophysiol. 39:* 996–1008.

Frantti, G. E., Willis, D. E., and Wilson, J. T. (1962). The spectrum of seismic noise. *Bull. Seismol. Soc. Am. 52:* 113–21.

Fraser, P. J. (1977). How morphology of semicircular canals affects transduction, as shown by response characteristics of statocyst interneurons in the crab *Carcinus maenas* (L.). *J. Comp. Physiol. 115:* 135–45.

Frishkopf, L. S., and Goldstein, M. H. (1963). Responses to acoustic stimuli from single units in the eighth nerve of the bullfrog. *J. Acoust. Soc. Am. 35:* 1219–28.

Gardner, E. (1950). Physiology of the movable joints. *Physiol. Rev. 30:* 127–76.

Gray, J. A. B., and Matthews, P. B. C. (1951). A comparison of the adaptation of the pacinian corpuscle with the accommodation of its own axon. *J. Physiol., Lond. 114:* 454–64.

Hartline, P. M. (1971). Mid-brain responses of the auditory and somatic vibration systems in snakes. *J. Exp. Biol. 54:* 373–90.

Henn, V., Cohen, B., and Young, L. R. (1980). *Visual–Vestibular Interaction in Motion Perception and the Generation of Nystagmus* (*Neurosci. Res. Progr. Bull.* vol. *18*, no. 4.). Cambridge, Massachusetts: Massachusetts Institute of Technology.

Horne, E. (1975). The contribution of different receptors to gravity orientation in insects. *Fortschr. Zool. 23:* 1–20.

Howse, P. E. (1962). The perception of vibration by the subgenual organ in *Zootermopsis angusticollis* Emerson and *Periplaneta americana* L. *Experientia 18:* 457–8.

Hudspeth, A. J. (1982). Extracellular current flow and the site of transduction by vertebrate hair cells. *J. Neurophysiol. 2:* 1–10.

Hudspeth, A. J., and Corey, D. P. (1977). Sensitivity, polarity, and conductance change in the response of vertebrate hair cells to controlled mechanical stimuli. *Proc. Natn. Acad. Sci. USA 76:* 1506–9.

Janse, C. (1982). Sensory systems involved in gravity orientation in the pulmonate snail *Lymnaea stagnalis. J. Comp. Physiol. 145:* 311–19.

Janse, C., and Sandeman, D. C. (1979a). The role of the fluid-filled balance organs in the induction of phase and gain in the compensatory eye reflex of the crab *Scylla serrata* during antennule rotation. *J. Comp. Physiol. 130:* 95–100.

Janse, C., and Sandeman, D. C. (1979b). The significance of canal-receptor properties for the induction of phase and gain in the fluid-filled balance organs of the crab *Scylla serrata. J. Comp. Physiol. 130:* 101–11.

Keidel, W. D. (1956). Vibrationsreception. Der Erschütterungssinn des Menschen. *Erlanger Forschr.* Reihe B, vol 2.

Keidel, W. D. (1968). Electrophysiology of vibratory perception. In *Contributions to Sensory Physiology*, vol. 3, ed. W. D. Neff, pp. 1–79. New York: Academic Press.

Koyama, H., Lewis, E. R., Baird, R. A., and Leverenz, E. L. (1982). Acute seismic sensitivity in the bullfrog ear. *Brain Res. 250:* 168–72.

Lewis, E. R., and Baird, R. A. (1981). Vibration sensitivity in the bullfrog inner ear. *J. Acoust. Soc. Am. 68:* S65–S66.

Lewis, E. R., Baird, R. A., Leverenz, E. L., and Koyama, H. (1982). Inner ear: dye injection reveals peripheral origins of specific sensitivities. *Science 215:* 1641–3.

Lewis, E. R., and Nairins, P. M. (1981). Seismic sensitivity in VIIIth nerve afferent fibers of the white-lipped frog. *Soc. Neurosci. Abstr. 7:* 148.

Loewenstein, W. R., and Mendelson, M. (1965). Components of receptor adaptation in a pacinian corpuscle. *J. Physiol., Lond. 177:* 377–97.

Lombard, R. E., and Straughan, I. R. (1974). Functional aspects of anuran middle ear structures. *J. Exp. Biol. 61:* 71–93.

Lowenstein, O., and Roberts, T. D. M. (1951). The localization and analysis of the responses to vibration from the isolated elasmobranch labyrinth. A contribution to the problem of the evolution of hearing in vertebrates. *J. Physiol. Lond. 114:* 471–89.

Lowenstein, O., and Saunders, R. D. (1975). Otolith-controlled responses from the first-order neurons of the labyrinth of the bullfrog (*Rana catesbeiana*) to changes in linear acceleration. *Proc. Roy. Soc. Lond. B 191:* 475–505.

Lowenstein, O., and Wersäll, J. (1959). A functional interpretation of the electron microscopic structure of the sensory hairs in the cristae of the elasmobranch *Raja clavata* in terms of directional sensitivity. *Nature 184:* 1807.

Maturana, H. R., and Sperling, S. (1963). Unidirectional response to angular acceleration recorded from the middle cristal nerve in the statocyst of *Octopus vulgaris. Nature 197:* 815–16.

McClary, A. (1966). Statocyst function in *Pomacea paludosa. Malacologia 3:* 419–31.

McLaren, J. W., and Hillman, D. E. (1979). Displacement of the semicircular canal cupula during sinusoidal rotation. *Neuroscience 4:* 2001–8.

Mill, P. J., ed. (1976). *Structure and Function of Proprioceptors in the Invertebrates.* London: Chapman & Hall.

Narins, P. M., and Lewis, E. R. (in preparation). Tuning properties of the exquisitely sensitive seismic afferent axons of the inner ear of *Leptodactylus albilabris.*

Olivio, R. F. (1970). Mechanoreceptor function in the razor clam. Sensory aspect of the foot withdrawal reflex. *Comp. Biochem. Physiol. 35:* 761–86.

Pringle, J. W. S. (1948). The gyroscopic mechanism of the halteres of Diptera. *Phil. Trans. Roy. Soc. Lond.,* Series B, *233:* 347–84.

Provins, K. A. (1958). The effect of peripheral nerve block on the application and execution of finger movements. *J. Physiol., Lond. 143:* 55–67.

Retzius, G. (1881). *Das Gehororgan des Wirbelthiere,* vol. 1. Stockholm: Samson & Wallin.

Roberts, T. D. M., and Murray-Smith, D. J. (1970). Method for the analysis of the neural mechanisms for postural adjustment. In *Principles and Practice of Bionics,* ed. H. E. von Gierke, W. E. Keidel and H. L. Oestreicher, pp. 371–87. Slough, England: Technical Services.

Sandeman, D. C. (1976). Spatial equilibrium in the arthropods. In *Structure and Function of Proprioceptors in the Invertebrates,* ed. P. J. Mill, pp. 485–527. London: Chapman & Hall.

Sandeman, D. C., and Okajima, A. (1972). Statocyst-induced eye movements in the crab *Scylla serrata.* I. The sensory input from the statocyst. *J. Exp. Biol. 57:* 187–204.

Schneider, W. (1950). Über den Erschütterungssinn von Käfern und Fliegen. *Z. vergl. Physiol. 32:* 287–302.

Schöne, H., ed. (1975a). *Mechanisms of Spatial Perception and Orientation as Related to Gravity (Fortschr. Zool.* vol. *23).* Stuttgart: Gustav Fischer Verlag.

Schöne, H. (1975b). On the transformation of the gravity input into reactions by statolith organs of the 'fan' type. *Fortschr. Zool. 23:* 120–7.

Schwartzkopff, J. (1974). Mechanoreception. In *The Physiology of Insecta,* vol. *2,* ed. M. Rockstein, pp. 273–352. New York: Academic Press.

Schwartzkopff, J. (1977). Comparative physiology of mechanoreception: origin and development of the field of research. *J. Comp. Physiol. 120:* 11–31.

Smith, J. J. B. (1968). Hearing in terrestrial urodeles: a vibration sensitive mechanism in the ear. *J. Exp. Biol. 48:* 191–205.

Stein, A. (1975). Attainment of positional information in the crayfish statocyst. *Fortschr. Zool. 23:* 109–19.

Takahata, M., and Hisada, M. (1979). Functional polarization of statocyst receptors in the crayfish *Procambarus clarkii* Girard. *J. Comp. Physiol. 130:* 201–7.

Talbot, S. A., and Gessner, U. (1973). *Systems Physiology.* New York: Wiley.

Talbot, W. H., Darian-Smith, I., Kornhuber, H. H., and Mountcastle, V. B. (1968). The sense of flutter-vibration: comparison of the human capacity with response patterns of mechanoreceptive afferents from the monkey hand. *J. Neurophysiol. 31:* 301–34.

Tautz, J. (1977). Reception of medium vibration by thoracic hairs of caterpillars of *Barathra brassicae* L. (Lepidoptera, Noctuidae). *J. Comp. Physiol. 118:* 13–31.

Thaler, G. J., and Brown, R. G. (1953). *Servomechanism Analysis.* New York: McGraw-Hill.

Tracy, D. (1975). Head movement mediated by halteres in the fly, *Musca domestica* during inertially guided flight. *Experientia 31:* 44–5.

Verillo, R. T. (1966). Specificity of a cutaneous receptor. *Perception and Psychophysics 1:* 149–53.

Vollrath, F. (1979). Vibrations: their signal function for spider kleptoparasite. *Science 205:* 1149–51.

Walcott, C., and van der Kloot, W. G. (1959). The physiology of the spider vibration receptor. *J. Exp. Zool. 141:* 191–244.

Wersäll, J., Flock, Å., and Lundquist, P.-G. (1965). Structural basis for directional sensitivity in cochlear and vestibular sensory receptors. *Cold Spring Harb. Symp. Quant. Biol. 30:* 115–32.

Weiderhold, M. L. (1977). Rectification in *Aplysia* statocyst receptor cells. *J. Physiol., Lond. 266:* 139–56.

Wilson, V. J., and Melvill Jones, G. (1979). *Mammalian Vestibular Physiology.* New York: Plenum.

Young, J. Z. (1959). The statocysts of *Octopus vulgaris. Proc. Roy. Soc. Lond. B152:* 3–27.

5.3

Topographic and non-topographic mapping of spatial sensory information. Predictions from Boring's formulation

P. R. BURGESS, ROBERT P. TUCKETT and
KENNETH W. HORCH

Information about stimuli that affect different parts of a sensory receptor sheet simultaneously must be signaled by different groups of neurons because the parameters of a stimulus that affect one part of the receptor sheet cannot be predicted from the parameters of a stimulus that affect some other part. For example, the depth of a skin indentation at one point on the body surface has no fixed relationship to the depth of an indentation at some other point, and so each must be signaled by separate neurons. Because of the presence of separate neuron groups for different parts of the receptor sheet, a change in the position of a stimulus on the receptor sheet is associated with a shift in the locus of neural activity in the central nervous system and this in turn is associated with an appropriate change in the perceived location of the stimulus on the body surface. Although a change in the depth of a skin indentation at only one site is associated with a change in the perceived location of a body part (the skin surface with respect to deeper tissues), the depth has only one value at any moment in time and so it is not required that perceived changes in skin indentation depth be associated with shifts in the locus of neural activity in the brain. Evidence is presented that a frequency code rather than a place code is used at the receptor level for signaling skin indentation depth. However, there are serious 'imperfections' in the frequency code because of the rate sensitivity and adaptation of the receptors. Tests on human subjects have shown them to have reliable depth information. This might be achieved by putting the receptor signals through an integrator (in the mathematical sense) within the central nervous system. If frequency codes are widely used by different animals for accurate position signaling, some such solution

611

must be widespread since rate sensitivity and adaptation are properties of mechanoreceptors in most species.

Signaling skin indentation depth

Proceeding from the conviction that not only lateral inhibition (Ratliff, 1965) but other mechanisms of information processing will prove to be common to animals that are distantly related phylogenetically, we will attempt to put this discussion of mammalian cutaneous mechanoreceptors into a general context. We will use a formulation made by Edwin Boring in 1935 as a point of departure for considering how cutaneous mechanoreceptors signal the depth of a skin indentation. Skin indentation depth is a spatial sensory experience; a change in indentation depth is felt as a change in the position of the skin surface with respect to the deeper tissues of the body. Making the most literal interpretation, we might expect a perceived change in skin depth to be associated with a shift in the locus of neural activity in the brain, particularly since other spatial sensory functions are known to be place coded within the central nervous system. Boring's formulation provides an interesting perspective on this question. As will become evident, it predicts that although a change in the position of a stimulator on the surface of the body is signaled with a place code, a frequency rather than a place code is used to signal the depth of a skin indentation as well as the position of other body parts. Our studies of receptors that signal skin indentation depth and joint angle support the idea that frequency codes are used to signal the position of body parts but at the same time point to certain difficulties with frequency codes.

Boring's formulation

In 1935 Edwin Boring published a paper in which he made certain explicit predictions for how sensory systems are organized. Figure 1 is taken from his paper and shows the essential features of his

Figure 1. This is Figure 2 from Boring's (1935) paper on sensory attributes and is an analogue for how sensory systems are organized. See text for further discussion. (Reproduced from *Philosophy of Science*, vol. 2, © 1935. The Williams and Wilkins Co., Baltimore.)

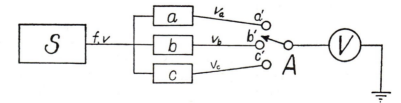

idea. Three different groups of neurons (a, b and c) are shown each extracting different information about the stimulus (S). V represents conscious sensory experience. The subject can deduce that the neuron groups are different because the information made available by any one neuron group cannot be predicted from the information provided by the other groups. Also, the subject must change the direction of his attention (A) to focus on the different types of information provided by each group of neurons. In the subsequent discussion we will attempt to show that Boring's formulation is a useful theoretical tool for understanding how the nervous system measures the position of different body parts. We will focus on the signaling of skin indentation depth (the position of the skin surface relative to the deeper tissues of the body) with some examples also taken from limb position sense (the relative position of the skeletal body parts). However, in order to make the arguments clear it is useful first to consider the signaling of stimuli that contact different parts of the cutaneous receptor sheet.

When are changes in the perceived location of an object associated with changes in the locus of neural activity in the central nervous system?

It is obvious that different groups of neurons are required to signal the depth (or any other parameter) of two (or more) stimuli that contact different areas of the skin simultaneously. This is because the depth of one indentation bears no necessary relationship to the depth of the other and hence it is easy to cause the depths of the two indentations to increase simultaneously or to diverge by independently varying the amplitude of the two stimuli. In addition, to obtain precise information about the depth of either stimulus, attention must be directed toward that stimulus, and such changes in the direction of attention provide another way to cause divergence in the perceived information from two stimulus sites. For similar reasons, separate neuron groups would be required for signaling the speed, force, direction, duration, size, etc., of multiple stimuli that contact different portions of the receptor sheet. This conclusion seems to be completely general and would apply to any device, biological or mechanical, with transducers distributed over its surface which could be programmed to report on stimuli that influence different portions of that surface.

At the level of perception in man and presumably at an equivalent level in other animals, a shift in the location of a single stimulator on the receptor sheet is associated with a change in the perceived location of the stimulus, as is appropriate since the position of the stimulus has in fact changed. Because of the requirement for separate neuron groups, these changes in perceived location are associated with changes in the locus of neural activity in the central nervous system. Place coding is the term commonly used to describe relationships of this sort.

Place coding may be defined as a code in which essential information is signaled by those members of a spatially distributed neuron population which are active. If, for example, a change in the position of a stimulus activated receptors that were differently located in the skin, place coding at the receptor level would be present. If, on the other hand, a previously stationary stimulus began to vibrate and so added activity from rapidly adapting receptors to that from the population of slowly adapting receptors already discharging, where both receptor types were in the same area of skin, this would not be an instance of place coding.

Boring's formulation predicts that shifts in the locus of neural activity on the peripheral receptor sheet will be associated with shifts in the locus of neural activity in the central nervous system. This was verified experimentally many years ago (Adrian, 1941; Woolsey, Marshall and Bard, 1942). In general, the peripheral shifts are in register with the central shifts so that one may say that the skin surface is topographically mapped into the central nervous system (see Appendix).

> *Are there shifts in the locus of neural activity in the central nervous system when the perceived position of a body part changes?*

Are shifts in the locus of central neural activity involved in signaling the depth of a localized skin indentation or the angle of a single joint? Our initial reaction was yes (Burgess, Wei, Clark and Simon, 1982) because changes in skin indentation depth or joint angle are associated with actual and perceived changes in the relative position of a body part. But, in fact, changes in the location of neural activity are not required in these cases. The depth of a particular patch of skin or the angle of an individual joint can have only one value at any moment in time and so in principle can be specified by one group of neurons occupying a single 'position' in neural space. The fact that a particular body part can occupy only one position at a given moment in time means that no change in direction of attention is required to appreciate the different depths of a single skin indentation or the various angles that a certain joint can occupy. This too is consistent with the idea that different circuits are not necessary for these sensory functions since changes in direction of attention are considered to reflect the switching of some 'high level' neural process from one group of central neurons to another. If only one group of neurons is used, then presumably the relative position of a body part is signaled by the level of activity in that neuron population, i.e., a frequency or interimpulse interval code is used.

Signaling of skin-indentation depth by cutaneous mechanoreceptors

Do cutaneous mechanoreceptors use a place code or a frequency code for signaling skin-indentation depth? This question can be approached by recording from individual mechanoreceptive afferents and examining their discharge as a function of skin-indentation depth. Figure 2 shows that receptors in the monkey's hand are recruited relatively early as a stimulator progressively indents the receptive field focus, especially when the rate of indentation is rapid. Since human subjects can judge indentation depth quite well at various depths and at indentation rates throughout the range from 0.2 to 16 mm s$^-$ (Burgess, Mei, Tuckett, Horch, Ballinger and Poulos, 1983), these data suggest that depth is not signaled by the recruitment order of receptors beneath the stimulator (a 'subsurface' place code). The principal alternative is that skin-indentation depth is signaled by a frequency or interimpulse-interval code.

Figure 3 shows the frequency of discharge as a function of indentation depth for a population of slowly-adapting receptors from the monkey's hand when the skin was indented at rates from 0.2 to 16 mm s^{-1}. It is the average discharge of the slowly-adapting receptors that is actually shown, these being the least rate-sensitive receptors in the skin of the hand. At each rate of indentation the discharge increases progressively with indentation depth so that a frequency signal for depth is present; but as the rate of indentation increases, the actual frequency at any given depth increases markedly. On the other hand, depth judgments by human subjects are relatively little affected by changes in skin indentation rate over this same range (Burgess et al., 1983). Such rate compensation presumably increases the practical utility of skin-depth information. Rate compensation also implies that the rate-sensitive signal from the receptors is somehow 'corrected' within the central nervous system.

One way that such a correction could be made is for the velocity-sensitive receptor discharge to be integrated (in the mathematical sense) by an appropriately designed neural circuit. The defining characteristic of a neural integrator is that excitation from one impulse persists so that it can add to the excitation produced by succeeding impulses, even though the integrator neuron(s) may have generated an impulse in the meantime. The rate of decay of the excitation produced by a particular impulse (the integrator leak) would have to be properly matched to the velocity-independent components of the receptors' output for the circuit to provide reliable depth information. Such an integration process could also help to compensate for the decline (adaptation) in the discharge of slowly adapting mechanoreceptors that occurs when the skin is steadily displaced; human subjects report little decrease in the perceived depth

Figure 2. Receptor recruitment profiles are shown for skin indentation over the center of the receptive field at 0.2, 0.4, 1.6, 4 and 16 mm s^{-1}. The total number of receptors recruited during an indentation increased as the indentation speed increased because more rapidly-adapting receptors were recruited; the numbers range from 118 at 0.2 mm s^{-1} to 176 at 16 mm s^{-1}. The recruitment threshold for a given receptor was calculated as the bin (130 μm indentation increment) in which its discharge frequency exceeded 5% of the maximal frequency occurring during the slowest indentation ramp (in the range of 0.2 to 16 mm s^{-1}) to which the receptor responded. The number of receptors whose threshold had been exceeded by a given indentation increment has been indicated with a point placed at the center of the bin for that increment. Most of the receptors were recruited during the first half of the 0.2-mm s^{-1} indentation and this tendency became more pronounced at higher velocities. (This is Figure 6 from Burgess et al., © 1983 Society for Neuroscience.)

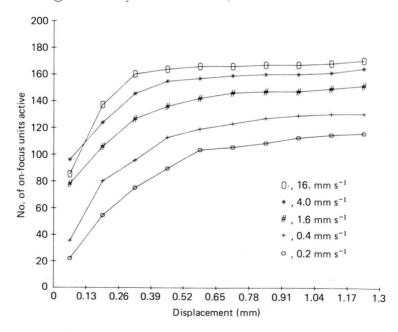

of a fingertip indentation for several seconds after the stimulus becomes steady (Mei, Tuckett, Poulos, Horch, Wei and Burgess, unpublished observations).

Conclusion

Evidence has been presented that skin-indentation depth is not signaled in the peripheral nervous system by a place mechanism but rather by a frequency or interimpulse-interval code. Thus as the depth of a skin indentation increases there is no evidence for a progressive shift in the locus of neural activity in the peripheral nervous system that can be utilized for full range depth coding. This is in accordance with Boring's formulation which predicts that a single circuit is sufficient for

Figure 3. Receptor-discharge frequency (ordinate) is shown as a function of skin-indentation depth (abscissa) when the skin of the receptive field focus was indented with triangular stimuli having velocities of 0.2, 0.4, 1.6, 4 and 16 mm s^{-1}. The average response for 78 slowly adapting receptors is presented during both the indentation and retraction phases of the stimuli. To produce the average slowly-adapting receptor response the numbers of impulses occurring in a particular bin (130-μm indentation increment) for each receptor were added together and divided by the total number of receptors in the population and the bin duration. Points are plotted at the bin center. The discharge frequency at any particular depth increases progressively as the rate of indentation increases. (This is Figure 8, from Burgess et al., © 1983 Society for Neuroscience.)

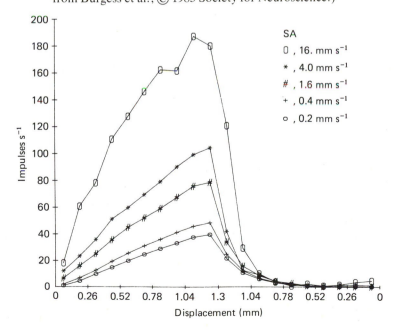

SA

0 , 16. mm s^{-1}
* , 4.0 mm s^{-1}
\# , 1.6 mm s^{-1}
+ , 0.4 mm s^{-1}
o , 0.2 mm s^{-1}

signaling the amount that any particular patch of skin has been indented; i.e., there need be no shift in the locus of neural activity in either the peripheral or central nervous system as indentation depth changes. However, signaling of skin depth has not been studied in the central nervous system and so it remains a possibility that the frequency signal in the periphery is converted into a place code within the central nervous system. There is evidence that joint angle in mammals is signaled over much of the range by a frequency code (Burgess et al., 1982), although there is a gross dichotomous place coding in the sense that receptors in agonist and antagonist muscles roughly divide up the range between them. Studies of mammalian sensory cortex have not revealed any evidence that the peripheral frequency coding of joint angle is converted into a place code within the central nervous system (Mountcastle and Powell, 1959; Gardner and Constanzo, 1981).

To what extent can these findings from mammals be generalized to other animals? Any animal with a compliant exterior might need to know the extent to which its body surface has been indented. Knowledge of the relative position of appendages or curvature of the body axis would appear to be essential for coordinated motor function in any animal. Knowledge of orientation with respect to the earth's surface is also likely to be important to many animals and Boring's formulation once again predicts that this information need not be topographically represented. If further investigation indicates that frequency coding is commonly used by different animals to signal accurately displacement of the body surface, joint angle and orientation to gravity, then the widespread existence of mechanoreceptor-rate sensitivity and adaptation (Thorson and Biederman-Thorson, 1974) suggests that we should be on the look out for central mechanisms that extract reliable position information from 'imperfect' receptor signals.

APPENDIX

Organization of sensory systems
Formal design requirements
(1) If spatially distinct portions of a sensory receptor sheet are used simultaneously to signal information that is 'different', each part of the receptor sheet that can be so utilized must be connected to a separate group of neurons, at least by the time the signals reach that part of the central nervous system where sensory information becomes available for symbolic or motor functions.

Different information is defined as sufficiently uncorrelated so that knowledge of how a stimulus affects one part of the receptor sheet does not allow a prediction concerning how some other part is affected. A conservative test for lack of correlation between stimulus parameters is to determine whether there are possible stimulus sequences in which the two stimulus parameters assumed or known to be signaled are positively correlated and other possible sequences in which the parameters are negatively correlated. For example, a stimulus sequence can be given in which the depths of two skin indentations at different sites on the body surface increase together and other stimulus sequences can be given in which the depth at one site increases while the depth at the other site decreases, etc. Nor must the stimulus parameters be of the same sort; an animal might be making depth discriminations at one site on the skin surface and thermal discriminations at another site. Again, since information about depth at one site cannot be used to predict information about temperature at another, separate groups of neurons are required for simultaneous processing of this information.

Separate groups of neurons have at least one neuron that is unshared. Thus neuron population A would differ from neuron population B if they differed by only one neuron. At the other extreme, groups A and B might have no neurons in common and be completely distinct. The formal requirement is only that the two populations should not be the same. In practice, one would expect that the neuron groups would be sufficiently distinct that the burden of signaling non-correlated information would not fall on a small fraction of the neurons involved.

> (2) If different information is signaled simultaneously from spatially distinct sources, each source must be represented by a separate group of neurons even if they do not engage different portions of a sensory receptor sheet.

In this case, the different groups of sensory neurons that signal non-correlated information for motor or symbolic functions may share common afferent channels in the more peripheral portions of the pathway. This may be the situation in the mapping of auditory space.

> (3) If different kinds of information are signaled simultaneously from the same location on a sensory receptor sheet, separate groups of neurons are required for each of these different kinds of information, at least at the level where the information is available for symbolic or motor functions.

This rule is meant to cover situations where different information can be signaled from the same general area either because there are different receptor types present there or because activity from the same receptors is treated differently within the central nervous system. An example of the former would be the simultaneous signaling of skin indentation depth and stimulator temperature from the same area of skin via specific mechanoreceptors and thermoreceptors which, although different receptor entities, may be one above the other in the skin. An example of a common carrier mechanism with different central decoders might be the signaling of indentation speed and indentation depth by the same mechanoreceptors, the latter signal being obtained from the time integral of the former.

Hypotheses

(1) The different groups of central neurons that represent different parts of a peripheral receptor sheet are in register with the peripheral sheet (neighbor relationships are preserved).

When this hypothesis is true it can be said that the peripheral receptor sheet is topographically mapped into the central nervous system. If the receptor sheet consists of a mosaic of different receptor types, in-register topography would be completely preserved if the different types of receptors had the same relative positions both on the receptor sheet and within the central nervous system; i.e., the central map would also be a mosaic of different receptor types. It is also possible for the different receptor types to be mapped into different parts of the central nervous system (thermoreceptors to one part, mechanoreceptors to another, etc.). According to hypothesis (1), the relative positions of the receptors in each of these separate representations would be maintained. Topographic mapping has the advantage that interactions, like lateral inhibition, between neighboring parts of a receptive field can be conveniently carried out and it is a regular feature of sensory organization.

(2) Frequency codes are used to signal the position of body parts. There is at least one population of neurons for each axis of movement that can be signaled independently.

This hypothesis, as is discussed in the present paper, must be considered only tentative.

This analysis was supported by grants from the National Science Foundation and the National Institutes of Health. We wish to thank Nelson Kiang, Max Mozell, Mark Konishi and Claudine Masson for helpful discussions during the conference and also Vicki Skelton for her help.

References

Adrian, E. D. (1941). Afferent discharges to the cerebral cortex from peripheral sense organs. *J. Physiol., Lond. 100:* 159–91.

Boring, E. G. (1935). The relation of the attributes of sensation to the dimensions of the stimulus. *Philos. Sci. 2:* 236–45.

Burgess, P. R., Mei, J., Tuckett, R. P., Horch, K. W., Ballinger, C. M., and Poulos, D. A. (1983). The neural signal for skin indentation depth. 1. Changing indentations. *J. Neurosci. 3:* 1572–85.

Burgess, P. R., Wei, J. Y., Clark, F. J., and Simon, J. (1982). Signaling of kinesthetic information by peripheral sensory receptors. *A. Rev. Neurosci. 5:* 171–87.

Gardner, E. P., and Constanzo, R. M. (1981). Properties of kinesthetic neurons in somatosensory cortex of awake monkeys. *Brain Res. 214:* 301–19.

Mountcastle, V. B., and Powell, T. P. S. (1959). Central nervous mechanisms subserving position sense and kinesthesis. *Bull. Johns Hopkins Hosp. 105:* 173–200.

Ratliff, F. (1965). *Mach Bands: Quantitative Studies on Neural Networks in the Retina.* San Francisco: Holden-Day.

Thorson, J., and Biederman-Thorson, M. (1974). Distributed relaxation processes in sensory adaptation. *Science 183:* 161–72.

Woolsey, C. N., Marshall, W. H., and Bard, P. (1942). Representation of cutaneous tactile sensibility in the cerebral cortex of the monkey as indicated by evoked potentials. *Bull. Johns Hopkins Hosp. 70:* 399–441.

5.4

Role of sensory information in the control of locomotion in fishes

B. L. ROBERTS

As a man walks along a mountain path he has continually to modify his stance and gait if he is to progress satisfactorily and yet retain his balance. This he does, subconsciously, by assessing the nature of the terrain over which he is walking, and the loading on his limbs, with sense organs located in skin, joints and muscles. In many cases these sense organs are complex structures that elicit powerful adaptive reflexes and play a clearly recognized role in the corrective coordination of locomotion. But do these sense organs contribute more than this to locomotion?

The problem of gravity compensation is faced by all terrestrial vertebrates as they move about and all have specific receptors and postural reflexes for this purpose. Aquatic animals like fishes, however, are supported by a dense medium and are relieved of this problem. Studies on the locomotion of these animals, therefore, could indicate other possible sensory contributions to locomotory control.

Although the overall equilibrium and pathway of a swimming fish are established by the brain, the basic form and rhythm of the body's undulatory motion is determined by the spinal cord. This is emphasized most clearly in the case of dogfish where it has been known for a long time that spinal preparations can perform continuous locomotory movements that are essentially of normal form. The present paper is based principally on experiments with this fish, but it is hoped that the ideas developed here may prove of more general utility.

Proprioceptors of fishes

Although all sensory systems in a fish must contribute to the regulation of locomotion it is evident that in a swimming spinal dogfish the only relevant receptors are proprioceptors in the body and fins. It was generally assumed that these are similar to the muscle spindles and tendon organs of mammals but subsequent histological study has failed to sustain this view. In all cases the stretch receptors identified so far are less developed than those found in other vertebrates.

Two forms of morphologically specialized terminals – the corpuscles of Wunderer and the endings of Poloumordwinoff – have been observed in the body of elasmobranch fishes. The intermuscular endings of the pectoral fins of skates and rays (Poloumordwinoff endings) consist of many beaded thin nerve fibres, derived from a single myelinated axon, that lie amongst fin muscle fibres. The endings are surrounded by Schwann cells that connect only loosely to adjacent muscle fibres (Bone and Chubb, 1975). These fibres are mostly of small diameter, receive multiple nerve endings, and are probably slow-contracting 'tonic' muscle fibres. A study of these endings by Ridge (1977) showed them to be slowly-adapting length and velocity receptors with qualitatively similar responses to the muscle spindles of frogs and reptiles. Undulatory movement of the pectoral fins is the principal form of locomotion in skates and rays and although no recordings have been taken from these endings while the pectoral fins are actually moving it seems likely that they could give specific information about length and tension changes during locomotion.

The corpuscles of Wunderer, found in the body of sharks, are located superficially within the dermis and deeper, on myotomal septa adjoining the vertebral column. They are encapsulated endings that consist of a whorl of fine unmyelinated fibres that terminate a large axon (Bone and Chubb, 1976); their physiological properties indicate that they are mechanoreceptors (Roberts, 1969c). Recordings taken from sensory nerves supplying the body wall of dogfish, bent in a way that simulates body locomotory movements, have shown that these receptors could provide information about body movement (Roberts, 1969b).

In contrast to the fairly complete picture in elasmobranch fishes, our knowledge of proprioceptors in bony fishes is very limited and there is no convincing description of a sensory supply to the body myotomes although stretch receptors have been observed in the extraocular muscles (Montgomery and Macdonald, 1980). However, recent studies have revealed the presence of specialized endings that are associated with mobile structures such as head barbels and modified fin rays (Ono, 1977, 1979, 1982) and free-nerve endings have been described in connective tissue interconnecting the fin bones of carp (Pac and Maly, 1971).

Although the majority of sensory elements lie at the periphery, and send information into the nervous system via the dorsal roots, it has to be recognized that some may pass in the ventral roots (Grillner, Perret and Zangger, 1976) and that elements within the central nervous system may even respond directly to mechanical stimulation (Grillner, McClellan and Perret, 1981).

Sensory action during locomotion

The significance of sensory information during locomotion can be assessed from recordings of sensory activity in moving animals and from observations on the effects of changes in, or the removal of, sensory inflow.

Sensory activity

Sensory recordings made during movement in the cat have now been obtained by several groups (see Loeb, 1981) and have revealed a variety of complex rhythmical patterns, originating from several receptors. In the dogfish, recordings from sensory nerves using suction electrodes in swimming preparations have shown that rhythmical bursts of sensory activity, presumably from Wunderer corpuscles, and time-locked to the movement, are passing into the spinal cord (Roberts and Williamson, unpublished).

Removal of sensory activity

Dorsal root rhizotomy ('deafferentation') has been carried out in elasmobranchs (Gray and Sand, 1936; Lissmann, 1946; Grillner et al., 1976) and teleosts (Gray, 1936; von Holst, 1936) but the results have led to conflicting interpretations. The studies by Gray and Sand (1936) and those by Grillner and his co-workers (1976) have shown that deafferented portions of the spinal cord of dogfish can produce organized movements that differ only slightly from the normal pattern. Lissmann (1946) found this to be the case only if spinal segments in other body regions were receiving some proprioceptive input, whereas Grillner et al. (1976) observed that motor discharges were of essentially normal pattern even in totally deafferented preparations. They did report, however, a very marked decline in the amplitude of these movements after deafferentation.

Pieces of the nervous system, as slices or *in vitro* preparations, are inevitably totally removed from sensory inflow but such preparations seldom exhibit organized spontaneous activity. However, the isolated spinal cord of the lamprey, if bathed in solutions containing L-DOPA or

D-glutamate, will produce regular motor activity, coordinated between and across segments, that differs little from that seen in the intact animal (Poon, 1980; Cohen and Wallen, 1980).

The presence of a steady motor rhythm, intrinsic to the central nervous system and underlying locomotion, is also revealed when recordings are made from motor nerves in preparations where body movement has been prevented by muscular paralysis. In spinal dogfish, for example, recordings from motor nerve endings made before and during curare-induced paralysis show that rhythmic motor discharges are still produced when locomotory-locked proprioceptive activity has been eliminated (Figure 1). The output is rhythmic and sustained and shows a rostro-caudal progression along the body and a strict alternation between opposite sides. Moreover, the output pattern is not fixed, for appropriate changes in burst duration and intersegmental lag are seen to accompany changes in cycle period. Nevertheless there are some differences between the motor outputs of swimming and immobilized fish. The most obvious is that the motor output is not always present

Figure 1. (A) Diagram of a spinal dogfish mounted in a head-holder in a tank of circulating seawater. The body is supported by a rod connected to a mechanotransducer and a d.c. motor (for oscillation experiments). Nerve recordings are obtained with a suction electrode from the sensory or motor branches of a spinal nerve. (B) Sample recordings from a motor nerve (top trace) and mechanotransducer in a swimming preparation and during curare paralysis.

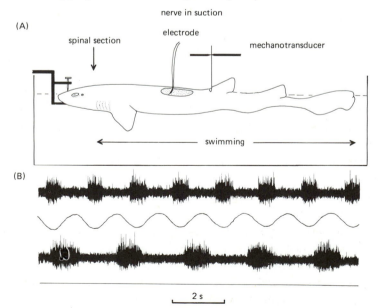

and, even when it is, the frequency in different specimens may vary considerably and is nearly always less than that obtained in recordings from free-moving fish. Numerous studies in other vertebrate and invertebrate preparations have revealed the presence of oscillating systems within the isolated central nervous system (Delcomyn, 1980). In invertebrates it is known that some of these rhythms result from the activity of 'pacemaker' neurons but it is more probable that for fishes the rhythm arises from the activity of neuronal networks. Whether these constitute a distinct 'spinal generator', distinguishable from other spinal neurons, however, remains to be seen.

The activity expressed in the *in vitro* spinal cord, or in curarized preparations, represents the free-running activity of a self-sustaining oscillator with its own natural period. Periodic inputs to the spinal cord, by way of dorsal roots or supraspinal pathways, can be expected to interact with this free-running oscillator.

Changes in sensory activity

Electrical stimulation of a sensory nerve, although a simple way of changing the pattern of sensory inflow during locomotion (e.g. Duysens, 1977), suffers from the disadvantage that many different fibres serving separate modalities may be excited simultaneously and so provide the nervous system with a quite inappropriate pattern of sensory activation. In the case of a swimming fish, moreover, stimulation of one sensory nerve, out of a total of 140 or so, will mimic the naturally occurring inflow in only the most basic manner. No studies of this type have been made in fish, but dorsal root stimulation in swimming tadpoles can result in either acceleration or deceleration of the motor rhythm (Stehouwer and Farel, 1981).

Changes in sensory activity can be brought about more satisfactorily in fishes if the size of body movements, and hence of the accompanying sensory feedback, is reduced. This has been done in spinal dogfish by injecting weak concentrations of curare intravenously so as to reduce muscular contractions rather than obtain muscular paralysis (Roberts and Williamson, unpublished). Undulatory movements continue, but with a reduced amplitude. The reduction in movement amplitude is accompanied by a parallel decline in the frequency of the motor output and, except when the amplitude is very small, the amplitude of lateral body movement and frequency of movement show a good linear correlation (Figure 2). Body amplitude, as assessed at one position, is of course only a very indirect measure of the actual sensory activity but this is, however, presumed to reflect the bending movements of the body.

The finding of a relationship between the size and frequency of movement emphasizes that the neural basis for locomotion in the spinal dogfish is not just an uncomplicated expression of a constant free-running oscillator, but reflects interactions between this oscillator and sensory inflow.

The interaction between the central and peripheral effects is further emphasized by the results of experiments in which forced oscillations are applied to the body of a spinal dogfish. When this is done to a free-swimming spinal preparation the frequency of the motor bursts seen in the electromyogram is modified by the applied oscillation, and oscillatory movements imposed on a non-swimming spinal preparation will actually initiate locomotion (Roberts, 1969c). Grillner and Wallen (1977) oscillated the tail of the dogfish *Squalus* and found that the motor

Figure 2. The relationship between the cycle period of the motor rhythm of a spinal dogfish and the amplitude of lateral body movement. A range of movement sizes was obtained by the intravenous injection of a low dosage of curare. $N = 100$; $R = -0.97$.

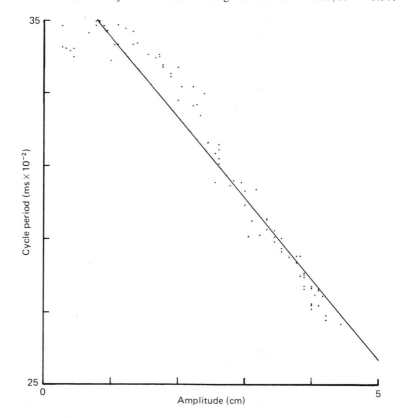

output in paralysed preparations could also be modified by the applied oscillation. The experiment illustrated in Figure 3 shows results of further experiments of this type (Roberts and Williamson, unpublished). Over a certain range of frequency of oscillation, usually extending from about one half to twice that of the free-running rhythm, the timing of the motor output recorded from a motor nerve follows exactly that of the applied oscillation. Outside this range the output is still synchronized to the input frequency but misses some input cycles or provides additional outputs. We believe that this loss of 1:1 synchronization results from interactions between the 'free-running' rhythm and the exogenous input. The input either occurs within the free-running rhythm at a time when motor activity is strongly suppressed or when there is sufficient time between inputs for 'free-running' motor bursts to be expressed.

The exogenous signals arising from body movement within the 'capture' range dominate endogenous pacemaking with respect not only to cycle initiation but also to burst duration. The effect on burst duration is seen most clearly in response to asymmetrical movements when the duration of the motor output can be less than predicted for a particular cycle period and determined by a change in the direction of movement.

Figure 3. The relationship between the cycle period of the lateral oscillation applied to a spinal dogfish paralysed with curare and the cycle period of the motor output recorded from a spinal nerve.

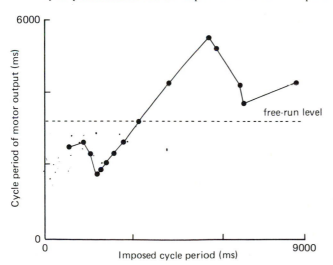

The contribution of sensory activity

It is evident that the activation of various sense organs during a sequence of locomotory movements can have several consequences for the final pattern of movement. Some of these effects are immediate and obvious while others exert a more subtle influence and have a longer time course.

Most direct actions can be described as 'reflex' and although this term is very imprecise it is universally understood to represent an element of behaviour where there is a fixed relationship between the stimulus and the response. The response is purposive in that the action is appropriately matched to the stimulus. For example, a mechanical stimulus applied to the teeth of a dogfish elicits a rapid jaw closure. The rapidity of this 'jaw-jerk' reflex, which is present in all vertebrates, requires a short-latency connection between the afferent fibres and the jaw-closing motoneurons (Roberts and Witkovsky, 1975). The 'startle response' of some teleost fishes, produced by a sudden visual or vibratory stimulus, is another example of a rapid reflex with a specialized neural circuit.

Other reflex responses may require more time as they involve longer circuits. A brief stimulus applied to the dorsal surface of the pectoral fin of the dogfish will elicit an elevating movement, but even the most rapid units do not respond until 30–40 ms after the stimulus has been presented (Paul and Roberts, 1979).

The longer the interval between the stimulus and the response, the more the stimulus should be seen as performing an initiating rather than a determining role. Thus, a brief pinch to the caudal fin of the spinal dogfish disrupts the steady activity of the lateral musculature and triggers an alternative motor pattern and activation of the extensive white musculature.

It is now clear that as well as these discrete effects sensory activity can have a variety of other influences on the central nervous system (Stein, Gordon, Oguztoreli and Lee, 1981). Overall, sensory activity appears to exert a tonic influence on spontaneous activity within the nervous system. The absence of rhythmic motor discharges from some immobilized dogfish, and the lengthening of the cycle periods of the motor rhythm seen in others, are findings that presumably reflect changes in the excitability of the neurons that produce the motor pattern resulting from sensory loss. In the intact fish, of course, this excitability is regulated not only by body proprioceptors but also by supraspinal influences. Stimulation at higher levels therefore can evoke locomotion (in the carp (Kashin, Feldman and Orlovsky, 1974); and sting ray (Leonard et al., 1979)).

A decline in the frequency of motor output, as observed after isolation of the nervous system from sensory inflow in *Scyliorhinus*, has been reported to follow isolation in walking (Pearson, 1972) and flying (Wilson and Gettrup, 1963) insects. The spinal-cord output of the dogfish *Squalus* however continues at around the normal frequency (Grillner et al., 1976) as does the motor output of the leech (Stent et al., 1978), sting ray (Droge and Leonard, 1979) and tadpole (Roberts, Kahn, Soffe and Clarke, 1981). The respiratory centre of the dogfish, when isolated from sensory inflow, discharges at frequencies higher than normal (Ballintijn and Roberts, unpublished).

Other responses seen in the dogfish motor system in relation to sensory activity indicate how the sensory inflow interacts with the spontaneous activity within the central nervous system. We have seen that the endogenous pacemaker can be overridden and the motor output reset to duplicate the exogenous sensory rhythm and this result indicates that the sensory input plays a modulating role in locomotory control. Similar modulating effects have been reported for some other motor systems. Thus, a change in the frequency of the treadmill belt will produce frequency modulation of walking in the high-decerebrate cat (Andersson, Forssberg, Grillner and Wallen, 1981), while Benchetrit (1980) has shown that the ventilation rate of a paralysed cat can be entrained to the frequency at which the lungs are artificially inflated.

The entrainment experiments in the dogfish also revealed a switching role for the sensory input, shortening or lengthening the duration of a motor burst. A similar switching action of sensory activity has been reported in other systems. During respiration in the mammal, for example, vagal stimulation presented during inspiration terminates that phase in a trigger-like fashion, and initiates expiration (Cohen and Feldman, 1977). Such a phase-switching action of sensory inflow has also been observed for vagal input in carp respiration (Ballintijn, Roberts and Luiten, 1983). In walking cats, flexion is prevented if the ankle extensor is still heavily loaded at the time when flexion should normally begin (Pearson and Duysens, 1976).

The free-running rhythm recorded from the dogfish spinal cord is surprisingly stable and shows no greater variation than would be expected if the sensory inflow were present (Williamson and Roberts, 1980). But this stability is not retained, in the absence of sensory activity, if the system is perturbed. Recordings taken from the nerve supplying the adductor mandibulae in dogfish paralysed with curare show that the motor rhythm underlying respiration has a steady free-running cycle period, somewhat faster than in the intact fish. A stimulus applied to the maxillary branch of the trigeminal nerve evokes a jaw-jerk reflex and, in this preparation, a marked increase in the rate of respiration, that continues for several cycles (Figure 4). However, if just one branchial branch of the vagus that supplies receptors in the gills is stimulated regularly, so as to entrain the respiratory rhythm then a stimulus presented to the maxillary nerve will elicit only the required jaw-jerk and does not modify respiration. The regular sensory input evidently plays a role in stabilizing the central oscillator (Ballintijn and Roberts, unpublished).

Central modification of sensory activity

We have discussed the way sensory input affects central neuronal networks but it is evident that the central networks can also modify the nature of the sensory input during locomotion. Good examples of this relationship are provided by the fusimotor supply to muscle spindles and the efferent innervation of the labyrinth and lateral-line organs. Some uncertainty remains about the role of the former during locomotion (see Matthews, 1981), but there is good evidence that lateral-line and labyrinthine efferent neurons become active in association with

Figure 4. Stabilization of motor output by rhythmic sensory input. A stimulus to maxillary branch of nerve V accelerates the rate of respiratory motor activity recorded from the mandibular branch of nerve V in a paralysed dogfish. This change is absent if the same stimulus is given while a branchial branch of the vagus is stimulated with brief stimulus trains every 950 ms. △, respiratory motor rhythm during rhythmic vagus stimulation; ●, respiratory motor rhythm when the vagus was unstimulated.

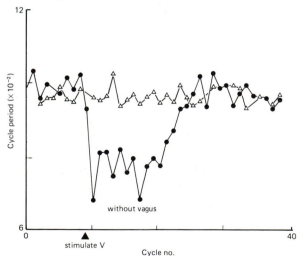

movements of the body (Roberts and Russell, 1972; Klinke and Galley, 1974) and that the lateral-line efferent neurons, located in the hind-brain, are activated in parallel with the circuits that initiate body movement (Russell, 1976).

As well as directly modifying sensory input at the periphery, central circuits can regulate the central action of sensory effects. This action may be continuous or vary according to the phase of various central programs. The 'state' of the spinal cord is clearly set by descending supraspinal influences as the dogfish swims steadily, with enhanced spinal activity, if descending inhibitory pathways are severed. Even in the intact fish there is evidence that the 'gain' of reflexes such as the pectoral fin reflex described previously is regulated by descending control, which in this case at least appears to be coordinated by cerebellar action (Paul and Roberts, 1979).

Other reflexes may vary cyclically in their expression. Thus a certain reflex response may be maximal during one phase of a locomotory cycle but be absent during the opposite phase when the same stimulus may then elicit responses from antagonistic muscles. Examples of such reflex reversal have been observed in walking cats, but it has also been reported in swimming dogfish (Wallen, 1980). It seems that these reversal effects are selected by both central and peripheral mechanisms (Rossignol, Julien and Gauthier, 1981).

Conclusion

It has become increasingly clear that the basic neural pattern required for locomotion is derived from within limited parts of the central nervous system. In some species central circuits are probably capable of developing most of the motor program, but in others influences from other parts of the nervous system and from sensory activity are normally essential.

This recent emphasis on the independence of the central nervous system in locomotion has tended to diminish the role played by proprioceptive information and to underestimate the integrity of the organism. In view of current ideas of corollary discharges and efferent supply of sense organs the distinction between 'central' and 'peripheral' events is becoming very blurred and, except for the initial element, it is difficult to determine just which component of the locomotory mechanism should be designated as 'sensory'.

The spinal cord neurons of fishes are able to generate bursts of motor discharges that provide the basis for undulatory motion. The role of proprioception seems to be to complement this action and to raise the excitability of the cord to appropriate levels, to stabilize the central circuits exposed to perturbations and to adapt the standardized output to changes in body form that result, for example, from body growth or the use of different muscle systems.

References

Andersson, O., Forssberg, H., Grillner, S., and Wallen, P. (1981). Peripheral feedback mechanisms acting on the central pattern generators for locomotion in fish and cat. *Can. J. Physiol. and Pharmac. 59:* 713–26.

Ballintijn, C. M., Roberts, B. L., and Luiten, P. G. M. (1983). Respiratory responses to stimulation of branchial vagus nerve ganglia of a teleost fish. *Respiration Physiol. 51:* 241–57.

Benchetrit, G. (1980). In Hugelin, A.: Does the respiratory rhythm originate from a reticular oscillator in the waking state? In *The Reticular Formation Revisited*, ed. J. A. Hobson and M. A. B. Brazier, pp. 261–74. New York: Raven Press.

Bone, Q., and Chubb, A. D. (1975). The structure of stretch receptor endings in the fin muscles of rays. *J. Mar. Biol. Ass. UK 55:* 939–43.

Bone, Q., and Chubb, A. D. (1976). On the structure of corpuscular endings in sharks. *J. Mar. Biol. Ass. UK 56:* 925–8.

Cohen, A. H., and Wallen, P. (1980). The neuronal correlate of locomotion in fish. *Expl Brain Res. 41:* 11–18.

Cohen, M. I., and Feldman, J. L. (1977). Models of respiratory phase switching. *Fedn Proc. 36:* 2367–74.

Delcomyn, F. (1980). Neural basis of rhythmic behaviour in animals. *Science 210:* 492–8.

Droge, M. H., and Leonard, R. B. (1979). Fictive locomotion in the stingray, *Dasyatis sabina*. *Soc. Neurosci. Abstr. 9:* 1229.

Duysens, J. (1977). Fluctuations in sensitivity to rhythm resetting effects during the cat's step cycle. *Brain Res. 133:* 190–5.

Gray, J. (1936). Studies in animal locomotion. IV. The neuromuscular mechanism of swimming in the eel. *J. Exp. Biol. 13:* 170–80.

Gray, J., and Sand, A. (1936). The locomotory rhythm of the dogfish (*Scyllium canicula*). *J. Exp. Biol. 13:* 200–9.

Grillner, S., McClellan, A., and Perret, C. (1981). Entrainment of the spinal pattern generators for swimming by mechano-sensitive elements in the lamprey spinal cord in vitro. *Brain Res. 217:* 380–6.

Grillner, S., Perret, C., and Zangger, P. (1976). Central generation of locomotion in the spinal dogfish. *Brain Res. 109:* 255–69.

Grillner, S., and Wallen, P. (1977). Is there a peripheral control of the central pattern generators for swimming in dogfish? *Brain Res. 127:* 291–5.

Kashin, S. M., Feldman, A. G., and Orlovsky, G. N. (1974). Locomotion of fish evoked by electrical stimulation of the brain. *Brain Res. 82:* 41–7.

Klinke, R., and Galley, N. (1974). Efferent innervation of vestibular and auditory receptors. *Physiol. Rev. 54:* 316–57.

Leonard, R. D., Rudomin, P., Droge, M. H., Grossman, A. E., and Willis, W. D. (1979). Locomotion in the decerebrate stingray. *Neurosci. Lett. 14:* 315–19.

Lissmann, H. W. (1946). The neurological basis of the locomotory rhythm in the spinal dogfish. II. The effect of deafferentation. *J. Exp. Biol. 23:* 162–76.

Loeb, G. E. (1981). Somatosensory unit input to the spinal cord during normal walking. *Can. J. Physiol. Pharmac. 59:* 627–35.

Matthews, P. B. C. (1981). Evolving views on the internal operation and functional role of the muscle spindle. *J. Physiol., Lond. 320:* 1–30.

Montgomery, J. C., and Macdonald, J. A. (1980). Stretch receptors in the eye muscles of a teleost fish. *Experientia 36:* 1176–7.

Ono, R. D. (1977). Histological evidence of stretch receptors in two marine teleost fishes. *Am. Zool. 17:* 652.

Ono, R. D. (1979). Sensory nerve endings of highly mobile structures in two marine teleost fishes. *Zoomorphologie 92:* 107–14.

Ono, R. D. (1982). Structure of tendon organs in fishes of the genus *Polymixia*. *Zoomorphology 99:* 131–44.

Pac, L., and Maly, J. (1971). Sensory nerve endings in the internal skeleton of the paired fins of some members of the carp family. *Folia Morphol. 19:* 411–15.

Paul, D. H., and Roberts, B. L. (1979). The significance of cerebellar function for a reflex movement of the dogfish. *J. Comp. Physiol. 134:* 69–74.

Pearson, K. G. (1972). Central programming and reflex control of walking in the cockroach. *J. Exp. Biol. 56:* 173–93.

Pearson, K. G., and Duysens, J. (1976). Function of segmental reflexes in the control of stepping in cockroaches and cats. In *Neural Control of Locomotion*, ed. R. Herman, S. Grillner, P. S. G. Stein and D. Stuart, pp. 519–38. New York: Plenum.

Poon, M. L. T. (1980). Induction of swimming in lamprey by L-DOPA and amino acids. *J. Comp. Physiol. 136:* 337–44.

Ridge, R. M. A. P. (1977). Physiological responses of stretch receptors in the pectoral fin of the ray, *Raja clavata. J. Mar. Biol. Ass. UK 57:* 535–41.

Roberts, A., Kahn, J. A., Soffe, S. R., and Clarke, J. D. W. (1981). Neural control of swimming in a vertebrate. *Science 213:* 1032–4.

Roberts, B. L. (1969a). The response of a proprioceptor to the undulatory movements of dogfish. *J. Exp. Biol. 51:* 775–85.

Roberts, B. L. (1969b). The co-ordination of the rhythmical fin movements of dogfish. *J. Mar. Biol. Ass. UK 49:* 357–425.

Roberts, B. L., and Russell, I. J. (1972). The activity of lateral-line efferent neurones in stationary and swimming dogfish. *J. Exp. Biol. 57:* 435–48.

Roberts, B. L., and Witkovsky, P. (1975). A functional analysis of the mesencephalic nucleus of the fifth nerve in the selachian brain. *Proc. Roy. Soc. Lond. B 190:* 473–95.

Rossignol, S., Julien, C., and Gauthier, L. (1981). Stimulus-response relationships during locomotion. *Can. J. Physiol. Pharmac. 59:* 667–74.

Russell, I. J. (1976). Central inhibition of lateral line input in the medulla of the goldfish by neurones which control active body movements. *J. Comp. Physiol. (A) 111:* 335–58.

Stein, R. B., Gordon, T., Oguztoreli, M. N., and Lee, R. G. (1981). Classifying sensory patterns and their effects on locomotion and tremor. *Can. J. Physiol. Pharmac. 59:* 645–55.

Stehouwer, D. J., and Farel, P. B. (1981). Sensory interactions with a central motor program in anuran larvae. *Brain Res. 218:* 131–40.

Stent, G. S., Kristan, W. B., Friesen, W. O., Ort, C. A., Poon, M., and Calabrese, R. L. (1978). Neuronal generation of the leech swimming movement. *Science 200:* 1348–57.

von Holst, E. (1936). Erregungsbildung und Erregungsleitung im Fischruckenmark. *Pflugers Archiv 235:* 345–59.

Wallen, P. (1980). On the mechanisms of a phase-dependent reflex occurring during locomotion in dogfish. *Expl Brain Res. 39:* 193–202.

Williamson, R. M., and Roberts, B. L. (1980). The timing of motoneuronal activity in the swimming spinal dogfish. *Proc. Roy. Soc. Lond. B211:* 119–33.

Wilson, D. M., and Gettrup, E. (1963). A stretch reflex controlling wing beat frequency in grasshoppers. *J. Exp. Biol. 40:* 171–85.

5.5

Effects of motor commands on sensory inflow, with examples from electric fish

C. C. BELL

Most talks at this conference have examined the effects of external sources of stimulation on sensory systems. But animals are not just passive receivers of environmental stimuli. They are active, and their movements, cries, or electric organ discharges can have strong effects on sensory receptors. von Holst and Mittelstaedt (1950) recognized the importance of this source of sensory input and termed it 'reafference' to distinguish it from afferent input caused by external sources. The latter was given the name 'exafference'.

von Holst and Mittelstaedt realized that an animal must always distinguish reafference from exafference or its behavior and knowledge will not fit the environment. These authors as well as Sperry (1950) were particularly concerned with voluntary movement and the sensory input it elicits. They asked how voluntary movement is even possible in the presence of stabilizing postural reflexes, since the reafference elicited by such movement must be very similar to the exafference evoked by destabilizing external stimuli. Why does the voluntary movement not elicit an opposing reflex? An earlier hypothesis held that there was a simple inhibition of the reflex or reafference by the voluntary motor command. However, both groups of authors were convinced by behavioral experiments that simple inhibition could not explain an animal's ability to turn voluntarily in the presence of stabilizing optomotor reflexes. Instead, they inferred that a negative image of the expected reafference, an image which can be excitatory, inhibitory or both, is elicited by the motor command and added to the actual reafference reducing it to zero. This command driven negative image was called an 'efference copy' by von Holst and Mittelstaedt and a 'corollary discharge' by Sperry.

The reafference resulting from a motor act may be undesirable for other reasons besides that of eliciting inappropriate reflexes. It may be confused with input from external sources, or it may disrupt the accurate sensing of such sources. A negative image of the expected reafference which eliminates such reafference from the sensory inflow allowing only the exafference to enter, would also be useful in such cases. This was of course the solution proposed first by Helmholtz (1867) and elaborated later by von Holst (1954) to explain why we are not disrupted by quick displacements of the visual world during saccadic eye movements.

'Efference copy' and 'corollary discharge' have been used in several different ways and there is now much confusion about the terms. McCloskey (1981) has recently reviewed the historical development of these concepts and suggests that 'efference copy' be used only where there is cancellation of the reafference by addition of a negative image of the expected input, with the exafference remaining after the cancellation. Thus, simple suppression of input would not qualify as an efference copy. He suggests, on the other hand, that 'corollary discharge' is a more general term to be used in referring to any effect of a motor command on sensation. He insists that the term be limited to effects on sensation. But current usage (e.g., Richmond and Wurtz, 1980; Zipser and Bennett, 1976) and the difficulty of establishing effects on sensation in animals would seem to require the inclusion of any physiological effect on a sensory-receiving area, whether such an effect has been shown to affect sensation or not. According to these modified definitions the generalized inhibition of lateral line activity which is associated with voluntary movements in fish and aquatic amphibians (Roberts and Russell, 1972; Russell, 1971) would qualify as a corollary discharge but not as an efference copy. Without efferent activity, lateral-line afferents would show a complex pattern of accelerations and decelerations during movement. This entire pattern is suppressed, not matched, by the efferent inhibition.

One problem with the efference copy mechanism is that the two major cases which it was meant to explain no longer seem to require such a mechanism. Thus, Mittelstaedt (1971) has recently stated that the behavioral results on insect optomotor reflexes obtained by him and von Holst can be explained without an efference copy and this has been confirmed by Reichardt and Poggio (1976). (Corollary discharges, however, do appear to be present, at least in related systems, e.g., Zaretsky, 1982.) Similarly, there is now much evidence against an efference copy cancellation mechanism as an explanation of the stability of the visual world during saccades (for discussion and references, see McCloskey, 1981). (Eye movement-related corollary discharges, however, are well established within the mammalian visual system, e.g., Richmond and Wurtz, 1980.)

A second problem with 'efference copy' is the name itself, a name which has caused much of the confusion regarding the concept. A negative image is not a copy. More importantly, the signal involved is not a negative image of the *efference* (the motor command), but of the expected *reafference*. In spite of these serious problems the term is used throughout the rest of this article because the concept remains important, and because there is at present no short and readily recognized alternative name.

von Holst and Mittelstaedt focused largely on the negative effects of reafference. But the sensory consequences of a motor act can also be highly informative and useful. Some examples may be given: (a) Motor acts are often controlled by the proprioceptive, tactile, or visual inputs they elicit. (b) An animal's movement through space induces parallax changes and optical flow patterns which provide information about the positions and forms of objects in the environment. (c) The moving human hand measures shapes, textures, and compliances. (d) In the specialized systems of echolocation and active electrolocation the motor acts, i.e., vocalizations or electrical discharges, elicit consequences which provide unique information about the environment. Corollary discharges which prepare the sensory-receiving areas for the expected reafference are probably involved in all these cases. However, the effects of such corollary discharges would certainly not be to nullify or reduce the reafference, but would involve instead 'evaluation', to use McKay's (1966) term. McKay has criticized the general applicability of an efference copy mechanism to problems of motor effects on sensory inputs. One basis of his criticism is the extraordinary, perhaps impossible, accuracy required of the efference copy to match reafferent input exactly, as for example in the cancellation of visual world movement during saccades. Another basis of his criticism is that, as described above, reafferent input is frequently informative, requiring a complex evaluative process rather than suppression.

As will be seen below, there is a different type of corollary discharge within each of the three subdivisions of the electrosensory system of mormyrid fish. These types correspond roughly to the major kinds of corollary discharge sketched above. In brief, there are: (a) a simple inhibition or suppression; (b) a negative image of expected reafference which can be excitatory or inhibitory, i.e., an efference copy; and (c) a facilitatory signal which may be part of an evaluative process similar to that described by McKay (1966).

Corollary discharges in the mormyrid electrosensory system

There are three types of electroreceptors in mormyrid fish; ampullary, knollenorgan and mormyromast. These receptors are morphologically and physiologically distinct. Each receptor type appears to have a separate role within the electrosensory system (see reviews by Bell, 1979; Bennett, 1971; Bullock, 1982; Heiligenberg, 1977; and Szabo and Fessard, 1974).

The *ampullary* type of receptor is seen in all electroreceptive fish and some amphibians (for the recent demonstration of ampullary receptors in amphibians, see Munz, Claas and Fritsch, 1982). The tonic discharge rate of these receptors depends on stimulus strength. Whether the rate is modulated up or down depends on stimulus polarity. The receptors respond well to the low-frequency (near d.c. to 20 Hz) electrical signals which are generated by aquatic animals and by non-biological sources. Ampullary receptors in mormyrids respond to the fish's own electric organ discharge (EOD) with a sequence of rate changes lasting about 80 ms. The amplitude of the response depends on water conductivity and probably on the proximity of large non-conducting surfaces. But in mormyrids at least the response is unaffected by smaller non-conducting objects near the receptor pore (Bell and Russell, 1978). Insensitivity of the ampullary EOD response to the presence or absence of objects suggests that these receptors are not important in mormyrids for the sensing of environmental conductances, i.e., that they are not important in active electrolocation. The main function of the ampullary receptors in mormyrids is probably to detect external sources of low-frequency electrical signals, a function which may be referred to as *low frequency passive electrolocation*.

A second type of electroreceptor, the *knollenorgans*, do not respond to low-frequency signals but only to high-frequency ones (300 Hz– 10 kHz). The most common environmental sources of such signals are the EODs of other electric fish. Knollenorgans have an extremely low threshold to an EOD or to an EOD-like pulse. The afferent fiber gives a single spike at a brief (1–3 ms) fixed latency to such a stimulus and once threshold is crossed the response is not much affected by intensity changes. Pulses at intensities many times that of threshold continue to yield a single spike with a latency which is only a fraction of a millisecond earlier than it was at threshold. Knollenorgan afferents respond to the fish's own EOD with the single fixed latency spike. The insensitivity to intensity changes means that the response will not vary with the small changes in EOD current caused by objects. Thus, like the ampullary receptors, the knollenorgan receptors probably do not have a role in active electrolocation (for further evidence, see below). Their exquisite sensitivity to other fishes' EODs, however, suggests a sensory role in a second important function of the electrosensory system, that of *communication*. Measured electrical thresholds of communication like behavioral responses, and the effects of lesions on central knollenorgan pathways, support this suggestion (see Szabo and Moller, 1983, this volume).

The third type of electroreceptors, *mormyromasts*, also respond only to pulses which contain high frequencies. Unlike knollenorgans, however, their response is exquisitely sensitive to intensity changes. Mormyromasts respond to the fish's own EOD with a brief burst of spikes lasting up to 20 ms. The response varies in both latency (2–9 ms) and spike number (1–10 spikes) when objects are placed near the receptor. Mormyromasts are therefore considered to be the receptors responsible for the third function of the system, *active electrolocation*.

Thus, the fish's own EOD generates three types of reafferent input. These inputs are different in form and significance. The responses of ampullary and knollenorgan receptors to the fish's own EOD convey little information and could, in fact, interfere with the sensing of the appropriate external signals. The reafferent mormyromast input, however, is critically important for it informs the fish about external conductances. Furthermore, it is only the mormyromast responses evoked by the fish's own EOD which are significant. Mormyromast responses caused by other sources such as the EODs of neighboring fish would be disruptive, just as unknown currents would be disruptive in measuring a resistance in an electrical circuit.

Electroreceptor afferents terminate in the electrosensory lobe of the medulla (formerly named the posterior lateral line lobe). Each receptor type terminates in a distinct region. In addition to peripheral input from receptors each region also receives a central input, a corollary discharge of the EOD motor command.

Experiments on the effects of the EOD motor command are done in the artificially-respired, curarized fish. Curare blocks not only ordinary neuromuscular junctions, but also the synapse between electro-motoneurons and electrocytes, silencing the electric organ. However, the synchronized discharge of the electromotoneurons which would normally elicit an EOD can still be recorded from the tail region. The synchronized volley is an indication of the EOD motor command and is referred to as the command signal. Different forms of electrical stimuli mimicking the EOD can be given after the command signal.

Using the above methods, Zipser and Bennett (1976) showed that the receiving cells in the knollenorgan region of the electrosensory lobe are strongly and completely inhibited by a corollary discharge associated with the EOD motor command. The inhibition is extremely brief, lasting only about three milliseconds. It occurs at exactly the time when the single spike of the knollenorgan response to the EOD would arrive at the cell in the uncurarized animal. Thus in the intact fish it completely blocks the further entry into the CNS of the EOD reafference. Such blocking is consistent with what was said above about the lack of information in the knollenorgan reafferent response and the lack of a role for knollenorgans in active electrolocation. Inhibition by the corollary discharge ensures that a system which is organized to sense small external signals will not be disrupted by a large reafferent volley arriving many times per second. The extreme brevity of the inhibition minimizes the time during which the system is insensitive to external signals. The corollary discharge in the knollenorgan region, unlike that in the ampullary region, does not appear to be plastic (see below). It remains the same, for example, in spite of hours in the absence of stimulation.

A corollary discharge could also be of use in the ampullary region where the reafferent input evoked by the EOD also appears to convey little information and could interfere with the sensing of external events. The simple inhibition seen in the knollenorgan area would not serve here, however. The ampullary response to the EOD can last 100 ms. Since the fish often discharges at rates above $10 s^{-1}$, inhibition for the duration of the response would reduce the system to minimal usefulness. Furthermore, the second-order cells are like the primary afferents and discharge tonically, the rate rising or falling according to stimulus polarity. The complete silencing of such cells would not signal a simple absence of input, but would signal (falsely) the presence of a strong stimulus of a particular polarity.

The problem of unwanted reafference is met in the ampullary zone by a corollary discharge which appears to convey a negative image or template of the expected input (Bell, 1982). The effect of the command is similar in duration to the reafferent response but always opposite in sign. For example, if the reafferent response is an acceleration-deceleration sequence, the effect of the command is a deceleration-acceleration sequence. When the two occur together the response of the secondary cells is nullified or reduced, thus reducing the disruptive effect of the fish's own EOD.

Most importantly, the effect of the command in the ampullary zone, unlike its effect in the knollenorgan region, is modifiable. As stated above, the effect of the command is opposite to the pattern of ampullary input which arrives during the 100 ms or so after the EOD command (and in the intact fish, the EOD). In the curarized fish this pattern of afferent input may be varied experimentally by changing the polarity, delay, amplitude, or spatial distribution of the stimulus. Such a stimulus change brings about a corresponding change in the effect of the command. Over a period of 10–20 min the effect of the command is altered to become the negative image of the new reafferent input pattern. Thus, the corollary discharge conveys an updatable template of the expected reafferent pattern to the secondary ampullary cells with each EOD motor command.

In the free-living fish the reafferent input pattern will vary with changes in water resistivity or with proximity to non-conducting boundaries. Modifiability of the efference copy assures that a good match is maintained between the efference copy and the reafference. Perhaps the absence of plasticity in the knollenorgan system is because the knollenorgans probably give the same response under all normal conditions. Furthermore, even if they should stop responding, the remaining inhibition caused by the corollary discharge is so brief that a mechanism for its removal would not confer a major advantage.

In the mormyromast receiving area the corollary discharge has a facilitatory effect on EOD-evoked reafferent input, rather than an inhibitory or suppressive one. This was first seen by Zipser and Bennett (1976). They showed that many mormyromast receiving cells in the electrosensory lobe were excited by a corollary discharge at the time when reafferent activity, elicited by the EOD, would arrive at these cells. Since 1976, Szabo, Enger and Libouban (1979) have shown a similar facilitatory effect of the EOD motor command on transmission through the electrosensory lobe. In each case the duration of the facilitation roughly matches the duration of mormyromast responses to the EOD. Facilitation or gating-on of the mormyromast EOD reafference by a corollary discharge is equivalent to suppression of receptor activity which could not have been evoked by the EOD. The latter is useful, as described above, in that mormyromast activity unrelated to the fish's own EOD is also irrelevant to active electrolocation and may be disruptive. Meyer and Bell (1982) have carried out behavioral studies on this gating which indicate that only afferent input arriving within a few tens of milliseconds after the command is treated as relevant for electrolocation. Work remains to be done in the mormyromast region and it is likely that the gate is only one step in a series of interactions with command-related signals that lead to the detection of environmental change and the evaluation of its significance.

In summary, the effects of the corollary discharge are different in the three regions. In the knollenorgan area there is a simple, brief and probably unmodifiable inhibition which blocks the reafferent signal. In the ampullary area there is a negative image of the expected reafference which may be excitatory or inhibitory, and which is modifiable. When added to the reafference, the effect is a suppression or reduction of the reafferent response. This effect of the command seems quite close to the efference copy concept of von Holst and Mittelstaedt (1950). In the mormyromast zone there is a facilitation of the reafferent response. In each case, the sign of the corollary discharge effect, whether suppression or facilitation, depends on the significance of the reafference for the fish. The timing and duration of the effect depends on the timing and duration of the reafference expected.

Conclusions

The idea of a variable efference copy or corollary discharge is not new. But in most cases such changes are considered to correspond to changes in the amplitude or pattern of the motor command sent to the effectors. Roberts and Russell (1972) showed, for example, that the amplitude of the efferent inhibition going out to the lateral line organs is larger with larger motor movements. In the ampullary zone of the electrosensory lobe, however, the changes in the efference copy are not related to changes in the associated motor output; that is constant. They are related instead to changes in the reafference or sensory consequences of the motor act. Such reafference-dependent modifiability could be important in other systems too. If the efference copy associated with a motor act is to be useful it must match the reafference. Thus if the reafference following a given motor command changes, due to muscle fatigue, growth, damage or some other reason, the efference copy should change too.

Here within the electrosensory system alone there are three very different effects of a corollary discharge signal. The variability among motor-sensory systems as a whole will certainly be larger still. In other systems, as in this one, the effect of a corollary discharge will depend on the form and significance of the expected reafference. If the reafference is disruptive or otherwise undesirable it may be suppressed by the corollary discharge. If the reafference conveys useful information then the corollary discharge will be part of an evaluative process, which may include facilitation.

The experimental work by the author was made possible by a grant from the U.S. National Science Foundation, BHS-7911956. Dr T. H. Bullock made many helpful criticisms of an early version of this paper.

References

Bell, C. C. (1979). Central nervous system physiology of electroreception, a review. *J. Physiol., Paris* 75: 361–79.

Bell, C. C. (1982). Properties of a modifiable efference copy in an electric fish. *J. Neurophysiol.* 47: 1043–56.

Bell, C. C., and Russell, C. J. (1978). Effect of electric organ discharge on ampullary receptors in a mormyrid. *Brain Res. 145:* 85–95.

Bennett, M. V. L. (1971). Electroreception. In *Fish Physiology*, ed. W. S. Hoar and D. J. Randall, pp. 493–574. New York: Academic Press.

Bullock, T. H. (1982). Electroreception. In *Annual Review of Neuroscience, 5:* 121–70. Palo Alto: Annual Reviews Inc.

Heiligenberg, W. (1977). Principles of electrolocation and jamming avoidance in electric fish. A neuroethological approach. In *Studies of Brain Function*, vol. 1, ed. V. Braitenberg, pp. 1–85. Berlin, Heidelberg, New York: Springer.

Helmholtz, H. L. F. von (1867). *Handbuch der physiologischen Optik*. vol. III. Leipzig: Leopold Voss.

Holst, E. von (1954). Relations between the central nervous systems and the peripheral organs. *Br. J. Anim. Behav. 2:* 89–94.

Holst, E. von, and Mittelstaedt, H. (1950). Das Reafferenzprinzip. *Naturwissenschaften 37:* 464–76.

McCloskey, D. I. (1981). Corollary discharges: motor commands and perception. In *Handbook of Physiology. The Nervous System*, vol. II, part 2, ed. V. B. Brooks, pp. 1415–47. Bethesda, MD.: Am. Physiol. Soc.

McKay, D. (1966). Cerebral organization and the conscious control of action. In *Brain and Conscious Experience*, ed. J. C. Eccles, pp. 422–45. New York: Springer.

Meyer, J. H., and Bell, C. C. (1983). Behavioural measurement of sensory gating by a corollary discharge. *J. Comp. Physiol. 151:* 401–6.

Mittelstaedt, H. 1971). Reafferenzprinzip-aplogie und Kritik. In *Vortrage der Erlanger Physiologentagung 1970*, ed. W. D. Keidel and K. H. Platlig. Berlin, Heidelberg, New York: Springer-Verlag.

Munz, H., Claas, B., and Fritzsch, B. (1982). Electrophysiological evidence of electroreception in the axolotl *Siredo mexicanum*. *Neurosci. Lett. 28:* 107–11.

Reichardt, W., and Poggio, T. (1976). Visual control of orientation behavior in the fly. Part I. A quantitative analysis. *Q. Rev. Biophys. 9:* 311–75.

Richmond, B. J., and Wurtz, R. H. (1980). Vision during saccadic eye movements. II. A corollary discharge to monkey superior colliculus. *J. Neurophysiol. 43:* 1156–67.

Roberts, B. L., and Russell, I. J. (1972). The activity of lateral line efferent neurones in stationary and swimming dogfish. *J. Exp. Biol. 57:* 435–48.

Russell, I. J. (1971). The role of the lateral line efferent system in *Xenopus laevis. J. Exp. Biol. 54:* 621–41.

Sperry, R. W. (1950). Neural basis of the spontaneous optokinetic response produced by visual inversion. *J. Comp. Physiol. Psychol. 43:* 482–9.

Szabo, T., Enger, P. S., and Libouban, S. (1979). Electrosensory systems in the mormyrid fish, *Gnathonemus petersii*: special emphasis on the fast conducting pathway. *J. Physiol., Paris 75:* 409–20.

Szabo, T., and Fessard, A. (1974). Physiology of electroreceptors. In *Handbook of Sensory Physiology*, vol. III/3: *Electroreceptors and other specialized receptors in other vertebrates*, ed. A. Fessard, pp. 60–124. Berlin: Springer-Verlag.

Szabo, T., and Moller, P. (1983). A neuroethological basis for electrocommunication. In *Comparative Physiology of Sensory Systems*, ed. L. Bolis, R. D. Keynes and S. H. P. Maddrell. Cambridge: Cambridge University Press.

Zaretsky, M. (1982). Quantitative measurements of centrally and retinally generated saccadic suppression in a locust movement detector neurone. *J. Physiol., Lond. 328:* 521–33.

Zipser, B., and Bennett, M. V. L. (1976). Interaction of electrosensory and signals in lateral line lobe of a mormyrid fish. *J. Neurophysiol. 39:* 713–21.

Index

acetylcholine, 575; and efferent transmission, 8, 181; and retinal inhibitory network, 346; and retinal neurotransmission, 423, 424
acetylcholinesterase (ACHE), 163, 164, 181
acetylcholintransferase, 181
adenylate cyclase in retina: and dopamine receptors, 421–2, 425, 442; and glucagon, 422, 425, 428–30; stimulation by neuropeptides, 422; and vasoactive intestinal peptide, 422, 425, 428–31
amacrine cells of retina, 373, 382; γ-aminobutyric acid in, 442; and retinal neuropeptides, 424, 426–7, 432–3, 434
amacrine cells of optic lobe, 348–9, 351
amino acid binding: and fish toxicant assessment, 289–90; to non-olfactory tissues, 289; by olfactory cilia, 293–4; to olfactory mucosa, 274–5; to olfactory receptors, 286–96, (and calcium ions) 263, (and specificity of sites) 295–6; at subcellular receptor sites, 292–5; to taste receptors, 287, 289, 292, 294
amino acids: chemospecificity of olfactory and gustatory responses, 268–70; and feeding behaviour, 275–8; levels in water, 257; molecular structure of, and olfactory and gustatory effectiveness, 270–1; and neurotransmission, 423, 424; olfactory bulbs' responses to, 265; olfactory receptors' responses to, 264, 266, 267–8; olfactory stimuli and cardiac response, 277; olfactory tract response to, 265; stimulus-induced release of, from lateral line, 7; taste sensitivity to, 266–7, (dose response) 268–9
γ-aminobutyric acid (GABA) in retina: activity of, 444–8, (compared to

glutamate-decarboxylase) 449–50; and neurotransmission, 424; and physiology, 397, 432–3; role of, 441, 442–3
ampullae of Lorenzini: electric field sensitivity, 541; electroreception mechanism, 510–14; neurophysiological responses of, 547–8; and orientation to earth's magnetic fields, 552–4; and orientation to motional electric fields, 544, (and biophysics of reception) 545–8
ampullary electroreceptors, 455; afferent central nervous pathways, 457–9, 478–80, (to torus semicircularis) 479, 482, 485; biased sensory epithelium, 520, 521; and corollary discharges, 642–3, 644; frequency modulation in, 520; functions of, 457, 478; mechanism of, in non-teleosts, 510–14; morphology and operation, 509, 511; roles of, 640; threshold level, 458; valvular projection area of, 465, 467, 468; see also ampullae of Lorenzini
anastomosis of Oort: efferent olivo-cochlear fibres in, 163, 169
antennae, insect, see olfactory receptors of insect antennae
ants: navigation by polarized skylight, 503; olfactory reception by, 248; retinal polarization analysers, 505
armadillo Chaetophractus villosus: olfactory bulb activity, 316–26, (and rhino-central rhythm) 316, 318–21, (and sinusoidal activity) 318, 319, 322–6, (and slow potentials) 318, 319
auditory systems: artificial song reception, 41–4; basal papilla morphology, 48–50; basilar membrane tuning, 206; bat-detection, 34, 35; directional hearing, 34; directional response and vector